ISBN 0-8373-5052-2

52 ADMISSION TEST SERIES

New RUDMAN'S QUESTIONS AND ANSWERS ON THE...

PCAT

PHARMACY COLLEGE ADMISSION TEST

How to qualify for admission to the Pharmacy Colleges of...

UNIVERSITY OF ILLINOIS
UNIVERSITY OF KENTUCKY
UNIVERSITY OF TENNESSEE
OREGON STATE UNIVERSITY
UNIVERSITY OF FLORIDA, GAINESVILLE
UNIVERSITY OF TORONTO
SOUTHEASTERN COLLEGE
PURDUE UNIVERSITY
UNIVERSITY OF UTAH
DALHOUSIE
FLORIDA A&M

...and a hundred others.

Intensive preparation for the examination including...

- Verbal Ability
- Quantitative Ability
- Biology
- Chemistry
- Reading Comprehension

NLC

NATIONAL LEARNING CORPORATION

National Learning Corporation

212 Michael Drive, Syosset, New York 11791
(516) 921-8888

PRINTED IN THE UNITED STATES OF AMERICA

PASSBOOK®

NOTICE

This book is *SOLELY* intended for, is sold *ONLY* to, and its use is *RESTRICTED* to *individual*, bona fide applicants or candidates who qualify by virtue of having seriously filed applications for appropriate license, certificate, professional and/or promotional advancement, higher school matriculation, scholarship, or other legitimate requirements of educational and/or governmental authorities.

This book is *NOT* intended for use, class instruction, tutoring, training, duplication, copying, reprinting, excerption, or adaptation, etc., by:

(1) Other Publishers
(2) Proprietors and/or Instructors of "Coaching" and/or Preparatory Courses
(3) Personnel and/or Training Divisions of commercial, industrial, and governmental organizations
(4) Schools, colleges, or universities and/or their departments and staffs, including teachers and other personnel
(5) Testing Agencies or Bureaus
(6) Study groups which seek by the purchase of a single volume to copy and/or duplicate and/or adapt this material for use by the group as a whole without having purchased individual volumes for each of the members of the group
(7) Et al.

Such persons would be in violation of appropriate Federal and State statutes.

PROVISION OF LICENSING AGREEMENTS. — Recognized educational commercial, industrial, and governmental institutions and organizations, and others legitimately engaged in educational pursuits, including training, testing, and measurement activities, may address a request for a licensing agreement to the copyright owners, who will determine whether, and under what conditions, including fees and charges, the materials in this book may be used by them. In other words, a licensing facility *exists* for the legitimate use of the material in this book on other than an individual basis. However, it is asseverated and affirmed here that the materials in this book *CANNOT* be used without the receipt of the express permission of such a licensing agreement from the Publishers.

NATIONAL LEARNING CORPORATION
212 Michael Drive
Syosset, New York 11791

Inquiries re licensing agreements should be addressed to:
The President
National Learning Corporation
212 Michael Drive
Syosset, New York 11791

PASSBOOK SERIES®

THE PASSBOOK SERIES® has been created to prepare applicants and candidates for the ultimate academic battlefield—the examination room.

AT SOME time in our lives, each and every one of us may be required to take an examination—for validation, matriculation, admission, qualification, registration, certification, or licensure.

BASED ON the assumption that every applicant or candidate has met the basic formal educational standards, has taken the required number of courses, and read the necessary texts, the PASSBOOK SERIES® furnishes the one special preparation which may assure passing with confidence, instead of failing with insecurity. Examination questions—together with answers—are furnished as the basic vehicle for study so that the mysteries of the examination and its compounding difficulties may be eliminated or diminished by a sure method.

THIS BOOK is meant to help you pass your examination provided that you qualify and are serious in your objective.

THE ENTIRE field is reviewed through the huge store of content information which is succinctly presented through a provocative and challenging approach—the question-and-answer method.

A CLIMATE of success is established by furnishing the correct answers at the end of each test.

YOU SOON learn to recognize types of questions, forms of questions, and patterns of questioning. You may even begin to anticipate expected outcomes.

YOU PERCEIVE that many questions are repeated or adapted so that you gain acute insights, which may enable you to score many sure points.

YOU LEARN how to confront new questions, or types of questions, and to attack them confidently and work out the correct answers.

YOU NOTE objectives and emphases, and recognize pitfalls and dangers, so that you may make positive educational adjustments.

MOREOVER, you are kept fully informed in relation to new concepts, methods, practices, and directions in the field.

YOU DISCOVER that you are actually taking the examination all the time: you are preparing for the examination by "taking" an examination, not by reading extraneous and/or supererogatory textbooks.

IN SHORT, this PASSBOOK®, used directedly, should be an important factor in helping you to pass your test.

Pharmacy College Admission Test
TABLE OF CONTENTS

for instructional use
from the official announcement

CALENDAR FOR 1994 – 1995 TESTS

	TEST DATES		
DEADLINES FOR RECEIPT OF:	Oct. 29, 1994	Feb. 18, 1995	Apr. 1, 1995
Application for Scheduled Saturday Testing Centers ($35.00)	Sept. 23, 1994	Jan. 13, 1995	Feb. 24, 1995
Late Application ($15.00)	Sept. 30, 1994	Jan. 20, 1995	Mar. 3, 1995
Request for a Special Testing Location ($100.00)	Sept. 16, 1994	Jan. 6, 1995	Feb. 17, 1995
Request for a Sunday Administration (No additional fee)	Sept. 16, 1994	Jan. 6, 1995	Feb. 17, 1995

Section I.
INTRODUCTION

The Candidate Information Booklet

This booklet contains complete information about the Pharmacy College Admission Test (PCAT). It explains how to apply for the test, describes the general content of the test, provides sample questions with answers, and tells you what happens after you have taken the test.

Your application can be found inside the envelope at the center of this booklet. Before you begin to fill in your application, be sure to look at the sample application provided in this booklet, and to read the guidelines for filling out your application correctly.

Read this booklet completely and carefully. You should not call or write The Psychological Corporation with questions until you have thoroughly read this booklet.

KEEP THIS BOOKLET FOR REFERENCE! It contains information you will need after you have applied for the test.

It is critical that you strictly adhere to all procedures and deadlines in this candidate information booklet.

The Psychological Corporation

Founded in 1921, The Psychological Corporation is the oldest commercial test publisher in the nation and is an acknowledged leader in the test development and publishing industry. The Psychological Corporation develops and publishes tests for college admissions, licensing and credentialing programs, and business, as well as materials for service providers in education, clinical psychology, and speech, language, and hearing.

The Psychological Corporation is a subsidiary of Harcourt Brace & Company, the world's leading educational publisher. More than 400 people work for The Psychological Corporation, most of them at the headquarters in San Antonio, Texas.

The American Association of Colleges of Pharmacy

The American Association of Colleges of Pharmacy (AACP) is the only organization representing the interests of pharmacy education and educators. The AACP is composed of approximately 3,000 faculty members from all 75 schools and colleges of pharmacy in the United States and Puerto Rico. The AACP and its members are committed to maintaining excellence in pharmaceutical education and to helping member schools prepare well-qualified graduates for entrance into the profession of pharmacy.

The Pharmacy College Admission Test Program

All correspondence and requests for information concerning the Pharmacy College Admission Test (PCAT) should be directed to:

Pharmacy College Admission Test (PCAT)
The Psychological Corporation
555 Academic Court
San Antonio, Texas 78204-2498
1-800-622-3231 or Fax 210-921-8861
Monday – Friday, 7:00 A.M. – 7:00 P.M. Central Time

When you write to The Psychological Corporation, always include in your letter: your name, address, social security number, and the name of the testing program your letter concerns.

DO NOT SEND YOUR APPLICATION OR FEE PAYMENTS TO THE ABOVE ADDRESS. SEE PAGE 7 FOR FEE PAYMENT ADDRESSES.

When you call The Psychological Corporation, you should keep a record of when you called, the name of the person you spoke to, and the information you were given. You should follow up any telephone conversation with a letter.

The policies, procedures, and fees in this candidate information booklet apply to all administrations of the Pharmacy College Admission Test (PCAT) that occur from September 1, 1994, to August 31, 1995. The application in this information booklet can be used to apply for tests given between September 1, 1994, and August 31, 1995, only.

By submitting your application, you agree to adhere to all policies and procedures in this information booklet.

Section II.
FEES AND SPECIAL SERVICES

ALL FEES MUST BE PAID BY MONEY ORDER. Your money order must display your name. Make your money order payable to THE PSYCHOLOGICAL CORPORATION. If you are applying from outside the United States, you must submit an international money order payable in U.S. dollars.

Do not send cash or personal checks.

All PCAT fee payments are deposited immediately upon receipt. Deposit of your fee payment does not constitute an agreement to grant you admission to the test. If your application does not meet the requirements described in this booklet, it will be returned for correction.

Your application with all required fees must be RECEIVED by the application deadline for the test date for which you are applying.

Send your application and fee payment by regular mail to the following address:

The Psychological Corporation
Pharmacy College Admission Test
P.O. Box 91581
Chicago, Illinois 60693

If you need to send your application and fee payment by overnight courier service, address it to:

The Psychological Corporation
c/o Continental Bank
P.O. Box 91581
840 S. Canal Street, 3rd Floor
Chicago, Illinois 60693

Test Fee – $35.00

Your Test Fee of $35 (with your **signed** application) registers you to take the test at a scheduled center. You must also pay this fee to be admitted to a testing center as a standby or to register for a special testing location. In addition, this fee covers your receiving a personal score report and having official score reports sent to one, two, or three colleges of pharmacy that you specify when you apply.

Optional Fees

Late Application Fee – $15.00

To apply after the regular deadline up to four weeks before the test, you must pay this fee in addition to the Test Fee.

Special Testing Location Fee – $100.00

To take your test at a location other than a scheduled testing center, you must pay the Special Testing Location Fee in addition to the Test Fee.

Standby Registration Fee – $25.00

If you do not pre-register to take your test, you must pay the Standby Registration Fee in addition to the Test Fee.

Additional Score Report Fee – $10.00 each

You must pay the Additional Score Report Fee for each score report beyond the three that your Test Fee covers and for any requested after you submit your application.

Handscoring Fee – $10.00

To have your electronically-scored answer sheet rescored by hand to confirm your reported score, you must pay the Handscoring Fee.

Cancelling Your Registration

If you know you will not be able to take a test that you have already registered for, you may request a cancellation of your registration. **Cancellations must be requested in writing and RECEIVED by The Psychological Corporation three weeks prior to the test date for which you are registered.**

Your cancellation request must include:

1. Your name, address and social security number;
2. The name of the test you are registered to take;
3. The date you are scheduled to test; and
4. Your signature.

Mail your cancellation request to the address shown on page 6 of this booklet.

If you comply with these requirements and your absence on the test day is verified, half of your application fee will be returned to you six to eight weeks after the **test** date. The remainder will be retained by The Psychological Corporation as a processing fee. Fees may NOT be applied to future test dates. Optional fees will not be refunded.

Refund Policy

Regardless of whether or not you actually take the test, certain costs are incurred by the Psychological Corporation for each application and must be recovered. After your application is received, it is checked for completeness and accuracy, optically scanned and read into a computer file, and carefully processed to ensure you have a seat at a test center. In addition, your admission ticket is printed and mailed, and materials are assembled and sent to your test center where a space is reserved for you. Because these labor and materials costs must still be recovered, except as noted in the cancellation policy above, **under no circumstances will test fees or optional fees be refunded or transferred to another test date.**

Special Testing Locations

The deadlines by which your application and fee payment for a special testing location must be received by The Psychological Corporation appear on the inside front cover of this booklet.

Special testing locations for the established testing dates may be arranged for candidates living more than 150 miles from a scheduled testing center.

To request a special testing location, submit the following:

1. The Test Fee;
2. The Special Testing Location Fee;
3. A written explanation to The Psychological Corporation; and
4. A completed application, with special attention to the following areas. On side 1 of your application, fill in the city and state where you wish to test and leave the test center number blank. On side 2, fill in the "Special Arrangements Needed" circle.

Requests for a special testing location should be mailed to the address shown on page 7 of this booklet.

In the written explanation, include the statement that you are requesting a special testing location, the address at which you will be residing on the test date for which you are applying, and your preferred testing location. Although your test will not necessarily be given at your preferred testing location, every attempt will be made to have it administered at your preferred location or within 75 miles of the address at which you will be residing on the test date for which you are applying.

A nonrefundable fee of $100, in addition to the Test Fee, is required of each candidate requesting a special testing location. **Fees in excess of $100 may be required for special testing locations in foreign countries. If you require a special testing location in a foreign country, call 1-800-622-3231 or 210-921-8798 for additional information.**

No arrangements for a special testing location will be made until your application, written request, and the entire fee have been received.

Sunday Administrations

For candidates whose religious convictions prohibit their testing on a Saturday, a special testing date on the Sunday following the scheduled test date may be arranged.

Each request for a Sunday administration must include:

1. A cover letter specifying that a Sunday administration is needed;
2. A letter on letterhead from your rabbi, pastor, or religious leader in support of your request for a Sunday test date;
3. Your completed application and fee payment.

Mail your request for a Sunday administration to the address on page 7 of this booklet.

There is no additional fee for Sunday test administrations. There is no standby admission to Sunday test administrations.

Application receipt deadlines for Sunday administrations appear on the inside front cover of this booklet.

Accommodations for Candidates with Disabilities

Requests for accommodations for candidates with disabilities must be received by The Psychological Corporation by the deadlines for application that appear on the inside front cover of this booklet.

If you need special accommodations because of a disability, **submit in one complete package:**

1. A completed application (with the circle in the "Special Arrangements Needed" box on side 2 filled in);
2. A current letter from a licensed physician, optometrist, social worker, or psychologist on his or her letterhead (including title, address, and telephone number) describing the nature of the functional limitation as it applies to taking a multiple-choice standardized test and the specific accommodations you will need for testing; and
3. Fee payment.

Mail your request for special accommodations to the address on page 7 of this booklet.

There is no additional charge for special accommodations for candidates with disabilities.

Section III.
APPLYING FOR THE TEST

To pre-register for the Pharmacy College Admission Test, you must complete an application and submit it together with fee payment so that they are received by The Psychological Corporation by the application receipt deadline. Application receipt deadlines appear on the inside front cover of this booklet.

When you have double-checked your application and are sure you have completed it correctly, mail it with a **money order** payable to The Psychological Corporation in the envelope in the center of this booklet. Your money order must display your name.

If you are applying from outside the United States, you must submit an **international** money order payable in U.S. dollars.

If your application is returned to you for correction and you cannot resubmit it with your fee payment in time to meet the deadline, you can report to a testing center as a standby candidate (see *How to Take the Test as a Standby*) or reapply for a later testing date. **Application deadlines will not be extended.**

Tips for Applying

- Choose a test date that will ensure that each institution to which you are applying will receive your scores before its application deadline. Score reports are mailed approximately four to six weeks after each test date.
- Apply early. Applications must be **received** by the deadlines. You may want to use an overnight courier service such as Federal Express if you are submitting your application close to a deadline. The address to use if mailing your application by overnight courier service is shown on page 7 of this booklet.
- **If you want confirmation that your application has been received by The Psychological Corporation, use a special form of mail, such as certified with return receipt or United Parcel Service with acknowledgment of delivery.**
- Carefully read and follow all directions in this booklet.
- Fill out your application completely. Only properly completed applications will be accepted.
- Use the application checklist to verify that you are submitting your application and fees correctly.
- **SIGN (DO NOT PRINT) YOUR APPLICATION. Unsigned applications will NOT be accepted.**
- Include a **money order** payable to The Psychological Corporation for the proper fee. **Personal checks will not be accepted.** Do not send cash.

How to Complete Your Application

The information you give on your application will be "read" by an optical scanner and recorded in a computer file. The optical scanner "sees" only the circles you fill in. The circles the scanner sees will determine where your admission ticket and score reports will be sent and the testing center and date to which you will be assigned.

You must use a black-lead, number 2 pencil (also called an HB pencil) to complete your application. The scanner cannot see marks made with ball-point pens, hard or colored lead pencils, felt-tip pens, or any writing instruments other than a black-lead, number 2 (or HB) pencil.

Filling in incorrect circles or using any writing instrument other than a black-lead, number 2 (HB) pencil may result in your admission ticket being sent to the wrong address, your scores being sent to the wrong schools, your being assigned to the wrong testing center, or your being scheduled for the wrong test date.

It is your responsibility to use a black-lead, number 2 (HB) pencil and to fill in the correct circles.

To complete side 1 of your application, you will print letters in boxes above columns of circles that contain letters and numbers. Then, under each box in which you print a letter or number, you will fill in the circle containing that letter or number. Make sure you fill in only one circle in each column.

Remember, the scanner that reads your application will see only the circles you fill in; it will not see the letters and numbers you print in the boxes.

Before you fill out your application, study the following example of a properly completed application, found on pages 16–17.

Then, remove the application from the envelope in the center of this booklet and turn it to side 1 so that the words "Pharmacy College Admission Test Application" appear at the top. Follow the steps below as you go along to make sure that you are filling out your application correctly. **It is important that you follow these steps and that the information on your application is correct; if not, processing may be delayed.**

1. LAST NAME, FIRST, M.I.

   Starting in the farthest left box, print your last name, one letter per box, skip a box, and print your first name, one letter per box, skip a box, and print your middle initial. If the number of letters in your name exceeds the number of boxes, print your full last name and use the remaining boxes to provide an abbreviated form of your first name and, if there is space, your middle initial.

   Beneath each box in which you have printed a letter, completely fill in the circle containing that letter.

2. NUMBER AND STREET, CITY, and STATE (PROVINCE)

   Your admission ticket and personal score report will be mailed to this address.

   In the boxes in these sections of your application, print your mailing address.

   If your mailing address contains an apartment number, be sure to include it.

   Abbreviate wherever possible, using appropriate abbreviations from *Appendix C – Postal Abbreviations.*

   Beneath each box in which you have printed a letter or number, completely fill in the circle containing the letter or number you printed in the box.

3. ZIP CODE

   a. For Applicants with U.S. Mailing Addresses:

      Print your 5-digit zip code beginning in the farthest left box. Leave the sixth (farthest right) box empty.

      Beneath each box in which you have printed a number, completely fill in the circle containing that number.

   b. For Applicants with Canadian Mailing Addresses:

      Print the 6 letters and numbers of your postal code in the boxes.

      Beneath each box in which you have printed a letter or number, completely fill in the circle containing that letter or number.

c. For Applicants with Mailing Addresses Outside the U.S. and Canada:

Print the abbreviation of your country in the boxes.

Do not fill in any circles.

Note: The address to which your admission ticket and personal score report will be mailed is determined by the circles you fill in. If you fill in incorrect circles under your name and address, your admission ticket and personal score report may be undeliverable.

4. CODE NUMBERS OF SCHOOLS TO RECEIVE SCORE REPORTS

In this section of your application, you will specify the schools to which you want your scores reported. If you leave the school codes blank when you submit your application you will be the only party to receive your scores.

School code numbers are listed in *Appendix B – Pharmacy College Code Numbers.*

To have your scores reported to any colleges, individuals, or organizations that do not appear on the Pharmacy College Code Numbers list in Appendix B, provide their full names and addresses on a separate 8 1/2″ by 11″ sheet of paper. **Include your name, address, social security number, and signature on the separate sheet.** Mail this sheet with your application.

On your application, you may specify up to 6 pharmacy colleges to which official score reports should be sent (but you are not required to have your scores reported to any colleges). Your Test Fee covers having official score reports sent to one, two, or three colleges that you specify when you apply.

Under A, print the 3-digit code number of the first college to which you want a report of your scores sent. Begin in the farthest left box.

Below each box, completely fill in the circle containing the number you printed in the box.

To have your scores reported to one or two additional colleges, complete sections B and C.

You may have your scores reported to up to three more colleges by completing sections 1, 2, and 3. In your fee payment, you must include the $10 Additional Score Report Fee for each official score report beyond the three covered by your Test Fee.

It is essential that you fill in the correct circles in this section. Filling in the wrong circles may result in your scores being reported to the wrong college or school.

To have your scores sent to more than six colleges, list on an 8 1/2″ by 11″ sheet of paper the school code number, school name, city, and state of each additional college to which your scores are to be sent. **Include your name, address, social security number, and signature on the sheet of paper.** Mail the list with your application. In your fee payment, you must include the $10 Additional Score Report Fee for each college beyond the three covered by your Test Fee.

Be sure you want your scores reported to the schools you list. Once you submit your application, these schools cannot be changed or deleted. However, you may request that your scores be sent to additional schools, and you can request at the time you take the test that your test not be scored.

Keep a record of the schools to which you are having your scores sent.

5. FEES

Moving to the right, calculate the fees you will submit with your application.

a. Examination Fee

After Examination Fee, print $35.

b. Additional Score Report Fee

Your personal score report and up to three official score reports requested now are covered by your Test Fee. There is a $10 fee for each additional score report. If you are requesting more than the three official score reports (and your personal score report), multiply the number of additional official score reports by $10 and print this amount after Additional Score Report Fee.

c. Special Testing Location Fee

If you are requesting a special testing location, print $100 after Special Testing Location Fee.

d. Standby Registration Fee

To be admitted to a testing center as a standby, you must take a completed application and fee payment to the center with you. If you will be reporting to a center as a standby, print $25 after Standby Registration Fee.

e. Miscellaneous Fees

The $15 Late Application Fee, if applicable, should be printed after Miscellaneous Fees.

f. Total

Add the fees you have printed, and print the total after Total.

6. TOTAL FEE

To the right of where you calculated your fees, under the words "TOTAL FEE," print in the boxes the total of the fees you are paying. Your money order must be made out for this amount. Applications received without fees will be returned.

If your total fee is less than $100, print a 0 in the farthest left box (for example, if the total fee you are paying is $35, you will print 035 in the boxes).

Under each box, completely fill in the circle containing the number you printed in the box.

7. TESTING CENTER INFORMATION

Scheduled testing center locations, their code numbers that you will specify on your application, and the dates on which each center will be open are listed in *Appendix A – Scheduled Testing Centers, Center Codes, and Test Dates.*

First, print the city and state (province) of the scheduled testing center location for which you are applying (or to which you will go as a standby). If you are requesting a special testing location, print the city and state (province) where you would like to take the test.

Then, in the boxes under the words "CENTER NUMBER," print the 3-digit testing center code number of that center. **Leave these boxes empty if you are requesting a special testing location.** Under each box, completely fill in the circle containing the number you printed in the box (if you are requesting a special location, do not fill in any of these circles). Be certain to use **testing center** code numbers, NOT **school** code numbers.

Remember, the circles you fill in will determine the testing center to which you are assigned (unless you are requesting a special location).

Note: Be sure that the test is scheduled for the date and center you select. You will not be allowed to change your test center after your application is submitted.

8. SOCIAL SECURITY NUMBER

Print your 9-digit social security number (leaving out the hyphens) in the boxes. Then, under each box, completely fill in the circle containing the number you printed in the box. If you do not provide your social security number, processing of your application may be delayed. If you do not have a social security number, leave this section blank.

Turn the application to side 2.

9. TELEPHONE NUMBER

   Print in the boxes the telephone number (including area code) at which you can be reached during the day. Under each box, completely fill in the circle containing the number you printed in the box.

10. TESTING DATE

    Completely fill in the circle to the right of the month in which your chosen test date occurs. Fill in only one circle.

Note: Be sure that the test is scheduled for the date and center you select. You will not be allowed to reschedule to another test date after your application is submitted.

11. SPECIAL ARRANGEMENTS NEEDED

    Completely fill in the circle if you require a special testing location, a Sunday administration, or special arrangements because of a disability.

12. PREVIOUS EXAMINATIONS

    Completely fill in the appropriate "NO" or "YES" circle. If you fill in the "YES" circle, print the month and year in which you most recently took the test.

13. CURRENT EDUCATIONAL STATUS

    Completely fill in the circle corresponding to your status at the time you are completing this application. If you are not presently enrolled, use the last year you completed.

14. YEARS COLLEGE CHEMISTRY

    Completely fill in the circle corresponding to the amount of chemistry course-time you have completed as of today. College level includes courses that are equivalent to college courses such as advanced placement courses.

15. YEARS COLLEGE BIOLOGY

    Completely fill in the circle corresponding to the amount of biology course-time you have completed as of today. College level includes courses that are equivalent to college courses such as advanced placement courses.

16. OPTIONAL INFORMATION

    You are not required to give this information, but we would appreciate your giving it. It will be used for research and planning only. Your specific responses will be kept strictly confidential and will not be reported to any individuals or institutions.

    To complete this section, completely fill in the circles to the right of the categories that accurately describe you.

17. DENIAL OF RELEASE

    Fill in the circle only if you do NOT want your name and address released for recruitment purposes.

18. SIGNATURE

    Read the agreement and then sign (do not print) your application. **IF YOU DO NOT SIGN YOUR APPLICATION, IT WILL BE RETURNED TO YOU.** If your application must be returned to you for your signature, you may not be able to resubmit it in time to meet the application deadline. Deadlines will not be extended.

PHARMACY COLLEGE ADMISSION TEST™ APPLICATION

LAST NAME, FIRST, M.I.: KING KIM P

NUMBER AND STREET: 107 OAK ST APT 5

CITY: JUNCTION CY

State Province: MT

ZIP CODE: 59405

CODE NUMBERS OF SCHOOLS TO RECEIVE SCORE REPORTS: A, B and C included in Examination Fee. Additional Score Reports available at $10.00 each. (See Candidate Information Booklet)

A	B	C	ADDITIONAL SCORE REPORTS 1	2	3
035	070	071	008		

FEES: Fee schedule in Candidate Information Booklet (Enter appropriate fees and total)

Examination Fee (including three Score Reports)	35.00
Additional Score Report Fee (number of reports x fee)	10.00
Special Location Fee	
Standby Registration Fee	
Miscellaneous Fees	
TOTAL	45.00

TOTAL FEE: 045

TESTING CENTER INFORMATION

City: BISMARCK, State: ND

Center Number: 734

SOCIAL SECURITY NUMBER: 470538029

Use a soft black lead pencil and fill in the appropriate circles like this: ●, not like this ✓ or ⊗ or ⊙.
DO NOT make any stray marks on this form.

TELEPHONE NUMBER

4	0	6	4	6	5	7	1	6	6
0	●	0	0	0	0	0	0	0	0
1	1	1	1	1	1	1	●	1	1
2	2	2	2	2	2	2	2	2	2
3	3	3	3	3	3	3	3	3	3
●	4	4	●	4	4	4	4	4	4
5	5	5	5	5	●	5	5	5	5
6	6	●	6	●	6	6	6	●	●
7	7	7	7	7	7	●	7	7	7
8	8	8	8	8	8	8	8	8	8
9	9	9	9	9	9	9	9	9	9

TESTING DATE

JAN	○	JUL	○
FEB	○	AUG	○
MAR	○	SEP	○
APR	○	OCT	○
MAY	○	NOV	●
JUN	○	DEC	○

SPECIAL ARRANGEMENTS NEEDED

If special testing arrangements are needed, such as Additional, Sunday, or Foreign centers, or if accommodations are needed for a disabled applicant, fill in this circle: ——→ ○

PREVIOUS EXAMINATIONS

Have you taken this examination before? No ○ Yes ●

If so, when? 11/95

Month / Year

CURRENT EDUCATIONAL STATUS

HIGH SCHOOL STUDENT	○
HIGH SCHOOL GRADUATE	○
COLLEGE: First Year	○
Second Year	○
Third Year	●
Fourth Year	○
COLLEGE GRADUATE	○

YEARS COLLEGE CHEMISTRY

None	○
Less than one	○
One	●
More than one	○

YEARS COLLEGE BIOLOGY

None	○
Less than one	○
One	●
More than one	○

OPTIONAL INFORMATION

SEX:	Male	○
	Female	●
RACE:	Asian	○
	Black	○
	Hispanic	○
	Native American	○
	White	○
	Other	●
AGE:	18 and under	○
	19	○
	20	○
	21–23	●
	24 and over	○
LINGUISTIC BACKGROUND (DOMINANT LANGUAGE OF HOME):	ENGLISH	●
	OTHER	○

DENIAL OF RELEASE

Schools of pharmacy may request your name and address for recruitment purposes. If you do NOT wish this information released, fill in this circle: ——→ ○

If using regular mail, return Application with appropriate fee in the envelope provided to:

The Psychological Corporation
Pharmacy College
Admission Test
P.O. Box 91581
Chicago, IL 60693

If using overnight courier, return Application with appropriate fee to:

The Psychological Corporation
c/o Continental Bank
P.O. Box 91581
840 S. Canal St., 3rd Floor
Chicago, IL 60693

I agree to adhere to all policies and procedures outlined in the current PCAT Candidate Information Booklet and attest that the information provided by me on this application is true to the best of my knowledge. I further certify that my own name and signature appear on this application.

X Kim P. King
SIGNATURE

APPLICATIONS WITHOUT A SIGNATURE WILL NOT BE PROCESSED.

Application Checklist

Review your application to make sure you have completed the following steps.

____ Filled in the correct circles under your name and address.

Filling in incorrect circles may result in your admission ticket and your personal score report being sent to the wrong address.

____ Filled in the correct circles under "Code Numbers of Schools to Receive Score Reports."

Filling in incorrect circles may result in your scores being sent to the wrong schools or being undeliverable.

____ Chosen a testing center that will be open on the test date you chose.

If you choose a date for which a center will not be open, your application will be returned to you for correction.

____ Filled in the correct circles under the boxes in which you printed the testing center code of the testing center you chose.

Filling in incorrect circles will result in your being assigned to the wrong testing center or your application being returned to you for correction.

____ Filled in the circle next to the month in which you want to test.

Filling in the incorrect circle or more than one circle will result in your being assigned to the wrong test date or your application being returned to you.

____ Calculated your fee payment correctly.

If you do not submit the correct fee payment, your application will be returned to you.

____ **Signed your application.**

IF YOU DO NOT SIGN YOUR APPLICATION, IT WILL BE RETURNED TO YOU.
If your application must be returned to you for your signature, you may not be able to resubmit it before the application deadline. Deadlines will not be extended.

Remember, it is your responsibility to fill in the correct circles.

It is advisable to keep a photocopy of your completed application for reference.

Send your application and fee payment by regular mail to the following address:

The Psychological Corporation
Pharmacy College Admission Test
P.O. Box 91581
Chicago, Illinois 60693

If you need to send your application and fee payment by overnight courier service, address it to:

The Psychological Corporation
c/o Continental Bank
P.O. Box 91581
840 S. Canal Street, 3rd Floor
Chicago, Illinois 60693

Address Changes

Your admission ticket and personal score report will be sent to you at the address you give on your application. If you believe that your admission ticket will not be properly delivered because of a change of address after you submit your application, please refer to the section on admission tickets in this booklet for the correct procedure for admission to the testing center.

When you take your test, you will be able to change the address to which your personal score report will be sent. Directions for changing the address will be provided at your testing center before the test begins.

How to Take the Test As a Standby

Standby registration will be available at **some** scheduled centers to accommodate individuals who need to take this test on an emergency basis. To find out which testing centers will be accepting standby candidates, call The Psychological Corporation at 1-800-622-3231. **This information will be available only during the week preceding the test date.** Telephones are staffed between 7:00 A.M. and 7:00 P.M. Central Time, Monday through Friday.

If the center of your choice will be accepting standbys, you will be given its reporting address.

To register as a standby at a center, you must:

1. Take a **completed application** to the center;
2. Take a **money order** for your **total fee payment**, including the $25 Standby Fee, to the center (no personal checks or cash will be accepted);
3. Take two forms of positive identification to the center — **at least one must be a photo ID with signature;**
4. Report to the center **NO LATER THAN 8:00 A.M.**; and
5. **Sign in** on the standby roster as soon as you arrive.

Admission of standbys to a testing center is never guaranteed. Centers that will accept standbys have limited space and are supplied with a limited number of testing materials for standby candidates.

As standbys report to a center, they sign in on a standby roster. Each standby must sign the roster personally. After all pre-registered candidates have been admitted to the center, standbys are admitted in the order in which they signed the roster. **Signing the roster does not guarantee your admission to the center.** If a center reaches its capacity before all standbys have been admitted, the remaining standbys will be turned away.

Admission Tickets

No less than three days before your test date, you should receive your admission ticket. This ticket will show the complete reporting address of your testing center, your reporting time, and your assigned ID number. When you report to your testing center, you must take your admission ticket with you and present it to gain admittance for testing.

When you receive your admission ticket, immediately inspect it to make sure it displays the correct test date and testing center. If either is incorrect, immediately call the Pharmacy College Admission Test Coordinator at 1-800-622-3231.

If you have not received your admission ticket by the Wednesday before your test date, call The Psychological Corporation's Pharmacy College Admission Test Coordinator at 1-800-622-3231 so that special arrangements can be made to have you admitted for testing.

Section IV.
AT THE TESTING CENTER

Test Day Schedule

The following schedule (in local time) will be observed at all testing centers.

- No later than 8:00 A.M. — Standby candidates report to testing centers
- No later than 8:30 A.M. — Pre-registered candidates report to testing centers
- 12:45 P.M. — Testing ends (approximately)

Admission to Testing

To be admitted to the test, pre-registered candidates must present their admission tickets and positive identification such as a driver's license or school identification card with photograph and signature. Photo ID credit cards are **NOT** acceptable.

Standby candidates must present two forms of identification. At least one form **must** be a photo ID with signature. Photo ID credit cards are **NOT** acceptable.

If you report to a center other than the one to which you were assigned, you will be treated as a standby, except that you will present your admission ticket instead of a completed application and you will not have to pay your Test Fee again. You will have to pay the Standby Registration Fee of $25 by money order. If you do not take your admission ticket with you, you will have to pay your Test Fee again (in addition to the Standby Registration Fee), and your original Test Fee will not be refunded. At 8:30 A.M., admission of pre-registered candidates to the testing room will begin. After all pre-registered candidates have been admitted, as many standbys will be admitted as there are space and materials to accommodate.

Pre-registered candidates arriving at the testing center after the capacity of the center has been reached because of the admission of standby candidates **will NOT be admitted** for testing and **will not be given refunds.**

No candidate will be admitted to the testing room after the administration has begun.

Testing Center Rules

- Take several sharpened number 2 pencils (also called HB pencils) with erasers to your testing center. For accurate scoring of your answer sheet, only number 2 (or HB) pencils can be used. Mechanical pencils and ink, felt-tip, or ball-point pens must NOT be used.
- If you are pre-registered, you must take your admission ticket to the testing center.
- If you go to a center as a standby, you must take to the testing center your completed application and fee payment by **money order** payable to The Psychological Corporation and displaying your name.
- You must take proper identification to your testing center. Pre-registered candidates must present positive identification such as a driver's license or school identification card with photograph and signature. Standby candidates must present **two** forms of identification; at least one of these **must** be a photo ID with signature. Photo ID credit cards are **NOT** acceptable.

- Arrive at your testing center on time. Testing will begin promptly. Latecomers (arriving after the test has begun) will not be admitted.
- You may not take calculators (including watch calculators), books, papers, or any reference materials into the testing room. You will be allowed to write in your test booklet.
- No food or beverages may be taken into the testing room.
- You may not ask questions about the test after the test begins.
- There will be a scheduled rest break approximately halfway through the test. Any examinee who leaves the testing room during the break must first receive permission from the examiner and will be escorted while outside the testing room.
- Visitors are not allowed in the testing room.
- Any candidate who gives or receives assistance during the test will be required to turn in all test materials immediately and leave the room. The candidate's answer sheet will not be scored. No fees will be refunded to the candidate.
- The Psychological Corporation reserves the right to cancel any test score if there is a nonstandard test administration.
- **It is of the utmost importance that all candidates carefully and completely follow all directions and regulations. Listen carefully to all instructions given by the examiner and follow the directions completely.**

No Score Option

During the test, you will be able to request that your test not be scored. How to request that your test not be scored will be explained before the test begins.

Note: If you request that your test not be scored, the request is irrevocable. Any later request to score your test and report your scores will NOT be honored.

Fees will not be refunded.

Testing Center Closings and Delayed Starting Times

Adverse conditions (such as extreme weather or a local power failure) or other circumstances at a testing center may make it necessary to cancel the administration of a test or to delay the beginning of testing from one to four hours at a particular center.

Do NOT call the testing center to which you are assigned or to which you plan to go as a standby to determine whether testing has been cancelled or delayed. This information can be provided only by The Psychological Corporation. To reach The Psychological Corporation on a Saturday test date, call 1-800-622-3231.

If you fail to appear for a test due to hazardous weather, you must notify The Psychological Corporation's Pharmacy College Admission Test Coordinator at 1-800-622-3231 no later than three days after the test date.

Section V.
AFTER THE TEST

How Your Test is Scored

Answer sheets are electronically scored, and the data are stored on computer files from which score reports are printed.

The Psychological Corporation understands the importance of your test results and uses many quality control procedures, both computerized and manual, during and after the scoring process to ensure the accuracy of scores.

The information on your score report is the only information available to you about your results. Because of the need to maintain test security, test booklets are not made available for review, and The Psychological Corporation does not provide a list of the questions you answered incorrectly or correctly. **Scores cannot be reported over the phone under any circumstances.**

Score Reporting

Approximately four to six weeks following the date of testing, you will be sent your personal score report, and the institutions to which you requested your scores be reported will be sent official score reports.

Do not attempt to send copies of your personal score report to schools to which you are applying. Schools will accept official score reports only.

How to Interpret Your Score Report

When you receive your score report, your scores will be reported as scaled scores and percentiles for each section of the test and for the test as a whole.

Different forms of any test may vary somewhat in difficulty. Because of the differences in difficulty between different forms of a test, the same raw scores on different forms are not necessarily equivalent. Using the statistical process of equating, it is possible to express scores in comparable terms across different forms of a test. Scaled scores are used for this purpose. The scale used for the PCAT ranges from approximately 100 to 300, with a mean of 200 (ie., a scaled score of 200 corresponds to the 50th percentile).

The percentile score indicates the percentage of applicants to colleges of pharmacy throughout the United States whose scores were lower than yours. For example, an examinee who earns a percentile score of 70 scored higher than 70 percent of other examinees.

An example of a personal score report with annotations appears in *Appendix D—Annotated Sample Personal Score Report.*

There is no passing or failing score set by The Psychological Corporation for this test. The extent to which test results are used in deciding whether or not a person will be admitted to a college of pharmacy varies from one school to another. Please consult the schools to which you are applying for information about their use of test scores. In general, test results are combined with other information, such as high school and undergraduate records, references, and the results of personal interviews.

Handscoring

After you receive your scores, you may request that your scores be verified by handscoring. There is a $10 fee for this service. However, the scoring methods used by The Psychological Corporation are highly reliable and accurate, and rarely does handscoring produce a change in a score.

To have your scores verified by handscoring, write to The Psychological Corporation and include:

1. The name of the test;
2. The date you took the test;
3. Your complete name, address, and social security number; and
4. A money order for $10 displaying your name.

Mail your request for handscoring to the address on page 7 of this booklet. Requests must be received within 60 days of your test date.

Replacement Score Reports

If you have not received your personal score report by six weeks after the date you tested, or if you receive a damaged score report, The Psychological Corporation will replace it at no cost to you.

If a school to which you had an official score report sent has not received it by six weeks after the date you tested, The Psychological Corporation will provide a replacement score report at no cost to you, providing you specified the proper school code when you applied. Mail your written request to the address on page 6 of this booklet.

Written requests for replacement score reports must be received by The Psychological Corporation no later than eight weeks after the test date. Requests after eight weeks must be accompanied by an Additional Score Report Fee.

Requesting Additional Score Reports

Score reports are available for five years after your test date. Scores older than five years will not be reported.

An Additional Score Report Fee of $10 must be paid **by money order for each score report you request** after you submit your application. When requesting additional score reports, you must provide the following information:

1. Your complete name as stated on your application, your address, and your social security number;
2. The name of the test you took;
3. The date you took the test;
4. The complete name and address to which each score report is to be sent; and
5. Your money order for the total fee.

Additional score reports normally will be mailed within two weeks of the receipt of your request by The Psychological Corporation.

To avoid duplication, you should keep a record of all schools to which you have your scores sent.

Mail your request to the address on page 7 of this booklet.

Cancellation of Scores by The Psychological Corporation

The Psychological Corporation is responsible for reporting scores that accurately reflect the performance of the examinee. For this reason, we adhere to a set of test administration and test security standards and review all test scores and administrative irregularities. The Psychological Corporation reserves the right to cancel any score it believes was obtained in a questionable manner.

When a score is cancelled, examinees will be given the opportunity to provide additional information about the situation. The examinee will also be given the option of retaking the test to verify scores. The Psychological Corporation will make no reimbursements for any expenses incurred by an examinee whose scores are cancelled.

All score cancellations are held in strict confidence. Reasons for score cancellations will not be disclosed to anyone except the examinee.

Section VI.
THE TEST

The Purpose of the Test

The Pharmacy College Admission Test is a specialized test which helps identify qualified applicants to pharmacy colleges by measuring general academic ability and scientific knowledge necessary for the commencement of pharmaceutical education.

Test Development

The Pharmacy College Admission Test (PCAT) is constructed specifically for colleges of pharmacy. The design and content of the PCAT are determined by the types of abilities, aptitudes, and skills deemed essential by colleges of pharmacy for success in the basic pharmacy curriculum, and by research concerning the kinds of tests that most accurately predict success in science-oriented courses, such as those included in pharmacy education. Periodic reviews of the test content are conducted with deans, faculty, and administrators in schools of pharmacy to ensure that the test items reflect curriculum changes in pharmacy schools.

Test Content

The Pharmacy College Admission Test consists of approximately 300 multiple-choice questions. Each question has four answer choices listed, only one of which is correct. The answer to each question can be derived independently of the answers to any other question.

You will have approximately three and one-half hours to complete the test (including a short rest break about halfway through the test).

The PCAT is divided into separate sections, each of which is timed separately. During the time allowed for each section, you will be permitted to work only on that section. You will not be allowed to go back to earlier sections or on to later sections. As you work on each section, it is advisable to answer first those questions which are easy for you, skipping over those questions to which you will need to return for further thought.

There are five content areas measured by the Pharmacy College Admission Test:

The **Verbal Ability** section measures general, nonscientific word knowledge using antonyms and analogies. There are approximately 50 questions in this section.

The **Quantitative Ability** section measures skills in arithmetic processes including fractions, decimals, and percentages, and ability to reason through and understand quantitative concepts and relationships, including applications of algebra (but not of trigonometry or calculus). There are approximately 65 questions in this section.

The **Biology** section measures knowledge of the principles and concepts of basic biology with major emphasis on human biology. There are approximately 50 questions in this section.

The **Chemistry** section measures knowledge of principles and concepts of inorganic and elementary organic chemistry. There are approximately 60 questions in this section.

The **Reading Comprehension** section measures ability to comprehend, analyze, and interpret reading passages on scientific topics. There are approximately 45 questions in this section.

Test-taking Strategies

- Be prepared physically and mentally. Get a good night's sleep the night before your test, eat what you consider a normal meal the morning of the test, and dress comfortably for the test.
- Heating and air conditioning systems may not be under the control of the test center staff; you may find the testing room to be unexpectedly warm or cool for the time of the year. Therefore, dress in a manner that will allow you to adapt to different room temperatures.
- Allow plenty of time to get to your testing center.
- Familiarize yourself with the test by reviewing the test content description and sample questions in this booklet. Most of the test involves knowledge, skills, and abilities accumulated over time, so cramming will probably not help. **The Psychological Corporation does not publish or recommend any study guides or materials for this test.**
- Answer as many questions as time allows. There is no penalty for guessing, so it is to your advantage to answer every question. When you are unsure which answer choice for a question is correct, eliminate as many wrong answers as you can. When you have second thoughts about your answer to a question, change your answer only if you have a good reason for doing so. Your "instinctive" response to a question is frequently correct.
- Do not dwell on questions that are unfamiliar or difficult since all questions count the same. In each section, answer questions about which you are confident, and return to answer the more difficult questions if time permits. Remember, however, that you may not return to earlier sections of the test. Going back to earlier sections (or working ahead) will result in your dismissal from the test.
- Work quickly, but carefully. Check regularly to make sure you are marking your answers in the correct place on the answer document.

Section VII.
SAMPLE TEST QUESTIONS AND ANSWERS

Sample Questions

The following sample questions are similar to those found in the test.

Verbal Ability

Directions: Choose the word that means the **opposite** or most nearly the opposite to the word in capitals.

1. IMPUDENT
A. Wise
B. Cautious
C. Respectful
D. Destructive

2. ASSUAGE
A. Harm
B. Oppress
C. Motivate
D. Intensify

Directions: Choose the word that **best** completes the analogy in capital letters.

3. PLANE : AIRPORT :: SHIP :
A. Pier
B. Berth
C. Depot
D. Station

4. INEPT : SKILL :: FLIMSY :
A. Power
B. Weight
C. Strength
D. Thickness

Quantitative Ability

Directions: Choose the one **best** answer to each of the following questions.

5. $.06(10^3) =$
A. 60
B. 600
C. 6000
D. 600,000

6. 40% of 20 = 25% of
A. 16
B. 32
C. 36
D. 64

7. $\sqrt{18} + \sqrt{32} =$
A. $2\sqrt{10}$
B. $5\sqrt{2}$
C. $7\sqrt{2}$
D. 14

8. Ten ml of pure acid must be added to what volume of water to make a solution containing 20% acid?
A. 30 ml
B. 40 ml
C. 50 ml
D. 60 ml

9. If $\log x = A$, then $\log x^2 =$
A. 2A
B. A^2
C. A + log 2
D. 2 log A

10. If two similar triangles have bases in the ratio of 2:3, what is the ratio of their areas?
A. 1:1.67
B. 2:3
C. 4:6
D. 4:9

Biology

Directions: Choose the **best** answer to each of the following questions.

11. In humans, the removal and storage of excess glucose from the blood is one of the primary functions of the
A. liver.
B. kidneys.
C. pancreas.
D. large intestine.

12. In a certain organism, red (R) color is dominant over white (r). In a cross between an RR and an rr individual, what percentage of the offspring will be red?
A. 25%
B. 50%
C. 75%
D. 100%

13. Which of the following graphs most accurately shows the relationship between the cell and the surrounding medium during osmosis?

A.

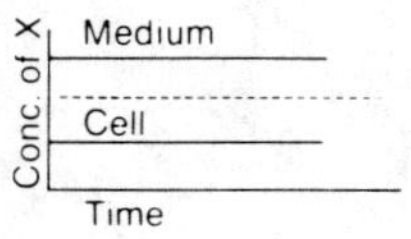

B.

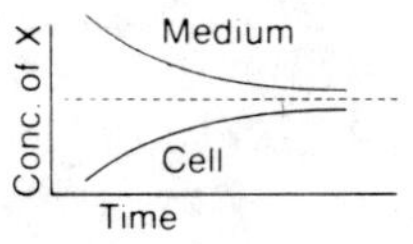

C.

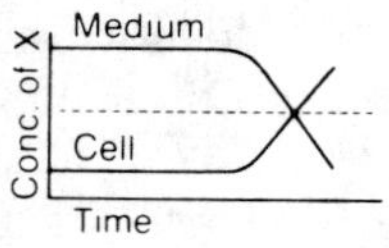

D.

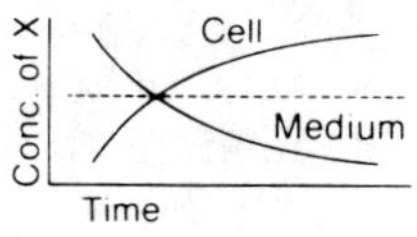

Chemistry

Directions: Choose the **best** answer to each of the following questions.

14. What volume of carbon dioxide would be produced if 5 liters of propane, C_3H_8, were burned in air according to the following equation?

$$C_3H_8 + 5O_2 \rightarrow 3CO_2 + 4H_2O$$

A. 1 liter
B. 3 liters
C. 15 liters
D. 30 liters

15. The fact that helium gas is monatomic is best explained by the
A. vacant 2s and 2p orbitals of the helium atom.
B. small diameter of the nucleus of the helium atom.
C. presence of a single proton in the nucleus of the helium atom.
D. relative magnitudes of attractive and repulsive forces between two helium atoms.

16. The equation, ${}^{40}_{19}K \rightarrow {}^{40}_{20}Ca + {}^{0}_{-1}e + v$, represents an example of the process called
A. alpha decay.
B. beta decay.
C. positron emission.
D. orbital electron capture.

Reading Comprehension

Directions: Read the following passage and then choose the one **best** answer to each of the questions following the passage.

Neomycin is a colorless antibiotic produced by certain strains of *Streptomyces fradiae*. The antibiotic is a polybasic, water-soluble substance. The neomycin complex consists of two isomeric substances, now recognized as neomycin B and neomycin C. Commercial neomycin is composed mainly of neomycin B and is usually in the form of a sulfate, a white amorphous powder. An A fraction was at first also described, but it was later found to be a degradation product. Neomycin is active against a great variety of Gram-positive cocci and rods, Gram-negative rods, and acid-fast bacteria, notably the tuberculosis organism. It is not active against anaerobic bacteria, fungi, most protozoa, rickettsiae, and viruses. Development of resistance to neomycin is slower than that to streptomycin. For subcutaneous injection of neomycin sulfate in mice, the LD_{50} or dosage at which 50 percent of the animals died is 165-250 mg/kg. The LD_{50} for intraperitoneal administration is about the same. Intravenously, neomycin is about five times as toxic. Orally, the LD_{50} is greater than 2800 mg/kg.

17. If neomycin is bought at a drugstore, it would most probably consist of a sulfate plus
- **A.** neomycin A.
- **B.** neomycin B.
- **C.** neomycin C.
- **D.** equal mixtures of neomycin B and C.

18. Neomycin would probably NOT be effective in treating
- **A.** athlete's foot.
- **B.** tuberculosis.
- **C.** infections of the skin caused by rod bacteria.
- **D.** infections of the skin caused by Gram-positive cocci.

19. Neomycin is LEAST toxic when it is administered by
- **A.** mouth.
- **B.** intraperitoneal injection.
- **C.** injection under the skin.
- **D.** injecting it into the veins.

Correct Answers

1. C	**5.** A	**9.** A	**13.** B	**17.** B
2. D	**6.** B	**10.** D	**14.** C	**18.** A
3. A	**7.** C	**11.** A	**15.** D	**19.** A
4. C	**8.** B	**12.** D	**16.** B	

Notes

APPENDIX A

Scheduled Testing Centers, Center Codes, and Test Dates

Use the following scheduled testing center code numbers to indicate your choice of testing center. Testing centers usually will be within 50 miles of the listed city. Your admission ticket will give the exact location of the testing center to which you are to report. **DO NOT** use these code numbers to specify colleges of pharmacy to which your scores are to be sent. Be sure the test is scheduled for the date and center you select.

Oct.	Feb.	Apr.	
			ALABAMA
	X		505 Auburn
	X	X	501 Birmingham
	X	X	504 Mobile
			ARIZONA
	X		510 Tempe
X	X	X	511 Tucson
			ARKANSAS
X	X		514 Fayetteville
X	X	X	513 Little Rock
X	X		766 State University (Jonesboro)
			CALIFORNIA
X	X	X	525 San Francisco
X	X	X	522 Los Angeles
			COLORADO
	X		527 Denver
			DISTRICT OF COLUMBIA
X	X	X	536 Washington
			FLORIDA
X	X	X	542 Gainesville
X	X	X	538 Miami
X			782 Pensacola
X	X	X	545 Tallahassee
X	X	X	544 Tampa
			GEORGIA
X	X	X	547 Athens
X	X	X	548 Atlanta
X			333 Cochran
		X	787 Savannah
X	X		332 Statesboro
			HAWAII
	X		551 Honolulu

Oct.	Feb.	Apr.	
			ILLINOIS
	X	X	556 Carbondale
X	X	X	555 Chicago
X	X		557 Urbana
			IOWA
X	X	X	567 Iowa City
			KANSAS
X	X	X	607 Kansas City
			KENTUCKY
X		X	575 Bowling Green
X	X	X	573 Lexington
X	X	X	574 Louisville
X			354 Murray
			LOUISIANA
X	X	X	577 New Orleans
		X	815 Shreveport
			MARYLAND
X	X	X	366 Catonsville (Baltimore)
			MASSACHUSETTS
X	X		587 Boston
			MICHIGAN
	X		593 Detroit
			MISSISSIPPI
	X		603 Jackson
X	X		833 University
			MISSOURI
X	X		834 Columbia
X	X		610 Springfield
	X		609 St. Louis
			NEBRASKA
	X		615 Omaha

Appendix A *(cont'd)*

Oct.	Feb.	Apr.	
			NEW JERSEY
	X	X	623 New Brunswick
			NEW YORK
	X		630 Albany
X	X	X	631 Buffalo
	X	X	634 New York*
	X	X	641 Syracuse
			NORTH CAROLINA
X	X	X	405 Chapel Hill/Durham
X	X	X	853 Charlotte
	X		407 Greenville
X			468 Wilmington
			NORTH DAKOTA
	X		734 Bismarck
X	X	X	736 Fargo
	X		737 Grand Forks
			OHIO
	X		646 Cincinnati
	X		647 Cleveland
	X	X	649 Columbus
			OKLAHOMA
X	X		658 Norman
			OREGON
	X		421 Ashland
X	X	X	422 Corvallis
	X	X	666 Portland
			PENNSYLVANIA
X	X	X	670 Philadelphia
X	X	X	674 Pittsburgh
			PUERTO RICO
X	X	X	746 Rio Piedras (San Juan)
			SOUTH CAROLINA
	X	X	684 Columbia
			TENNESSEE
X	X	X	688 Knoxville
X	X	X	689 Memphis
X	X	X	692 Nashville

*New York test sites may be located in any of the five boroughs.

Oct.	Feb.	Apr.	
			TEXAS
	X	X	865 Austin
		X	696 Dallas
X	X	X	700 Houston
	X		701 Lubbock
		X	703 San Antonio
			UTAH
	X		707 Salt Lake City
			VIRGINIA
X	X	X	710 Blacksburg
X	X	X	712 Richmond
			WASHINGTON
		X	718 Seattle
			WEST VIRGINIA
	X		720 Charleston
X	X	X	883 Morgantown
			WISCONSIN
X	X	X	886 Madison
	X		724 Milwaukee
	X		460 Wausau
			CANADA
	X		952 Bathurst, NB
	X		975 Charlottetown, PE
	X		954 Corner Brook, NF
X	X	X	956 Halifax, NS
	X		958 Kingston, ON
	X		959 London, ON
	X		960 Montreal, PQ
	X	X	957 Ottawa, ON
	X		961 Owen Sound, ON
	X		967 St. Catharines, ON
	X		979 St. John, NB
	X	X	963 St. John's, NF
	X		970 Sault Ste. Marie, ON
	X	X	964 Sudbury, ON
	X		978 Sydney, NS
	X	X	971 Thunder Bay, ON
		X	980 Timmins, ON
	X	X	965 Toronto, ON
	X		973 Windsor, ON

APPENDIX B

Pharmacy College Code Numbers

It is essential that you give on your application the correct **code numbers** of the schools to which you want your scores reported.

ALABAMA
001 Auburn University, Auburn
002 Samford University, Birmingham

ARIZONA
003 The University of Arizona, Tucson

ARKANSAS
004 University of Arkansas Medical Center, Little Rock

CALIFORNIA
005 University of California, San Francisco
007 University of Southern California, Los Angeles
006 University of the Pacific, Stockton

COLORADO
008 University of Colorado, Boulder

CONNECTICUT
009 The University of Connecticut, Storrs

DISTRICT OF COLUMBIA
010 Howard University, Washington

FLORIDA
011 Florida Agricultural & Mechanical University, Tallahassee
077 Nova Southeastern University, Health Professions Division
012 University of Florida, Gainesville

GEORGIA
079 George College
013 Mercer University, Atlanta
014 University of Georgia, Athens

IDAHO
015 Idaho State University, Pocatello

ILLINOIS
016 University of Illinois, Chicago
040 Chicago College of Pharmacy, Downers Grove

INDIANA
017 Butler University, Indianapolis
018 Purdue University, Lafayette

IOWA
019 Drake University, Des Moines
020 The University of Iowa, Iowa City

KANSAS
021 The University of Kansas, Lawrence

KENTUCKY
080 Morehead State University
022 University of Kentucky, Lexington

LOUISIANA
023 Northeast Louisiana University, Monroe
024 Xavier University of Louisiana, New Orleans

MARYLAND
025 University of Maryland, Baltimore

MASSACHUSETTS
026 Massachusetts College of Pharmacy, Boston
027 Northeastern University, Boston

MICHIGAN
028 Ferris State College, Big Rapids
029 The University of Michigan, Ann Arbor
030 Wayne State University, Detroit

MINNESOTA
031 University of Minnesota, Minneapolis

MISSISSIPPI
032 The University of Mississippi, University

MISSOURI
033 St. Louis College of Pharmacy, St. Louis
034 University of Missouri-Kansas City, Kansas City

MONTANA
035 University of Montana, Missoula

NEBRASKA
036 Creighton University, Omaha
037 The University of Nebraska Medical Center, Omaha

NEW JERSEY
038 Rutgers-The State University, New Brunswick

NEW MEXICO
039 University of New Mexico, Albuquerque

Appendix B *(cont'd)*

NEW YORK

042 Long Island University, College of Pharmacy and Health Sciences, Brooklyn

043 St. John's University, Jamaica

044 State University of New York at Buffalo, Buffalo

045 Union University, Albany College of Pharmacy, Albany

NORTH CAROLINA

076 Campbell University, Buies Creek

041 Campbell University School of Pharmacy

046 The University of North Carolina, Chapel Hill

NORTH DAKOTA

047 North Dakota State University, Fargo

OHIO

048 Ohio Northern University, Ada

049 The Ohio State University, Columbus

051 The University of Toledo, Toledo

050 University of Cincinnati, Cincinnati

OKLAHOMA

052 Southwestern State College, Weatherford

053 University of Oklahoma, Health Sciences Center, Oklahoma City

OREGON

054 Oregon State University, Corvallis

PENNSYLVANIA

055 Duquesne University, Pittsburgh

056 Philadelphia College of Pharmacy & Science, Philadelphia

057 Temple University of the Commonwealth System of Higher Education, Philadelphia

058 University of Pittsburgh, Pittsburgh

PUERTO RICO

059 University of Puerto Rico, Medical Science Campus, San Juan

RHODE ISLAND

060 University of Rhode Island, Kingston

SOUTH CAROLINA

061 Medical University of South Carolina, Charleston

062 University of South Carolina, Columbia

SOUTH DAKOTA

063 South Dakota State University, Brookings

TENNESSEE

064 University of Tennessee, Memphis

TEXAS

065 Texas Southern University, Houston

078 University of Houston, Downtown Campus

066 University of Houston, Houston

067 The University of Texas, Austin

UTAH

068 University of Utah, Salt Lake City

VIRGINIA

069 Virginia Commonwealth University, Richmond

WASHINGTON

070 University of Washington, Seattle

071 Washington State University, Pullman

WEST VIRGINIA

072 West Virginia University, Morgantown

WISCONSIN

073 University of Wisconsin, Madison

WYOMING

074 University of Wyoming, Laramie

CANADA

281 Dalhousie University, Halifax

075 Memorial University of Newfoundland, St. John's

275 The University of Alberta, Edmonton

276 University of British Columbia, Vancouver

282 University of Manitoba, Manitoba

277 University of Montreal, Montreal

280 University of Saskatchewan, Saskatoon

278 University of Toronto, Toronto

PHILIPPINES

379 University of the Philippines, Diliman, Quezon City

APPENDIX C

Postal Abbreviations

Street and City

APARTMENT..............APT	EAST........................E	NORTH ....N	SOUTH.....................S
AVENUE ....AVE	FORT ....FT	PARK.......................PK	STATION ....STA
BOULEVARD ....BLVD	GARDEN ....GDN	PARKWAY.............PKWY	STREET...................ST
BOX.........................BX	HEADQUARTER.........HQ	PIKE.........................PI	TERRACE ....TER
CIRCLE....................CIR	HEIGHTS...............HTS	PLACE......................PL	TRAIL ....TRL
CITY........................CY	HIGHWAY.............HWY	POINT ....PT	TRAILER...............TRLR
COLLEGE.................CLG	JUNCTION ....JCT	PORT......................PRT	TURNPIKE............TPKE
COMMUNITY..........CMTY	LAKE.....................LK	POST OFFICE ....PO	UNIVERSITY...........UNIV
COUNTY ....CNTY	LANE.....................LN	ROAD ....RD	WAY....................WAY
COURT ....CT	MOUNT..................MT	ROUTE....................RTE	WEST ....W
DRIVE......................DR	MOUNTAIN ....MTN	SCHOOL..................SCH	

State and Province

ALABAMA.................AL	KENTUCKY ....KY	OHIO ....OH	ALBERTA ....AB
ALASKA...................AK	LOUISIANA ....LA	OKLAHOMA...............OK	BRITISH COLUMBIA.....BC
ARIZONA ....AZ	MAINE ....ME	OREGON...................OR	LABRADOR ....LB
ARKANSAS................AR	MARYLAND............MD	PENNSYLVANIA ....PA	MANITOBA ....MB
CALIFORNIA..............CA	MASSACHUSETTS ......MA	PUERTO RICO..............PR	NEW BRUNSWICK ......NB
CANAL ZONE ....CZ	MICHIGAN...............MI	RHODE ISLAND ....RI	NEWFOUNDLAND ....NF
COLORADO ....CO	MINNESOTA ....MN	SOUTH CAROLINA ....SC	NORTHWEST TERRITORIES..........NT
CONNECTICUT............CT	MISSISSIPPI ....MS	SOUTH DAKOTA...........SD	NOVA SCOTIA ....NS
DELAWARE ....DE	MISSOURI..............MO	TENNESSEE ....TN	ONTARIO ....ON
DIST. OF COLUMBIA......DC	MONTANA ....MT	TEXAS.......................TX	PRINCE EDWARD IS .....PE
FLORIDA ....FL	NEBRASKA ....NE	UTAH.......................UT	QUEBEC ....PQ
GEORGIA..................GA	NEVADA ....NV	VERMONT..................VT	SASKATCHEWAN........SK
HAWAII.....................HI	NEW HAMPSHIRE.......NH	VIRGIN ISLANDS VI	YUKON TERRITORY .....YT
IDAHO......................ID	NEW JERSEY............NJ	VIRGINIA ....VA	
ILLINOIS IL	NEW MEXICO ....NM	WASHINGTON ....WA	
INDIANA ....IN	NEW YORK ....NY	WEST VIRGINIA ....WV	
IOWA.......................IA	NORTH CAROLINA......NC	WISCONSIN................WI	FOREIGN.................FR
KANSAS....................KS	NORTH DAKOTA ....ND	WYOMING ....WY	

Notes

APPENDIX D

Annotated Sample Personal Score Report

THE PSYCHOLOGICAL CORPORATION®
555 ACADEMIC COURT
SAN ANTONIO, TEXAS 78204-0952 MAIL TO: 604.2/PCA2

(1) PHARMACY COLLEGE ADMISSION TEST

(2) ADDITIONAL SCHOOL TRANSCRIPTS MAY BE REQUESTED UNTIL FEBRUARY 2000

	(4) SCALED Score	(5) %ile *	
(3) VERBAL ABILITY	169	11	(6) TAKEN FEBRUARY 1995
READING COMPREHENSION	188	30	(7) FIRST EXAMINATION
BIOLOGY	178	18	
CHEMISTRY	162	4	
QUANTITATIVE ABILITY	176	23	
COMPOSITE	175	11	

(8) Transcripts sent to these school codes:
0077 0011 0012

ID - 930225O5152 PG - 604.2 TD - 9502

(9) AGEE ANNE D 604.2
3150 SW 55 AVE 3
MIAMI, FL 33145

*See candidate information booklet for explanation.

(10) THIS IS NOT AN OFFICIAL SCHOOL TRANSCRIPT

600-33-01

Explanation of the Annotated Personal Score Report

(1) Gives the name of the test.

(2) Specifies the last month and year that score reports from this administration will be available. Score reports may be requested until five years after a test date.

(3) Gives the names of the sections of this test.

(4) Listed below this heading are the scaled scores the examinee earned on each section of this test. A composite scaled score is also given for the test as a whole. Different forms of any test may vary somewhat in difficulty. Because of differences in difficulty between different forms of a test, the same raw scores on different forms are not necessarily equivalent. Using the statistical process of equating, it is possible to express scores in comparable terms across different forms of a test. Scaled scores are used for this purpose. The scale ranges from approximately 100 to 300 with a mean of 200 (i.e., a scaled score of 200 is equivalent to the 50th percentile).

(5) Listed below this heading are the examinee's percentiles for each section of this test. A composite percentile is also given which shows how well the examinee performed on the test as a whole. Percentiles for this test were determined by administering the test to applicants to colleges of pharmacy throughout the United States. Statistical analysis of the percentage of examinees earning each scaled score was used to determine the percentile corresponding to each scaled score.

(6) Gives the month and year the test was taken.

(7) Shows whether this was the first time this examinee took this test or whether the examinee has taken it at least once before.

(8) Gives the code numbers of the schools to which official score reports have been sent.

(9) Gives the examinee's name (last name first) and address as they appear in The Psychological Corporation's records. Also shown are your unique ID number, the test program number, and the test date for the scores reported.

(10) Shows this is a personal score report.

Notes

PHARMACY CAREERS

In asking, "Shall I study pharmacy?" you are really asking a series of questions:

Who are the pharmacists?

What personal qualifications should I have to become a pharmacist?

What about women as pharmacists?

What are the educational requirements?

What would I study?

Where would I work?

What would I do as a pharmacist?

What is the present and future outlook for employment and advancement?

Once these and other questions are answered to your satisfaction, you are prepared to give an honest answer to your basic question—Shall I study pharmacy?

If you have a sincere interest in people and health, you really should consider pharmacy as a career. Modern pharmacy offers outstanding opportunity for professional service and personal achievement.

Professional Commitment

Pharmacy's ultimate goal is to render pharmaceutical care. Pharmaceutical care focuses pharmacists' attitudes, behaviors, commitments, concerns, ethics, functions, knowledge, responsibilities, and skills on the provision of drug therapy with the goal of achieving definite outcomes toward the improvement of a patient's quality of life. These outcomes of drug use are: 1) cure of a disease; 2) elimination or reduction of symptoms; 3) arresting or slowing a disease process; 4) prevention of disease; 5) diagnosis of disease; and 6) desired alterations in physiological processes, all with minimum risk to patients. Pharmacists are professionals, uniquely prepared and available, committed to public service and to the achievement of this goal.

Professional Prospects

The practice of pharmacy is a vital part of total health care. More people are receiving health care than ever before, and this trend will continue. Young men and women in pharmacy will face new challenges, expanded responsibilities, and an ever-increasing growth in opportunities. An expanding need for pharmacists is shown by listing some of society's growth factors. These include a longer life span; a greater demand for drugs, especially among the older age groups; a broader range of specific drugs for more diseases; a larger number of preventive medicines; increased opportunities for home health care; growth of health insurance and medical-care prepayment plans; more interest in obtaining prompt and proper medical attention; burgeoning population; greater demand for more hospitals, nursing homes, and extended care facilities; and the emphasis on research by the pharmaceutical industry and government. These factors combine to point out the short-range prospects as well as long-range opportunities for pharmacists; the profession is ever becoming more important to society.

These, then are the prospects. Next, let's look at "who should study pharmacy?" You may have noted already that young men and women are invited to consider careers in pharmacy. Every area of pharmacy that we will be discussing has women in practice. They use the same professional skills, call on the same fund of scientific knowledge, hold the same responsibilities, and earn the same respect as their male counterparts.

Nearly 30% of the nation's pharmacists are women; they currently represent over 60% of the students enrolled in pharmacy schools.

Community Pharmacy

Nearly everyone is familiar with community pharmacists and the pharmacy in which they practice. The pharmacy size and type of practice may vary. Community pharmacies may be large or small establishments, owned by individuals or operated by chains; located on quiet streets or on busy city corners, in professional health centers or in bustling shopping centers. Depending on local as well as professional needs, the pharmacies range from those where patrons find a complete line of needed items for health, beauty, and comfort to those that concentrate their activities exclusively in the supply of medicines and sickroom needs.

Pharmacists staffing these pharmacies make up the bulk of practitioners. Six out of every ten—almost 120,000 men and women—practice in community pharmacies.

You probably visit the community pharmacist more often than you do any other member of the health team. Americans make over five billion trips a year to pharmacies; the pharmacist has an opportunity to see at least one member of every family in his community every week. He or she talks to people when they are healthy and when they are sick, when they are "just browsing" or when they are concerned with an emergency, when they ask for their needs and when they are seeking advice or information. Pharmacists are playing an increasing role in the "wellness" movement, especially through counseling about preventive medicine. According to one estimate, pharmacists get more than two billion inquiries a year from their patrons.

Pharmacists are primary dispensers of medicines and health supplies. They make available thousands of items used in health care, ranging from the drugs and chemicals used in compounding prescription medication to sickroom supplies. Pharmacists also serve the community as a prime source of information on health topics. They help patrons maintain their health and well-being by giving them the health information they need, or by telling them where they can get the help they should have.

Advances in the use of computers in pharmacy practice now allow pharmacists to spend more time educating patients and maintaining and monitoring patient records. As a result, patients have come to depend on the pharmacist as an "answer man" of the highest caliber.

Pharmacists, despite the variety of tasks performed in and out of the community pharmacy, basically are specialists in the science of drugs. They must understand drug composition, chemical and physical properties, manufacture and uses, activity in the normal body as well as in the person who is ill, and must be familiar with tests for purity and for strength. Pharmacists are well prepared to compound medicines and to dispense prescription orders written by physicians, dentists, and other prescribers. More and more prescribers rely on pharmacists for information about various drugs, their availability and their activity, just as patrons do when they ask about nonprescription medicines.

If pharmacists want to combine their professional talents with the challenge of the fast-moving retail pharmacy business, they often consider management positions in chain pharmacy practice or ownership of their own pharmacy. In chain practice, career paths usually begin at the store level with subsequent advancement to positions at the district, regional, and corporate levels. Many chain companies have management development programs in marketing operations, legal affairs, third party programs, computerization, and pharmacy affairs.

Independent retail practice offers the opportunity for pharmacists to be "their own boss." The spirit of entrepreneurism and motivation has enabled many pharmacists to successfully own their pharmacy or, through establishing consultation services, own their own pharmacy practice.

Hospital Pharmacy

As society moves toward a concept of total health care, there is increasing emphasis on provision of that care through organized health care settings. As a result, increasing numbers of pharmacists practice in large and small hospitals, nursing homes, extended care facilities, neighborhood health centers, and health maintenance organizations.

Hospital pharmacists, as members of the health care team along with physicians and nurses, have a unique opportunity for direct involvement with patient care. The clinical skills and knowledge received by pharmacy students today make this individual an authoritative source of drug information for physicians, nurses, and patients.

In addition to direct patient care involvement, pharmacists in hospitals are responsible for systems of total control of drug distribution, designed to assure that each patient receives the appropriate medication, in the correct form and dosage, at the correct time. Many hospital pharmacists maintain records on each patient, using them not only to fill medication orders but also to screen for drug allergies and adverse drug effects.

Contemporary hospital pharmacy practice includes a number of highly specialized areas, such as nuclear pharmacy, drug and poison information, and intravenous therapy. In addition, clinical pharmacy practitioners provide specialized services in adult medicine, pediatrics, oncology, ambulatory care, and psychiatry. The nature and size of the hospital helps to determine the extent to which these specialized services are needed. Because of the diversity of activities involved in pharmacy departments, there is also an ever increasing demand for management expertise, including finance and budgeting, personnel administration, systems development, and planning.

About 38,000 registered pharmacists work on a full- or part-time basis in hospitals or nursing homes. As hospital pharmacists continue to become more involved in providing patient-oriented services, the demand for practitioners in this area of pharmacy continues to grow.

The Pharmaceutical Industry

Another area for a pharmaceutical career is represented by the industry that produces chemicals, prescription and nonprescription drugs, and other health products.

Pharmacists are employed in the pharmaceutical industry in the areas of marketing, research and product development, quality control, sales, and administration.

In the production of pharmaceutical products, industry employs pharmacists, as well as engineers, chemists, and biologists. Many pharmacists have gone on to obtain postgraduate degrees in order to meet the technical demands and scientific duties required in pharmaceutical manufacturing.

Pharmacists interested in sales and administration can combine their interests with their technical background in pharmacy by serving as medical service representatives. These representatives call on physicians, dentists, veterinarians, and on other pharmacists to explain the uses and merits of the products their firms produce. Experienced and successful medical service representatives with administrative abilities often rise to supervisory or executive posts in the ever-growing pharmaceutical industry.

Pharmacists also are employed as salesmen, supervisors, and administrators in wholesale drug firms. Since there are fewer wholesale drug firms than there are community and hospital pharmacies, the opportunities are fewer. It is true, nonetheless, that many of the leading figures in wholesaling and pharmaceutical manufacturing entered those fields as pharmacists, previously having practiced in community and hospital pharmacies.

Academic Pharmacy

Almost 3,000 full-time faculty members work in the nation's 75 colleges and schools of pharmacy; approximately one-third of these are women. In general, all participate in teaching, research, and public service. Some faculty are involved in patient care. Others, such as department chairs and deans, serve as consultants for local, state, national, and international agencies' organizations. Many are leaders in their communities.

To join the faculty at a college of pharmacy almost without exception requires a graduate-level doctorate or professional degree. Such additional education as residencies and postdoctoral fellowships may also be desirable.

While most pharmacists who complete graduate school exercise the option to teach, there currently are shortages of faculty creating an array of excellent professional opportunities. Clinical pharmacy faculty have significant responsibility for patient care in addition to their work in teaching and research. These academicians often are called educator/practitioners, and they serve as role models for pharmacy students and residents in many practice settings. Faculty in disciplines other than clinical pharmacy usually are not directly involved in patient care or clinical research. Instead, the basic sciences are mainly concerned with "bench" research that depends on sophisticated instrumentation, analytical methods, and animal models. Pharmacy administration research often uses survey methods and statistical analyses to solve complex problems of drug utilization review, marketing, management, and other practice issues.

To paraphrase one current pharmacy faculty member, "perhaps no other job in pharmacy has such far-reaching effects on the profession as that of an educator. It is in academia that one can excite individuals about pharmacy and lay the groundwork for continuing advances in the field."

Other Specialized Fields in Pharmacy

Pharmacists use their basic educational backgrounds in a host of federal and state positions. At the federal level, pharmacists hold staff and supervisory posts in the United States Public Health Service, the Veterans Administration, the Food and Drug Administration, and in all branches of the armed services. Some of these posts provide commissioned officer status; others come under civil service.

At the state level there are agencies charged with regulating the practice of pharmacy to preserve and protect the public health. These legal boards governing pharmacy practice usually have pharmacists employed as full-time executive officers. Also, one or more inspectors, frequently pharmacists, are employed by each state pharmacy board. As more state health agencies consolidate their purchases, a pharmacist is often engaged as a purchaser of medical and pharmaceutical supplies for the entire state.

Nearly every state has an active pharmaceutical association which employs a full-time executive officer, usually a graduate of a college of pharmacy. Several national professional associations are also guided by pharmacists with interest and special talents in organizational work.

You may know other pharmacists who are engaged in highly specialized tasks. There are pharmacists in advertising, packaging, technical writing, magazine editing, and science reporting. There are pharmacists with legal training serving as patent lawyers or as experts in pharmaceutical law. There are pharmacists in America's space laboratories and aboard ships such as *S.S. Hope*; others direct giant manufacturing firms or specialize in medicinal plant cultivation.

By now, it should be clear to you that this diversity of pharmacy is one of its chief strengths. And, in diversity lies your opportunity. In the United States, over 140,000 pharmacists practice in community, or hospital pharmacies, or long-term and ambulatory care facilities. The remainder follow one or another of the special fields you have just reviewed. The prospects for immediate employment and for long-term career growth, have never been better. Today's pharmacy graduates have a greater variety of careers open to them than the graduates of past years. The opportunity for success in any of these fields is wide open for the man or women with ability, education, and imagination.

Personal Qualifications

As you think about your place in pharmacy, you must also think about your qualifications to meet pharmacy's demands for judgment, dependability, and conscientious performance. You must be good at detail and willing to check and doublecheck your own work. As with others on the health care team, your decisions and actions involve human life and well-being. Your need for careful attention to your work, your decisions, and the results of your actions cannot be overemphasized. Accuracy, neatness, orderliness and cleanliness must be your guidelines.

Since pharmacists, by law, are entrusted with the proper storage, handling, and dispensing of dangerous and habit-forming drug substances, they must be absolutely scrupulous in handling and dispensing them. Their ethical standards must be high, and they must use fact and good judgment in answering the questions people ask them.

Experts in drugs and chemicals, it follows that pharmacists need a good education in scientific subjects and should have curiosity and a willingness to learn. The pharmacist needs some background in the principles of management; should have an interest in these subjects and the desire to maintain the records, legal and otherwise, required for pharmacy practice. Most importantly, pharmacists must enjoy working with people, be able to meet them and be willing to serve them in a variety of circumstances.

Let's look now at what you need to prepare yourself for the study of pharmacy.

Preparation for Study

Students enrolled in colleges of pharmacy study for a minimum of five years after graduation from high school. There are accredited programs at 75 colleges and schools of pharmacy in the U.S. and Puerto Rico; several of them offer a required or optional six-year program of study.

All pharmacy colleges operate under one of three plans: (1) One year of preprofessional education preceding admission to the professional curriculum; (2) Two years of preprofessional education followed by professional studies; (3) An integrated curriculum with all years of study in the professional college. Where preprofessional education is required for admission, the first year or two of study may be taken in any approved junior college or university.

In high school the student should take an academic curriculum in preparation for entrance to college. Grades should be good—colleges of pharmacy do not judge an applicant solely by high school marks, but these certainly are an important factor.

If you are considering a career in pharmacy, you should write to the pharmacy college of choice (See page 9 for names and addresses) or to several colleges and ask for details about entrance requirements. These vary from college to college, so the best way to avoid disappointment is to make sure that high school and preprofessional college courses are carefully planned.

A sound basic education in math and science courses is an essential part of preparation for the study of pharmacy. Also, good written and verbal communication skills are important in both the study and practice of pharmacy. Since courses of study taken in college by pharmacy students may not demand many classes in literature, history, government, or social studies, you may want to get a good background in one or more of these fields from high school or preprofessional schooling. Foreign languages are not generally required for admission but may be needed later by students who pursue graduate studies. Contrary to popular opinion, the study of Latin in high school is not needed for admission to pharmacy school.

High school science courses are helpful in preparing students for the many science courses studied in pharmacy college. Biology, chemistry, physics, and mathematics are especially desirable. Beyond this, a good student with a strong background in nonscientific college preparatory subjects will be in a favorable position for succeeding in the study of pharmacy. Of course, if you have completed high school and are now enrolled in a community or liberal arts college, you will have credits in and exposure to many of the courses discussed above. It is important that preprofessional students arrange their course work to meet the requirements of the college of pharmacy in which they plan to enroll. Early consultation with the dean or admissions officer is important. If your decision to study pharmacy is not yet firm, you can still have your program checked by the pharmacy school; this advice can be helpful when you do make application for admission.

Colleges of pharmacy, in considering applicants for admission, often give attention to the relative position of a student in their class—near the top, in the middle group, or near the bottom. Although colleges of pharmacy are interested in enrolling students who have demonstrated the ability to do good work in school, they are also interested in students who demonstrate potential for good academic work and contribution to the profession.

Many colleges, both preprofessional and professional, require education tests for admission including the Pharmacy College Admission Test (PCAT)* and/or various college entrance exam scores (i.e. SAT or ACT) as criteria for entrance. The PCAT can be taken either in high school or college. The results are one of several factors usually considered in the admission of each student.

The variations in admission requirements and procedures among the colleges of pharmacy make it necessary for you to inquire concerning the situation at the college you wish to enter. In some cases your high school counselor or college advisor may have the necessary information. You may wish to refer to one or more of the publications listed on page 27 of this booklet, or inquiries may be sent directly to the dean of the pharmacy college selected. Schools will be pleased to supply you with details concerning admission or other information in which you may be interested.

*administered by The Psychological Corp.
555 Academic Court
San Antonio, Texas 78204
(512) 554-8198

Pharmaceutical Education

With all this as preparation, let's turn now to education in the pharmaceutical sciences.

Colleges of pharmacy award two professional degrees in pharmacy, the Bachelor of Science in Pharmacy (B.S. Pharmacy) and the Doctor of Pharmacy (Pharm.D.). Both of these degrees qualify the student to take the State Board of Pharmacy Licensing Examination, a requirement to practice pharmacy in any state. Including preprofessional college study, the minimum educational program for a B.S. in Pharmacy is five academic years; and for the Pharm.D. degree, it is six academic years when offered as the first professional degree. Both the B.S. Pharmacy and the Pharm.D. curricula are designed to produce a scientifically and technically competent pharmacist who can apply this training in such a manner as to provide maximum health care services to patients. Because the Pharm.D. program is of greater length, it often provides the opportunity for students to gain greater experience in patient-centered learning experiences and in working in close cooperative relationships with health practitioners. It is the goal of all pharmacy schools to prepare pharmacists who can support expanded responsibilities in the clinical use of drugs and assist in the provision of rational drug therapy.

The Pharm.D. degree is the highest university or college degree awarded in pharmacy for completion of academic preparation for practice. At some schools the Pharm.D. is offered as the only professional degree in pharmacy, at other schools a student may elect to enroll in either the B.S. Pharmacy or the Pharm.D. program, and some schools require a B.S. Pharmacy prior to enrolling in the Pharm.D. program. Write the pharmacy school in which you are interested to determine what professional degree programs they offer.

After graduating from pharmacy school an increasing number of students are seeking residency training in institutional pharmacy practice. Over two hundred pharmacy residency programs are offered in 185 hospitals throughout the United States. These residency programs may be taken in general pharmacy practice, clinical pharmacy practice, or other specialty areas depending upon personal interests and specific career requirements. Completion of a pharmacy residency is sometimes a requirement for employment in hospital pharmacy practice or in clinical faculty positions at pharmacy schools. In some cases, residencies in community practice settings also are available.

Students also have the opportunity to complete advanced study (graduate work) at many colleges of pharmacy. Graduate study in one of the specialized areas of pharmacy may qualify the student for a master of science (M.S.) or doctor of philosophy (Ph.D.) degree. These advanced degree programs require an undergraduate degree at least at the bachelor's level prior to enrollment; however, the undergraduate degree need not be in pharmacy. The M.S. and Ph.D. degrees are research degrees and do not qualify the student to be a licensed pharmacy practitioner unless the student has also earned a B.S. Pharmacy or Pharm.D.

If you examine several pharmacy college catalogs you will notice that courses are similar but not identical. There are no rigid rules on curriculum enforced on colleges, but a common core of subjects is found in every college of pharmacy. You will find that certain colleges emphasize certain subjects, and thus place less emphasis on others. Since you will certainly be examining catalogs of colleges that interest you, the following discussion will touch largely on the core of subjects common to most colleges of pharmacy.

Our earlier descriptions of community pharmacy and of the various specialities should have conveyed the idea that the profession of pharmacy blends science, technical art, and human relationships in a unique fashion. Basic to the science in pharmacy are contributions from three broad fields—biology, chemistry, and mathematics. So courses in these basic sciences are required in pharmacy curricula.

Mathematics is an important tool in most scientific courses, so two or more semesters of college mathematics are usually required. In addition, a pharmacist uses math a great deal in dispensing prescriptions, in determining proper drug dosage levels, in preparing formulas of many types, in management procedures, and in certain chemical calculations. Hence, additional instruction is given in the various kinds of weights and measures used in pharmacy, in calculating doses of drugs given to persons of different ages and weights, in figuring the amount of material to use for a solution, and in many other operations included under pharmaceutical calculations.

Instruction in physics is usually given because the principles are basic to many pharmaceutical practices. In addition, physics has a close relationship to chemistry; both sciences are needed in order to understand the behavior and properties of matter. The fineness of powdered drugs, the transfer of heat, the behavior of gases, the formation and decay of radioactive isotopes—these and other phenomena of pharmacy can be well understood only through knowledge of the principles of physics.

Many medical substances are pure chemicals, so the importance to pharmacists of a knowledge of chemistry is easy to see. From simple table salt to substances so complex that their formulas are not completely known, pharmacists are continually dealing with chemicals. They must know how to handle and store them, as some are dangerous; how to analyze them to determine their purity; and how to dissolve them, combine them, package them, and preserve them—as well as many additional factors involving chemicals. Small wonder then that pharmacy students study the principles of the common divisions of chemistry and finish off this study with several courses in pharmaceutical chemistry. Here the principles of basic chemistry are applied in the study of medicinal products.

In addition to chemical medicines, many drugs come from plants and animals. Moreover, the practical use of nearly all medicinal substances is within or upon the body of man or animal. Hence, as a background to knowledge of natural drugs and the actions of drugs in the body, the study of a number of courses in biology is included in the educational program of the pharmacy student. Some of the courses offered in the biological sciences include biology, botany, zoology, physiology, microbiology, and biochemistry.

Courses in the basic sciences, mathematics, psychology, sciology, and English are usually given in the preprofessional years, but some may be scheduled throughout the curriculum. These social sciences provide the student a better ability to understand people and to deal effectively as a health professional in society.

Professional Courses

The professional curriculum is composed of six of the courses in six major areas of instruction.

Pharmaceutical chemistry, already mentioned, emphasizes the application of chemical know-how to pharmacy. Some of the courses deal with chemicals used as medicines—their use, nature, preparation and preservation. In other courses, attention is given to the processes and tests used to determine the purity and strength of a chemical or its pharmaceutical form. The pharmacy student learns, for example, how to find out if aspirin is pure, or how to determine how much vitamin C is contained in a particular solution or tablet.

Pharmacognosy deals with the nature and sources of "natural drugs"—those obtained from plants or animals, either directly or indirectly. For example, with a drug such as quinine, this study involves the source, the commercial production, the marketing, the chief pure chemicals contained in the drug, and the uses made of the drug and its derivatives.

Pharmacology is concerned with understanding the action of drugs in the body. Attention is given to the effects of various doses of each medicinal substance and to the different ways in which medicine can be introduced into the body. The effects of poisons and the means to overcome them are studied in toxicology. Generally animal tests are required to learn the strength of drugs. Physicians know a great deal about pharmacology and toxicology; yet as the expert in drugs the pharmacist must have this knowledge to even a greater extent.

Education in modern business management is important for graduates who plan to enter community pharmacy and some institution practices. This area is commonly designated pharmacy administration. Instruction frequently includes principles of basic economics, accounting, management, computer applications, marketing, merchandising, and legal phases of the profession of pharmacy. Courses in pharmacy administration are especially helpful to pharmacists who become executives in pharmacies, hospitals, service wholesale houses, or manufacturing concerns.

All colleges of pharmacy offer a variety of courses in pharmacy practice. These courses are designed to give an appreciation of the background and nature of the profession, to familiarize students with the many skilled processes used in pharmacy, to introduce the various forms of medicines, and to teach them how to dispense medication accurately and skillfully. Instruction in pharmacy practice again emphasizes the fact that pharmacy blends science and technology, and that throughout the professional services of the pharmacist there is always a responsible relationship both to the patient and the physician.

Laboratory instruction may be of some concern to you. Instruction in the basic sciences and in the professional areas (except for most of the administration courses) includes some laboratory work. This laboratory work is both traditional and clinical. It explores various scientific phenomena, as well as studies the clinical application of the principles of pharmaceutical sciences.

Clinical pharmacy is that area within the pharmacy curriculum which deals with patient care, with emphasis on drug therapy. Clinical pharmacy seeks to develop a patient-oriented attitude in the student. The education of pharmacists to meet the needs of society can be attained only through a careful blending of theoretical course work and clinical experiences. The clinical component of the pharmacy curriculum varies from school to school; however, the basic objectives are the same. Some of these objectives are (1) to help students become more aware of the general methods of diagnosis and patient care specifically related to drug therapy, (2) to develop students' communication skills for effective interaction with patients and with practitioners of other health professions, (3) to help students develop a patient awareness in the practice of pharmacy, (4) to enable students to integrate the knowledge acquired in course work prior to clinical exposure, and to apply it to the solution of real problems, and (5) to develop students' awareness of their responsibility for monitoring the drugs taken by patients.

Working Conditions

You have, by now, been given answers or general responses to many of your general questions. Let's take some others.

How many hours a week does a pharmacist work?

What is the pay?

Is there much chance for advancement?

There is no single answer to the first question. You may have read that there are over 200 potential careers on the health care team. The pharmacist is one of the leading members of the team, along with the physician, the dentist, and the nurse. As health care workers, this team is prepared to render service when it is needed. As we said earlier, pharmacy has a special appeal to those who want to serve their community and society.

Your own experience tells you that emergencies do not wait; pharmaceutical service may be required at 2:00 A.M. as well as 2:00 P.M. As a result, pharmacists expect to make their services available to the public at hours other than those you might think of as "normal" for professional people. Except for the true emergency where time isn't measured for time's sake, the pharmacist's work week probably averages around forty-eight hours. In hospitals and long-term care facilities, pharmacists average forty to forty-four hours a week.

Despite our desire to be specific, we must generalize. Salaries are not uniform in all parts of the country. All pharmacists in the same community may not receive like salaries. Better prepared, better informed, more skillful, and more experienced pharmacists will naturally command better salaries than beginners. However, surveys have shown that two years after college the pharmacist has among the highest starting salaries of college graduates in the United States. Future salary progress, of course, depends on ability and experience.

The easiest of this series of questions concerns opportunity for advancement. Most owners of pharmacies started their careers as pharmacists working for someone else. Many had no money other than their weekly salary. From such starts, many have become owners of one or more pharmacies or have sometimes developed chains of pharmacies. Not only does this apply to opportunities for community pharmacy, the same is true for other fields in pharmacy. Of course, you generally do not "own" a hospital or nursing home pharmacy, but staff pharmacists do become directors of pharmacy services. Medical service representatives have risen in their organizations to lead their firms. Distinguished scientists move to major roles in research administration. Civil servants and commissioned officers rise to policy and command positions.

The rewards will be many: a well-paying profession accompanied by the sense of service, pride, and recognition.

No country in the world has more colleges of pharmacy than the United States. Nor does any country have as many different kinds of pharmacy colleges. Some of them are in our largest cities, others are in small towns. A few colleges are independent institutions, while the vast majority are parts of universities, state colleges, municipal institutions of higher education, or of denominational universities. Almost every state has at least one college of pharmacy.

Students who are considering pharmacy frequently ask, "Where can I study pharmacy?" Some also want an answer to, "What college is the best one?"

The first question is answered easily. The colleges of pharmacy are listed beginning on page 9. The American Council on Pharmaceutical Education periodically examines these colleges to accredit the pharmacy program.

A nonaccredited pharmacy program may be legally recognized by the board of pharmacy in the state in which it is located, but graduates of the college who wish to practice pharmacy in any other state will probably be denied permission to do so.

There is no satisfactory answer to the question, "What college is the best one?" Due to institutional policy and faculty strength, one college may be unusually strong in administration courses, a second one in chemistry, a third in pharmacology. Or, a college may be good in almost all of the basic and professional fields. One college may offer the student advantages in extracurricular activities, and another may be especially strong in emphasis on ethical values. College A may have a brand new building, but College B in the old building may have superior equipment. College C may have a faculty with an outstanding research or public service reputation.

A better question from the thoughtful prospective pharmacy student is, "Everything considered, what is the best college of pharmacy for me?" You will want to investigate several possible college choices.

A visit to one or more colleges of pharmacy is a valuable means for learning firsthand something about the college and about tuition and other costs. As a pharmacy student you will spend considerable money and at least three years at the college of pharmacy. Since education is an investment for a lifetime, visits to colleges in which you are interested are very important.

A visit with the dean, admissions officer or faculty members at the college(s) of pharmacy you are considering will be particularly helpful. If you are currently enrolled in a two- or four-year college and are just beginning to explore career options, you should make it a point to talk with the health professions advisor at your campus. These individuals are excellent sources of information.

Other contacts include practicing pharmacists and state pharmaceutical associations (any pharmacist has the address).

Expenses

"What is all of this going to cost?" is certainly an important question. How much it will cost depends on where you enroll, how far it is from your home town, and the extent to which public dollars are used to support the institution.

One thing should be stressed. Every dollar you spend on your education is a dollar well invested. The returns in direct salary benefits and in other less tangible gains will be far in excess of your initial investment. You should know, also, that it is possible today for nearly every student who meets academic and personal qualifications to get as much education as they desire.

The next section describes general sources of financial aid. The admissions officers of the colleges of pharmacy will be happy to describe additional scholarship or loan sources available at their colleges.

Practicing pharmacists who have attended various colleges also can be helpful in giving their impressions of the institutions. Other alumni can also help if the college is part of a larger institution. Frequently high school counselors, science teachers, and principals can give information about one or more specific colleges.

All colleges publish catalogs and frequently additional literature which will gladly be furnished on request. It would be to your advantage to study your possible choices in terms of area, at least, and then request catalogs to study and compare.

The End of the Beginning

This booklet, "Shall I Study Pharmacy?" was prepared to help you answer the question for yourself. It contains general answers to some questions, specific answers to others. You also may have noted that some other questions, obvious to you, were not even considered. This is as it should be. "Shall I Study Pharmacy?," as we noted earlier is but one of a series of questions that thousands of young men and women ask every year. You have begun to get answers to basic questions in this publication. Others, specific and general alike, will be answered for you in still other publications.

You will note that we did not discuss legal requirements for practice. This information can be obtained from the board of pharmacy for the state where you have an interest. We did not discuss dormitory living or other housing, social activities, honorary or professional sororities or fraternities, athletics or other extracurricular activities, or professional societies or other interest groups. Each college of pharmacy catalog you will examine will point out these specifics; some of the sources that follow also will be helpful to you.

Publications

If you think that pharmacy may be for you, or if you still seek answers to other questions, here is a list of sources of information that you should read:

Pharmacy School Admission Requirements and Graduate Program Guidebook
Published by:
American Association of Colleges of Pharmacy
Price: $20.00 each (Payment must accompany order)

Opportunities in Pharmacy Careers
by Fred B. Gable
Published by:
National Textbook Co.
4255 W. Touhy Avenue
Lincolnwood, IL 60646
Price: $6.95 pprbk.; $9.95 hdbk.

Employment Outlook for Pharmacists From Occupational Outlook Handbook
Bureau of Labor Statistics
Superintendent of Documents
U.S. Government Printing Office
Washington, D.C. 20402
Price: $8.50

Pharmacy: Career Planning and Professional Opportunities
Edited by T. Donald Rucker
Published by:
Health Administration Press
School of Public Health
The University of Michigan
102 E. Horan St.
Ann Arbor, Michigan 48109
Price: $24.00

The Pfizer Guide: Pharmacy Career Opportunities
Published by:
Mark Powley Associates, Inc.
15 Meigs Avenue
Madison, CT
Available free.

Sources of Financial Aid

The American Association of Colleges of Pharmacy, itself, does not administer any student assistance programs. Most loan and scholarship programs are administered by the financial aid office on each college campus. The aid officers, therefore, are the most reliable sources of current and complete information regarding financial assistance for students interested in studying pharmacy. The following outline of sources of financial aid only generally discusses the types of programs available. You are advised to write directly to the financial aid office identified in the pharmacy school's catalog for specific information and application forms.

Federal Scholarships and Loans

- Pell Grants and Supplemental Educational Opportunities Grants—federal scholarships available for the neediest undergraduate students.
- College Work Study Program—a combination of federal and local school funds used to pay salaries for students who work on campus.
- National Direct Student Loan Program—a campus-based, low-interest bearing loan program for undergraduate students.
- Stafford Loan Program and Parent Loans for Undergraduate Students—educational loan programs administered by local banking institutions.
- Health Education Assistance Loans and Health Professions Student Loans—federal loan programs for which pharmacy students are currently eligible.

State Scholarships and Loans

Consult your high school counselor, college advisor, or write the state department of education to find out what financial assistance may be available from your state.

College Scholarships and Loans

Pharmacy colleges also administer student financial assistance funds provided by local or state pharmaceutical associations and their auxiliaries, practicing pharmacists, drug manufacturers and wholesalers, memorial funds and foundations, alumni associations, local chapters of pharmaceutical organizations and fraternities, as well as general university funds allocated for this purpose. For further information about aid which may be available, write to the college of pharmacy of your choice.

Prepharmacy students may be eligible to receive similar assistance from the community colleges or universities they plan to attend before entering professional schools.

Sources of Assistance

We recommend working closely with your high school or college advisors who can sometimes be the best source of information about grants or scholarships which go beyond federal and state programs. You also should look outside of the health professions for support—you may be able to compete successfully for economically or academically awarded scholarships from private groups and associations.

Finally, if you cannot find outside grant or scholarship support and decide to seek loan support, you may wish to contact NARD (representing independent retail pharmacists) regarding its loan program. Information can be obtained from NARD, 205 Daingerfield Road, Alexandria, Virginia 22314.

The Next Step

As you evaluate your financial and educational options it is important to remember that pharmacy graduates are among the most sought after of health professionals. The career options are numerous, salaries outstanding and commitment rewarding. Any investment in a pharmaceutical education will guarantee you an excellent future.

Contact one or more of the colleges or schools listed on the following pages. You will find the admissions personnel and other faculty members anxious to answer your questions about pharmacy and about their institution's programs.

UNITED STATES COLLEGES AND SCHOOLS OF PHARMACY

ALABAMA

School of Pharmacy
Auburn University
Auburn University, AL 36849-5501
(205) 844-4740

School of Pharmacy
Samford University
800 Lakeshore Drive
Birmingham, AL 35229
(205) 870-2820

ARIZONA

College of Pharmacy
The University of Arizona
Tucson, AZ 85721
(602) 626-1427

ARKANSAS

College of Pharmacy
University of Arkansas for Medical Sciences
4301 West Markham—Slot 522
Little Rock, AR 72205-7122
(501) 686-5557

CALIFORNIA

School of Pharmacy S-926
University of California
San Francisco, CA 94143-0446
(415) 476-1225

School of Pharmacy
University of the Pacific
3601 Pacific Avenue
Stockton, CA 95211
(209) 946-2561

School of Pharmacy
University of Southern California
1985 Zonal Avenue
Los Angeles, CA 90033-1086
(213) 342-1369

COLORADO

School of Pharmacy
University of Colorado
Box 297
Boulder, CO 80309-0297
(303) 492-6278

CONNECTICUT

School of Pharmacy
The University of Connecticut
Box U-92, 372 Fairfield Road
Storrs, CT 06269-2092
(203) 486-2129

DISTRICT OF COLUMBIA

College of Pharmacy & Pharmacal Sciences
Howard University
2300 4th Street, N.W.
Washington, DC 20059
(202) 806-6530

FLORIDA

College of Pharmacy & Pharmaceutical Sciences
Florida Agricultural and Mechanical University
P.O. Box 367
Tallahassee, FL 32307
(904) 599-3593

College of Pharmacy
Southeastern University of the Health Sciences
1750 NE 168th Street
North Miami Beach, FL 33162-3097
(305) 949-4000

College of Pharmacy
University of Florida
Box J-484, Health Science Center
Gainesville, FL 32610-0484
(904) 392-9713

GEORGIA

Southern School of Pharmacy
Mercer University
3001 Mercer University Drive
Atlanta, GA 30341
(404) 986-3300

College of Pharmacy
The University of Georgia
Athens, GA 30602
(404) 542-1911

IDAHO

College of Pharmacy
Campus Box 8288
Idaho State University
Pocatello, ID 83209-8288
(208) 236-2175

ILLINOIS

College of Pharmacy
University of Illinois at Chicago
P.O. Box 6998 M/C 874
Chicago, IL 60680-6998
(312) 996-7240

Chicago College of Pharmacy
Chicago College of Osteopathic Medicine
555 31st Street
Downers Grove, IL 60515-1235
(708) 971-6417

INDIANA

College of Pharmacy
Butler University
4600 Sunset Avenue
Indianapolis, IN 46208
(317) 283-9322

School of Pharmacy and Pharmacal Sciences
Purdue University
West Lafayette, IN 47907-0708
(317) 494-1357

IOWA

College of Pharmacy
Drake University
28th and Forest
Des Moines, IA 50311
(515) 271-2172

College of Pharmacy
The University of Iowa
Iowa City, IA 52242
(319) 335-8794

KANSAS

School of Pharmacy
University of Kansas
2056 Malott
Lawrence, KS 66045-2500
(913) 864-3591

KENTUCKY
College of Pharmacy
University of Kentucky
Rose Street-Pharmacy Bldg.
Lexington, KY 40536-0082
(606) 257-2738

LOUISIANA
School of Pharmacy
Northeast Louisiana University
700 University Avenue
Monroe, LA 71209-0470
(318) 342-1600

College of Pharmacy
Xavier University of Louisiana
7325 Palmetto Street
New Orleans, LA 70125
(504) 483-7424

MARYLAND
School of Pharmacy
University of Maryland
20 North Pine Street
Baltimore, MD 21202-1180
(410) 328-7650

MASSACHUSETTS
Massachusetts College of Pharmacy
and Allied Health Sciences
179 Longwood Avenue
Boston, MA 02115
(617) 732-2800

College of Pharmacy and Allied Health
Professions
Northeastern University
360 Huntington Avenue
Boston, MA 02115
(617) 437-3321

MICHIGAN
College of Pharmacy
Ferris State University
901 South State Street
Big Rapids, MI 49307
(616) 592-2254

College of Pharmacy
The University of Michigan
Ann Arbor, MI 48109-1065
(313) 764-7312

College of Pharmacy and Allied Health
Professions
Wayne State University
105 Shapero Hall
Detroit, MI 48202-3489
(313) 577-1574

MINNESOTA
College of Pharmacy
University of Minnesota
5-130 Health Sciences Unit F
308 Harvard Street, S.E.
Minneapolis, MN 55455-0343
(612) 624-1900

MISSISSIPPI
School of Pharmacy
The University of Mississippi
University, MS 38677-9814
(601) 232-7265

MISSOURI
St. Louis College of Pharmacy
4588 Parkview Place
St. Louis, MO 63110-1088
(314) 367-8700

School of Pharmacy
University of Missouri-Kansas City
5005 Rockhill Road
Kansas City, MO 64110-2499
(816) 235-1607

MONTANA
School of Pharmacy & Allied Health
Sciences
University of Montana
Missoula, MT 59812-1075
(406) 243-4621

NEBRASKA
School of Pharmacy and Allied Health
Professions
Creighton University
California at 24th Street
Omaha, NE 68178
(402) 280-2950

College of Pharmacy
University of Nebraska
600 S 42nd St.
Omaha, NE 68198-6000
(402) 559-4333

NEW JERSEY
College of Pharmacy
Rutgers University
The State University of New Jersey
Post Office Box 789
Piscataway, NJ 08855-0789
(908) 932-2666

NEW MEXICO
College of Pharmacy
University of New Mexico
Albuquerque, NM 87131-1066
(505) 277-2461

NEW YORK
Arnold & Marie Schwartz College of
Pharmacy and Health Sciences
Long Island University
75 DeKalb Avenue at University Plaza
Brooklyn, NY 11201
(718) 488-1000

College of Pharmacy and Allied Health
Professions
St. John's University
Grand Central & Utopia Parkways
Jamaica, NY 11439
(718) 990-6275

School of Pharmacy
University at Buffalo
C126 Cooke-Hochstetter Complex
Buffalo, NY 14260
(716) 636-2823

Albany College of Pharmacy
Union University
106 New Scotland
Albany, NY 12208
(518) 445-7211

NORTH CAROLINA
School of Pharmacy
Campbell University
Post Office Box 1090
Buies Creek, NC 27506
(919) 893-4111

School of Pharmacy
University of North Carolina
at Chapel Hill
CB#7360 Beard Hall
Chapel Hill, NC 27599-7360
(919) 966-1121

NORTH DAKOTA
College of Pharmacy
North Dakota State University
Box 5055
Fargo, ND 58105
(701) 237-7456

OHIO
College of Pharmacy
Ohio Northern University
Ada, OH 45810
(419) 772-2275

College of Pharmacy
The Ohio State University
500 West 12th Avenue
Columbus, OH 43210-1291
(614) 292-2266

College of Pharmacy
University of Cincinnati-Medical Center
Mail Location #4
Cincinnati, OH 45267
(513) 558-3784

College of Pharmacy
The University of Toledo
2801 West Bancroft Street
Toledo, OH 43606
(419) 537-2019

OKLAHOMA
School of Pharmacy
Southwestern Oklahoma
State University
100 Campus Drive
Weatherford, OK 73096
(405) 774-3105

College of Pharmacy
University of Oklahoma
P.O. Box 26901
Oklahoma City, OK 73190-5040
(405) 271-6484

OREGON
College of Pharmacy
Oregon State University
Pharmacy Bldg
Corvallis, OR 97331-3507
(503) 737-3424

PENNSYLVANIA
School of Pharmacy
Duquesne University
Pittsburgh, PA 15282
(412) 434-6380

School of Pharmacy
Philadelphia College of Pharmacy and
Science
600 South 43rd Street
Philadelphia, PA 19104-4495
(215) 596-8870

School of Pharmacy
Temple University
3307 North Broad Street
Philadelphia, PA 19140
(215) 221-4990

School of Pharmacy
University of Pittsburgh
1106 Salk Hall
Pittsburgh, PA 15261
(412) 648-8579

PUERTO RICO
School of Pharmacy
University of Puerto Rico
GPO Box 5067
San Juan, PR 00936-5067
(809) 758-2525 Ext. 5400

RHODE ISLAND
College of Pharmacy
University of Rhode Island
Kingston, RI 02881-0809
(401) 792-2761

SOUTH CAROLINA
College of Pharmacy
Medical University of South Carolina
171 Ashley Avenue
Charleston, SC 29425-2301
(803) 792-3115

College of Pharmacy
University of South Carolina
Columbia, SC 29208
(803) 777-4151

SOUTH DAKOTA
College of Pharmacy
South Dakota State University
Box 2202C
Brookings, SD 57007-0197
(605) 688-6197

TENNESSEE
College of Pharmacy
University of Tennessee
847 Monroe Ave., Suite 238
Memphis, TN 38163
(901) 528-6036

TEXAS
College of Pharmacy & Health Sci-
ences
Texas Southern University
3100 Cleburne
Houston, TX 77004
(713) 527-7164

College of Pharmacy
University of Houston
4800 Calhoun
Houston, TX 77204-5511
(713) 749-4106

College of Pharmacy
University of Texas at Austin
Austin, TX 78712-1074
(512) 471-1737

UTAH
College of Pharmacy
University of Utah
Salt Lake City, UT 84112
(801) 581-6731

VIRGINIA
School of Pharmacy
Virginia Commonwealth University
MCV Campus—Box 581
410 North 12th Street
Richmond, VA 23298-0581
(804) 786-7346

WASHINGTON
School of Pharmacy
University of Washington
T-341 Health Science Center SC-69
Seattle, WA 98195
(206) 543-2030

College of Pharmacy
Washington State University
Pullman, WA 99164-6510
(509) 335-8664

WEST VIRGINIA
School of Pharmacy
West Virginia University
Health Sciences Center
Morgantown, WV 26506
(304) 293-5101

WISCONSIN
School of Pharmacy
University of Wisconsin-Madison
425 North Charter Street
Madison, WI 53706
(608) 262-1416

WYOMING
School of Pharmacy
University of Wyoming
P.O. Box 3375
Laramie, WY 82071-3375
(307) 766-6120

Graduate Programs in Pharmaceutical Sciences

General Information

A Brief History

Graduate work in pharmacy in America had its beginnings at the University of Wisconsin, but did not flourish until the professional pharmacy curriculum provided a sufficient academic foundation for graduate study (the four-year BS in pharmacy became the norm in 1935). Several factors were responsible for the development of graduate work: (1) the evolution of the pharmaceutical industry, (2) the expectation by parent universities that schools of pharmacy have faculty educated and trained, in part, with faculties in other disciplines, (3) student desires to pursue a graduate education, and (4) the realization of pharmacy faculty that research and scholarly activity are both stimulating and obligatory to the enhancement of the profession.

Unlike many other professions, entry into pharmacy practice traditionally has been accessible at the baccalaureate (undergraduate) level. Doctoral level education began within specific disciplines of the pharmaceutical sciences; graduates of Ph.D. programs may or may not be pharmacy graduates. Beginning with that first University of Wisconsin program, there was a steady increase in both the number of colleges and schools of pharmacy offering graduate programs and the numbers of students seeking an advanced degree. Early surveys of the American Association of Colleges of Pharmacy (AACP) indicate that in 1965 there were 661 students enrolled in doctoral programs in the pharmaceutical sciences at 44 schools. By 1970 that figure had risen to 994. In 1975 enrollments dropped slightly to 980, climbing to 1,191 by 1980. By 1985 enrollments had increased to 1,502.

A Current Snapshot

According to the most recent AACP enrollment survey, 2,524 students were enrolled in graduate programs in the pharmaceutical sciences: 1,850 in Ph.D. programs (73 percent) and 674 in master of science programs (27 percent).

Over the years, graduate programs have remained strongly male dominated. The past several years, however, have seen the ratio of women pursuing masters and doctoral degrees increase upward, now tallying 37 percent. Although not approaching the 62 percent enrollment level women currently hold in entry level pharmacy programs, it appears that women increasingly will continue to seek careers in which postgraduate coursework is necessary.

Black, Hispanic and American Indians comprise four percent of Ph.D. and M.S. students. Foreign born students (nonpermanent U.S. residents) comprise 43 percent of the graduate student population.

Sixty-one (61) colleges and schools of pharmacy offer graduate programs in the pharmaceutical sciences. Data provided in the fall of 1990 indicate 205 graduate programs are offered: 41 M.S., 130 M.S. and Ph.D., and 26 Ph.D. Forty-eight (48) schools offer Ph.D. and/or M.S. programs in medicinal/pharmaceutical chemistry/pharmacognosy; 40 offer programs in pharmacology; 15 offer programs in the pharmaceutical sciences; 44 offer programs in pharmaceutics; 32 offer programs in pharmacy administration; and 18 offer programs in pharmacy practice.

Based on projections provided by the schools, graduate student tuition for public schools will average $2,475 for in-state residents in 1991/92; private college tuitions will average $8,348. Over seventy percent of the schools reporting indicate fee waivers are granted for all or some residents and 79 percent of the schools waived fees for all or some nonresidents. The median level of support for Ph.D. students receiving full support in 1989 was $8,850 for teaching assistantships and $4,500 for research assistantships. The median fellowship stipend for Ph.D. students was $10,000 and the median residency stipend was $12,468.

Demographic information for graduate students enrolled in fall 1989 reflect that 58 percent had previously earned a pharmacy degree and, of that group, 82 percent were pursuing their graduate degree at that same institution; 42 percent were U.S. citizens; and English is the second language for 33 percent of M.S. and Ph.D. students.

Admissions data indicate that 51.1 percent of applicants selected for graduate programs in 1991 came from an applicant pool considered "highly selective." Graduate Record Examination median scores for fall 1989 graduate enrollees across all disciplines were: 500 verbal; 650 quantitative; and 580 analytical.

Why Consider a Graduate Degree in the Pharmaceutical Sciences?

A graduate degree provides almost limitless options in the pursuit of scientific interests as well as excellent opportunities to attain a position of leadership in academia, industry or government. If you are willing to invest the time and the commitment to attain a graduate degree, you will find opportunities available to:

- contribute to the medical knowledge base by performing basic research in an area of your choice;
- interact with a myriad of professionals in the sciences and other disciplines;
- help assure an ongoing supply of health professionals through teaching;
- design and develop drug products;
- perform multidisciplinary work; and,
- exercise scientific and managerial control over projects of personal interest.

If you like to make a difference, pursuing a graduate degree could be exactly the right choice for you. The result of earning a masters or doctoral degree in any of the pharmaceutical science disciplines couples the challenge of independent research with personal interests and talents which will expand your career and the pharmacy profession.

Candidate Characteristics and Qualifications

Graduate degree candidates come from a variety of backgrounds:

- pharmacy students enrolled in professional programs, pharmacists with a B.S. or Pharm.D. degree;
- individuals with degrees in chemistry, biology or other sciences;
- men, women, minorities.

If you fall somewhere within these categories, you are a candidate for a graduate program in the pharmaceutical sciences.

Graduate programs are demanding and require additional years of intense study and research. Such an undertaking is certainly not for everyone. But men and women who enjoy the sciences or health systems management and policy, who are looking for professional advancement, intellectual challenge and an expanded earning potential, should actively consider and pursue a graduate degree in the pharmaceutical sciences.

It is important to remember that we practice our careers for 30 to 40 years or more. From that perspective, the investment of time to earn a graduate degree is relatively minor compared to the long-term benefits a graduate degree provides.

Women, blacks, Hispanics and American Indians have proven to be exceptionally motivated and productive graduate students. Currently over a third of pharmacy's graduate students are women. Since professional enrollments of women pharmacy students have surpassed 60 percent, pharmacy educators are currently focusing a great deal of attention on attracting qualified women to their graduate programs.

A little over 10 percent of pharmacy's graduate students are minorities. While this level is on a parity with professional program enrollments, pharmacy educators and employers consider it entirely too low. Minorities considering going on to graduate programs in the pharmaceutical sciences will find themselves in particular demand.

What is a Graduate Program in the Pharmaceutical Sciences?

There simply is no one answer to this question. The true benefit of graduate level work is that it is almost completely individualized. Graduate programs, therefore, take on the characteristics of the students currently in them.

A masters program typically consists of:

- approximately one year of coursework (minimum number of credit hours usually set by department/school/university;
- an independent research project;
- a written thesis describing the completed research; and
- oral defense of the research.

A doctoral program typically consists of:

- approximately one more year of coursework (minimum number of credit hours set by department/school/university -- usually two times the requirements of a masters program);
- an independent, original research project (research for a Ph.D. is more complex and intense than what is required for masters);
- written dissertation; and
- oral defense of the dissertation.

There are several attractive characteristics of graduate programs:

- you will work closely with your advisor on research projects.
- as analytical skills develop, you will increasingly be able to explore your specific research interests in more depth; and,
- you will spend time in the classroom with a small number of fellow candidates. Through intense and highly interactive learning experiences, strong camaraderie grows, as will your self-confidence and the cadre of academicians and professionals with whom you will be associated for the remainder of your career.

Perhaps the biggest adjustment you will have to make when entering a graduate program is to the cultural and social environment in which you will be living and working as a graduate student. These years often are ones of personal sacrifice in terms of time, temporarily lost earning potential and energy. Students considering graduate school must consider these negatives, but should not lose sight of the positives--the gratification in terms of accomplishment, personal and professional growth, and enhanced career potential. And perhaps the most important factor of survival is the strong support system which naturally evolves in any community of graduate students.

Graduate Student Financial Support

Generally, U.S. citizens can obtain financial support to defray tuition, fees and living expenses. The usual forms of financial support are assistantships, fellowships and tuition waivers. These funds are drawn from college and university resources as well as from grant support of individual faculty members. Financial aid in the form of loans, grants and scholarships based on need and academic accomplishment also is available from federal and state government and from private sources. For example, the American Foundation for Pharmaceutical Education currently supports over 60 graduate students with various scholarship and fellowship grants. The Pharmaceutical Manufacturers Association Foundation also supports a number of discipline specific fellowships. Admissions officers and contacts at each pharmacy school can provide full information about available financial support.

A Guide to Selecting a Graduate Program in the Pharmaceutical Sciences

Graduate programs in the pharmaceutical sciences need to be investigated rigorously because no two are alike. While perhaps confusing, this diversity is good on two counts: first, students are allowed, in fact encouraged, to find a program that is closely aligned with their individual interests; and, second, once your degree is in hand, you will possess individually developed, uniquely marketable skills with which to move into your desired career path.

The following tips are offered to help you identify the best graduate program for you.

The academic factors. Besides evaluating written material available through the colleges and schools you may be considering, you should interview current students about their experiences--social and academic. Look at policies concerning credits, off-campus learning opportunities, typical modes of instruction and relative strengths of the various programs. And then ask a few additional questions...

How good is the program for you?

- How is an advisor chosen? Do you have free choice? What system allows you the opportunity to gather information in order to make that decision?
- Does the work promise to be in an area in which you are interested? How much flexibility is there in the program for elective coursework?
- Is there a spirit of interdisciplinary cooperation within the faculty?
- How much time do advisors devote to their graduate students? How will you know you are making appropriate progress through your program? What are the feedback mechanisms?
- Will the faculty member who will be your major advisor be taking any sabbatical time during your tenure in the program?
- What is the nature of faculty members' work in the lab, the classroom, and the field?
- Will postgraduate work be necessary for you to obtain a position in the field you are considering?
- What access do advisors have to job markets, both within and outside the academic community, that might help you network as you approach graduation?

Does the program enjoy a national reputation?

- Does the faculty, in general, have a national reputation? What about the individual who might be your advisor?
- Are faculty members currently publishing in refereed journals, presenting research findings or being invited to make presentations at national and international meetings? Do they contribute to the body of knowledge in the specialty area?
- Are there cross-campus relationships among the faculty? Are there opportunities to work with graduate students from other disciplines?
- Is the program well-funded through a good balance of university, public and private support?

The outcome factors.

- What is the average length of time it has taken the most recent ten graduates to complete their program?
- What is the school/program attrition rate?
- Will the program prepare you for the specific career you have chosen, or will the program provide you an opportunity to sample various research experiences if you have not yet settled on a specific career?
- How many individuals have graduated from the program in the past five years and what are they now doing career-wise? Salary-wise?

The personal factors.

- What kinds of academic and personal support are available?
- What, if any, are the health risks associated with your proposed area of study?
- Is the geographic location of the college convenient considering your family ties and commitments?
- Is the nature of the campus and community such that you can make yourself relatively comfortable and highly productive for the next few years?
- What are the costs and quality of available housing?
- Will your spouse be able to find suitable employment?

The cost factors. Make sure you know what is available and what eligibility criteria exists. Then ask,

- Are there application fees?
- How will you be supported?
- Does your faculty advisor have sufficient and secure funding to see you through your program?
- Does the college have a fall back pool of funds to help support you should your advisor's funding end?
- What will your responsibilities be as a teaching assistant? Is training in education and teaching techniques available?
- If loans are to be one source of your funds, just what will your payback obligation be after earning your degree?
- Is moonlighting necessary to make ends meet? and if so, is it allowed?
- Are there funds to support travel to scientific meetings?

Resources

This publication, we hope, helps plant the seed or nurture your interest in a graduate program. Please take the next step and start asking additional questions. Carefully review the information contained in the following sections of this publication, which should provide sufficient information for you to begin in earnest the process of sifting through your graduate program options.

Once into the process, you may find the following organizations useful as you seek more specific information about career opportunities or support.

American Association of Pharmaceutical Scientists
1650 King Street
Alexandria, Virginia 22314

American Foundation for Pharmaceutical Education
618 Somerset Hall
P.O. Box 7126
North Plainfield, New Jersey 07060

American Pharmaceutical Association
2215 Constitution Avenue, N.W.
Washington, D.C. 20037

National Pharmaceutical Council
1894 Preston White Drive
Reston, Virginia 22091

Pharmaceutical Manufacturers Association Foundation
1100 15th Street, N.W.
Washington, D. C. 20005

The American Foundation for Pharmaceutical Education and the Pharmaceutical Manufacturers Association Foundation particularly may be contacted to obtain a list of funding support programs each organization provides for graduate students.

Each college and school of pharmacy has available information specific to its graduate programs and faculty beyond what you will find in this publication. In addition, most libraries and faculty members generally have a copy of the following materials which also are useful to prospective graduate students: Peterson's *Guide to Graduate Programs*; and, the American Chemical Society's *Directory of Graduate Research*.

A visit to the school for personal interviews with faculty members and students is strongly recommended. There is no better way to get a feel for the environment in which you would be living and working.

Don't overlook the excellent resource of current graduate students--at your university or within programs you are considering. These are individuals who, a few years before, were in your shoes. You will learn a great deal from their experiences and you will find them anxious to help you avoid the mistakes they may have made and to help you ask the questions they forgot to ask.

And, finally, without a doubt the most important resources available to you are the faculty members at your school. These men and women best know you and your potential, they are active in their discipline and, while likely not familiar with every graduate program, they can find information for you through their network of colleagues.

So...Is a graduate program in the pharmaceutical sciences an option for you? That, of course, is for you to decide. We hope, though, this publication helps you successfully sort through the evaluation and decision making process and that, ultimately, your answer will be YES.

ACADEMIC PHARMACY'S VITAL STATISTICS

Institutions and Programs

- There are 75 U.S. colleges and schools of pharmacy. Seventy-three (73) have accredited first professional degree programs, one has programs in candidate accreditation status, and one has programs in precandidate status. A few Pharm.D. programs have not yet been accredited by the American Council on Pharmaceutical Education (ACPE).

- Twenty-one (21) programs are in private institutions and 54 are in publicly-supported universities.

- There are three independent and free-standing pharmacy schools, all private. The remaining 72 schools are university affiliated.

- Sixty-two (62) schools offer the B.S. in pharmacy. Twenty-six (26) of these schools also offer the Pharm.D. degree as a first professional degree. Thirteen (13) schools offer the Pharm.D. as the only first professional degree program. Forty-seven (47) schools offer the Pharm.D. as a post-B.S. degree.

- Sixty-one (61) schools offer 205 graduate programs in the pharmaceutical sciences at the M.S. and/or Ph.D. level.

- There are 2,829 full-time, 581 part-time, and 1,234 adjunct/volunteer pharmacy faculty members at the 75 schools and colleges of pharmacy.

Pharmacy Students

- Pharmacy student enrollment ranged from 123 to 1132 students per school in fall 1990. Schools report an application to enrollment rate of 2.7:1.

- Total full-time pharmacy student enrollment was 29,797 in fall 1990: 24,252 in B.S. programs and 5,545 in entry-level Pharm.D. programs. The number of full-time students already holding a B.S. in pharmacy who were enrolled in Pharm.D. programs was 536.

- Over 62 percent of the total students were women and over 11 percent were minority students: black (7.0 percent), Hispanic (4.0 percent) and American Indian (less than 1 percent).

- Pharmacy school student enrollment peaked in 1975--having increased 56 percent since 1970. Enrollment declined steadily between 1975 and 1983. A 27.8 percent increase in enrollment, however, occurred between fall 1984 and fall 1990 (including a fall 1990 0.8 percent increase). Attrition (tracking enrollees through to graduation) over the past nine years appears to have averaged about 14 percent per class.

- Total fall 1990 full-time graduate student enrollment was 2,610: 1,926 students in Ph.D. programs and 684 in M.S. programs. Forty (40) percent of full-time graduate students were women. The total Ph.D. enrollment made up of U.S. educated pharmacists was, in fall 1990, 27.2 percent (a decline from an average of 32 percent over the past several years).

- In 1989-90, 6,956 (4,175 female and 2,781 male) entry-level degrees were awarded (a 6.0 percent increase over 1988-89), consisting of 6,010 B.S. and 946 Pharm.D. degrees. In addition, 302 post-B.S. Pharm.D. degrees were awarded (a 36.0 percent increase over 1988-89).

- In 1989-90, 273 (181 male, 92 female) Ph.D. degrees were awarded (a 4.9 percent decrease over 1988-89). M.S. degrees awarded decreased 1.5 percent from 391 in 1988-89 to 385 (202 male, 183 female) in 1989-90.

(over)

Sources: AACP's institutional, faculty, and student databases track on an annual basis the status of pharmacy's academic enterprise. Data in "Academic Pharmacy's Vital Statistics" publication are reflective of the Association's Roster of Faculty and Professional Staff, Pharmacy School Admission Requirements, and profiles of pharmacy students and faculty.

Programs in Pharmacy

The following inventory represents programs offered by the 75 U.S. colleges and schools of pharmacy. To ascertain the current accreditation status of each program, contact the individual college or school or The American Council on Pharmaceutical Education, 311 West Superior Street, Suite 512, Chicago, Illinois 60610; 312/664-3575.

Sixty-two schools offer the B.S. in pharmacy as a first professional degree:

Auburn University
Samford University (AL)
Colorado, University of
Connecticut, University of
Howard University (DC)
Florida A & M University
Southeastern University of the Health Sciences (FL)
Florida, University of
Georgia, University of
Chicago College of Pharmacy (IL)
Butler University (IN)
Purdue University (IN)
Drake University (IA)
Iowa, University of
Kansas, University of
Kentucky, University of
Northeast Louisiana University
Xavier University of Louisiana
Maryland, University of
Massachusetts College of Pharmacy and Allied Health Sciences
Northeastern University (MA)
Ferris State University (MI)
Wayne State University (MI)
Minnesota, University of
Mississippi, University of
St. Louis College of Pharmacy (MO)
Missouri-Kansas City, University of
Montana, University of
Creighton University (NE)
Rutgers University (NJ)
New Mexico, University of
Arnold & Marie Schwartz College of Pharmacy and Health Sciences (NY)
St. John's University (NY)
New York at Buffalo, State University of
Albany College of Pharmacy (NY)
North Carolina at Chapel Hill, University of
Ohio Northern University
Ohio State University
Cincinnati, University of (OH)
Toledo, University of (OH)
Southwestern Oklahoma State University
Oklahoma, University of
Oregon State University
Duquesne University (PA)
Philadelphia College of Pharmacy and Science (PA)
Temple University (PA)
Pittsburgh, University of (PA)
Puerto Rico, University of
Rhode Island, University of
South Carolina, Medical University of
South Carolina, University of
South Dakota State University
Texas Southern University
Houston, University of (TX)
Texas at Austin, University of
Utah, University of
Virginia Commonwealth University
Washington, University of
Washington State University
West Virginia University
Wisconsin, University of
Wyoming, University of

Twenty-six of these schools also offer the doctor of pharmacy (Pharm.D.) as a first professional degree:

Samford University (AL)
Howard University (DC)
Florida A & M University
Southeastern University of the Health Sciences (FL)
Florida, University of
Georgia, University of
Butler University (IN)
Purdue University (IN)
Kansas, University of
Kentucky, University of
Xavier University of Louisiana
Maryland, University of
Ferris State University (MI)
Minnesota, University of
St. Louis College of Pharmacy (MO)
Missouri-Kansas City, University of
Creighton University (NE)
Rutgers University (NJ)
North Carolina at Chapel Hill, University of
Ohio Northern University
Oklahoma, University of
Philadelphia College of Pharmacy and Science (PA)
South Carolina, University of
Texas at Austin, University of
Utah, University of
Wisconsin, University of

Thirteen schools offer only the Pharm.D. as a first professional degree:

Arizona, University of
Arkansas, University of
California-San Francisco, University of
Pacific, University of the (CA)
Southern California, University of
Mercer University (GA)
Idaho State University
Illinois at Chicago, University of
Michigan, University of
Nebraska, University of
Campbell University (NC)
North Dakota State University
Tennessee, University of

Forty-seven schools offer the Pharm.D. as a post-B.S. in pharmacy degree:

Auburn University (AL)
Samford University (AL)
Pacific, University of the (CA)
Southern California, University of
Howard University (DC)
Southeastern University of the Health Sciences (FL)
Georgia, University of
Idaho State University
Illinois at Chicago, University of
Purdue University (IN)
Drake University (IA)
Iowa, University of
Kansas, University of
Kentucky, University of
Xavier University of Louisiana
Maryland, University of
Massachusetts College of Pharmacy and Allied Health Sciences
Northeastern University (MA)
Ferris State University (MI)
Michigan, University of
Wayne State University (MI)
Minnesota, University of
Mississippi, University of
Creighton University (NE)
Rutgers University (NJ)
St. John's University (NY)
New York at Buffalo, State University of
Albany College of Pharmacy (NY) and Allied Health Sciences
Campbell University (NC)
North Carolina at Chapel Hill, University of
North Dakota State University
Ohio State University
Cincinnati, University of (OH)
Toledo, University of (OH)
Oklahoma, University of
Duquesne University (PA)
Philadelphia College of Pharmacy and Science (PA)
Temple University (PA)
Rhode Island, University of
South Carolina, Medical University of
South Carolina, University of
Texas Southern University
Texas at Austin, University of
Utah, University of
Virginia Commonwealth University
Washington, University of
Wisconsin, University of

How to Take a Test

You have studied hard, long, and conscientiously.

With your official admission card in hand, and your heart pounding, you have been admitted to the examination room.

You note that there are several hundred other applicants in the examination room waiting to take the same test.

They all appear to be equally well prepared.

You know that nothing but your best effort will suffice. The "moment of truth" is at hand: you now have to demonstrate objectively, in writing, your knowledge of content and your understanding of subject matter.

You are fighting the most important battle of your life—to pass and/or score high on an examination which will determine your career and provide the economic basis for your livelihood.

What extra, special things should you know and should you do in taking the examination?

Before the Test

Your Physical Condition Is Important

If you are not well, you can't do your best work on tests. If you are half asleep, you can't do your best either. Here are some tips:

1. Get about the same amount of sleep you usually get. Don't stay up all night before the test, either partying or worrying—DON'T DO IT.
2. If you wear glasses, be sure to wear them when you go to take the test. This goes for hearing aids, too.
3. If you have any physical problems that may keep you from doing your best, be sure to tell the person giving the test. If you are sick or in poor health, you really cannot do your best on any test. You can always come back and take the test some other time.

At the Test

Examination Techniques

1. Read the *general* instructions carefully. These are usually printed on the first page of the examination booklet. As a rule, these instructions refer to the timing of the examination; the fact that you should not start work until the signal and must stop work at a signal, etc. If there are any *special* instructions, such as a choice of questions to be answered, make sure that you note this instruction carefully.

2. When you are ready to start work on the examination, that is as soon as the signal has been given, read the instructions to each question booklet, underline any key words or phrases, such as *least, best, outline, describe*, and the like. In this way you will tend to answer as requested rather than discover on reviewing your paper that you *listed without describing,* that you selected the *worst* choice rather than the *best* choice, etc.

3. If the examination is of the objective or so-called multiple-choice type, that is, each question will also give a series of possible answers: A, B, C, or D, and you are called upon to select the best answer and write the letter next to that answer on your answer paper, it is advisable to start answering each question in turn. There may be anywhere from 50 to 100 such questions in the three or four hours allotted and you can see how much time would be taken if you read through all the questions before beginning to answer any. Furthermore, if you come across a question or a group of questions which you know would be difficult to answer, it would undoubtedly affect your handling of all the other questions.

4. If the examination is of the essay-type and contains but a few questions, it is a moot point as to whether you should read all the questions before starting to answer any one. Of course if you are given a choice, say five out of seven and the like, then it is essential to read all the questions so you can eliminate the two which are most difficult. If, however, you are asked to answer all the questions, there may be danger in trying to answer the easiest one first because you may find that you will spend too much time on it. The best technique is to answer the first question, then proceed to the second, etc.

5. Time your answers. Before the examination begins, write down the time it started, then add the time allowed for the examination and write down the time it must be completed, then divide the time available somewhat as follows:
   - **a.** If 3 ½ hours are allowed, that would be 210 minutes. If you have 80 objective-type questions, that would be an average of about 2 ½ minutes per question. Allow yourself no more than 2 minutes per question, or a total of 160 minutes, which will permit about 50 minutes to review.
   - **b.** If for the time allotment of 210 minutes, there are 7 essay questions to answer, that would average about 30 minutes a question. Give yourself only 25 minutes per question so that you have about 35 minutes to review.

6. The most important instruction is *to read each question* and make sure you know what is wanted. The second most important instruction is to *time yourself properly* so that you answer every question. The third most important instruction is to *answer every question*. Guess if you have to but include something for each question, Remember that you will receive no credit for a blank and will probably receive some credit if you write something in answer to an essay question. If you guess a letter, say "B" for a multiple-choice question, you may have guessed right. If you leave a blank as the answer to a multiple-choice question, the examiners may respect your feelings but it will not add a point to your score. Some exams may penalize you for wrong answers, so in such cases *only*, you may not want to guess unless you have some basis for your answer.

7. Suggestions

   a. Objective-Type Questions

      (1) Examine the question booklet for proper sequence of pages and questions.
      (2) Read all instructions carefully.
      (3) Skip any question which seems too difficult; return to it after all other questions have been answered.
      (4) Apportion your time properly; do not spend too much time on any single question or group of questions.
      (5) Note and underline key words—*all, most, fewest, least, best, worst, same, opposite.*
      (6) Pay particular attention to negatives.
      (7) Note unusual option, e.g., unduly long, short, complex, different or similar in content to the body of the question.
      (8) Observe the use of "hedging" words—*probably, may, most likely, etc.*
      (9) Make sure that your answer is put next to the same number as the question.
      (10) Do not second guess unless you have good reason to believe the second answer is definitely more correct.
      (11) Cross out original answer if you decide another answer is more accurate; do not erase, *until* you are ready to hand your paper in.
      (12) Answer all questions; guess unless instructed otherwise.
      (13) Leave time for review.

b. Essay-Type Questions

(1) Read each question carefully.

(2) Determine exactly what is wanted. Underline key words or phrases.

(3) Decide on outline or paragraph answer.

(4) Include many different points and elements unless asked to develop any one or two points or elements.

(5) Show impartiality by giving pros and cons unless directed to select one side only.

(6) Make and write down any assumptions you find necessary to answer the question.

(7) Watch your English, grammar, punctuation, choice of words.

(8) Time your answers; don't crowd material.

8. Answering the Essay Question

Most essay questions can be answered by framing the specific response around several key words or ideas. Here are a few such key words or ideas:

M's: manpower, materials, methods, money, management

P's: purpose, program, policy, plan, procedure, practice, problems, pitfalls, personnel, public relations

a. Six basic steps in handling problems:

(1) preliminary plan and background development

(2) collect information, data and facts

(3) analyze and interpret information, data and facts

(4) analyze and develop solutions as well as make recommendations

(5) prepare report and sell recommendations

(6) install recommendations and follow up effectiveness

b. Pitfalls to Avoid

(1) *Taking Things for Granted*
A statement of the situation does not necessarily imply that each of the elements is necessarily true; for example, a complaint may be invalid and biased so that all that can be taken for granted is that a complaint has been registered

(2) *Considering only one side of a situation*
Wherever possible, indicate several alternatives and then point out the reasons you selected the best one.

(3) *Failing to indicate follow up*
Whenever your answer indicates action on your part, make certain that you will take proper follow-up action to see how successful your recommendations, procedures, or actions turn out to be.

(4) *Taking too long in answering any single question*
Remember to time your answers properly.

EXAMINATION SECTION

VERBAL ANALOGIES

The verbal-analogy type question is now a staple component of tests of general and mental ability, scholastic aptitude, professional qualification, and civil service examinations. This question-type is also being used for achievement testing.

The verbal analogy is considered an excellent measure for evaluating the ability of the student to reason with and in words. It is not, primarily, a test of vocabulary *per se*, for very rarely are the words that are used in this type of question difficult or abstruse in meaning (as they are, for example, in the same-opposite or sentence-completion type). Rather, they are everyday terms and phrases descriptive of materials and actions familiar to all of us.

The verbal analogy is a test of *word relationships* and *idea relationships*, involving a neat and algebraic-like arrangement in ratio (proportion) form not of numbers but of words. Some testers see in this type of question the development on the verbal (linguistic or qualitative) side of the same logical reasoning as occurs on the mathematical (numerical or quantitative) side in number problems. This type of question is ranked just after the reading-comprehension type in difficulty. However, it constitutes by far the most fascinating and challenging area in aptitude testing.

In general, three levels of ability are involved in answering the verbal analogy question.

First, and easiest in this connection, is the ability to understand the meanings of the words used in the question (understanding).

Second, and more difficult , is the ability to comprehend the relationship between the subject-, or question-, pair of words (the process of logical reasoning).

Third, and most difficult of all, is the ability to select from the five (pairs of) choices given, that choice which bears the same relationship to (within) itself as the subject words bear to one another. This involves analysis, comparison, and judgment (the process of evaluation).

In the verbal-analogy type of question, two important symbols are employed, which must be thoroughly understood beforehand. These are the colon(:), which is to be translated into words, when reading the question, in the same way as its mathematical equivalent, that is, "is to"; and the double colon (::), which is to be translated as "in the same way as." Thus, the analogy, BURGLAR: PRISON :: juvenile delinquent : reformatory, is to be read, A burglar is to a prison in the same way as a juvenile delinquent is to a reformatory. Or, reading for meaning, we could say instead, "A burglar is punished by being sent to a prison in the same way as a juvenile delinquent is punished by being sent to a reformatory."

SAMPLE QUESTIONS AND EXPLANATIONS

DIRECTIONS: Each question in this part consists of a pair of words in capital letters, which have a certain relationship to each other, followed *either* by a third word in capital letters and five lettered words in small letters (1 blank missing) OR by five lettered pairs of words in small letters (2 blanks missing). Choose *either* the letter of the word that is related to the third word in capital letters OR of the pair of words that are related to each other in the same way as the first two capitalized words are related to each other, and mark the appropriate space on your answer sheet.

1. EROSION : ROCKS :: DISSIPATION : ________
A. character B. temperance C. penance D. influence
E. sincerity
2. MUNDANE : SPIRITUAL :: SECULAR : ________
A. scientist B. clerical C. pecuniary D. municipal
E. teacher
3. ANARCHY : LAWLESSNESS :: ________ : ________
A. autocracy : peace B. disturbance : safety
C. government : order D. confusion : law
E. democracy : dictatorship
4. UMBRELLA : RAIN :: ________ : ________
A. roof : snow B. screen : insects
C. sewer : water D. body : disease
E. gong : dinner

EXPLANATION OF QUESTION 1

Item A, character, is correct.

Erosion is a geological development that wears away Rocks. This is an example of a cause-effect relationship -- a concrete relationship.

Dissipation wears away character (Item A) in the same way --however, this is an abstract relationship.

But the comparison is apt and appropriate. This is a usual, general type of analogy whose difficulty is compounded by the fact that a concrete relationship is compared with an abstract one.

Item B, temperance (moderation), is merely one aspect of character.

Item C, penance (repentance), bears no relationship to dissipation in the sense of the subject words.

Item D, influence, and Item E, sincerity, may or may not be affected by dissipation.

This question is an example of a one-blank analogy, that is, only one word is to be supplied in the answer (a subject pair and a third subject word being given in the question itself).

EXPLANATION OF QUESTION 2

Item B, clerical, is correct.

Mundane means worldly, earthly. The opposite of this word is spiritual -- unworldly, devout, eternal. This is a relationship of opposites.

Secular means worldly, earthly, temporal. It is a synonym for mundane What is needed as the answer is an opposite equal in meaning to spiritua

A. A scientist may or may not be worldly or spiritual. At any rate, an adjective is needed as an answer, and scientist is a noun.

B. Clerical ("pertaining to the clergy") denotes, usually, apiritual or religious qualities. It is an adjective. This is the correct answer.

C. Pecuniary refers to money, and may, therefore, be regarded as a synonym for secular.

D. Municipal refers to municipalities or cities, and has no standing here as an answer.

E. A teacher may or may not be worldly or spiritual. At any rate, just as for A. scientist, it is a noun and not an adjective, which is needed as an answer here.

EXPLANATION OF QUESTION 3

Item C, government : order, is correct.

Anarchy, or no government, is characterized by lawlessness while a government is characterized by order. This is an example of an object (situation) : characteristic relationship.

Item A, autocracy : peace, is incorrect since very often autocracy (absolute monarchy or rule by an individual) is characterized by war.

Item B, disturbance : safety, is manifestly untrue.

Item D, confusion : law, is likewise untrue.

Item E, democracy : dictatorship, bears no relationship to the meaning conveyed by the subject pair.

This is an example of a two-blank analogy, that is, a pair of words is to be supplied. This is the more difficult type of analogy, and the one most frequently encountered on advanced-level examinations.

EXPLANATION OF QUESTION 4

Item B, screen : insects, is correct.

By means of an umbrella, one keeps the rain off his person just as a screen keeps insects out of the house. This is an example of an object: assists relationship.

Item A, roof : snow, is not correct since a roof keeps out many other things as well, e.g., light, heat, rain, insects, etc.

Item C, sewer : water, is incorrect since a sewer keeps water in or water flows through and in a sewer.

Item D, body : disease, is incorrect since often disease enters and destroys the body.

Item E, gong : dinner, is incorrect since the gong merely summons to dinner but does not keep anyone away.

As can be discerned from the examples above, there are many possible relationships on which word analogies may be formed. Some of these will be listed and illustrated below. However, the important point is not to ponder over labels and attempt to peg the relationships thereby. This is as unnecessary as it is time-consuming. The real object, or the real method, is to examine and to fully comprehend the relationship expressed in the subject pair and *then* to select as the correct answer that item which *most approximately* is in greatest consonance with all or most of the aspects of the given relationship.

TYPES AND FORMS OF ANALOGY QUESTIONS

Some or all of the following types of analogies or relationships are to be encountered on examinations.

1. PART : WHOLE
   Example: LEG : BODY :: wheel : car
2. CAUSE : EFFECT
   Example: RAIN : FLOOD :: disease : epidemic
3. CONCRETE: ABSTRACT
   Example: ROAD : VEHICLE :: life : person
4. WORD : SYNONYM
   Example: VACUOUS : EMPTY :: seemly : fit
5. WORD : ANTONYM
   Example: SLAVE : FREEMAN :: desolate : joyous

6. OBJECT : MATERIAL
   Example: COAT : WOOL :: dress : cotton
7. OBJECT : DEFINITION
   Example: ASSEVERATE : AFFIRM :: segregate : separate
8. OBJECT : SEX
   Example: COLT : MARE :: buck : doe
9. TIME : TIME
   Example: DAY : NIGHT :: sunrise : sunset
10. DEGREE : DEGREE
    Example: HAPPY : ECSTATIC :: warm : hot
11. OBJECT : TOOL
    Example: STENCIL : TYPEWRITER :: thread : needle
12. USER : TOOL
    Example: FARMER : HOE :: dentist : drill
13. CREATOR : CREATION
    Example: ARTIST : PICTURE :: poet : poem
14. CATEGORY : TYPE
    Example: RODENT : SQUIRREL :: fish : flounder
15. PERSON (ANIMAL,ETC.) : CHARACTERISTIC
    Example: MONSTER : FEROCITY :: baby : helplessness
16. OBJECT : CHARACTERISTIC
    Example: PICKLE : SOUR :: sugar : sweet
17. PERSON : FUNCTION
    Example: TEACHER : EDUCATION :: doctor : health
18. INSTRUMENT : FUNCTION
    Example: CAMERA : PHOTOGRAPHY :: ruler : measurement
19. WORD : GRAMMATICAL FORM
    Example: WE : I :: they : he
20. SYMBOL : ATTITUDE
    Example: SALUTE : PATRIOTISM :: prayer : religion
21. REWARD : ACTION
    Example: MEDAL : BRAVERY :: trophy : championship
22. OBJECT : ASSISTS
    Example: WATER : THIRST :: food : hunger
23. OBJECT : HINDERS
    Example: NOISE : STUDY :: rut : car
24. PERSON : RELATIONSHIP
    Example: FATHER : SON :: uncle : nephew
25. OBJECT : LOCALE
    Example: SHIP : WATER :: airplane : air
26. OBJECT : METHOD
    Example: DOOR : KEY :: safe : combination
27. QUALITY : PROFUSION
    Example: WIND : TORNADO :: water : flood
28. QUALITY : ABSENCE
    Example: FORTITUDE : COWARDICE :: carefully : casually
29. SIZE : SIZE
    Example: BOAT : SHIP :: lake : sea
30. GENUS : SPECIES
    Example: RODENT : RAT :: canine : wolf

There are other relationships, but these will suffice to show some of those more frequently occurring.

SUGGESTIONS FOR ANSWERING THE VERBAL ANALOGY QUESTION (APTITUDE)

1. Always keep in mind that a verbal analogy is a relationship of likeness between two things, consisting in the resemblances not, usually, of the things themselves but of two or more of their attributes, functions, circumstances, or effects. Therefore, in the one-blank or two-blank questions, you are not looking so much for similarity in structure (although this may prove to be a factor, too), as you are for a relationship in the <u>functioning</u> of the subject words.

2. How do we proceed to answer the verbal-analogy type question? *First,* discover for yourself in a meaningful way the exact relationship existing between the subject words. Whether you are able to label or tag this relationship is not so important (as we have said before) as to <u>understand</u> the relationship that exists. The logical *second* and *final* step is to examine the possible answers given and to ascertain which of these possibilities, on the basis of *meaning, order,* and *form,* bears a similar relationship to the subject pair.

3. For the analogy in question, the subject words (i.e., the question words given in the first part of the analogy) need not be of the same class, type, order, or species as the object words (i.e., the answer-words or fill-ins). For example, in the analogy, BUCCANEER:SAILOR :: fungus : plant, the subject words (in capital letters) are types of people, the object words (in small letters) refer to types of things. However, the analogy that exists is on the basis of a descriptive relationship between these two different sets of words. (The first word in each pair constitutes the depredatory or despoiling form of the second, which is the general category name.) Thus, it is actually the <u>total</u> effect of the *first pair* on each other that is being compared with the <u>total</u> effect of the *second pair* on each other: *this is what really counts,* and not the individual components of each pair.

4. The order of the object words must be in the same sequence as the order of the subject words. For example, the analogy, INAUGURATION : PRESIDENT :: ordination : priest, is correct. But, INAUGURATION : PRESIDENT :: priest : ordination, would be incorrect. Watch for this <u>reversal</u> of order in word sequence; it is a common source of entrapment for the uninitiated.

5. Likewise, it is necessary to check to see that the parts of speech used in the analogy are the same, and occur in the same sequence. For example, if the subject pair contains a noun and an adjective in that order, the object pair <u>must</u> contain a noun and an adjective in *that* order. Thus, MOTHER : GOOD :: murderer : bad, is correct. But, MOTHER : GOOD :: murderer : badly, is incorrect.

6. The best way to answer the analogy question -- one-blank or two-blanks -- is to study intensively the relationship contained in the given pair. Having fully comprehended this relationship and, perhaps, having "labeled" it, proceed to scan the possible answers, choosing the most likely one. This will save time, and avoid needless trial and error.

VERBAL ANALOGIES — 2 BLANKS

EXAMINATION SECTION

DIRECTIONS FOR THIS SECTION:

Each question in this part consists of two capitalized words which have a certain relationship to each other, followed by five lettered pairs of words in small letters. Choose the letter of the pair of words which are related to each other in the SAME way as the words of the capitalized pair are related to each other. *PRINT THE LETTER OF THE CORRECT ANSWER IN THE SPACE AT THE RIGHT.*

TEST 1

1. DISCRETE : ABRIDGED :: ________ : ________ 1. ...
   A. quotes : parentheses B. decimal : fraction
   C. separation : partition D. hyphenated : abbreviated
   E. separated : slang
2. COURT : DESERT :: ________ : ________ 2. ...
   A. boar : camel B. diversion : pachyderm C. fig : forest
   D. droll : dromedary E. plant : person
3. RECORDS : FILE :: ________ : ________ 3. ...
   A. stipend : income B. wall : plug C. socket : bulb
   D. stocks : bonds E. savings : bank
4. FURROW : PLOW :: ________ : ________ 4. ...
   A. sign : street B. route : avenue C. orbit : earth
   D. ring : bull E. crash : aeroplane
5. FAMILY : CHILDREN :: ________ : ________ 5. ...
   A. party : guests B. clan : crest C. flag : country
   D. club : members E. feline : cat
6. RECIDIVISTIC : PRUDENT :: ________ : ________ 6. ...
   A. period : proper B. cadence : credo
   C. impoverished : wealthy D. depraved : respectful
   E. decadent : circumspect
7. PARTITION : SERIES :: ________ : ________ 7. ...
   A. enclosing : parietal B. division : rescission
   C. septum : spectrum D. wall : ghastly
   E. fencing : parading
8. SEISMOGRAPH : EARTHQUAKE :: ________ : ________ 8. ...
   A. barometer : temperature B. thermometer : pressure
   C. fluoroscope : tuberculosis
   D. lubritorium : laboratory E. x-ray : pulsation
9. ELECTRICITY : ILLUMINATION :: ________ : ________ 9. ...
   A. gravity : force B. water : power C. sieve : straining
   D. stroke : brush E. atomic : bomb
10. DEMEANOR : CHARACTER :: ________ : ________ 10. ...
    A. innate : temperament B. distinguished : personified
    C. singer : song D. tenor : type E. aspect : acuity
11. INSTINCT : BEAST :: ________ : ________ 11. ...
    A. reason : rationale B. mind : brain C. thought : process
    D. intelligence : man E. rattle : snake
12. ROMANTIC : PRACTICAL :: ________ : ________ 12. ...
    A. weak : strong B. inspired : clumsy C. quixotic : realistic
    D. light : heavy E. surface : depth
13. REPRESSION : AWARENESS :: ________ : ________ 13. ...
    A. passivity : activity B. sleep : dream
    C. forget : remember D. coma : comatose
    E. unconscious : conscious
14. PREDISPOSITION : RELATIONSHIP :: ________ : ________ 14. ...
    A. prepossession : prediction B. atom : combination

C. impartiality : partiality D. predilection : affinity
E. affiliation : preponderance

15. STORM : HURRICANE :: ________ : ________ 15. ...
A. disease : germ B. fear : panic C. ship : sank
D. courage : hero E. solitude : hermit

16. SUPPLY : DEMAND :: ________ : ________ 16. ...
A. cost : market B. price : value C. wholesale : retail
D. net : worth E. tax : article

17. CAMOUFLAGE : GUERRILLA :: ________ : ________ 17. ...
A. radar : instrument B. painter : anonymity
C. cocoon : butterfly D. costume : masquerader
E. color : ship

18. LENS : CAMERA :: ________ : ________ 18. ...
A. toe : foot B. beacon : lighthouse C. eye : mind
D. head : body E. vision : thought

19. CRUTCHES : MOVEMENT :: ________ : ________ 19. ...
A. windows : houses B. defect : myopic
C. glasses : vision D. teeth : braces
E. telescope : astronomer

20. MILES : AUTOMOBILES :: ________ : ________ 20. ...
A. sea : fathoms B. suits : divers C. knots : ships
D. gasoline : aeroplane E. milligram : gram

21. NOMINATION : CONVENTION :: ________ : ________ 21. ...
A. judge : sentence B. panel : member C. verdict : jury
D. criminal : crime E. policeman : arrest

22. FACET : GEM :: ________ : ________ 22. ...
A. intelligence : test B. father : son
C. brilliance : genius D. heredity : environment
E. constellation : star

23. ABSTRUSE : OBTUSE :: ________ : ________ 23. ...
A. concave : convex B. erudition : profundity
C. dull : translucent D. abstract : realistic
E. recondite : opaque

24. TURNSTILE : SUBWAY :: ________ : ________ 24. ...
A. ticket : aeroplane B. price : goods C. desk : office
D. door : taxicab E. porthole : ship

25. CAGE : CANARY :: ________ : ________ 25. ...
A. walls : jail B. warden : prison C. cell : inmate
D. jungle : lion E. patient : hospital

TEST 2

1. PSEUDONYM : ASSUMED NAME :: ________ : ________ 1. ...
A. nomenclature : title B. appellation : given name
C. nom de plume : pen name D. surname : first name
E. title : aristocrat

2. PECK : BUSHEL :: ________ : ________ 2. ...
A. dram : ton B. rod : pound C. gill : fathom
D. gallon : cord E. ounce : inch

3. ABDICATE : KING :: ________ : ________ 3. ...
A. track : train B. derail : engineer C. execute : warden
D. crash : aeroplane E. revolution : anarchist

4. SECURE : WITHDRAW :: ________ : ________ 4. ...
A. anchor : anchorite B. ship : mausoleum C. sailor : salacious
D. secrete : drop E. article : manufacturer

5. MATHEMATICAL : VERBAL :: ________ : ________ 5. ...
   A. numbers : equation B. quotient : proportion
   C. ratio : analogy D. fraction : word
   E. computation : anagram
6. SEASONING : THYME :: ________ : ________ 6. ...
   A. space : season B. hybrid : herb C. measure : mite
   D. predict : plant E. time : season
7. VOLATILE : TACITURN :: ________ : ________ 7. ...
   A. planet : position B. mercurial : saturnine
   C. Mercury : Saturn D. mood : fluid C. undependable : stolid
8. HEAD : AX :: ________ : ________ 8. ...
   A. pine : cone B. close : call C. cylinder : engine
   D. chair : rung E. angle : line
9. BEAM : SEARCHLIGHT :: ________ : ________ 9. ...
   A. tank : oil B. flame : welder C. torch : fire
   D. film : projector E. forest : timber
10. CONSPIRE : CABAL :: ________ : ________ 10. ...
    A. scheme : expedite B. contrivance : contrive
    C. machinate : plot D. conspiracy : intrigue
    E. object : plan
11. LAW : PROMULGATION :: ________ : ________ 11. ...
    A. voting : election B. interview : census
    C. decision : declaration D. battle : war E. idea : action
12. MEMBER : SOCIETY :: ________ : ________ 12. ...
    A. molecule : amoeba B. growth : osmosis
    C. cell : organism D. disease : parasite E. leg : foot
13. HIPPOCRATIC OATH : PHYSICIAN :: ________ : ________ 13. ...
    A. fealty : fief B. citizenship : alien
    C. allegiance : citizen D. contract : marriage
    E. covenant : treaty
14. SKIS : SNOW :: ________ : ________ 14. ...
    A. cork : water B. rain : umbrellas C. clouds : sky
    D. shoes : feet E. parachutes : air
15. TASTE : SMELL :: ________ : ________ 15. ...
    A. touch : hand B. sight : hearing C. ears : eyes
    D. hearing aid : eyeglasses E. aural : oral
16. SORCERY : PRESTIDIGITATOR :: ________ : ________ 16. ...
    A. magic : demonology B. witchcraft : entomologist
    C. conjure : spirit D. astrology : astrologist
    E. fetishism : palmist
17. YOUTH : IMPULSIVE :: ________ : ________ 17. ...
    A. juvenile : puerile B. characteristic : degree
    C. adolescence : childhood D. soil : erosion
    E. age : senile
18. SATISFACTION : DISQUIETUDE :: ________ : ________ 18. ...
    A. chaos : satisfaction B. doubt : security
    C. dissatisfaction : friction
    D. civilization : jungle E. complacent : restive
19. GASLIGHT : ELECTRICITY :: ________ : ________ 19. ...
    A. jet : aeroplane B. fiction : science C. loud : gift
    C. obsolete : extant E. horse : carriage
20. HYPOTHETICAL : FORMULATED :: ________ : ________ 20. ...
    A. method : science B. irrational : deranged
    C. insanity : sanity D. vagary : rationality
    E. animal : machine

21. OATH : PERJURY :: ________ : ________ 21. ...
A. truth : oath B. perfidy : imposture C. promise : renege
D. inviolability : swear E. inaccuracy : falsity
22. PROSAIC : AESTHETIC :: ________ : ________ 22. ...
A. dull : beautiful B. lethargic : ambitious
C. behavior : feeling D. humorous : brilliant
E. judicious : sensitivity
23. OPERATION : SURGEON :: ________ : ________ 23. ...
A. philately : necromancer B. student : study
C. pyromaniac : fire D. embezzlement : thief
E. murderer : homicide
24. BEIGE : BROWN :: ________ : ________ 24. ...
A. primary : secondary B. hue : value
C. shade : color D. yellow : gold E. red : pink
25. CLOTH : DESIGNER :: ________ : ________ 25. ...
A. clay : model B. statue : sculptor C. brush : palette
D. paint : artist E. painting : canvas

TEST 3

1. RUPEE : INDIA :: ________ : ________ 1. ...
A. peseta : Cuba B. drachma : Hong Kong
C. escudo : Spain D. franc : France
E. krona : Czechoslavakia
2. REDUCTION : REMOVAL :: ________ : ________ 2. ...
A. abate : abstruse B. dwindle : inattentive
C. decree : summarize D. diminution : difficult
E. contraction : abstraction
3. STYLIZED : FACTUAL :: ________ : ________ 3. ...
A. question : fact B. abstract : equation
C. rhetorical : pragmatical D. florid : dogma
E. doctrinaire : philosophy
4. REFLECTOR : SIGHT :: ________ : ________ 4. ...
A. color wheel : rotation B. vision : eyeglasses
C. mirror : image D. compendium : exhibit
E. spectrum : spectacles
5. GENE : GENDER :: ________ : ________ 5. ...
A. corporeal : body B. paper : wood
C. factor : characteristic D. composition : author
E. ventricle : heart
6. STRONGHOLD : MUNICIPALITY :: ________ : ________ 6. ...
A. state : capital B. citadel : city C. fortress : command
D. protected : protector E. strategic : locale
7. HYDROGEN : WATER :: ________ : ________ 7. ...
A. organic : compound B. dextrose : glucose
C. coal : carbon D. liquid : solid E. pure : impure
8. ARRAY : MEDITATION :: ________ : ________ 8. ...
A. image : idea B. spectrum : speculation
C. varying : thought D. sequence : continuous
E. reflecting : reflect
9. BUDDHISM : MOHAMMEDANISM :: ________ : ________ 9. ...
A. Islamic : Utopia B. Hindu : Arabian
C. heaven : center D. nirvana : mecca E. fantasy : reality
10. NOTICE : APPEASE :: ________ : ________ 10. ...
A. pacific : pacify B. placard : placate

C. poster : propaganda D. agreement : compromise
E. place : please

11. WEEK : MONTH :: ________ : ________ 11. ...
A. month : day B. foot : inch C. hour : clock
D. vacation : holiday E. Sunday : July

12. CANOE : RIVER :: ________ : ________ 12. ...
A. element : vehicle B. ride : winter C. ice : skate
D. sleigh : snow E. hounds : ranger

13. MINERAL : REPTILE :: ________ : ________ 13. ...
A. lizard : lair B. ocean : amphibian C. stone : snake
D. mummy : body E. water : goldfish

14. MAN : BEE :: ________ : ________ 14. ...
A. domestic : habitat B. abode : hiatus
C. domicile : hive D. ant : hill E. sanctuary : wilderness

15. PATIENT : PHYSICIAN :: ________ : ________ 15. ...
A. jury : judge B. audience : actor C. client : attorney
D. customer : store E. adviser : advised

16. PIANO : SCALE :: ________ : ________ 16. ...
A. violin : music B. range : singer
C. instrument : octave D. one : seven E. stanza : poem

17. MAN : BROTHER :: ________ : ________ 17. ...
A. death : dishonor B. homicide : fratricide
C. father : son D. murder : man E. child : murder

18. ARM : HEAD :: ________ : ________ 18. ...
A. leg : temple B. brain : foot C. hole : bullet
D. head : neck E. break : concussion

19. SEW : CLOTH :: ________ : ________ 19. ...
A. staple : machine B. sharpener : pencil
C. stamp : letter D. clip : paper E. stamp : mail

20. PAPER : BODY :: ________ : ________ 20. ...
A. break : crack B. arm : cast C. bruise : heal
D. tear : wound E. rip : mend

21. PLUCK : CHICKEN :: ________ : ________ 21. ...
A. wood : fire B. goat : milk C. skin : snake
D. fur : bear E. feather : ostrich

22. SAIL : BOAT :: ________ : ________ 22. ...
A. pinwheel : toy B. pilot : controls C. wing : aeroplane
D. fender : automobile E. ski shoes : skis

23. VIBRATION : LIGHT :: ________ : ________ 23. ...
A. sound : reflection B. symphony : color wheel
C. intensity : pitch D. music : color
E. rhyme : harmony

24. REBELLION : GOVERNMENT :: ________ : ________ 24. ...
A. motion : meeting B. discord : partisan
C. dissent : group D. disbanding : party
E. commitment : withdrawl

25. GREGARIOUSNESS : ASCETICISM :: ________ : ________ 25. ...
A. denial : acceptance B. austere : sensuous
C. monastery : monk D. conviviality : seclusion
E. secluded : remote

TEST 4

1. BURY : DISINTER :: ________ : ________ 1. ...
A. inhale : exhale B. inhume : exhume

C. corporeal : spirit D. autopsy : funeral
E. burial : cremation

2. INVOLUNTARY : VOLUNTARY :: ________ : ________ 2. ...
A. criminal : soldier B. export : import C. illegal : legal
D. deportation : expatriation E. punishment : crime

3. IGNITE : FIRE :: ________ : ________ 3. ...
A. water : flood B. ax : tree C. incite : revolt
D. mass : riot E. flame : gasoline

4. LEDGER : BOOKKEEPER ________ : ________ 4. ...
A. fort : cavalry B. compass : direction
C. log : captain D. deck : crew
E. biography : historian

5. SPACE : TIME :: ________ : ________ 5. ...
A. locale : situation B. geography : history
C. navigation : course D. individual : ancestry
E. dimension : depth

6. STRAITS : GIBRALTAR :: ________ : ________ 6. ...
A. island : coast B. ocean : Atlantic C. peninsula : Malta
D. cape : Africa E. Danube : river

7. HERD : CATTLE :: ________ : ________ 7. ...
A. sled : snow B. team : dogs C. race : horse
D. people : group E. sheep : flock

8. ELECT : GOVERNOR :: ________ : ________ 8. ...
A. office : appoint B. administer : administration
C. position : order D. inauguration : president
E. deputize : deputy

9. COMBINATION : SAFE :: ________ : ________ 9. ...
A. raise : window B. key : door C. nail : picture
D. hanger : coat E. latch : key

10. SALT : SHAKER :: ________ : ________ 10. ...
A. minute : time B. bottle : milk C. sand : hourglass
D. sun dial : sun E. ship : ocean

11. STORY : SENTENCE :: ________ : ________ 11. ...
A. poem : rhyme B. chant : paean C. hymn : note
D. brushstroke : painting E. song : music

12. LOOSE : DISCIPLINE :: ________ : ________ 12. ...
A. lazy : perfect B. individual : political
C. dinner : banquet D. order : disorder
E. lax : protocol

13. CREST : CLAN :: ________ : ________ 13. ...
A. judge : robe B. road : sign C. insignia : army
D. fairy : wand E. king : scepter

14. PENULTIMATE : ULTIMATE :: ________ : ________ 14. ...
A. among : between B. first : second
C. perfect : excellent D. better : best
E. more : many

15. WORSEN : WITHDRAW :: ________ : ________ 15. ...
A. regress : egress B. down : up C. fantasy : reality
D. swing : gate E. retrogress : digress

16. CEREMONY : CORRECT :: ________ : ________ 16. ...
A. manner : might B. rite : right C. kinsman : kind
C. inauguration : irate E. sworn : swerve

17. CHALLENGE : CONTEST :: ________ : ________ 17. ...
A. sprint : pistol B. fencing : sport C. hat : ring
D. insult : duel E. sword : rapier

18. WORM : SNAKE :: ________ : ________ 18. ...
A. shark : whale B. lion : tamer C. cat : mouse
D. cat : panther E. shark : carnivorous

19. INDIFFERENCE : UNDERSTANDING :: ________ : ________ 19. ...
A. sympathy : identification B. peasant : worker
C. apathy : empathy D. peon : peonage
E. happiness : sadness

20. INCIPIENT : RUDIMENTARY :: ________ : ________ 20. ...
A. disappearing : appearing B. plant : seed
C. inchoate : embryonic D. unknown : unseen
E. death : birth

21. SEASONING : HERB :: ________ : ________ 21. ...
A. saccharine : sugar B. candy : dextrose
C. condiment : thyme D. synthetic : genuine
E. natural : manufactured

22. SIMULATED : GENUINE :: ________ : ________ 22. ...
A. semi-precious : precious B. bullion : gold
C. pretense : fraud D. rhinestone : diamond
E. private : general

23. FLOWER : PETAL :: ________ : ________ 23. ...
A. sprout : potato B. seed : plant C. tree : branch
D. root : earth E. moss : stone

24. DESERT : OCEAN :: ________ : ________ 24. ...
A. illness : death B. parch : thirst C. abundance : surfeit
D. suffocation : evaporation E. dehydrate : drown

25. STANZA : CHAPTER :: ________ : ________ 25. ...
A. art : fiction B. meter : rhyme C. narration : style
D. poetry : prose E. clause : sentence

TEST 5

1. DOGMATIC : VACILLATORY :: ________ : ________ 1. ...
A. absolute : relative B. all : few C. certain : decisive
D. affinity : infinity E. pure : contaminated

2. LINE : CURVE :: ________ : ________ 2. ...
A. perimeter : parallel B. hypotenuse : rectangle
C. earth : equator D. diameter : circumference
E. semi-circle : circle

3. BOWL : BALL :: ________ : ________ 3. ...
A. up : down B. hemisphere : globe
C. concave : convex D. earth : cave
E. bulging and curved : hollow and curved

4. WIND : CYCLONE :: ________ : ________ 4. ...
A. river : ocean B. exhaust : fume C. suffocate : drown
D. water : deluge E. pressure : atmosphere

5. LION : JUNGLE :: ________ : ________ 5. ...
A. faun : deer B. plant : flower C. fauna : flora
D. seaweed : octopus E. cow : milk

6. SUBTERRANEAN : SURFACE :: ________ : ________ 6. ...
A. road : sea B. league : fathom C. ship : car
D. depth : distance E. diver : driver

7. IMPASSIVE : INFLATED :: ________ : ________ 7. ...
A. pain : noise B. enthusiasm : exuberance
C. stoical : bombastic D. mediocre : outstanding
E. hermit : pedant

8. PRODUCT : MULTIPLICATION :: ________ : ________ 8. ...
A. multiplication : table B. add : arithmetic
C. part : whole D. words : sentence E. sum : addition

9. DECIMAL : COMMA :: ________ : ________ 9. ...
A. sum : fraction B. number : word C. letter : fraction
D. period : sentence E. clause : ratio

10. ANARCHIST : PATRIOT :: ________ : ________ 10. ...
A. iconoclast : chauvinist B. agnostic : heretic
C. soldier : revolutionary D. topple : government
E. Loyalist : Tory

11. SPEED : SOUND :: ________ : ________ 11. ...
A. linear : dimension B. fathom : ocean C. time : hour
D. velocity : light E. force : gravity

12. SUBURB : CITY :: ________ : ________ 12. ...
A. peasant : peon B. prince : pauper
C. provincial : urban D. capital : state
E. town : country

13. VELOCITY : WIND :: ________ : ________ 13. ...
A. economy : gross national product
B. element : temperament C. variable : constant
D. same : change E. fluctuation : rate

14. WIRE : TELEPHONE :: ________ : ________ 14. ...
A. refrigerator : freezer B. bookcase : book
C. telephone : dial D. bureau : drawer
E. ribbon : typewriter

15. TRAIN : DEPOT :: ________ : ________ 15. ...
A. cow : barn B. traveler : destination
C. baseball : home plate D. bus : terminal
E. field : hangar

KEYS (CORRECT ANSWERS)

TEST 1	TEST 2	TEST 3	TEST 4	TEST 5
1. D	1. C	1. D	1. B	1. A
2. D	2. A	2. E	2. D	2. D
3. E	3. B	3. C	3. C	3. C
4. C	4. A	4. E	4. C	4. D
5. D	5. C	5. C	5. B	5. C
6. E	6. E	6. B	6. B	6. E
7. C	7. B	7. B	7. B	7. C
8. C	8. C	8. B	8. E	8. E
9. B	9. D	9. D	9. B	9. B
10. D	10. C	10. B	10. C	10. A
11. D	11. C	11. E	11. C	11. D
12. C	12. C	12. D	12. E	12. C
13. E	13. C	13. C	13. C	13. C
14. D	14. E	14. C	14. D	14. E
15. B	15. B	15. C	15. A	15. D
16. B	16. D	16. C	16. B	
17. D	17. E	17. B	17. D	
18. C	18. E	18. E	18. D	
19. C	19. D	19. D	19. C	
20. C	20. D	20. D	20. C	
21. C	21. C	21. C	21. C	
22. C	22. A	22. C	22. D	
23. E	23. D	23. D	23. C	
24. D	24. C	24. C	24. E	
25. C	25. D	25. D	25. D	

VERBAL ANALOGIES — 2 BLANKS

EXAMINATION SECTION

DIRECTIONS FOR THIS SECTION:

Each question in this part consists of two capitalized words which have a certain relationship to each other, followed by five lettered pairs of words in small letters. Choose the letter of the pair of words which are related to each other in the SAME way as the words of the capitalized pair are related to each other. *PRINT THE LETTER OF THE CORRECT ANSWER IN THE SPACE AT THE RIGHT.*

TEST 1

1. PRESS : NATION :: ________ : ________ 1. ...
   A. village : reputation B. gossip : hamlet
   C. gossip : newspaper D. truth : story E. chapter : book
2. INK : BLOTTER :: ________ : ________ 2. ...
   A. spore : sponge B. water : sponge C. water : wet
   D. pen : pencil E. margin : hole
3. DEMOCRACY : AUTOCRACY :: ________ : ________ 3. ...
   A. leisure class : aristocracy B. freedom : tyranny
   C. tyranny : nobility D. mob : despot E. poverty : wealth
4. GESTATION : BIRTH :: ________ : ________ 4. ...
   A. seedling : towering oak B. ponder : puzzle
   C. hypothesis : premise D. solution : crystallization
   E. answer : question
5. KNOWLEDGE : RUDIMENTS :: ________ : ________ 5. ...
   A. sophistication : ingenuity B. virtuoso : tyro
   C. end : beginning D. complexity : elementary
   E. bellicosity : ingenuousness
6. UNSHACKLE : FETTERS :: ________ : ________ 6. ...
   A. pardon : prisoner B. slake : thirst C. devour : food
   D. loose : tight E. vent : ire
7. INDOLENCE : CURSORILY :: ________ : ________ 7. ...
   A. determination : flatteringly
   B. error : not thoroughly C. ardor : elusively
   D. perfunctory : diligently E. zeal : assiduously
8. ANCIENT : OLD :: ________ : ________ 8. ...
   A. demented : vexed B. peremptory : positive
   C. ineluctable : indefeasible
   D. celibate : without relatives E. generosity : parsimony
9. RECUPERATION : VACATION :: ________ : ________ 9. ...
   A. refugee : homeland B. redress : lawsuit
   C. bail : sentence D. cajole : jailor E. joy : sorrow
10. WATER : JUG :: ________ : ________ 10. ...
    A. disillusionment : life B. acid : carboy
    C. destructiveness : railway
    D. solution : mineral E. discipline : army
11. DOCK : SHIP :: ________ : ________ 11. ...
    A. lair : fox B. home : parent C. station : train
    D. whistle : cab E. haven : refugee
12. POEM : EPIC :: ________ : ________ 12. ...
    A. scenery : play B. mustache : face C. drape : window
    D. setting : ring E. art : cubism
13. DAWN : DAY :: ________ : ________ 13. ...
    A. fight : might B. telegram : event
    C. harbinger : spring D. tail : comet
    E. spring : winter

14. CULMINATE : TERMINATE :: _______ : _______ 14. ...
A. start : finish B. pinnacle : climax
C. maturity : homestretch D. baptism : birth
E. meridian : setting

15. RAFTERS : ROOF :: _______ : _______ 15. ...
A. ribs : umbrella B. roof : rafters C. garret : house
D. spokes : hub E. skeleton : frame

16. UNCLE : NIECE :: _______ : _______ 16. ...
A. aunt : nephew B. father : daughter C. nephew : niece
D. mother : daughter-in-law E. minor : adult

17. FINS : FEET :: _______ : _______ 17. ...
A. water : air B. gills : lungs C. mouth : ears
D. tail : feathers E. wings : arms

18. SAND : POWDER :: _______ : _______ 18. ...
A. sawdust : flour B. bread : wood C. table : chair
D. sky : water E. rain : snow

19. CAKE : COOKIES :: _______ : _______ 19. ...
A. pie : dessert B. salad : dressing
C. steak : lamb chops D. chicken : egg E. bread : biscuit

20. PENCIL : PEN :: _______ : _______ 20. ...
A. baseball bat : baseball B. pencil : eraser
C. wall : brick D. broom : mop E. water : wash

21. BEAT : MEASURE :: _______ : _______ 21. ...
A. pedometer : hydrometer
B. daylight saving : standard time
C. chronometer : calendar D. sun-dial : candle power
E. chronicle : anachronism

22. PROLOGUE : EPILOGUE :: _______ : _______ 22. ...
A. coda : prelude B. elephant : tail C. glossary : appendix
D. alpha : omega E. plot : denouement

23. DECADE : YEAR :: _______ : _______ 23. ...
A. year : month B. month : day C. minute : second
D. hour : minute E. millennium : century

24. COOL : FRIGID :: _______ : _______ 24. ...
A. turgid : horrid B. tepid : torrid C. livid : lurid
D. pool : placid E. tumid : turbid

25. SPLASH : INUNDATE :: _______ : _______ 25. ...
A. crawl : creep B. freeze : jell C. freshen : clean
D. drizzle : drench E. drift : swim

TEST 2

1. ACKNOWLEDGMENT : RUMOR :: _______ : _______ 1. ...
A. affirmation : report B. testify : certify
C. probably : possible D. reputation : gossip
E. servility : dependability

2. SAGACITY : EXPERIENCE :: _______ : _______ 2. ...
A. failure : timorousness B. study : mastery
C. heredity : wisdom D. smarting : ointment
E. experiment : hypothesis

3. CRISIS : DISEASE :: _______ : _______ 3. ...
A. prelude : interlude B. emergency : decision
C. coup d'état : revolution D. apex : flight
E. climax : battle

4. CAPRICIOUS : VAGARY :: ______ : ______ 4. ...
A. unstable : stability B. aberrant : constancy
C. variable : wind D. inconstant : vacillation
E. vacillating : steadfastness

5. MIND : PREJUDICE :: ______ : ______ 5. ...
A. crime : sex B. sun : shade C. sky : cloud
D. ugly : thought E. knowledge : obtuse

6. SLIM : OBESE :: ______ : ______ 6. ...
A. cow : pig B. state : nation C. mountain : sea
D. tremendous : prodigious E. terse : turgid

7. WHEEL : HUB :: ______ : ______ 7. ...
A. earth : axis B. state : nation C. mountain : sea
D. earth : sun E. orbit : firmament

8. IMPURITIES : FILTER :: ______ : ______ 8. ...
A. water : faucet B. failures : examination
C. remedies : petition D. quality : denier E. wheat : chaff

9. MEDICINE : DOSE :: ______ : ______ 9. ...
A. vegetables : portion B. oatmeal : spoon
C. bread : loaf D. water : glass E. fish : vitamins

10. PITCH : ROOF :: ______ : ______ 10. ...
A. altitude : hill B. grade : mountain
C. shingles : roof D. depth : valley E. height : hill

11. REPETITION : MONOTONY :: ______ : ______ 11. ...
A. callowness : inexperience B. attempt : achievement
C. dissipation : depravity D. familiarity : recognition
E. interest : boredom

12. CALAMITY : DISTRESS :: ______ : ______ 12. ...
A. war : victory B. triumph : exultation
C. tidings : jubilation D. emergency : desolation
E. news : gratification

13. OINTMENT : BURN :: ______ : ______ 13. ...
A. pain : agony B. sympathy : sorrow
C. powder : face D. water : fire
E. medicine : doctor

14. DUSK : DAWN :: ______ : ______ 14. ...
A. callow : mature B. light : murky
C. diurnal : nocturnal D. moon : sun E. fall : rise

15. TABLE : LEGS :: ______ : ______ 15. ...
A. government : army B. men : men C. manuscript : thesis
D. legislature : judiciary E. religion : rites

16. MANY : FEW :: ______ : ______ 16. ...
A. myriad : sparse B. major : minor C. minority : plurality
D. plethora : innumerable E. predominant : sporadic

17. KING : MONARCHY :: ______ : ______ 17. ...
A. leader : executive B. clansman : tribe
C. pope : papacy D. president : democracy
E. queen : aristocracy

18. SQUARE : CIRCLE :: ______ : ______ 18. ...
A. acre : rod B. rectangle : oval C. sphere : cube
D. cube : sphere E. hexagon : pentagon

19. DECADE : CENTURY :: ______ : ______ 19. ...
A. dime : dollar B. time : number C. little : much
D. penny : dime E. decalogue : trilogy

20. ORNITHOLOGIST : BIRDS :: ______ : ______ 20. ...
A. philologist : language B. biologist : cells

C. pediatrician : feet D. botanist : animals
E. etymologist : insects

21. DEER : VENISON :: _______ : _______ 21. ...
A. lion : jackal B. beef : stew C. hog : pork
D. mutton : sheep E. lamb : chops

22. INNUENDO : ASSERTION :: _______ : _______ 22. ...
A. suggestion : recommendation B. implicit : explicit
C. state : hint D. allusion : insinuation
E. indirect : devious

23. VOLUME : BOOKLET :: _______ : _______ 23. ...
A. genuine : synthetic B. tome : epitaph
C. synopsis : compendium D. exposition : precis
E. obese : slender

24. TOWER : DUNGEON :: _______ : _______ 24. ...
A. virtue : disgrace B. building : foundation
C. citadel : vault D. prop : cornice E. head : foot

25. TRANSLATE : PARAPHRASE :: _______ : _______ 25. ...
A. intrinsic : extrinsic B. communicate : express
C. hews : hearsay D. literal : free
E. simile : metaphor

TEST 3

1. ANCHOR : SHIP :: _______ : _______ 1. ...
A. stopper : door B. sound : whisper C. length : inch
D. weight : paper E. cork : bottle

2. KING : PURPLE :: _______ : _______ 2. ...
A. sum : gold B. soldier : whisper C. soldier : khaki
D. grass : green E. cork : bottle

3. HORSE : CENTAUR :: _______ : _______ 3. ...
A. fish : mermaid B. fish : nymph C. horse : man
D. crocodile : dragon E. shark : whale

4. POOR : FRUGAL :: _______ : _______ 4. ...
A. rich : gorgeous B. wealth : prosperous
C. well-to-do : heedless D. prosperous : prodigal
E. lachrymose : indolent

5. INTEMPERATE : CRITICAL :: _______ : _______ 5. ...
A. deference : thought B. anger : spite
C. emotion : reason D. devotion : fondness
E. fulmination : recrimination

6. PRICES : SUBSIDY :: _______ : _______ 6. ...
A. steel : girder B. apex : climax C. tree: trunk
D. society : law E. ceiling : pillar

7. GOVERNMENT : ORDER :: _______ : _______ 7. ...
A. hierarchy : peace B. disturbance : problem
C. anarchy : chaos D. oppression : confusion
E. dictator : democrat

8. GRUMBLE : SCOWL :: _______ : _______ 8. ...
A. laugh : smile B. express : restrain C. cry : sigh
D. lament : condole E. entice : endow

9. FLEETNESS : RUNNER :: _______ : _______ 9. ...
A. paint : artist B. imagination : artist
C. grace : chess-player D. suppleness : acrobat
E. strength : detective

10. HAND : WRIST :: ______ : ______ 10. ...
A. angle : elbow B. compound sentence : conjunction
C. leg : knee D. ribs : breastbone
E. simile : metaphor

11. MÉTIER : CALLING :: ______ : ______ 11. ...
A. heresy : hexapla B. purveyor : overseer
C. minion : dominion
D. hierarchy : organization of officials according to rank
E. administration : oligarchy

12. SIDEREAL : STARRY :: ______ : ______ 12. ...
A. bovine : piglike B. discrepant : discordant
C. perspicuous : ambiguous D. browsing : carousing
E. declivitous : narrow

13. DUB : DRESS :: ______ : ______ 13. ...
A. acerbate : retaliate B. deprecate : depreciate
C. cavil : carp D. cadge : lie E. comprise : constrain

14. EIDOLON : IMAGE :: ______ : ______ 14. ...
A. tarantella : dance of the spiders B. covert : bevy
C. argot : dragon D. nexus : link E. efflux : effluvium

15. DECUMAN : TENTH :: ______ : ______ 15. ...
A. consummate : inchoate B. plethoric : insufficient
C. callow : mature D. crepuscular : glimmering
E. decumbent : lambent

16. DECOCT : PREPARE BY BOILING :: ______ : ______ 16. ...
A. eviscerate : thin out B. skulk : hulk
C. demean : conduct oneself D. concoct : evict
E. rescind : abstain

17. HONORARIUM : FEE :: ______ : ______ 17. ...
A. fatuity : crassness B. canard : hoax
C. torpor : trudgen D. trull : trumpet
E. truffle : trousseau

18. FRICATIVE : FORCED :: ______ : ______ 18. ...
A. voracious : veracious B. clamorous : glamorous
C. adipose : fatty D. vaunted : truckle
E. bellicose : mangy

19. ASSEVERATE : AFFIRM :: ______ : ______ 19. ...
A. enervate : give impetus to B. roil : convulse
C. impugn : call in question D. essay : assay
E. digest : diffuse

20. ZEITGEIST : SPIRIT OF THE TIME :: ______ : ______ 20. ...
A. nimbus : atmosphere B. lintel : vertical support
C. atoll : treeless plain D. cloak : cloister
E. cloisonné : filigree-work

21. FUSTY : MUSTY :: ______ : ______ 21. ...
A. tractable : spineless B. maudlin : fuddled
C. climacteric : released D. donative : illative
E. fictile : fictive

22. ADUMBRATE : OUTLINE :: ______ : ______ 22. ...
A. derogate : detract B. reticulate : reformulate
C. obtrude : obtest D. obvert : obviate
E. abrogate : validate

23. SEQUESTER : SET APART :: ______ : ______ 23. ...
A. obliquity : defamatory language
B. junto : hunt C. scourge : dereliction
D. noblesse oblige : obligation of generous behavior associated with high rank E. colander : calendar

24. ANOMALOUS : ABNORMAL :: _____ : _____ 24. ...
A. dulcet : tame B. cavalier : finical
C. feigned : restricted D. recondite : elementary
E. esoteric : abstruse

25. ASPERSE : DISCREDIT :: _____ : _____ 25. ...
A. inveigh : impound B. inculpate : exculpate
C. lampoon : satirize D. accede : exceed
E. condone : condign

TEST 4

1. INCONGRUITY : DISCREPANT :: _____ : _____ 1. ...
A. incoherent : unconsolidated B. unfit : absurd
C. slacken : looseness D. instrument : orchestra
E. dissonance : discordant

2. LOAF : LOITER :: _____ : _____ 2. ...
A. doze : somnolence B. vegetate : dormant
C. slumber : hibernate D. dawdler : truant
E. eater : opium

3. HALLUCINATION : ILLUSION :: _____ : _____ 3. ...
A. phantom : apparition B. phantasm : phantasmagorical
C. fancy : visual D. error : deceptive E. ghost : appear

4. PARKING : OFFENSE :: _____ : _____ 4. ...
A. tort : wrong B. smuggle : contraband
C. breach : violation D. void : marriage
E. annulment : invalidation

5. SEMBLANCE : ADAPTATION :: _____ : _____ 5. ...
A. imitate : duplication B. mimicking : parrot
C. satirize : parody D. counterfeit : forgery
E. echo : mountain

6. OBLATION : IMMOLATION :: _____ : _____ 6. ...
A. bemusement : inaptness B. babbling : idiocy
C. fatuity : inanity D. shallowness : asininity
E. thralldom : freedom

7. BOWER : PERGOLA :: _____ : _____ 7. ...
A. orchard : vineyard B. market : agriculture
C. greenhouse : gardening D. wine : apple
E. fertilizer : vintage

8. FURROW : MOAT :: _____ : _____ 8. ...
A. carve : chisel B. trench : ditch C. engraving : offset
D. slit : seam E. etch : wrinkle

9. JOINTURE : APPANAGE :: _____ : _____ 9. ...
A. quarry : prey B. sporting : blood
C. contest : play D. divert : entertain E. chase : animal

10. GHOULISH : SPIRITS :: _____ : _____ 10. ...
A. devilish : ghoulish B. demoniacal : fabulous
C. hobgoblin : spook D. fiendish : incubi
E. gnome : salamander

11. LISTLESS : MOTIVATING :: _____ : _____ 11. ...
A. effective : effectual B. active : thinking
C. enervating : stimulating D. cold : hot
E. energizing : forcible

12. MATURATION : INCIPIENCE :: _____ : _____ 12. ...
A. fertility : fruition B. materialism : existentialism

C. senescence : youth D. imbecile : moron
E. field marshal : lieutenant

13. CURSORY : CONSUMMATE :: ______ : ______ 13. ...
A. pompous : pomposity B. archaic : archeological
C. signature : calligraphy D. diffident : sanguine
E. alto : contralto

14. DECEIT : FURTIVE :: ______ : ______ 14. ...
A. affluence : parsimony B. notoriety : flagrant
C. generosity : altruism D. perennial : decennial
E. subterfuge : clandestine

15. WOOF : WARP :: ______ : ______ 15. ...
A. windmill : water B. smokestack : chimney
C. forest : meadow D. ledge : minaret
E. supine : horizontal

16. DOCTOR : TREATMENT :: ______ : ______ 16. ...
A. thief : theft B. electors : president C. pirate : ship
D. nun : ministration E. boss : efficiency

17. DILEMMA : PUZZLE :: ______ : ______ 17. ...
A. guess : choose B. oracle : treacle
C. maturation : condensation
D. sphinx : enigma E. portent : foretell

18. PUNCTURE : INCISE :: ______ : ______ 18. ...
A. precipice : precipitous B. engulf : convulse
C. holocaust : flagrant D. burn : wound
E. seethe : smolder

19. LANGUAGE : WORDS :: ______ : ______ 19. ...
A. science : experiments B. arithmetic : numbers
C. center : arc D. social science : history
E. spelling : phonetics

20. ACQUIT : CRIME :: ______ : ______ 20. ...
A. prescription : sickness B. repent : sin
C. release : bail D. presentment : jury
E. exonerate : charge

21. DECADE : CENTURY :: ______ : ______ 21. ...
A. multitude : myriads B. second : hour
C. youth : senescence D. dime : dollar E. penny : dime

22. BROKER : INVESTOR :: ______ : ______ 22. ...
A. doctor : nurse B. executive : subordinate
C. student : teacher D. merchant : marine
E. attorney : client

23. PUNGENT : BITTER :: ______ : ______ 23. ...
A. refreshing : refreshment B. flabby : flaccid
C. brusque : brisk D. acute : acerb
E. morbid : morbidity

24. UNCTUOUS : SMOOTH :: ______ : ______ 24. ...
A. terse : succinct B. cowardly : obsequious
C. stalwart : pusillanimous
D. valiant : verve E. viscous : suave

25. NERVOUS : DEPRESSED :: ______ : ______ 25. ...
A. intensive : extensive B. fabulous : large
C. physical : mental D. exultant : gratified
E. insane : neurotic

TEST 5

1. CHESS : PIECES :: ________ : ________ 1. ...
   A. cards : bridge B. Mah Jongg : tiles
   C. Russian roulette : dice D. tennis : court
   E. letters : scrabble
2. MOOSE : NORTH AMERICA :: ________ : ________ 2. ...
   A. camel : South America B. beaver : Egypt
   C. mosquito : malaria D. elk : Asia
   E. Australia : kangaroo
3. PROCESS : PARTICIPANT :: ________ : ________ 3. ...
   A. vote : voter B. election : elector C. choice : chosen
   D. president : people E. primary : privilege
4. PUNGENT : PERCEPTIVE :: ________ : ________ 4. ...
   A. poignant : sentient B. biting : feeling
   C. sensitive : emotional D. keen : piercing
   E. arouse : display
5. CARBOLIC ACID : MILK :: ________ : ________ 5. ...
   A. poison : emetic B. catalyst : venomous
   C. infect : defect D. arsenic : anecdote
   E. nicotine : cigarette
6. CONIC : FUNNEL :: ________ : ________ 6. ...
   A. triangular : obelisk B. cylindrical : column
   C. hexagonal : star D. cyanic : bluish
   E. rhombus : parallelogram
7. MONSOON : WIND :: ________ : ________ 7. ...
   A. river : overflowing B. raining : excessively
   C. flood : rain D. cyclone : hurricane
   E. earthquake : volcano
8. ELEMENT : SUPPORT :: ________ : ________ 8. ...
   A. tire : puncture B. gas : leak C. clay : mold
   D. fire : andiron E. paper : perforate
9. IODINE : CHLORINE :: ________ : ________ 9. ...
   A. calcium : enamel B. copper : penny C. carbon : diamond
   D. pure : impure E. cobalt : nickel
10. EXPERIMENT : CATALYST :: ________ : ________ 10. ...
    A. travel : interfere B. business : expediter
    C. manuscript : publisher D. hasten : rush
    E. energy : expend

KEYS (CORRECT ANSWERS)

TEST 1	TEST 2	TEST 3	TEST 4	TEST 5
1. B	1. A	1. D	1. E	1. B
2. B	2. A	2. C	2. C	2. D
3. B	3. E	3. A	3. A	3. B
4. D	4. D	4. D	4. A	4. A
5. B	5. C	5. C	5. D	5. A
6. E	6. E	6. E	6. A	6. B
7. E	7. A	7. C	7. A	7. C
8. B	8. B	8. A	8. B	8. D
9. B	9. A	9. D	9. A	9. E
10. B	10. B	10. C	10. D	10. B
11. C	11. C	11. D	11. C	
12. E	12. B	12. B	12. C	
13. C	13. B	13. C	13. D	
14. E	14. E	14. D	14. E	
15. A	15. E	15. D	15. D	
16. B	16. A	16. C	16. D	
17. B	17. C	17. B	17. D	
18. A	18. B	18. C	18. E	
19. E	19. A	19. C	19. B	
20. D	20. A	20. A	20. E	
21. C	21. C	21. B	21. D	
22. D	22. B	22. A	22. E	
23. E	23. D'	23. D	23. D	
24. B	24. C	24. E	24. A	
25. D	25. D	25. C	25. D	

ANTONYMS/OPPOSITES

COMMENTARY

The opposite-type question is one step further removed in difficulty from the synonym-type. Its greater difficulty is readily discernible when one considers that in order to answer as to the opposite, one must first know what the word means -- that is, the synonym. Thus, a transitional stage in the thought process (the same) is skipped over, and one is compelled forthwith to move on to the next stage (the opposite) in the same amount of time allotted.

For this type of vocabulary question, it is not sufficient for the candidate to have merely a general knowledge of the meanings of words. It will be necessary for him to know their meanings with power and discrimination.

In the questions presented, the items or choices will be very closely related so that only a sure and precise understanding will lead to the correct answer. To the uninitiated, i.e., the candidate with average word-power, any one of the choices presented in the question will seem acceptable and each, in turn, will present individual difficulty, leading to uncertainty, confusion, and loss of time on a test for which definite time limits are assigned. Therefore, it is most important that the candidate reinforce his accustomed incidental learning of the meanings of words by directed, purposeful study and overlearning of vocabulary.

The opposite type of question is usually attended by the following directions:

DIRECTIONS: Each question in this part consists of a word in capital letters, followed by five words numbered 1 through 5. Choose the number of the word that is most nearly OPPOSITE in meaning to the word in capital letters, and mark the appropriate space on your answer sheet.

SUGGESTIONS FOR ANSWERING THE OPPOSITE (ANTONYM)-TYPE QUESTION

1. Since this is an aptitude test, whose validity rests upon its ability to measure your power to reason with words, please accept without reservation the reality that the antonym answer is at best an approximation and not, in most cases, a true opposite. It is up to you to choose the MOST NEARLY correct answer or BEST answer (of the choices offered). Do not anticipate finding literal or exact opposite meanings used in these questions. This is how and where your ability to think, to reason, and to select will be shown.

2. Be alert concerning the part of speech of the subject word and question items. In all cases, the correct answer should be of the same part of speech (e.g., an adjective) as the subject or question word (e.g., an adjective). This is a quick and easy test

or method to eliminate some of the given possibilities in the question. (Violations of this rule in previous examinations have proved to be exceptional.)

3. Beware of choosing as an opposite a word which is broader or more limited in scope than the subject word. For example, in the question below:

ECONOMICAL 1. deistic 2. liberal 3. lavish 4. frugal 5. amicable,

the correct answer is 3. lavish, not 2. liberal. The reason for this is that while liberal is opposed to economical, it is too moderate in scope, denoting a quality not so adequately described as by the word, lavish, which is on the extreme opposite end of the word-pole in relation to the subject word, economical.

4. The opposite, to be correct, must be in the same state, that is, active or passive, transitive or intransitive, as the subject word. This is really a continuation of the thought contained in (3) above. Thus. in the question:

ENTICE 1. detract 2. repelled 3. decoy 4. repulse 5. negate,

the correct answer is 4. repulse, not 2. repelled, since the latter word is in the past tense, while the subject word is in the present tense.

5. Should the question call for an opposite, be sure that you do not make the usual mistake of seizing upon a synonym which you readily recognize in the question group, when an antonym is called for. This is a favorite device of the examiners - to throw in ready synonyms in order to test the alertness and perspicacity of the candidate.

6. You should make time on this type of question. A strong and confident facility in vocabulary should enable you to recognize synonyms at once; antonyms should cause you to think, but, nevertheless, should take just a little longer than the synonym question. Perhaps, it is an axiom to state that if you cannot handle this type of question quickly and efficiently, you will not do well on the aptitude test as a whole.

7. The best way to answer the opposite type of question is to scan the possible answers and to decide immediately upon the correct one. This presupposes strength and maturity of vocabulary. Only where the meaning of the word has little or no connotation for the candidate should he attempt, by trial and error, to examine each possible answer in turn.

The formula then is: scan and answer.

ANTONYMS/OPPOSITES

EXAMINATION SECTION

DIRECTIONS FOR THIS SECTION: Each question below consists of a word printed in capital letters, followed by five words or phrases lettered A through E. Choose the lettered word or phrase that is *most nearly* OPPOSITE in meaning to the word in capital letters. *PRINT THE LETTER OF THE CORRECT ANSWER IN THE SPACE AT THE RIGHT.*

TEST 1

1. ABEYANCE A. revival B. following orders C. temporary inactivity D. adjournment E. concealment 1. ...
2. ACADEMIC A. unseasoned B. scholarly C. practical D. attainable E. superficial 2. ...
3. AFFECTATION A. histrionics B. conquetry C. shield D. airs E. ingeniousness 3. ...
4. AFFILIATE A. thread B. honor C. cut away D. associate oneself E. feign 4. ...
5. ALLEGE A. deny B. declare C. arouse D. arrest E.conjure 5. ...
6. ALLEVIATE A. moderate B. assign C. tax D. antagonize E. deceive 6. ...
7. ANIMOSITY A. hatred B. affection C. sprightliness D. animalism E. contempt 7. ...
8. APATHY A. hatred B. indifference C. policy D. cowardice E. fervor 8. ...
9. APPAL A. pierce B. apportion C. dismay D. attach E. gratify 9. ...
10. AUTHENTIC A. severe B. gracious C. mendacious D. reliable E. supreme 10. ...
11. BRISK A. large B.fragile C.alert D.flagging E.tolerant 11. ...
12. BRUSQUE A. keen B. smooth C.menacing D.quick E.abrupt 12. ...
13. CALUMNIOUS A. disastrous B.quartz-like C.laudatory E.slanderous E.querulous 13. ...
14. CANDID A. straightforward B. evasive C. profound D. pleasant E. contrite 14. ...
15. CAROUSE A. cajole B. revel C. decay D. induce E.abstain 15. ...
16. CELIBATE A. chaste B. spouseless C. pertaining to funerals D. relic E. conjugal 16. ...
17. CLEMENCY A. weather condition B. climbing plant C. type of cloud D. rigor E. mercy 17. ...
18. COMMODIOUS A. inutile B. spacious C. ordinary D. interchangeable E. useful 18. ...
19. COMPETENT A. equivalent B. compact C. adequate D. based on rivalry E. maladroit 19. ...
20. COMPLICITY A. deceit B. antipathy C. partnership in wrong D. collusion E. delight in society 20. ...
21. CONSTERNATION A. dissapointment B.dismay C.disapproval D.distrust E. intrepidity 21. ...
22. CONTAMINATE A. include B. expurgate C. pollute D. adjacent E. reflect upon 22. ...
23. CORROBORATE A. withdraw B. terminate C. disavow D. confirm E. correlate 23. ...
24. COSMIC A. funny B.vast C.greasy D.childish E.finite 24. ...
25. CRITERION A. standard B. anomaly C. judgment D. analysis E. probability 25. ...

TEST 2

1.	CRUCIAL	A. pending B. conditional C. critical D. un- D. unreasonable E. unessential	1. ...
2.	CULPABILITY	A. misprint B. blame C. felony D.impeccability E. whitewash	2. ...
3.	DAUB	A. alarm B.delay C.depict D.stupefy E.smear	3. ...
4.	DELINEATE	A. crack B.blotch C.do twice D.make of linen E. describe	4. ...
5.	DEVIATING	A. conspiring B. depressing C. indirect D. unswerving E. turning	5. ...
6.	DILAPIDATED	A. lonely B. integral C. ruined D. sequestered E. old-fashioned	6. ...
7.	DILATORY	A. reclining B. spiteful C. expeditious D. praiseworthy E. procrastinating	7. ...
8.	DISPATCH	A. curb B.argue C.send off D.mend E.receive	8. ...
9.	DOCILE	A. parasitic B.ungovernable C.mournful D.teach-able E. compliant	9. ...
10.	DRIFT	A. meaning B. tendency C. riot D. motion E. procession	10. ...
11.	DUALITY	A. unity B. falsity C. biformity D. perversity E. intactness	11. ...
12.	DUBIOUS	A. questionable B. categorical C. sufficient D. pleasant to the ear E. composed	12. ...
13.	DURABLE	A. flimsy B. permanent C.ugly D.timely E.callous	13. ...
14.	ECCENTRIC	A. peculiar B. convergent C. ecliptic D. eclectic E. pragmatic	14. ...
15.	EMBELLISH	A. defraud B. deface C. represent symbolically D. point up E. review	15. ...
16.	EMBRYONIC	A. accelerated B. many-colored C. rudimentary D. undeveloped E. perfected	16. ...
17.	ENIGMATIC	A. cognitive B. fraudulent C. odious D. magical E. puzzling	17. ...
18.	EPIGRAMMATIC	A. pointed B. national C. ungrammatical D. scabrous E. concise	18. ...
19.	FANATICISM	A. perplexity B. indifference C. endurance D. flatulence E. excessive enthusiasm	19. ...
20.	FORMIDABLE	A. menacing B. conventional C.loathsome D. apprehensive E. resolute	20. ...
21.	GAWKY	A. gaudy B.clumsy C.meager D.elegant E.straight-forward	21. ...
22.	GENESIS	A. gender B.origin C.outcome D.inception E. exodus	22. ...
23.	HILARITY	A. celerity B. mirth C. despondence D. abandon E. covetousness	23. ...
24.	HOSTILE	A. singular B. convincing C. poisonous D. stimulating E. amicable	24. ...
25.	HYBRID	A. mongrel B. eugenic C. exaggerated D. dwarfed E. homogenous	25. ...

TEST 3

1.	IMPEDIMENT	A. accusation B. hindrance C. succor D. admission E. inhibition	1. ...
2.	IMPERVIOUS	A. incomparable B. impenetrable C. inhuman D. trackless D. dissoluble	2. ...
3.	INCREDIBLE	A. hard to believe B. skeptical C. bad beyond correction D. indisputable D. illogical	3. ...

4.	INGENIOUS	A. frank B. deceitful C. ingenuous D. subversive E. clever	4. ...
5.	INTEGRITY	A. honesty B. opprobrium C. humor D. courage E. knowledge	5. ...
6.	INTIMIDATE	A. to defy B. to make afraid C. to come without invitation D. to weary E. to make less fearful	6. ...
7.	INTROSPECTION	A. bending backwards B. insertion C. performation D. self examination E. extroversion	7. ...
8.	JOSTLE	A. trip B. elbow C.bully D.rob E. quail	8. ...
9.	LAVISH	A. niggardly B.extravagant C.prodigal D. convalescent E. plain	9. ...
10.	LENIENCY	A. transparent substance B. stringency C. fickleness D. forbearance E. decay	10. ...
11.	MERCENARY	A. egoistic B. pestilential C. altruistic D. greedy E. venal	11. ...
12.	MEDIOCRE	A. yellow B. boundless C. ordinary E. eminent E. tiny	12. ...
13.	NOVELTY	A. modernism B. pseudonym C. relic D. innovation E. quaintness	13. ...
14.	OBSOLETE	A. antiquated B. polite C. neglected D. rectangular E. vernal	14. ...
15.	ONSLAUGHT	A. furious attack B. murder C. repulse D. adventure E. severe punishment	15. ...
16.	OUST	A. evict B. banish C. injure D. admit E. cry out	16. ...
17.	PALATABLE	A. toothsome B. savory C. soft D. intolerable E. vindictive	17. ...
18.	PALLID	A. wretched B. funereal C. ghastly D.spectral E. vivid	18. ...
19.	PALTRY	A. consequential B. pitiable C. grandiloquent D. prevalent E. petty	19. ...
20.	PARABLE	A. analogy B. pattern C. phenomenon D. fable E. allegory	20. ...
21.	PARAPHRASE	A. restate B. convey C. reword D. articulate E. translate	21. ...
22.	PARCH	A. swab B. saturate C.desiccate D.sponge E. scorch	22. ...
23.	PATHOLOGICAL	A. morbid B. virulent C.salubrious E.diseased E. implied	23. ...
24.	PERMEATE	A. enfilade B. traverse C. pervade D.infiltrate E. block	24. ...
25.	PERPETUATE	A. obliterate B. punish C. preserve D.flourish E. enshrine	25. ...

TEST 4

1.	PERTINENT	A. appropriate B. awkward C. obstinate D. abusive E. irrelevant	1. ...
2.	PONDER	A. reflect B. hazard C. argue D. reject E. consider	2. ...
3.	POLLUTE	A. spread B. foul C. stain D. decontaminate E. rebut	3. ...
4.	POSTHUMOUS	A. hastily B. extant C. inappropriate D. happening after one's death E. unawakened	4. ...

5. PREDILECTION A. maintenance B. negotiation C. investment D. inclination E. evulsion 5. ...

6. PRETEXT A. reason B. fact C. excuse D. opinion E. illusion 6. ...

7. PRODIGAL A. perturbing B.wasteful C. venal D. large E. wandering 7. ...

8. REFUTE A. disobey B. disprove C. remove D. affirm E. strike out 8. ...

9. RELENTLESS A. compassionate B. unmoved by pity C. confident D. unexciting E. graceful 9. ...

10. RETICENT A. backward B.rash C.timid D.reserved E. gushing 10. ...

11. SEDENTARY A. soothing B. calm C. migratory D. aged E. stationary 11. ...

12. SKEPTICISM A. cynicism B. simplicity C. critical state of mind D. distortion E. chariness 12. ...

13. SMUG A. uncomplaisant B. adjacent C. self-satisfied D. hazy E. cozy 13. ...

14. SPASMODIC A. continuous B. intermittent C. feverish D. gradual E. momentary 14. ...

15. STILTED A. formal B. subdued C. deprived D. archaic E. facile 15. ...

16. SUCCINCT A. superfluous B. concise C. pithy D. succulent E. colloquial 16. ...

17. SURREPTITIOUS A. stealthy B.surprising C.authorized D. affected E. unobserved 17. ...

18. SUSCEPTIBLE A. aggressive B. impotent C. cowering D. unimpressionable E. hesitant 18. ...

19. TANTRUM A. symbol B. tranquility C. commiseration D. conundrum E. display of temper 19. ...

20. TATTERS A. finery B.gossip C.sails D.riches E. rags 20. ...

KEYS (CORRECT ANSWERS)

TEST 1

1.	A	11.	D
2.	E	12.	B
3.	E	13.	C
4.	C	14.	B
5.	A	15.	E
6.	D	16.	E
7.	B	17.	D
8.	E	18.	A
9.	E	19.	E
10.	C	20.	B

21. E
22. B
23. C
24. E
25. B

TEST 2

1.	E	11.	A
2.	D	12.	B
3.	C	13.	A
4.	B	14.	D
5.	D	15.	B
6.	B	16.	E
7.	C	17.	A
8.	A	18.	E
9.	B	19.	B
10.	E	20.	B

21. D
22. C
23. C
24. E
25. E

TEST 3

1.	C	11.	C
2.	E	12.	D
3.	D	13.	C
4.	C	14.	E
5.	B	15.	C
6.	A	16.	D
7.	E	17.	D
8.	E	18.	E
9.	A	19.	A
10.	B	20.	C

21. E
22. B
23. C
24. E
25. A

TEST 4

1.	E	11.	C
2.	B	12.	B
3.	D	13.	A
4.	B	14.	A
5.	E	15.	E
6.	B	16.	A
7.	C	17.	C
8.	D	18.	D
9.	A	19.	B
10.	E	20.	A

ANTONYMS/OPPOSITES
EXAMINATION SECTION

DIRECTIONS FOR THIS SECTION: Each question below consists of a word printed in capital letters, followed by five words or phrases lettered A through E. Choose the lettered word or phrase that is *most nearly* OPPOSITE in meaning to the word in capital letters. *PRINT THE LETTER OF THE CORRECT ANSWER IN THE SPACE AT THE RIGHT.*

TEST 1

1. CELERITY — A. torpor B. felicity C. fame D. acrimony E. temerity — 1. ...
2. APATHETIC — A. stoical B. amative C.lissome D.finical E. redolent — 2. ...
3. FLACCID — A. cold B. sterile C. brave D. stiff E. whimsical — 3. ...
4. INGENUOUS — A. foolish B. intelligent C. wily D. indigent E. native — 4. ...
5. AMENABLE — A. prayerful B.conciliatory C.pliant D. truculent E. mendacious — 5. ...
6. PARSIMONIOUS — A. benevolent B.worldly C.scoffing D. ungrammatical E. grudging — 6. ...
7. INDIGENOUS — A. caustic B.factitious C.exotic D.opulent E. sophisticated — 7. ...
8. SAPIENT — A. distasteful B.animalistic C.ignorant D. jejune E. zestful — 8. ...
9. TENUOUS — A. substantial B.decadent C.salubrious D. illogical E. slender — 9. ...
10. ZENITH — A. acme B.nadir C.pentacle D.azimuth E.apogee — 10. ...
11. RESTIVE — A. overactive B.refractory C.compliant D. uneasy E. listless — 11. ...
12. ADAMANT — A. primeval B.laudatory C.polite D.yielding E. intractable — 12. ...
13. DISCRETE — A. continuous B.separate C.foolish D.tactful E. serrated — 13. ...
14. SANGUINE — A. bloody B.diffident C.happy D.pale E. confident — 14. ...
15. PLACATE — A. retaliate B.confuse C.wander D.nettle E. condone — 15. ...
16. FATUOUS — A. inane B.stout C.witty D.empty E.vacuous — 16. ...
17. INNOCUOUS — A. toxic B.guileful C.gullible D.criminal E. culpable — 17. ...
18. DEARTH — A. demise B.copiousness C.nativity D.distaste E. lack — 18. ...
19. RESPITE — A. affirmation B.intermission C.continuance D. colloquy E. fairness — 19. ...
20. LACONIC — A. turgid B.replete C.tearful D.negligent E. draconic — 20. ...
21. ANIMADVERSION — A. censure B.distaste C. spirituality D. bestiality E. approbation — 21. ...
22. NOISOME — A. boisterous B. beneficial C. villous D. pallid E. noxious — 22. ...
23. EXPURGATE — A. cleanse B. harden C. improve D. deflect E. smirch — 23. ...
24. ATAVISM — A. progression B.favoritism C.inclination D. cannibalism E. reversion — 24. ...
25. ATTRITION — A. appeasement B.capitulation C.wearing away D. calming down E. aggrandizement — 25. ...

TEST 2

1. FABRICATE A. consume B. furrow C. construct D. materialize E. delete 1. ...
2. COMMAND A. mandate B. consummation C. correlation D. commitment E. supplication 2. ...
3. DISSIPATE A. sip B. amass C. disturb D. outdistance E. disperse 3. ...
4. UNBIASED A. unfair B. unreasonable C. uniform D. equitable E. disquieting 4. ...
5. SATURNINE A. buoyant B. gloomy C. aspiring D. incongruous E. splenetic 5. ...
6. PROFITABLE A. preferable B. chagrined C. ruinous D. lucrative E. profligate 6. ...
7. GENERATING A. generous B. originating C. degenerating D. terminating E. ingenuous 7. ...
8. SANCTION A. safety B. performance C. injunction D. sanctuary E. permission 8. ...
9. PROBABLE A. perchance B. imprudent C. unlikely D. perilous E. unsavory 9. ...
10. FRUITION A. exposure B. harvest C. frustration D. neglect E. attainment 10. ...
11. RANCOROUS A. benign B. confusing C. satiated D. complex E. malicious 11. ...
12. AVARICIOUS A. munificent B. rapacious C. analogous D. perverse E. atonal 12. ...
13. UNIQUE A. uniform B. single C. utilitarian D. senescent E. unitary 13. ...
14. PROCURE A. decline B. reap C. forfeit D. effect E. contrive 14. ...
15. RAVENOUS A. birdlike B. hungry C. rancid D. venial E. sated 15. ...
16. INNOCUOUS A. mixed B. pernicious C. defiled D. harmless E. diffused 16. ...
17. PERMEATE A. smooth B. pulverize C. obstruct D. pollute E. penetrate 17. ...
18. AXIOM A. adage B. proof C. precept D. dictum E. hearsay 18. ...
19. RELEVANT A. immaterial B. pertinent C. relenting D. capable E. released 19. ...
20. POTENT A. secretive B. powerful C. restive D. puissant E. enervated 20. ...
21. AMELIORATE A. improve B. embitter C. alter D. mellow E. impair 21. ...
22. IMPENDING A. pendulous B. impeding C. fortuitous D. imminent E. looming 22. ...
23. LATENT A. tricky B. hidden C. pompous D. overt E. hateful 23. ...
24. DISCERNMENT A. concern B. obtuseness C. distance D. sickness E. acumen 24. ...
25. SUAVE A. genuine B. captive C. gauche D. bland E. captious 25. ...

TEST 3

1. WORLDLY A. trifling B. secular C. mundane D. unworthy E. impractical 1. ...
2. BEG A. seek B. implore C. convert D. vaunt E. donate 2. ...
3. ERUDITE A. impolite B. learned C. correct D. illiterate E. contrite 3. ...
4. CURSORY A. protracted B. persistent C. evanescent D. superficial E. gentle 4. ...

5. ENIGMATIC A. evident B.enormous C.lucid D.abstruse E. sphinxlike 5. ...
6. PROSCRIBE A. banish B.condemn C.diagnose poorly D. transcend E. prescribe 6. ...
7. TURBID A. limpid B.muddy C.moody D.settled E.turgid 7. ...
8. PERSPICACITY A. keenness B. penetration C. rudeness D. discernment E. insensibility 8. ...
9. CONTIGUOUS A. contagious B. adjoining C. intolerant D. unconnected E. uncontaminated 9. ...
10. ASSUAGE A. intensify B. coagulate C. alleviate D. congeal E. molest 10. ...
11. PROTAGONIST A. enemy B. participant C. champion D. protector E. patron 11. ...
12. VIRULENT A. vehement B. virtuous C. deadly D. reparatory E. virile 12. ...
13. PROLIX A. tiresome B. exciting C. wordy D. terse E. pompous 13. ...
14. LEVITY A. lengthiness B. glumness C. lenience D. frivolity E. lewdness 14. ...
15. METICULOUS A. careful B. approximate C. untrue D.metallic E. indiscriminate 15. ...
16. ANALOGOUS A. tantamount B. extracurricular C. distinctive D. presumptuous E. cavernous 16. ...
17. VICARIOUS A. inconsiderate B. direct C. fraudulent D. substitute E. prestigious 17. ...
18. ABROGATION A. promulgation B. repeal C. extension D. investigation E. postponement 18. ...
19. HOMOGENEOUS A. manly B. assorted C. creamy D. similar E. parallel 19. ...
20. ARRAIGN A. accuse B. convict C. disentangle D. disarrange E. discharge 20. ...
21. ABJURE A. remove B. disavow C. acknowledge D.imagine E. entreat 21. ...
22. INTESTATE A. relating to inner parts B. legally devised C. shipped from one place to another D. subject to taxation E.not disposed of by will 22. ...
23. ANCILLARY A. deterrent B.temporary C.auxiliary D. approved E. additional 23. ...
24. EXTRANEOUS A. foreign B. accidental C. mixed D. indigenous E. adventitious 24. ...
25. DISPARAGE A. divide B. dismiss C. depreciate D.discourage E. dignify 25. ...

TEST 4

1. FUGACIOUS A. pugnacious B. tenacious C. mendacious D. settled E. migratory 1. ...
2. THRASONICAL A. treasonable B. gingival C. vainglorious D. unassuming E. lyrical 2. ...
3. PELAGIC A. terrestrial B. aquatic C. noncontagious D. polemical E. epigrammatic 3. ...
4. FUSCOUS A. importunate B. chaste C. radiant D. fractious E. amenable 4. ...
5. CREPUSCULAR A. glimmering B. crackling C. pussy D.mutable E. distinct 5. ...

6. NOISOME — A. attractive B.noxious C.inoffensive D. winsome E. noiseless — 6. ...

7. PEJORATIVE — A. appreciative B. acceding C. ultimate D. alliterative E. conceding — 7. ...

8. JEJUNE — A. valiant B.vital C.graceful D.senile E. incipient — 8. ...

9. FULGENT — A. divergent B.lambent C.unresplendent D. cogent E. indigent — 9. ...

10. LENITIVE — A. laxative B. provocative C. menial D. incursive E. malevolent — 10. ...

11. IRREFRAGABLE — A. breakable B. desirable C. tractable D. inconclusive E. refutable — 11. ...

12. INCHOATE — A. chaotic B. disclosed C. coherent D. infatuated E. complete — 12. ...

13. MINATORY — A. vanishing B. nugatory C. myriad D. malignant E. propitious — 13. ...

14. AMBIENT — A. wandering B. pandering C. transient D. remote E. hostile — 14. ...

15. EUPHEMISTIC — A. euphuisticB. grating C. masochistic D. palpable E. insolent — 15. ...

16. FACTIOUS — A. fractious B. fictitious C. scrupulous D. seemly E. disinterested — 16. ...

17. FRIABLE — A. unseasoned B. palatable C. renascent D. indestructible E. adhesive — 17. ...

18. HEGEMONY — A. thraldom B.testimony C. followership D. necromancy E. obligation — 18. ...

19. IMMANENT — A. illative B. imminent C. emanating D. unessential E. clement — 19. ...

20. INDEFEASIBLE — A. defensible B. abrogable C. disputable D. deferential E. execrable — 20. ...

21. EQUIVOCAL — A. ambiguous B. ambivalent C. equitable D. esoteric E. unquestionable — 21. ...

22. LIVID — A. lurid B. discolored C. unrestrained D. rubicund E. ghastly — 22. ...

23. MOIETY — A. impiety B. notoriety C. unity D.harmony E. inconsistency — 23. ...

24. PEREMPTORY — A. dogmatic B. authoritarian C. indecisive D. conciliatory E. whimsical — 24. ...

25. VENIAL — A. mercenary B. venous C. purulent D. aberrant E. loathsome — 25. ...

KEYS (CORRECT ANSWERS)

TEST 1

1.	A	11.	C
2.	B	12.	D
3.	D	13.	A
4.	C	14.	B
5.	D	15.	D
6.	A	16.	C
7.	C	17.	A
8.	C	18.	B
9.	A	19.	C
10.	B	20.	A
		21.	E
		22.	B
		23.	E
		24.	A
		25.	E

TEST 2

1.	A	11.	A
2.	E	12.	A
3.	B	13.	A
4.	A	14.	C
5.	A	15.	E
6.	C	16.	B
7.	D	17.	C
8.	C	18.	E
9.	C	19.	A
10.	C	20.	E
		21.	B
		22.	C
		23.	D
		24.	B
		25.	C

TEST 3

1.	E	11.	A
2.	E	12.	D
3.	D	13.	D
4.	A	14.	B
5.	C	15.	E
6.	E	16.	C
7.	A	17.	B
8.	E	18.	A
9.	D	19.	B
10.	A	20.	E
		21.	C
		22.	B
		23.	A
		24.	D
		25.	E

TEST 4

1.	D	11.	E
2.	D	12.	E
3.	A	13.	E
4.	C	14.	D
5.	E	15.	B
6.	C	16.	E
7.	A	17.	D
8.	B	18.	A
9.	C	19.	D
10.	B	20.	B
		21.	E
		22.	D
		23.	C
		24.	C
		25.	E

ANTONYMS/OPPOSITES

EXAMINATION SECTION

DIRECTIONS FOR THIS SECTION: Each question below consists of a word printed in capital letters, followed by five words or phrases lettered A through E. Choose the lettered word or phrase that is *most nearly* OPPOSITE in meaning to the word in capital letters. *PRINT THE LETTER OF THE CORRECT ANSWER IN THE SPACE AT THE RIGHT.*

TEST 1

1. ACRID	A. smoky B. withered C. sharp D. mild E. acerb	1. ...
2. ALLERGY	A. extreme sensitivity B. distaste C. sleepiness D. suppressed desire E. unsusceptibility	2. ...
3. AMBIGUOUS	A. acoustic B. ambivalent C. equivocal D. imitating E. succinct	3. ...
4. AMELIORATE	A. bring together B. settle a dispute C. worsen D. improve E. amend	4. ...
5. AUGMENT	A. sever B. disperse C. increase D. diminish E. argue	5. ...
6. BANAL	A. sarcastic B. trite C. novel D. futuristic E. sagacious	6. ...
7. BEATIFY	A. make lovely B. desecrate C. make happy D. restore E. hallow	7. ...
8. BOURGEOIS	A. middle-class citizen B. capital letters C. swollen streams D. nobility E. peasant	8. ...
9. BROMIDE	A. vegetable B. petty bribe C. pamphlet D. skin abrasion E. epigram	9. ...
10. BRING	A. fetch B. transfer C. relate D. suggest E. dispatch	10. ...
11. CAPRICIOUS	A. fickle B. fault-finding C. sneering D. dominating E. resolve	11. ...
12. CASUAL	A. watery B. fated C. fortuitous D. aromatic E. moving	12. ...
13. CHOLERIC	A. dignified B. high-tempered C. gloomy D. unexcitable E. caustic	13. ...
14. CIRCULAR	A. muscular B. oblique C. grouped D. pivotal E. incongruous	14. ...
15. CIRCUMVENT	A. succor B. reserve C. fortify D. surround E. delude	15. ...
16. COMPASSIONATE	A. pitiful B. merciful C. ruthless D. reluctant E. pietistic	16. ...
17. COMPLIANCE	A. violation B. regulation C. attendance D. submission E. conformance	17. ...
18. CONDIGN	A. punishable B. scheming C. undeserved D. merited E. condemn	18. ...
19. CONDONE	A. demand payment B. express sympathy C. forget D. revenge E. forgive	19. ...
20. COPE	A. fail in striving B. contend on equal terms C. plug with soft material D. crown with laurel E. compare with others	20. ...
21. DECOROUS	A. unseemly B. proper C. low cut D. in groups of ten E. deteriorating	21. ...
22. DESPONDENT	A. powdery B. bent C. optional D. artificial E. elated	22. ...
23. DESULTORY	A. pompous B. methodical C. rambling D. oppressively hot E. cursory	23. ...

24. DETONATE — A. explode B. deafen C. muffle D. fizzle out E. destroy — 24. ...

25. DISCIPLE — A. impostor B. follower C. antagonist D. paragon E. colleague — 25. ...

TEST 2

1. DISCREET — A. cautious B. chary C. prudent D. distinct E. temerarious — 1. ...

2. DISINTER — A. dig up from a grave B. lack interest C. interrupt D. inject between muscles E. entomb — 2. ...

3. DOGGEREL — A. trivial verse B. small canine species C. stubborn behavior D. sophisticated poetry E. manger — 3. ...

4. DOLE OUT — A. squander B. distribute piecemeal C. control D. deny alms E. hoard — 4. ...

5. DOMINEERING — A. dictatorial B. pliant C. considerate D. unsympathetic E. recreant — 5. ...

6. ELEGY — A. inheritance B. burnt offering C. violin obbligato D. dirge E. paean — 6. ...

7. ELICIT — A. concoct with alcohol B. draw out C. compel approval D. request sharply E. ignite — 7. ...

8. EMOLLIENT — A. salve B. monument C. tariff charge E. extra tip E. abrasive — 8. ...

9. ENCORE — A. intermission B. termination C. heart of the matter D. repetition E. variation — 9. ...

10. ENERVATE — A. stumble B. devitalize C. stimulate D. rejoice E. impede — 10. ...

11. EXPIATION — A. reprobation B. clarification C. failure D. atonement E. interpretation — 11. ...

12. FABULOUS — A. wealthy B. impressionistic C. realistic D. legendary E. fictional — 12. ...

13. FAIRWAY — A. airplane landing field B. golf greensward C. captain's private quarters D. entrance to ferry slip E. coppice — 13. ...

14. FEASIBLE — A. garish B. festive C. theoretical D. practicable E. pertinent — 14. ...

15. FIERY — A. vehement B. irritable C. restive D. gay E. indifferent — 15. ...

16. FLORID — A. flowing B. livid C. blotchy D. ruddy E. over-heated — 16. ...

17. FLOUT — A. move B. mock C. obey D. defy E. flog — 17. ...

18. FOREGO — A. prosecute B. align C. renounce D. look forward E. over-heated — 18. ...

19. FURTIVE — A. fleeing B. hairy C. glancing D. stealthy E. ingenuous — 19. ...

20. GARBLE — A. substantiate B. garnish C. mutilate D. unravel E. embroider — 20. ...

21. GARRULOUS — A. talkative B. quarrelsome C. snarling D. laconic E. ungainly — 21. ...

22. GOSSAMER — A. sleezy B. dusty C. gauzy D. unbreakable E. zephyr-like — 22. ...

23. GOURMAND — A. greedy eater B. epicure C. hungry person D. ascetic E. fried pumpkin shell — 23. ...

24. GRIEVOUS — A. rutty B. gratifying C. sorrowful D. vicious E. unmentionable — 24. ...

25. GRIMACE	A. happy smile B. fruit sherbet C. twisting of the countenance D. fine quality silk E. sneer	25. ...

TEST 3

1. HEINOUS	A. criminal B. elevated C. inhuman D. flagrant E. moderate	1. ...
2. HUE	A. tint B. shade C. tone D. tinge E. etiolation	2. ...
3. IMMUNITY	A. protection against accident B. exemption C. freedom from disease D. dispensation E. tendency	3. ...
4. IMPLICIT	A. directly stated B. understood though not expressed C. omitted entirely by chance D. stated but not for publication E. inherent	4. ...
5. IMPUTE	A. insult B. contradict C. ascribe D. question E. refer	5. ...
6. INCIPIENT	A. tasteless B. criminal C. beginning D. diseased E. terminal	6. ...
7. INGENUOUS	A. guileful B. naive C. frank D. uncertain E. jealous	7. ...
8. INIQUITOUS	A. awesome B. unequal C. wicked D. present everywhere E. exemplary	8. ...
9. INTERMITTENT	A. continuing without break B. occurring at intervals C. persistently noisy D. gradually subdued E. intermediate	9. ...
10. INTRANSIGENT	A. utterly fearless B. irreconcilable C. invalid D. not transferable E. tractable	10. ...
11. INTREPID	A. fearful B. uneasy C. dauntless D. stumbling E. insistent	11. ...
12. INURE	A. maim B. entice C. deplete D. toughen E. endure	12. ...
13. INVOKE	A. provoke B. denounce C. slanderous D. address in prayer E. evoke	13. ...
14. NOSTALGIA	A. homesickness B. inertia C. gloominess D. nasal catarrh E. wanderlust	14. ...
15. OCCULT	A. abstract B. manifest C. secret D. oriental E. acute	15. ...
16. ONEROUS	A. unwanted B. impossible C. delicate D. burdensome E. facile	16. ...
17. OPULENT	A. expensive B. oily C. crafty D. profuse E. jejune	17. ...
18. ORDINANCE	A. excess weight B. anarchy C. law D. military supplies E. mound of filth	18. ...
19. ORTHOGRAPHY	A. correct accent B. choice of words C. misspelling D. derivation of words E. clear enunciation	19. ...
20. PAROCHIAL	A. limited in range B. sacred C. stubborn D. objective E. easily manageable	20. ...
21. PEREMPTORY	A. trifling B. compliant C. arbitrary D. binding E. camouflaged	21. ...
22. PERVADE	A. pass along B. escape quietly C. convince at length D. to be diffused throughout E. confine	22. ...
23. PERVERSITY	A. cruelty B. miserliness C. conformity D. adherent E. miserliness	23. ...
24. PHLEGMATIC	A. stolid B. figurative C. aphasic D. sentient E. substantial	24. ...
25. POIGNANT	A. melancholy B. soothing C. doubtful D. keen E. reluctant	25. ...

TEST 4

1. PRODIGIOUS — A. extraordinary B. commonplace C. profound E. prehistoric E. infinitesimal — 1. ..
2. PUERILE — A. childish B. mature C. feverish D. immaculate E. pusillanimous — 2. ..
3. PUNCTILIOUS — A. offensively frank B. willing to admit blame C. sarcastically polite D. precise in conduct E. indiscriminate — 3. ..
4. RAZE — A. torture B. erect C. salvage D. destroy E. prorogue — 4. ..
5. RECESSIVE — A. inclined to go back B. relating to slavery C. moving forward D. modest E. allemorphic — 5. ..
6. RENEGADE — A. turncoat B. loyalist C. habitual drunkard D. confirmed criminal E. one who kills a king — 6. ..
7. RENASCENCE — A. unwinding B. restoration C. unscrewing D. detraining E. perdition — 7. ..
8. RESPITE — A. pardon B. re-trial C. stay D. vengeance E. continuation — 8. ..
9. SALIENT — A. hidden B. salty C. floating D. prominent E. flagrant — 9. ..
10. SATELLITE — A. falling star B. attentive follower C. adversary D. flint spark E. fellow captive — 10. ..
11. SCRUPULOUS — A. niggardly B. abusive C. conscientious D. unprincipled E. guilty — 11. ..
12. SINEWY — A. callused B. enervated C. springy D. slimy E. brawny — 12. ..
13. SKEPTIC — A. agnostic B. suave C. ingenious D. credulous E. faithful — 13. ..
14. SPARE — A. forbear B. forego C. reserve D. control E. squander — 14. ..
15. SPORADIC — A. isolated B. incessant C. dissipated D. involuntary E. discrete — 15. ..

KEYS (CORRECT ANSWERS)

TEST 1

1.	D	11.	E
2.	E	12.	B
3.	E	13.	D
4.	C	14.	B
5.	D	15.	A
6.	C	16.	C
7.	B	17.	A
8.	E	18.	C
9.	E	19.	D
10.	E	20.	A
		21.	A
		22.	E
		23.	B
		24.	C
		25.	C

TEST 2

1.	E	11.	A
2.	E	12.	C
3.	D	13.	E
4.	A	14.	C
5.	B	15.	E
6.	E	16.	B
7.	D	17.	C
8.	E	18.	A
9.	B	19.	E
10.	C	20.	A
		21.	D
		22.	D
		23.	D
		24.	B
		25.	A

TEST 3

1.	B	11.	A
2.	E	12.	C
3.	E	13.	B
4.	A	14.	E
5.	B	15.	B
6.	E	16.	E
7.	A	17.	E
8.	E	18.	B
9.	A	19.	C
10.	E	20.	D
		21.	B
		22.	E
		23.	C
		24.	D
		25.	B

TEST 4

1.	E
2.	B
3.	E
4.	B
5.	C
6.	B
7.	E
8.	E
9.	A
10.	C
11.	D
12.	B
13.	D
14.	E
15.	B

EXAMINATION SECTION

TEST 1

DIRECTIONS: Each question or incomplete statement is followed by several suggested answers or completions. Select the one that BEST answers the question or completes the statement. *PRINT THE LETTER OF THE CORRECT ANSWER IN THE SPACE AT THE RIGHT.*

1. Assuming that the series will continue in the same pattern, the NEXT number in the series 3, 5, 11, 29,... is 1.____
   A. 41 B. 47 C. 65 D. 83

2. To check the correctness of a division example, 2.____
   A. multiply the quotient by the divisor and add the remainder
   B. multiply the remainder by the quotient and add the dividend
   C. multiply the dividend by the divisor and add the remainder
   D. multiply the quotient by the dividend and add the remainder

3. If $(4\sqrt{2})^2$ = n, the value of n is 3.____
   A. 8 B. 36 C. 32 D. 16

4. The list price of a radio is $128. If the dealer gets successive discounts of 25% and 10%, the net price to the dealer is 4.____
   A. $83.20 B. $93.00 C. $86.40 D. $96.00

5. A salesman, after deducting his commission of 6%, remits $2491 to his company. The gross amount of the sale amounted to 5.____
   A. $2809 B. $2650 C. $2640 D. $2341.54

6. The factors of $x^{2n}-1$ are 6.____
   A. (x^n+1), (x^n-1)
   B. (x^2+1), (x^n-1)
   C. $(x^{2n}+1)$, $(x-1)$
   D. (x^2-1), (x^n)

7. $16\frac{1}{2} \div \frac{1}{4}$ may be CORRECTLY expressed as 7.____
   A. $(\frac{1}{4} \times 16) + (\frac{1}{4} \times \frac{1}{2})$
   B. $4\sqrt{16.5}$
   C. $(4 \times 16) + (4 \times \frac{1}{2})$
   D. $\frac{1}{4}$ times 33/2

8. An automobile traveled 7 hours at an average speed of 50 miles per hour. It averaged only 40 miles per hour on the return trip. The average speed per hour, to the NEAREST mile, for the round trip was 8.____
   A. 46 miles per hour
   B. 44 miles per hour
   C. 43 miles per hour
   D. 47 miles per hour

9. If the edges of a cube are increased by 2 inches, 9.___
   A. the volume is increased by 8 cubic inches
   B. the area of each face is increased by 4 square inches
   C. the diagonal of each face is increased by 2 inches
   D. the sum of the edges is increased by 24 inches

10. Each of the following numbers in the base three system is equivalent to an odd number in the base ten system EXCEPT 10.___
   A. 12 three
   B. 21 three
   C. 101 three
   D. 111 three

11. In a number system using the base 10, the value represented by the digit 3 in the number 5,386 is 11.___
   A. $3(10)^2$ B. $3(10)$ C. $3(10)^3$ D. $(10)^2$

12. John can do a job in 6 days. Harry can do the same job in 8 days. It takes Tom 12 days to do the job. If all three work together, how long will it take them to finish the job? 12.___
   A. 6 days B. $1\frac{3}{4}$ days C. $2\frac{2}{3}$ days D. 4 days

13. If the same number is added to both the numerator and denominator of a proper fraction, the 13.___
   A. value of the fraction is decreased
   B. value of the fraction is increased
   C. value of the fraction is unchanged
   D. effect of the operation depends on the original fraction

14. The equation $6 \times (7+2) = 6 \times 7 + 6 \times 2$ illustrates the 14.___
   A. Distributive Law of multiplication with respect to addition
   B. Associative Law for addition
   C. Commutative Law for multiplication
   D. Associative Law for multiplication

15. On a blueprint, $\frac{1}{4}$ inch equals 1 foot. The actual length in feet of a steel bar represented on the blueprint by a line $3\frac{3}{8}$ inches long is 15.___
   A. $3\frac{3}{8}$ ft. B. $6\frac{3}{4}$ ft. C. $12\frac{1}{2}$ ft. D. $13\frac{1}{2}$ ft.

16. The accepted form for expressing 1958 in Roman numerals is 16.___
   A. MDCDLVIII B. CMMLVIII C. MCMLVIII D. MCMLIIX

17. Two prime numbers whose sum is 32 are 17.___
   A. 7, 25 B. 11, 21 C. 13, 19 D. 17, 15

18. The pair of fractions in which the value of the second fraction is one-half the value of the first is 18.___
   A. $\frac{1}{32}$ $\frac{1}{16}$
   B. $\frac{3}{7}$ $\frac{6}{14}$
   C. $\frac{6}{16}$ $\frac{3}{8}$
   D. $\frac{8}{22}$ $\frac{2}{11}$

19. The time, 3 hours, 58 minutes after 10:56 A.M. is 19.___
A. 4:45 P.M. B. 2:54 P.M. C. 4:15 P.M. D. 2:15 P.M.

20. The part of the total quantity represented by a 24 degree sector of a circle is 20.___
A. $6\frac{2}{3}\%$ B. 12% C. $13\frac{1}{3}\%$ D. 24%

KEY (CORRECT ANSWERS)

1. D
2. A
3. C
4. C
5. B

6. A
7. C
8. B
9. D
10. C

11. A
12. C
13. B
14. A
15. D

16. C
17. C
18. D
19. B
20. A

SOLUTIONS TO PROBLEMS

1. The plan of the series is to multiply the difference between the two preceding numbers by 3 and then add the product to the immediately preceding number. Thus, the difference between 11 and 29 is 18; 18 multiplied by 3 is 54; 54 added to 29 equals 83. (Ans. D)

2. By inspection. Thus, $7 \div 3 = 2\frac{1}{3}$ or 2R1. The number 7 is the DIVIDEND, 3 is the DIVISOR, and 2R1 is the QUOTIENT, of which 1 is the REMAINDER. (Ans. A)

3. $4\sqrt{2} \times 4\sqrt{2} = 16 \times 2 = 32$ (Ans. C)

4. \$128 × .25 = \$32
   \$128 − \$32 = \$96
   \$96 × .10 = \$9.60
   \$96 − \$9.60 = \$86.40

   (Ans. C)

   Work:
   $$\begin{array}{r} 128 \\ \times .25 \\ \hline 640 \\ 256 \\ \hline 32.00 \end{array}$$

5. \$2491 ÷ .94 = \$2650 (Gross Amount)

   (Ans. B)

   Work:
   $$\begin{array}{r} 2650 \\ .94\overline{)249100.} \\ 188 \\ \hline 611 \\ 564 \\ \hline 470 \\ 470 \\ \hline 0000 \end{array}$$

6. By inspection. (Ans. A)

7. $16\frac{1}{2} \div \frac{1}{4} = \frac{16\frac{1}{2}}{1} \div \frac{1}{4} = \frac{\frac{16\frac{1}{2}}{1}}{\frac{1}{4}} = \frac{16\frac{1}{2}}{1} \times \frac{4}{1} = (4 \times 16) + (4 \times \frac{1}{2})$

   (Ans. C)

8. Total distance for the round trip was 700 miles. (7 hours × 50 mph = 350 miles, going; return trip also = 350. 350 + 350 = 700.
   Time for return trip − 350 miles ÷ 40 mph = $8\frac{3}{4}$ hours.

   Total time for the trip was $15\frac{3}{4}$ hours. (7 hours + $8\frac{3}{4}$ hours = $15\frac{3}{4}$ hours).

   Therefore, 700 miles ÷ $15\frac{3}{4}$ hours = 44^{+} mph, average speed for the round trip.

   Work
   $700 \div 15\frac{3}{4} = 700 \div 63/4$

   $700 \times 4/63 = 2800/63 = 44^{+}$

   $$\begin{array}{r} 44 \\ 63\overline{)2800} \\ 252 \\ \hline 280 \\ 252 \\ \hline 28 \end{array}$$

   (Ans. B)

9. By inspection. A cube is a regular body with six square faces or twelve edges. (Ans. D)

10.

	Base Ten	
A.	$1 \times 10 + 2$	ODD NUMBER
B.	$2 \times 10 + 1$	ODD NUMBER
C.	$1 \times 10^2 + 0 + 1$	EVEN NUMBER
D.	$1 \times 10^2 + 1 \times 10 + 1$	ODD NUMBER

(Ans. C)

11. The digit 3, in this number system, represents the value 300 or $3(10)^2$. (Ans. A)

12. John can do 1/6 of the job in one day.
Harry can do 1/8 of the job in one day.
Tom can do 1/12 of the job in one day.

Then, $\frac{1}{6} + \frac{1}{8} + \frac{1}{12} = \frac{4}{24} + \frac{3}{24} + \frac{2}{24} = \frac{9}{24}$ (of the job in one day if all three work together).

$\frac{24}{9} = 2\frac{6}{9} = 2\frac{2}{3}$ days. (Ans. C)

13. Let us assume that the proper fraction is ½. Then, adding the number 2 to both the numerator and the denominator, we have:

$$\frac{1+2}{2+2} = \frac{3}{4}$$

(Ans. B)

14. The Distributive Law of Multiplication states:
If the sum or difference of two or more numbers is multiplied by a third number, the product may be found by multiplying each of the numbers separately by the multiplier and connecting the results by the proper signs.
<u>EXAMPLE</u>: By arithmetic, $4(3+2) = 4\times3+4\times2$
By algebra, $a(b+c) = ab+ac$

(Ans. A)

15. $3\frac{3}{8} \div \frac{1}{4} = \frac{27}{8} \div \frac{1}{4} = \frac{27}{\cancel{8}_2} \times \frac{\cancel{4}^1}{1} = 13\frac{1}{2}$ (Ans. D)

16. By inspection. (Ans. C)

17. By inspection. A prime number is a number that has no factors except itself and 1. (Ans. C)

18. 8/22 = 4/11; 2/11 is one-half the value. (Ans. D)

19. 10:56 A.M. + 3 hrs, 58 min. = 13 hrs. + 114 min. = 14 hrs. + 54 min. = 2:54 P.M. (Ans. B)

20. $24'' \div 360'' = 6\frac{2}{3}\%$

(Ans. A)

Work:

```
       .066
360)24.00
    21 60
     2 400
     2 160
       240
```

TEST 2

DIRECTIONS: Each question or incomplete statement is followed by several suggested answers or completions. Select the one that BEST answers the question or completes the statement. *PRINT THE LETTER OF THE CORRECT ANSWER IN THE SPACE AT THE RIGHT.*

1. If -13 is subtracted from 1, the result is 1.___
   A. 14 B. 12 C. -12 D. -14

2. 2.___

$$\begin{array}{r} 32 \\ 45 \\ \underline{12} \\ 89 \end{array}$$

   When we add the tens column in the above example as 3+4+1 equals 8, we are applying
   A. the law of commutation B. the law of association
   C. the law of distribution D. the law of likeness

3. A man drove 240 miles south at the rate of 60 miles per hour. On the return trip, he drove at the rate of 40 miles per hour. The average rate per hour for the round trip was 3.___
   A. 55 B. 50 C. 48 D. 45

4. A teacher made the following drawing on the chalkboard 4.___

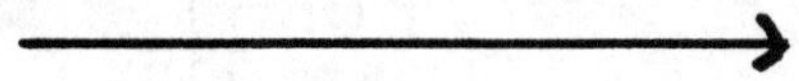

   She properly identified this as a
   A. line B. ray
   C. line segment D. vertex

5. One secretary can address a set of envelopes in 20 minutes. Her partner takes 30 minutes to do the same job. If they both work on the job at their usual rates, the work will be completed in 5.___
   A. 25 minutes B. 15 minutes
   C. 12 minutes D. 10 minutes

6. Of the following progressions, the one that is geometric is 6.___
   A. 1,4,9,16 B. 3,6,12,24
   C. 1,5,9,13 D. 2,4,6,8

7. The area of the figure to the right is 7.___
   A. 12π
   B. $2\pi6$
   C. 144π
   D. 36π

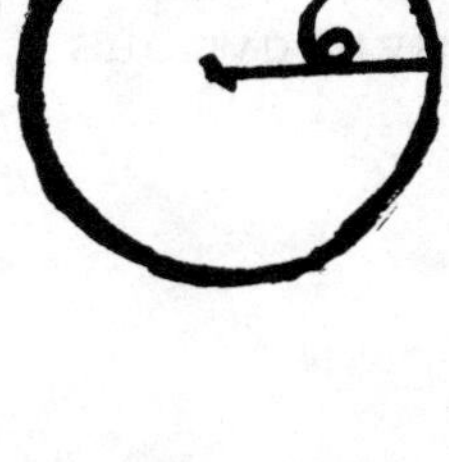

8. The number of prime numbers between 30 and 50 is 8.____
A. 4 B. 5 C. 6 D. 7

9. If it costs a cents for the first 10 words and b cents for each additional word, a formula for finding the cost c of sending a telegram is 9.____
A. c = a+b(n-10) B. c = a+10+bn
C. c = a+b(10-n) D. c = a+10(b-n)

10. A right triangle can also be 10.____
A. isosceles B. obtuse
C. equilateral D. equi-angular

11. At a clearance sale, a table was offered at a discount of 40%. If the price during the sale was $82.50, the original list price was 11.____
A. $115.00 B. $137.50 C. $155.00 D. $206.25

12. The median of the set 39.2, 38.7, 36.4, 39.2, 31.0 is 12.____
A. 38.7 B. 39.2 C. 36.9 D. 36.4

13. A mixture contains 7 ounces of acid and 28 ounces of water. When 7 ounces of water are added, the percentage of acid in the new mixture is 13.____
A. 50% B. 20% C. $16\frac{2}{3}$% D. 25%

14. The CORRECT way to write .0625 as a percent is 14.____
A. $62\frac{1}{2}$% B. .625% C. $.06\frac{1}{4}$% D. $6\frac{1}{4}$%

15. Ten to the zero power (10^0) is 15.____
A. 10 B. 1 C. $\frac{1}{110}$ D. 100

16. If a half-pound package of bacon contains twelve slices, the average weight of a slice of bacon in this package is 16.____
A. $\frac{1}{2}$ ounce B. $\frac{2}{3}$ ounce C. $\frac{3}{4}$ ounce D. 1 ounce

17. The square root of a number is 17.____
A. one of two equal factors of the number
B. the number multiplied by itself
C. the equal factors of the number
D. the number raised to the second power

18. Each of the following statements concerning sets is true EXCEPT: 18.____
A. When sets can be placed in one-to-one correspondence, they have the same number property
B. Addition of whole numbers can be taught by the union of sets
C. If the elements of two sets can be placed in one-to-one correspondence, the sets are equivalent
D. The term "equal sets" and "equivalent sets" are synonymous

19. A snapshot measures $3\frac{1}{2}$ inches by $2\frac{1}{4}$ inches. If this picture is enlarged so that the larger side is $17\frac{1}{2}$ inches long, the length of the shorter side is 19.___

A. $5\frac{3}{4}$" B. $4\frac{3}{8}$" C. $11\frac{1}{4}$" D. $9\frac{1}{4}$"

20. Fifty equally spaced markers are placed on a level highway so that the distance between the first and tenth markers is 90 meters. 20.___
How many meters are in the distance between the first and the last marker?
A. 441 B. 450 C. 490 D. 500

KEY (CORRECT ANSWERS)

1.	A	6.	B	11.	B	16.	B
2.	C	7.	D	12.	A	17.	A
3.	C	8.	B	13.	C	18.	D
4.	B	9.	A	14.	D	19.	C
5.	C	10.	A	15.	B	20.	C

SOLUTIONS TO PROBLEMS

1. 1 - (-13) = 1 + 13 = 14 (Ans. A)

2. The distributive property of multiplication with respect to addition is stated thus:

   For every number a, every number b, and every number c,
   a(b+c) = ab + ac or ab + ac = a(b+c)
   In the tens column, 3 = 30 = 3 (10)
   4 = 40 = 4 (10)
   1 = 10 = 1 (10)
   Thus, when we add the tens column as 3+4+1 equals 8, we are applying the law of distribution. (Ans. C)

3. Going: 240 (miles) ÷ 60 (m.p.h.) = 4 hours
   Returning: 240 (miles) ÷ 40 (m.p.h.) = 6 hours
   Total time: 4 hours + 6 hours = 10 hours
   Average time for round trip: 480 (miles) ÷ 10 (hours) = 48 m.p.h.
   (Ans. C)

4. By inspection. A ray is determined by its end point, together with any one of its other points. An angle is the set of points on two rays (its sides) with a common point (its vertex). (Ans. B)

5. One secretary does the job in 20 minutes or 1/20 in one minute. Her partner does the job in 30 minutes or 1/30 in one minute. Then, 1/20 + 1/30 = 50/600 = 1/12 of the job in one minute, working together. Therefore, it will take them 12 minutes to complete the work. (Ans. C)

6. 3, 6, 12, 24

   3 × 2 = 6
   6 × 2 = 12
   12 × 2 = 24

   The progression is geometric. (Ans. B)

7. Area of a circle = πr^2 or $\frac{1}{4}\pi D^2$.
   Therefore, $\pi \times 6 \times 6 = 36\pi$
   (Ans. D)

8. A prime number is a number that has no factors except itself and 1. The following series shows all the prime numbers up to 60:

   1, 2, 3, 5, 7, 11, 13, 17, 19, 23, 29, 31, 37, 41, 43,

   47, 53, 59

   Notice that 2 is the only even prime number. All other even numbers are divisible by 2. Note that there are five (5) prime numbers between 30 and 50. (Ans. B)

9. By inspection. (Ans. A)

10. The base angles of an isosceles triangle are equal. If the right triangle has two equal angles (of 45^0 each), the triangle is an isosceles triangle. (Ans. A)

11. Sale price of \$82.50 = 60% of the original list price.

Then, $\frac{\$82.50}{6/10} = \$82.50 \times \frac{10}{6} = \frac{\$825}{6} = \$137.50$

(Ans. B)

12. By inspection.
The median is the middle number in a given sequence of numbers. Thus, the median of the set is 38.7. This can be readily seen by rearranging the numbers in descending order: 39.2, 39.2, 38.7, 36.4, 31.0.
Do NOT confuse "median" with "average."
(Ans. A)

13. 7(acid) + 28(water) + 7(water) = 42 ounces
The percentage of acid is now 7/42 = 1/6 = $16\frac{2}{3}$%. (Ans. C)

14. By inspection. (Ans. D)

15. Any number other than zero raised to the zero power equals 1. (Ans. B)

16. A half-pound = 8 ounces.
Then $\frac{8 \text{ ounces}}{12 \text{ slices}} = \frac{2}{3}$ ounce.
(Ans. B)

17. By inspection. (Ans. A)

18. The addition and subtraction properties of equality imply that sets may have the same solution set and be equivalent sets but they are not equal sets.
(Ans. D)

19. Let x = the length of the shorter side.

$3\frac{1}{2}:2\frac{1}{4} = 17\frac{1}{2}:x$
$3\frac{1}{2} \times x = 2\frac{1}{4} \times 17\frac{1}{2}$
$3\frac{1}{2}x = 9/4 \times 35/2$
$7/2x = 9/4 \times 35/2$
$7/2x = 315/8$
$28x = 315$
$x = 315/28$
$x = 11\frac{1}{4}$

Work:

```
      11.25
28)315.00
   28
    35
    28
     70
     56
     140
     140
```

(Ans. C)

20. There is a distance of 10 meters between each marker. From the first marker to the last represents 49 markers in distance, which equals (49)(10) = 490 meters. (Ans.C)

TEST 3

DIRECTIONS: Each question or incomplete statement is followed by several suggested answers or completions. Select the one that BEST answers the question or completes the statement. *PRINT THE LETTER OF THE CORRECT ANSWER IN THE SPACE AT THE RIGHT.*

1. In the United States Olympic tryouts, trackmen competed in the 100 meter dash. Approximately how many yards did they run? 1.____
   A. 90 B. 100 C. 110 D. 120

2. Mrs. Ward opened a savings account with $500.00 in a bank which paid 4% a year, compounded semi-annually. How much interest did her money earn at the end of 1 year? 2.____
   A. $2.00 B. $20.00 C. $20.20 D. $22.00

3. A boy and his father played 26 games of checkers. For every game the boy lost, he gave his father 5 cents. For every game the boy won, his father gave him 8 cents. When all the games were played, neither had won nor lost anything. The number of games the boy won is 3.____
   A. 12 B. 10 C. 13 D. 16

4. If n is b greater than r, the one of the following that is NOT true is 4.____
   A. n-b = r
   B. n = b+r
   C. n-r = b
   D. n+b = r

5. Of the following, the one that has NO meaning is 5.____
   A. $\frac{4}{0}$ B. 4^0 C. $\frac{0}{4}$ D. .4

6. A can do a piece of work in 6 days. B is 50% more efficient. The number of days it takes B to do the work is 6.____
   A. 9 B. 3 C. 2 D. 4

7. A class of 20 students got an average of 80% on a test. On the same test, another class of 30 students got an average of 70%. The average for all the students in both classes is 7.____
   A. 74% B. 75% C. $76\frac{1}{3}$% D. $73\frac{1}{3}$%

8. The numerator and denominator of a fraction are in the ratio of 3 to 4. If 4 is added to the numerator and subtracted from the denominator, the value of the resulting fraction is $\frac{4}{3}$. The numerator of the original fraction is 8.____
   A. 12 B. 9 C. 3 D. 4

9. If it takes b hours to walk a certain distance at the rate of 3 miles an hour, the number of hours it takes to return the same distance at 4 miles an hour is 9.___

A. $\frac{4}{3}$ B. $\frac{4b}{3}$ C. $\frac{3b}{4}$ D. $\frac{3}{4}$

10. The perimeter of a rectangle is 20 inches and its length is 6 inches. The area of the rectangle in square inches is 10.___

A. 20 B. 24 C. 60 D. 48

11. If a and b are integers, $\frac{a}{b}$ is 11.___

A. always an integer B. never an integer
C. sometimes an integer D. always a proper fraction

12. The population of a town of 8,000 people increased 200% in the last ten years. The population now is 12.___

A. 16,000 B. 32,000 C. 24,000 D. 20,000

13. $2^3 \times 2^{-1} + 2^0$ is equal to 13.___

A. 5 B. 6 C. -16 D. 8

14. If the denominator of a fraction is multiplied by 2, the value of the fraction is 14.___

A. multiplied by 2 B. divided by 2
C. increased by 2 D. decreased by 2

15. The diameter of a circle is equal to the side of a square. The ratio of the area of the circle to the area of the square is 15.___

A. $\frac{\pi}{2}$ B. $\frac{2}{\pi}$ C. $\frac{2}{1}$ D. $\frac{11}{14}$

16. The price of a coat was reduced 10%. To restore it to its original price, we would have to increase the new price by 16.___

A. 10% B. 9% C. $11\frac{1}{9}$% D. 11%

17. Of the following, the one that is NOT equivalent to $\frac{1}{2}$% is 17.___

A. $\frac{1}{200}$ B. .005 C. $.001\frac{1}{2}$ D. .05

18. The ratio of $\frac{1}{3}$ to 100 may be expressed as 18.___

A. $\frac{3}{100}$ B. $\frac{1}{300}$ C. $33\frac{1}{3}$ D. $\frac{100}{3}$

19. What percent of a dollar is 25 cents? 19.___

A. $\frac{1}{4}$ B. 25 C. 0.25 D. 4

20. A bar of chocolate costs 5 cents when purchased in a candy store and 6 cents when purchased at a newsstand. What percent of the candy store price is the newsstand price? 20.___

A. .12% B. 1% C. 12% D. 120%

KEY (CORRECT ANSWERS)

1. C	11. C
2. C	12. C
3. B	13. A
4. D	14. B
5. A	15. D
6. D	16. C
7. A	17. D
8. A	18. B
9. C	19. B
10. B	20. D

SOLUTIONS TO PROBLEMS

1. 1 meter = 1.094 yd. (= 3.281 ft.)
   1 meter = APPROXIMATELY $1\frac{1}{10}$ yd.

   $100 \times 1\frac{1}{10} = 110$ yards. (Ans. C)

2. Interest at end of six months ($\frac{1}{2}$ year):
   $500 × .02 = $10.00
   Total in bank, $510
   Interest at end of second six-month period:
   $510 × .02 = $10.20
   Total interest at end of year:
   $10 + $10.20 = $20.20
   (Ans. C)

3. Let x = number of games the boy won.
   Then, 26-x = number of games his father won.
   Therefore, $.08 \times x = .05(26-x)$
   $.08x = 1.30 - .05x$
   $.13x = 1.30$
   $x = 10$
   (Ans. B)

4. Given: n = b+r. Then, by identity, item B is true, and, by transposition, items A and C are true, but item D is NOT true.
   (Ans. D)

5. The multiplicative property of 0, shown in $0 \times 4 = 4 \times 0 = 0$, states that when one of the factors of a product is 0, the product itself is 0.
   This multiplicative property of 0 affects the use of 0 as a divisor. The fraction $\frac{4}{0}$ has NO value or is indefinite in value. A consequence of the multiplicative property of 0 is that you may not divide by 0.
   (Ans. A)

6. A can do $\frac{1}{6}$ of the work in 1 day. B can do $\frac{1}{4}$ of the work in 1 day. (Since he is 50% more efficient, he does $\frac{1}{6} + \frac{1}{12} = \frac{3}{12} = \frac{1}{4}$ of the work each day.) If B can do $\frac{1}{4}$ of the work each day, it will take him 4 days to do the work.
   (Ans. D)

7. 20 × .80 = 16 (total of scores for first class)
   30 × .70 = 21 (total of scores for second class)
   37 (total score)
   37 ÷ 50 = 74%

   <u>Work</u>:

   $$50\overline{)37.00}\quad .74$$
   $$\underline{35\ 0}$$
   $$2\ 00$$

   (Ans. A)

8. Let 3x = numerator
Let 4x = denominator
Then, $\frac{3x+4}{4x-4} = \frac{4}{3}$

$9x + 12 = 16x - 16$
$7x = 28$
$x = 4$
The numerator, 3x, = 12.
(Ans. A)

9. By inspection.
Rate × time = distance
$3 \times b = 3b$ (distance)
To return the same distance, 3b, divide 3b by 4 or $\frac{3b}{4}$.

(Ans. C)

10. A rectangle is a parallelogram with all of its angles right angles and its opposite sides equal. Since the perimeter (the length of the outer boundary of a two-dimensional figure) is 20 inches and its length is 6 inches, then the width must be 4 inches (6 + 6 + 4 + 4 = 20). Area of a rectangle = bh (base × altitude). Then, 6" × 4" = 24 sq. in. (Ans. B)

11. (1) Let a = b
Let b = 3
Then, $\frac{6}{3} = 2$ (an integer)
(2) Let a = 4
Let b = 8
Then, $\frac{4}{8} = \frac{1}{2}$ (a fraction)
(Ans. C)

12. Increase: 8000 × 2(200%) = 16,000
The population now is: 8,000 + 16,000 = 24,000
(Ans. C)

13. $2^3 = 2 \times 2 \times 2 = 8$

$2^{-1} = \frac{1}{2^1} = \frac{1}{2}$

$2^0 = 1$

Then, $8 \times \frac{1}{2} + 1 = 4 + 1 = 5$
(Note 1: 2^{-1} represents a negative exponent.)
(Note 2: 2^0 represents a number that is its own reciprocal. The only number with this property is 1.)
(Ans. A)

14. Let ½ = the fraction.
Then, $\frac{1}{2 \times 2} = \frac{1}{4}$, which equals ½ the value of the fraction.
(Ans. B)

15. Area of a circle = $\frac{1}{4}\pi d^2$
Area of a square = s^2

π(pi) = $\frac{22}{7}$; $\frac{22}{7} \times \frac{1}{4} = \frac{22}{28} = \frac{11}{14}$.

The ratio of the area of the circle, to the area of the square,

$= \dfrac{\frac{11}{14}d^{2\,1}}{d^2_1(s^2=d^2)} = \dfrac{\frac{11}{14}}{1} = \dfrac{11}{14}$

(Ans. D)

16. If the original price = 100%, then the reduction of 10% left 90%, the new price.
10% of 90% = $\frac{1}{9}$ or 11 $\frac{1}{9}$%.

We would have to increase the new price by 11 $\frac{1}{9}$% to restore it to its original price.
(Ans. C)

17. A. 1/200 = .005 = $\frac{1}{2}$%
B. .005 = 1/200 = $\frac{1}{2}$%
C. .001/2 = .005 = $\frac{1}{2}$%
D. .05 = 5/00 = 5%

(Ans. D)

18. $\frac{1}{3} : 100 = \dfrac{\frac{1}{3}}{100} = \frac{1}{3} \times \frac{1}{100} = \frac{1}{300}$. (Ans. B)

19. 25/100 = $\frac{1}{4}$ or 25%
(Ans. B)

20. $\frac{.06}{.05}$ =

```
         1.20
    05./06.00
        05
        10
        10
        00
```

(Ans. D)

TEST 4

DIRECTIONS: Each question or incomplete statement is followed by several suggested answers or completions. Select the one that BEST answers the question or completes the statement. *PRINT THE LETTER OF THE CORRECT ANSWER IN THE SPACE AT THE RIGHT.*

1. $(-0.2)^4$ is equal to 1.___
   A. -0.16 B. .0016 C. .016 D. 0.16

2. A = {a,b,c,d,e} 2.___
   B = {a,d,e,g}
   AUB is
   A. {d,e} B. {2a,b,c,2d,2e,g}
   C. {a,b,c,d,e,g} D. {b,c,g}

3. Of the following, the one that applies the associative law for multiplication is 3.___
   A. 3(6+2) = 18+6 B. 6(3) + 6(7) = 6(10)
   C. 8 × 4 = 4 × 8 D. $\frac{1}{2}$(8×9) = 4 × 9

4. The positive root of $x^2+5x-36 = 0$ is 4.___
   A. 4 B. 9 C. 12 D. 3

5. The SMALLEST of 3 consecutive numbers is n. The average of these 3 integers is 5.___
   A. $\frac{n+2}{3}$ B. n+1 C. $\frac{3(n+1)}{2}$ D. $\frac{3n}{3}$

6. The star diagram 6.___
   ***   ****
   ***   ****
   may be used to demonstrate the truth of
   A. 3 × 4 = 4 × 3
   B. 2+(3×4) = 2x(3+4)
   C. 2 × (3+4) = (2 × 3) + (2 × 4)
   D. 2 × (3×4) = 2 × 3 × 4

7. Consider the number 52,754. The digit 2, in the decimal system of numeration, does NOT represent 7.___
   A. two thousand B. two hundred tens
   C. twenty hundreds D. twenty thousands

8. The number of pounds of one-dollar-a-pound coffee needed to mix with 80 pounds of 70¢ a pound coffee to make a mixture worth 84¢ a pound is 8.___
   A. 70 B. 80 C. 95 D. 65

9. The star diagram *** | **** | ***** may be used to demonstrate 9.___
   A. 3 × 4 = 4 × 3
   B. 3 × 4 × 5
   C. 3 × (4+5) = 3 × 4 + 3 × 5
   D. (3+4) + 5 = 3 + (4+5)

10. $8 \times 3\frac{1}{2} = 8 \times (3+\frac{1}{2}) = (8 \times 3) + (8 \times \frac{1}{2}) = 24 + 4 = 28$ 10.____
The above is an example of
A. associative property
B. commutative property
C. the property of one
D. distributive property of multiplication with respect to addition

11. A man is paid at the rate of 6 dollars an hour for a 40-hour week, and time and a half for overtime. One week he earned $294.00. The number of hours he worked overtime was 11.____
A. $3\frac{3}{4}$ B. 6 C. $7\frac{1}{2}$ D. 9

12. Two planes start at 11 A.M. from two airports 1800 miles apart, and fly toward each other at average rates of 200 and 250 miles per hour. The time at which they pass each other will be 12.____
A. 4:30 P.M. B. 2:30 P.M.
C. 2 P.M. D. 3 P.M.

13. If Y is 2,851, 1% of Y is 13.____
A. 28.51 B. 285.1 C. 2.851 D. .2851

14. A statement TRUE of all prime numbers is that they 14.____
A. have no divisors B. are not even
C. are not odd D. are not composite

15. Mr. Jones got a loan for a sum of money, and at the time of repayment he owed $75.00 in interest. Mr. Brown borrowed three times the amount of money Mr. Jones had borrowed at the same rate of interest for twice as long a time. How much interest does Mr. Brown pay? 15.____
A. $150.00 B. $225.00 C. $300.00 D. $450.00

16. The perimeter of a rectangle whose length is a and whose width is b is 102 inches. The diagonal is 39 inches. Of the following, the equations which should be used to find the dimensions of the rectangle are 16.____
A. $a+b = 51,\ a^2+b^2 = 39$
B. $a+b = 51,\ a^2+b^2 = (39)^2$
C. $a+b = 102,\ a^2+b^2 = 39$
D. $2(a+b) = 102,\ a+b = (39)^2$

17. The factors have been listed for the following numbers. One set of factors is incomplete. It is 17.____
A. factors for 42: 1,2,3,6,7,14,21,42
B. factors for 18: 1,2,3,6,9,18
C. factors for 12: 1,2,3,4,12
D. factors for 105: 1,3,5,7,15,21,35,105

18. A number of coats were placed on sale at $72.00 each. This was 80% of the original price. The original price was 18.____
A. $80.00 B. $90.00 C. $78.00 D. $85.00

19. The CORRECT solution for 2.59 × .015 is 19.___
A. 3.885 B. 38.85 C. .03885 D. .3885

20. One of the equations demonstrates both the commutative and the associative properties for addition: 20.___
A. (4+3) + 2 = 4 + (3+2) B. 18 + 57 = 57 + 18
C. (5+6) + 7 = 6 + (5+7) D. 3 + 4 + 5 = (3+4) + 5

KEY (CORRECT ANSWERS)

1. B	11. B
2. C	12. D
3. D	13. A
4. A	14. D
5. B	15. D
6. C	16. B
7. D	17. C
8. A	18. B
9. D	19. C
10. D	20. C

SOLUTIONS TO PROBLEMS

1. (1) $-0.2 \times -0.2 = .04$
   (2) $.04 \times -.02 = -.008$
   (3) $-.008 \times -0.2 = .0016$

   (Ans. B)

2. This question concerns the arithmetic of sets or union. The union of two sets consists of all of the elements of both sets, but no element is listed more than once.
   In the given example, the union of the sets A = {a,b,c,d,e} and B = {a,d,e,g} may be called set C.
   Then, A U B = C
   {a,b,c,d,e} U {a,d,e,g} = {a,b,c,d,e,g}

   (U is read "cup.")

   (Ans. C)

3. The associative property of multiplication states: For every number a, every number b, and every number c, a(bc) = (ab)c.
   Item D, $\frac{1}{2}(8 \times 9) = 4 \times 9$, illustrates this law.
   (Ans. D)

4. The equation is of degree two and called a quadratic equation. To obtain its roots, factor the left member and find the numbers for which at least one of these factors is zero.
   $x^2 + 5x - 36 = 0$
   (1) Factor the left member. $(x+9)(x-4) = 0$
   (2) Set each factor equal to zero. $x+9 = 0$ | $x-4 = 0$
   (3) Solving the resulting linear equations. $x = -9$ | $x = 4$

   (4) Put the equation into standard form. $x^2 + 5x = 36$
   (5) Check each apparent root in this equation.

$(-9)^2 + 5(-9) = 36$	$(4)^2 + 5(4) = 36$
$81 - 45 = 36$	$16 + 20 = 36$
$36 = 36$	$36 = 36$

   The positive root is 4.
   (Ans. A)

5. If the smallest of the 3 consecutive numbers is n, then the next number is n+1, and the third number is n+2.

   Graphic sequence:
   $$\begin{array}{r} n \\ n+1 \\ \underline{n+2} \\ \text{Adding} \quad 3n+3 \end{array}$$
   Dividing by 3 (the number of numbers) $\frac{3n+3}{3} = n+1$

   (Ans. B)

6. By inspection.
The star diagram demonstrates the commutative property of multiplication, which states that for every number a, and every number b, ab = ba.
(Ans. C)

7. By inspection.
It represents each of items A, B, and C, but not D.
(Ans. D)

8. Let x = total number of pounds of coffee in the mixture.
Then, x-80 = number of pounds of one-dollar-a-pound coffee needed.
Therefore, $1(x-80) + .70(80) = .84(x)$

$$x - 80 + 56 = .84x$$

$$x - 24 = .84x$$

(Transposing) $.16x = 24$

$$x = \frac{24}{.16}$$

$$x = 150$$

150 - 80 = 70 (number of pounds of one-dollar-a-pound coffee needed)
(Ans. A)

9. By inspection.
The star diagram demonstrates the associative property of addition, which states that for every number a, every number b, and every number c, a + (b+c) = (a+b) + c
(Ans. D)

10. The distributive property of multiplication with respect to addition may be stated as follows:
For every number a, every number b, and every number c, a(b+c) = ab + ac OR ab + ac = a(b+c)
(Ans. D)

11. $6 × 40 = $240 for a forty-hour week
$294 - $240 = $54 overtime
$6 × 1½ = $9 an hour overtime pay
Then, $54 ÷ $9 = 6 hours (worked overtime)
(Ans. B)

12. Plane A flies at average rate of 200 miles per hour.
Plane B flies at average rate of 250 miles per hour.
In 4 hours, Plane A will have flown 800 miles and passed the 1000-mile mark.
In 4 hours, Plane B will have flown 1000 miles and passed the 1000-mile mark.
The time at which they will pass each other will be, therefore, 3 P.M.
(Ans. D)

13. 1% = .01
    2,851 × .01 = 28.51
    (Ans. A)

14. A prime number is an integer greater than one, having no positive integral factor other than itself and one.
    (Ans. D)

15. "Mr. Brown borrowed three times the amount of money Mr. Jones had borrowed at the same rate of interest."
    Therefore, 3 × \$75.00 = \$225.00.
    "For twice as long a time."
    Therefore, 2 × \$225.00 = \$450.00.
    (Ans. D)

16. Since the perimeter is 102, then the two sides, a+b, = 51. The diagonal in a rectangle forms two right triangles. In any right triangle, the square of the length of the hypotenuse equals the sum of the squares of the length of the other two sides. (The hypotenuse of a right triangle is the longest side and is opposite the right angle.)
    Thus, $a^2+b^2 = (39)^2$ is correct.
    (Ans. B)

17. An additional factor for 12 is 6.
    (Ans. C)

18. \$72 = .80 or 8/10 of the original price.
    \$72 = 8/10

    Then, $\$\overset{9}{\cancel{72}} \times \frac{10}{\underset{1}{\cancel{8}}} = \$90$

    (Ans. B)

19. By inspection, it can be seen that the answer must contain five decimal places. Only C fulfills this requirement.

    Work:

$$\begin{array}{r} 2.59 \\ \times .015 \\ \hline 1295 \\ 259 \\ \hline .03885 \end{array}$$

    (Ans. C)

20. In arithmetic, when you add two numbers, you get the same sum no matter what order you use in adding them. This commutative property of addition may be stated thus:
    For every number a, and every number b, a + b = b + a.
    In arithmetic, you are free to choose any adjacent pair in addition, for the answer is the same. This associative property of addition may be stated thus:
    For every number a, every number b, and every number c, a + (b+c) = (a+b) + c.
    (Ans. C)

TEST 5

DIRECTIONS: Each question or incomplete statement is followed by several suggested answers or completions. Select the one that BEST answers the question or completes the statement. *PRINT THE LETTER OF THE CORRECT ANSWER IN THE SPACE AT THE RIGHT.*

1. A customer paid $7.68 for 8 gallons of gasoline and 2 quarts of oil. The next customer paid $7.64 for 9 gallons of the gasoline and 1 quart of the oil. The cost of gasoline per gallon was 1.___
   A. 76¢ B. 72¢ C. 70¢ D. 80¢

2. In solving equations involving multiplication, the pupils will discover the MOST important property is 2.___
   A. the commutative property
   B. the associative property
   C. the distributive property
   D. closure

3. A dealer sells radios for $38 and $75. If he sells 10 more of the $38 sets than the $75 sets and takes in $832, the number of $38 sets that he sells is 3.___
   A. 16 B. 20 C. 15 D. 14

4. A high school has n classes, of which b classes are mathematics classes. The ratio of mathematics classes to non-mathematics classes is 4.___
   A. $\frac{b}{n-b}$ B. $\frac{b}{b-n}$ C. $\frac{n-b}{n}$ D. $\frac{b}{n}$

5. In the addition of counting numbers, zero is 5.___
   A. the identity element B. the additive inverse
   C. a binary operation D. the reciprocal

6. A motorist left his home at 8 A.M., traveling at the rate of 32 miles per hour. At 10 A.M., a neighbor followed, traveling at the rate of 48 miles per hour. The time at which the neighbor overtook the motorist was 6.___
   A. 12 M B. 2 P.M. C. 3:30 P.M. D. 4 P.M.

7. If $\underline{a}$ represents Mary's age, and $\underline{b}$ represents John's age, the sum of their ages three years ago is expressed as 7.___
   A. (a+b) - 3 B. (a+3) - (b+3)
   C. (a-3) + (b-3) D. (a-b) 3

8. A cake is divided equally among 3 boys and 2 girls. The girls' share compared with that of the boys' share is 8.___
   A. $\frac{1}{3}$ B. $\frac{2}{5}$ C. $\frac{2}{3}$ D. $\frac{3}{2}$

9. A \$30,000 house is assessed at 75% of its value. The tax rate is \$4.36 per \$1000 of assessed valuation. The amount of the tax on the house is 9.____
   A. \$98.10 B. \$123.60 C. \$150.40 D. \$172.80

10. A radio was sold for \$50.20, which represented a price arrived at after a discount of 20% on the list price. This discount accounted for a saving to the buyer of 10.____
   A. \$10.04 B. \$12.55 C. \$16.75 D. \$22.75

11. Each of the following is equal to one million EXCEPT 11.____
   A. $100 \times 100 \times 100$ B. 1000^2
   C. $100^2 \times 10^3$ D. 10^6

12. A child who says that 7×6 is 42 because 36 and 6 is 42 is applying 12.____
   A. the distributive principle
   B. the associative principle
   C. higher decade addition
   D. the commutative principle

13. Each of the following statements is true concerning "$\frac{3}{4}$" EXCEPT 13.____
   A. 3/4 is a fractional number
   B. 3/4 is a rational number
   C. 3/4 may be represented as a non-repeating decimal
   D. 3/4 belongs to the set of integers

14. The prime factors of 6xy are 14.____
   A. 6, x, y B. 3x, 2y
   C. 2x, 3y D. 3, 2, x, y

15. Successive discounts of 40% and 10% are equivalent to a single discount of 15.____
   A. 44% B. 46% C. 48% D. 50%

16. 3/4 of the members of a committee passed a resolution by a vote of 28 to 14. The percent of the entire committee that voted against the resolution was 16.____
   A. 50 B. $66\frac{2}{3}$ C. 75 D. 25

17. A dealer paid x dollars for a chair and sold it at a profit for y dollars. The ratio of the profit to the selling price was 17.____
   A. $\frac{y-x}{x}$ B. $\frac{y-x}{y}$ C. $\frac{y}{x}$ D. $\frac{x-y}{y}$

18. Blocks in the shape of 2-inch cubes are piled together to form a cube which measures 8 inches on the side. The number of smaller blocks used is 18.____
   A. 16 B. 64 C. 256 D. 512

19. The price of a 1-pound can of coffee increased from 80¢ to 93¢. The percent of increase was 19.____
   A. $8\frac{1}{8}$ B. 14 C. $16\frac{1}{4}$ D. $32\frac{1}{2}$

20. Tom is now twice as old as Alice. The only statement about their ages which is NOT true is: 20.___
   A. In 5 years, Tom will be twice as old as Alice
   B. In 5 years, the sum of their ages will be 10 more than the sum of their present ages
   C. Alice's present age is one-third of the sum of their present ages
   D. Two years ago, the difference between their ages was the same as it will be two years hence

---

KEY (CORRECT ANSWERS)

1. A	11. C
2. C	12. A
3. D	13. D
4. A	14. D
5. A	15. B
6. B	16. D
7. C	17. B
8. C	18. B
9. A	19. C
10. B	20. A

SOLUTIONS TO PROBLEMS

1. Step 1: Let x = cost of 1 gallon of gasoline
   Let y = price of 1 quart of oil

   Step 2: $8x + 2y = \$7.68$
   $9x + y = \$7.64$

   Step 3: $8x + 2y = \$7.68$
   $18x + 2y = \$15.28$ (multiplying by 2)

   $-10x = -\$7.60$ (subtracting)
   $10x = \$7.60$
   $x = .76$ (cost of 1 gallon of gasoline)
   ($y = .80$) (cost of 1 quart of oil)
   (Ans. A)

2. If the sum or difference of two or more numbers is multiplied by a third number, the product may be found by multiplying each of the numbers separately by the multiplier and connecting the results by the proper signs.
   EXAMPLE:
   By arithmetic, $4(3+2-1) = 4 \times 3 + 4 \times 2 - 4 \times 1$
   $4(4) = 12 + 8 - 4 = 16$

   By algebra, $a(b + c + d) = ab + ac + ad$.
   (Ans. C)

3. Let x = number of 75-dollar sets sold.
   Therefore, x + 10 = number of 38-dollar sets sold.
   Then, $75(x) + 38(x+10) = 832$
   $75x + 38x + 380 = 832$
   $113x = 452$
   $x = 4$
   $x + 10 = 14$ (the number of 38-dollar sets sold)
   (Ans. D)

4. By inspection.
   (Ans. A)

5. For example, in the addition of

   $$\begin{array}{r} 4 \\ 40 \\ \underline{400} \end{array},$$

   the 0 in 40 helps us to show the place value of the 4. Similarly, the value of the 4 is shown in the number 400.
   (Ans. A)

6. By 10 A.M., when the neighbor began to follow, the motorist who had left home at 8 A.M. would have traveled 64 miles (32 mph × 2 hrs.). Then, hour by hour, the two would have traveled the following distances:

11 A.M.	Motorist:	96 miles (32 mph × 3 hrs)
	Neighbor:	48 miles (48 mph × 1 hr)
12 A.M.	Motorist:	128 miles (32 mph × 4 hrs)
	Neighbor:	96 miles (48 mph × 2 hrs)
1 P.M.	Motorist:	160 miles (32 mph × 5 hrs)
	Neighbor:	144 miles (48 mph × 3 hrs)
2 P.M.	Motorist:	192 miles (32 mph × 6 hrs)
	Neighbor:	192 miles (48 mph × 4 hrs)

   (Ans. B)

7. By inspection.
(Ans. C)

8. By inspection.
$2/5 : 3/5 = 2 : 3 = 2/3$
(Ans. C)

9. \$30,000 × .75 = \$22,500 (assessed valuation)
\$22,500 ÷ \$1000 = \$22.50 (number of \$1000's of assessed valuation)
Then, \$22.50 × 4.36 = \$98.10
Work:

```
  $22.50
 × 4.36
  13500
  6750
 9000
98.1000
```

(Ans. A)

10. Let x = the list price.
Then, $x \times .20 = x - 50.20$
$.20x = x - 50.20$
(transposing) $-.80x = -50.20$
$-x = \frac{50.20}{.80}$
$x = \$62.75$
\$62.75 - \$50.20 = \$12.55 (saving to the buyer)
(Ans. B)

WORK

```
        62.75
.80)50.20.00
    48 0
     2 20
     1 60
       60 0
       56 0
        4 00
        4 00
```

11. Item A: 100 × 100 × 100 = 1,000,000
Item B: 1000^2 = 1000 × 1000 = 1,000,000
Item C: 100^2 = 100 × 100 = 10,000
10^3 = 10 × 10 × 10 = 1,000
∴ 10,000 × 1000 = 10,000,000
Item D: 10^6 = 10 × 10 × 10 × 10 × 10 × 10 = 1,000,000
(Ans. C)

12. 7 × 6 = 6 × 6 + 6.
(See also answer to question 2.)
(Ans. A)

13. An integer is one of the numbers 0, 1, 2, 3, 4, etc.; a whole number as distinguished from a fraction or a mixed number. (Ans. D)

14. By inspection.
A number that has no factors except itself and 1 is a prime number. If a factor of a number is prime, it is called a prime factor. (Ans. D)

15. Let \$100 be the original price.
Then, \$100 × .40 = \$40 (discount) or \$60 (new price) (\$100 - \$40)
Then, \$60 × .10 = \$6 (discount) or \$54 (new price) (\$60 - \$6)
\$100 × .46 = \$46 (discount) or \$54 (new price) (\$100 - \$46)
(Ans. B)

16. 3/4 of the members = 28 + 14 = 42.
Therefore, total membership = $\frac{42}{\frac{3}{4}} = 42 \times \frac{4}{3} = 56$

14 (against) : 56 (total membership) = 1 : 4
(Ans. D)

17. By inspection.
(Ans. B)

18. 8 in. ÷ 2 in. = 4 cubes
4 × 4 × 4 = 64 (smaller blocks used)
(Ans. B)

19. 93¢ - 80¢ = 13¢

$\frac{.13}{.80} = 16\frac{1}{4}\%$

(Ans. C)

Work:

$$\begin{array}{r} .1625 \\ .80\overline{)\,13.000} \\ 8\,0 \\ \hline 5\,00 \\ 4\,80 \\ \hline 200 \\ 160 \\ \hline 400 \\ 400 \\ \hline \end{array}$$

20. Let 10 = age of Alice
Therefore, 20 = age of Tom.

Item A: Tom = 20 + 5 = 25
Alice = 10 + 5 = 15
FALSE. Tom is NOT twice as old as Alice.

Item B: Tom = 20 + 5 = 25
Alice = 10 + 5 = 15
40
40 - 30 (sum of their present ages) = 10
TRUE.

Item C: Sum of their present ages = 30 (20+10)
Alice's present age, 10, is 1/3 of the sum of their present ages, 30.
TRUE.

Item D: Tom, 2 years ago = 20 - 2 = 18
Alice, 2 years ago = 10 - 2 = 8
18 - 8 = 20 - 10
10 = 10
TRUE.

(Ans. A)

NOTES

NOTES

NOTES

EXAMINATION SECTION

TEST 1

DIRECTIONS: Each question or incomplete statement is followed by several suggested answers or completions. Select the one that BEST answers the question or completes the statement. *PRINT THE LETTER OF THE CORRECT ANSWER IN THE SPACE AT THE RIGHT.*

1. In the number system with base 5, the value of the repeating decimal, .232323...., expressed as a common fraction, is 1.____
   A. $\frac{44}{344}$ B. $\frac{14}{24}$ C. $\frac{23}{44}$ D. none of these

2. The number 122, base 4, is added to the number 212, base 3. Their sum, when expressed in the base 5, is written 2.____
   A. 2,314 B. 334 C. 144 D. 49

3. If 13^{62} is multiplied out, the units digit in the final product is 3.____
   A. 1 B. 3 C. 7 D. 9

4. On a $10,000 order, a merchant has a choice between three successive discounts of 20%, 20%, and 10%, and three successive discounts of 40%, 5%, and 5%. 4.____
   By choosing the better offer, he can save
   A. $330 B. $345 C. $360 D. $400

5. An article was sold for $21.00 more than it cost. 5.____
   If the marked price of this article was 150% of its cost price, and if it was sold at a discount of 30%, then its cost price was
   A. $19.09 B. $70 C. $210 D. $420

6. If the statement $202_b = (13_b) \cdot (13_b)$ is true in a number system whose base is b, and b is a natural number, then b is equal to 6.____
   A. 5 B. 6 C. 7 D. 8

7. A rope 10 yards long is divided into three lengths so that the shortest is equal to the difference in the lengths of the two others. 7.____
   Then the LONGEST piece is what part of the whole rope?
   A. 1/4 B. 1/2 C. 2/3 D. 3/4

8. Assume that a storekeeper reduces his profit on all merchandise in the store from 40% of the cost to 33 1/3% of the cost. 8.____
   If an article originally sold for $14.70, what would its new selling price be?
   A. $9.80 B. $10.78 C. $11.76 D. $14.00

9. The numbers 314 and 1011 are written in two different bases. Each number contains the largest digit available on its base.
The sum of these two numbers, if written in base 3, is 9.____
A. 10112 B. 1211002 C. 20220 D. 1011111

10. An automobile covered the first 60 miles of its journey in 1 hour 30 minutes and the next 87 miles in 2 hours.
The AVERAGE speed, in miles per hour, for the total trip is 10.____
A. 41 3/4 B. 42 C. 58 4/5 D. 73 1/2

11. If the radius of a circle is increased 50%, the area is INCREASED ____%. 11.____
A. 50 B. 125 C. 200 D. 225

12. Assuming the use of α as a symbol for *ten* and β for *eleven*, the number 283_{ten}, when written in the duodecimal system of numeration, is represented by 12.____
A. 1β7 B. 1α7 C. 21β D. 21α

13. A owns a house worth $10,000. He sells it to B at a 10% profit. B sells the house back to A at a 10% loss.
Then, among the following, which is CORRECT? 13.____
A. A comes out even. B. A makes $100.
C. A makes $1,100. D. B loses $1,000.

14. If the length and width of a rectangle are each doubled, the area is increased by 14.____
A. 100% B. 200% C. 300% D. 400%

15. The list price of an article is $500. On this article, one dealer offers successive discounts of 10% and 20%, while another offers a single discount of 30%.
As a result of these offers, what will the difference be in the selling price of the article be? 15.____
A. No difference B. $5
C. $10 D. $15

16. Of a group of pupils, 1/3 walk home, 3/8 of the remaining members go home by bus, and the other 35 use bicycles to go home.
How many pupils are there in the group? 16.____
A. 64 B. 84 C. 120 D. 280

17. A merchant paid $90 for a desk.
At what price should he mark it if he wishes to offer his customers a 10% discount and still make a profit of 20% on the cost? 17.____
A. $108 B. $112 C. $116 D. $120

18. If 16 men require 24 cases of rations for 10 days, then at the same rate of consumption, the number of days that 27 cases of rations will last for 12 men is 18.____
A. 12 B. 15 C. 18 D. 21

19. A man deposits $1,000 in a new account which earns interest at 4% compounded quarterly from the day of deposit.
How much must he deposit in this account three months later in order that the account will contain exactly $2020 six months from the day of the initial deposit?
A. $940 B. $980 C. $990 D. $1,000 19.___

20. The integer 5x327y, where x and y stand for missing digits, is divisible by 9.
Which of the following could the sum of x and y be?
A. 5 B. 9 C. 10 D. 11 20.___

KEY (CORRECT ANSWERS)

1. B
2. C
3. D
4. B
5. D

6. C
7. B
8. D
9. A
10. B

11. B
12. A
13. C
14. C
15. C

16. C
17. D
18. B
19. D
20. C

SOLUTIONS TO PROBLEMS

1. $.232323\ldots_{\text{base }5} = \left(\frac{2}{5} + \frac{3}{25} + \frac{2}{125} + \frac{3}{625} + \frac{2}{3125} + \frac{3}{15625} \ldots\right)_{\text{base }10} =$ .541632, which approaches $\frac{13}{24}$. (Ans. B)

2. $122_{\text{base }4} = 26_{\text{base }10}$. $212_{\text{base }3} = 23_{\text{base }10}$. Sum $= 49_{\text{base }10}$, which is $144_{\text{base }5}$. (Ans. C)

3. $13^1 = 13$, $13^2 = 169$, $13^3 = 2197$, $13^4 = 28561$, $13^5 = 371293$, etc. The last digit is of a cyclic nature and has the pattern 3, 9, 7, 1, 3, 9, 7, 1, 3, 9, 7, 1, etc. for consecutive powers of 13.
Now, 13^{62} would end in the same digit as 13^2 which is 9. (Ans. D)

4. Under the first option, the merchant would pay (\$10000)(.8)(.8)(.1) = \$5760; but under the second option, he would pay (\$10000)(.6)(.95)(.95) = \$5415. This represents a savings of \$345. (Ans. B)

5. Let c = cost. Then, c+21 = selling price and 1.50c = marked price. Since the article was sold at a 30% discount (off the marked price), c + 21 = .70(1.50c). Solving, c = \$420. (Ans. D)

6. $202_7 = (2)(7^2) + 2 = 100$ and $13_7 = 10$. Now, $202_7 = (13_7)(13_7)$.

   (Ans. C)

7. Let x = shortest piece, y = second piece. Then, 10 - x - y = longest piece. Now, x = (10-x-y) - y. Thus, x + y = 5. Then, 10 - x - y must equal 5, and this represents $\frac{1}{2}$ the length of the rope. (Ans. B)

8. Let x = cost. Then, 14.70 = (1.40)(x) and x = 10.50. The new selling price is (10.50)(133 1/3%) = \$14.00. (Ans. D)

9. $314_{\text{base }5} = (3)(25) + (1)(5) + 4 = 84$

   $1011_{\text{base }2} = (1)(8) + (0)(4) + 1(2) + 1 = 11$

   The sum = 95, which is $10112_{\text{base }3}$. (Ans. A)

10. Average speed = total distance/total time = 147/3.5 = 42 mph. (Ans. B)

11. If R = original radius, area = πR^2. If new radius = 1.5R, new area = $\pi(1.5R)^2 = 2.25\pi R^2$. The area increased $1.25\pi R^2$, which represents a 125% increase. (Ans. B)

12. __ __ __ The leftmost placeholder represents $12^2 = 144$. Since 283 ÷ 144 = 1 with remainder of 139, the first dash = 1. The second dash represents 12, and 139 consists of 11 12's with remainder of 7. Thus, the symbol for 11, β, occupies the second dash. 7 must occupy the rightmost dash. The final answer = 1β7. (Ans. A)

13. A sells the house to B for ($10,000)(1.10) = $11,000. Then, B sells the house to A for ($11,000)(.90) = $9,900. A nets $1,100. (Ans. C)

14. Let L = length, w = width, so that area = Lw. The new length and width are 2L and 2w, and so the new area = 4Lw. The increase in area is 3Lw, which represents 300%. (Ans. C)

15. Successive discounts of 10% and 20% would mean that the final price is (.80)(.90)($500) = $360. A single discount of 30% would yield a final price of (.70)($500) = $350. The difference is $10. (Ans. C)

16. Let x = number of students. Then, $x - \frac{1}{3}x - \frac{3}{8}x = 35$. $\frac{7}{24}x = 35$. Solving, x = 120. (Ans. C)

17. Let x = marked price. Sale price = .90x, and this price will be 120% of $90. Thus, .90x = (1.20)(90) = 108. Solving, x = $120. (Ans. D)

18. For 10 days, 12 men would require x rations. $\frac{12}{x} = \frac{16}{24}$.

Then, x = 18. Now, if 18 rations last 10 days, 27 rations will last y days. $\frac{18}{10} = \frac{27}{y}$. Solving, y = 15. (Ans. B)

19. In three months, his account will grow to $\$1000(1.01)^1 = \$1010$. If he deposits x dollars, $(1000+x)(1.01)^1 = 2020$. Solving, x = $1000. (Ans. D)

20. Since the sum of all digits = a multiple of 9, 5+x+3+2+7+y = a multiple of 9. Thus, 17 + x + y = a multiple of 9, and so x+y could be 10. (Ans. C)

TEST 2

DIRECTIONS: Each question or incomplete statement is followed by several suggested answers or completions. Select the one that BEST answers the question or completes the statement. *PRINT THE LETTER OF THE CORRECT ANSWER IN THE SPACE AT THE RIGHT.*

1. Which of the following lengths: (A) 2.990 in., (B) 2.998 in., (C) 3.002 in. may be accepted for a part designed to be 3 inches long if a .003 inch tolerance is permitted? 1.____
   A. A and B *only*
   B. A and C *only*
   C. B and C *only*
   D. A, B, and C

2. The number 478 (base 10), when changed to base 5 notation, becomes 2.____
   A. 3
   B. 2390
   C. 3403
   D. 11102

3. If an article costs $36, the price at which it should be marked to allow a discount of 10% and still make a profit of 20% on the actual selling price is 3.____
   A. $40
   B. $46
   C. $50
   D. $54

4. Of the following pairs, the one which is composed of two equivalents is 4.____
   A. 1/2 = .5%
   B. 1.01 = 110%
   C. .0001/4 = .0025%
   D. .02/3 = .062/3%

5. A man needs $8000 for the purchase of a business. A loan is available at 6% interest, discounted in advance. The amount he must borrow, to the nearest dollar, to net $8000 repayable at the end of six months is 5.____
   A. $8240
   B. $8247
   C. $8480
   D. $8511

6. Of the following, the one which is CLOSEST to the result of the computation of $\frac{(.846)^2 \sqrt[3]{18.7}}{3.42}$ is 6.____
   A. .5555
   B. 5.555
   C. 55.55
   D. 555.5

7. Which one of the following is NOT a perfect number? 7.____
   A. 28
   B. $2^{k-1}(2^{k-1})$ (where k is prime)
   C. 15
   D. 6

8. The product of the highest common factor and the lowest common multiple of 18 and 24 is 8.____
   A. *equal* to the product of 18 and 24
   B. *equal* to the quotient of 24 and 18
   C. *greater* than the product of 18 and 24
   D. *equal* to half the product of 18 and 24

9. Which one of the following is NOT a characteristic of all *groups*? 9.____
   A. Associative law B. Commutative law
   C. Closure D. An inverse element

10. Of the following, the set of numbers arranged in ascending order of values is 10.____
    A. 114_{five}, 122_{three}, 10110_{two}
    B. 122_{three}, 10110_{two}, 114_{five}
    C. 10110_{two}, 122_{three}, 114_{five}
    D. 10111_{two}, 114_{five}, 122_{three}

11. All of the following numbers are congruent to -14 modulo 4, EXCEPT 11.____
    A. -8 B. -6 C. 2 D. 6

12. The product of .00000149 and .0000000006 written in scientific notation is 12.____
    A. 8.94×10^{-16} B. 8.94×10^{-17}
    C. 8.94×10^{-18} D. 8.94×10^{-19}

13. If an airplane is flying with a ground speed of 200 miles per hour, the number of seconds required for it to travel a ground mile is 13.____
    A. 1/18 B. 3 1/3 C. 18 D. 60

14. When 148, a numeral to the base 10, is expressed as a numeral to the base 7, it becomes 14.____
    A. 103 B. 231 C. 301 D. 321

15. When 231 and 332, numerals expressed to the base 4, are expressed to the base 10, the sum of the two then would be 15.____
    A. 107 B. 563
    C. 1225 D. none of these

16. The arithmetic mean of the measures 4.18, 4.23, 4.15, 4.17, 4.09 is CLOSEST to which one of the following? 16.____
    A. 4.15 B. 4.16 C. 4.17 D. 4.18

17. Of the following pairs, the one containing two equivalent values is 17.____
    A. .0375, 3 3/4% B. 2.75, .02 3/4%
    C. .8 1/3%; 1/12 D. .0125%, .01 1/4

18. Assume that a gasoline tank was half full, and the gasoline was used until the tank is only 1/8 full. If the tank is then filled to capacity by putting in 21 gallons, the capacity of the tank, in gallons, is 18.____
    A. 24 B. 42
    C. 56 D. none of these

19. The smallest subdivision on a certain accurately calibrated instrument is .01 inch. Assuming no human errors in use, the possible error of measurement in using the above instrument is 19.___
   A. .001"   B. .005"   C. .010"   D. .050"

20. The number 1011 to the base 2, if expressed to the base 10, would be 20.___
   A. 11   B. 14   C. 22   D. 38

KEY (CORRECT ANSWERS)

1. C	11. A
2. C	12. A
3. C	13. C
4. D	14. C
5. B	15. A
6. A	16. B
7. C	17. A
8. A	18. A
9. B	19. B
10. B	20. A

SOLUTIONS TO PROBLEMS

1. $3 \pm .003 = 2.997$ to 3.003. Only choices B and C are acceptable. (Ans. C)

2. In base 5, the name of the columns are units, 5's, 25's, 125's, etc. reading from right to left. Since $478 \div 125$ gives 3 with remainder 103, the leftmost digit = 3. Then, $103 \div 25$ gives 4 with remainder 3; so the next digit = 4. Now, $3 \div 5$ gives 0 with remainder 3; thus the next digit = 0 and the rightmost digit = 3. The number is 3403. (Ans. C)

3. Let x = marked price. With a discount of 10%, the selling price = $.90x$. To realize a profit of 20% on the selling price, $.90x - 36 = .20(.90x)$. Solving, $x = \$50$. (Ans. C)

4. $\frac{1}{2} = 50\% \neq .5\%$, $1.01 = 101\% \neq 110\%$, $.000\frac{1}{4} = .00025 \neq .0025\%$,

   and $.0\frac{2}{3} = .0\overline{6}\ \frac{2}{3} = .06\frac{2}{3}\%$. (Ans. D)

5. Let x = amount borrowed. Then, $.97x = 8000$, and x is approximately \$8247. (Ans. B)

6. The expression is approximated by $\frac{(.7)(2.6)}{3.4}$, which is about .54. Thus, .5555 is the closest given approximation. (Ans. A)

7. 15 is not a perfect number since the sum of all its factors (except 15) $= 1 + 3 + 5 = 9 \neq 15$. (Ans. C)

8. Highest common factor = 6, and the lowest common multiple is 72. Now, $(72)(6) = 432$, which equals $(18)(24)$. (Ans. A)

9. A group need not be commutative. If it has this property, it is called Abelian. (Ans. B)

10. $122_{three} = 9 + (2)(3) + 2 = 17$, $10110_{two} = 16 + 4 + 2 = 22$,

    and $114_{five} = 25 + 5 + 4 = 34$. (Ans. B)

11. -8 is NOT congruent to -14 modulo 4 since $-8 - (-14)$ is not a multiple of 4. (Ans. A)

12. $(1.49 \times 10^{-6})(6 \times 10^{-10}) = 8.94 \times 10^{-16}$. (Ans. A)

13. 200 mi/hr = 1 mi/$\frac{1}{200}$ hr. $\frac{1}{200}$ hr. $= (\frac{1}{200})(3600) = 18$ seconds.

    (Ans. C)

14. $148_{base\ 10} = 301_{base\ 7}$, since $301_{base\ 7} = (3)(49) + 1$.
(Ans. C)

15. $231_{base\ 4} = 2(16) + 3(4) + 1 = 45_{base\ 10}$
$332_{base\ 4} = 3(16) + 3(4) + 2 = 62_{base\ 10}$
Their sum = 107. (Ans. A)

16. The arithmetic mean of the 5 numbers = $\frac{20.82}{5}$ = 4.164, which rounds off to 4.16. (Ans. B)

17. .0375 is equivalent to 3.75%, which equals 3 3/4%. (Ans. A)

18. 21 gallons represents $\frac{7}{8}$ of the tank's capacity. Thus, the tank's capacity is $(21)(\frac{8}{7}) = 24$ gallons. (Ans. A)

19. The error of measurement = $(\frac{1}{2})(.01) = .005$ inches. (Ans. B)

20. $1011_{base\ 2} = 8 + 2 + 1 = 11_{base\ 10}$. (Ans. A)

TEST 3

DIRECTIONS: Each question or incomplete statement is followed by several suggested answers or completions. Select the one that BEST answers the question or completes the statement. *PRINT THE LETTER OF THE CORRECT ANSWER IN THE SPACE AT THE RIGHT.*

1. If the integers 6 and 3 are interchanged in the number 2635 now expressed to the base seven, the quantity expressed to the base 10 by which the number is reduced is 1.____
   A. 21 B. 30
   C. 147 D. none of these

2. A number of the form $an^4 + bn^2 + cn + d$, where a = 4, b = 2, c = 2, d = 1 and n = 10, is divisible by 2.____
   A. 2 B. 5 C. 7 D. 9

3. Of the following, the set in which all are units which may be used for measuring a one-dimensional object is 3.____
   A. meter, liter, decimeter, kilometer
   B. meter, kilometer, decimeter, millimeter
   C. liter, decimeter, kilometer, millimeter
   D. meter, liter, millimeter, decimeter

4. To arrange the following ruler measurements in order of increasing lengths, the CORRECT arrangement should be 4.____

   $A = \frac{27}{32}$ in., $B = \frac{7}{8}$ in., $C = \frac{51}{64}$ in., $D = \frac{13}{16}$ in.

   A. B, D, A, C B. D, C, A, B
   C. C, D, A, B D. C, A, D, B

5. The ratio of 3'6" to 6" is BEST expressed as 5.____
   A. 1 to 7 B. 3.6" to 6"
   C. 6" to 42" D. 7 to 1

6. A layout of a rectangular foundation for a building is drawn to scale. The 72-foot length of the foundation is represented on the drawing by a line 27 inches long. The length, in inches, of the line needed to represent the 45-foot width of the foundation is 6.____

   A. $16\frac{7}{8}$ B. $17\frac{1}{4}$ C. $17\frac{7}{8}$ D. $18\frac{3}{8}$

7. A circle graph is to be made to show the parts of the total city budget allocated to each department; the total budget is 2 billion, 100 million dollars. If 630 million dollars is allocated for education, the number of degrees on the circle graph which would represent the amount for education is CLOSEST to 7.____
   A. 30 B. 54 C. 84 D. 108

8. The screw which advances the thimble of a micrometer has 40 threads to the inch.
If the thimble is turned exactly 3 threads, the micrometer will be opened by _____ inches. 8.____
A. 0.025 B. 0.075 C. 0.340 D. 0.750

9. A voltmeter scale is divided into ten major divisions, each of which is divided into five minor divisions. Full-scale deflection occurs when 30 volts are across the meter. The number of volts indicated when the needle is on the second minor division beyond the sixth major division is 9.____
A. 6.4 B. 16.4 C. 18.6 D. 19.2

10. The number of rectangular cards 11 inches long and 8 inches wide that can be cut from a sheet 33 inches long and 27 inches wide with a minimum of waste is 10.____
A. 6 B. 9 C. 10 D. 12

11. Of the following four fractions, the one that is CLOSEST in value to $\sqrt{5}$ is 11.____

A. $2\frac{1}{10}$ B. $2\frac{1}{5}$ C. $2\frac{1}{8}$ D. $2\frac{1}{2}$

12. During a transfer of oil from one tank to another, $1\frac{1}{2}$ gallons were lost through leaks in the hose. This represented 0.3 percent of the capacity of the first tank. The capacity of this tank, in gallons, is 12.____
A. 50 B. 200 C. 450 D. 500

13. Using six number punches with digits 1, 2, 3, 4, 5, and 6, the number of differently numbered tags that can be made with three-digit numbers on each tag is 13.____
A. 120 B. 216 C. 278 D. 556

14. A junior high school class studying the metric system came to the following conclusions. Of these, it is INCORRECT to conclude that a(n) 14.____
A. basketball player can be 2 meters tall
B. football player can weigh 100 kilograms
C. track star can run 2 kilometers in 1 minute
D. automobile gasoline tank can hold 80 liters of gasoline

15. The product of 32,000,000 and .000028 is 15.____
A. 8.96×10^{-2} B. 896×10^{-2}
C. 8.96×10^{2} D. 896×10^{2}

16. Which of the following is its own multiplicative inverse? 16.____
I. -1 II. 0 III. +.1 IV. +1

A. I, IV B. II, IV C. III, IV D. IV *only*

17. If 1 inch ≈ 2.5 centimeters, then the number of yards in a kilometer can be found by computing the fraction 17.___

A. $\frac{36\times100{,}000}{2.5}$ B. $\frac{1000}{2.5\times36}$

C. $\frac{100{,}000}{2.5\times36}$ D. $\frac{2.5\times36\times100}{1000}$

18. A man invested \$120,000 in a new business enterprise. The first year, he lost $37\frac{1}{2}$% of the original investment. The next year, he made a profit of 40% of his net worth at the beginning of that year. His net worth at the end of the second year was what percent of his original investment? 18.___

A. $62\frac{1}{2}$ B. 75 C. $87\frac{1}{2}$ D. $97\frac{1}{2}$

19. The arithmetic mean (average) of a set of 50 numbers is 38. If two numbers 45 and 55 are discarded, the mean of the remaining set of numbers is 19.___

A. 36.5 B. 37.0 C. 37.24 D. 37.5

20. Which of the following numbers is 26^9? 20.___

A. 5,011,849,549,824 B. 5,429,503,678,976
C. 5,847,157,808,128 D. 5,638,330,743,552

KEY (CORRECT ANSWERS)

1. D	11. B
2. D	12. D
3. B	13. B
4. C	14. C
5. D	15. C
6. A	16. A
7. D	17. C
8. B	18. C
9. D	19. D
10. B	20. B

SOLUTIONS TO PROBLEMS

1. $2635_{\text{base }7} = (2)(343) + (6)(49) + (3)(7) + 5 = 1006_{\text{base }10}$ and

   $2365_{\text{base }7} = (2)(343) + (3)(49) + (6)(7) + 5 = 880_{\text{base }10}$.

   The amount reduction is 126. (Ans. D)

2. The number's value is $4 \times 10^4 + 2 \times 10^2 + 2 \times 10 + 1 = 40{,}221$. Since the sum of the digits of this number is divisible by 9, then so must the number be divisible by 9. (Ans. D)

3. All four of the units meter, kilometer, decimeter, and millimeter are linear measurements. Thus, they can be used to measure one-dimensional objects. (Ans. B)

4. Convert all fractions to like demonimators: $A = \frac{54}{64}$ in., $B = \frac{56}{64}$ in., $C = \frac{51}{64}$ in., $D = \frac{52}{64}$ in. Thus, in increasing length, the arrangement is C, D, A, B. (Ans. C)

5. Change 3'6" to 42". Then, 42" to 6" = 7 to 1. (Ans. D)

6. Let x = required line. Then $\frac{27}{x} = \frac{72}{45}$, and $x = 16\frac{7}{8}$ in. (Ans. A)

7. The ratio of 630 million to 2 billion, 100 million is 630 to 2100 $= \frac{3}{10}$. $(\frac{3}{10})(360°) = 108°$. (Ans. D)

8. $3 \div 40 = .075$ inches. NOTE correction of problem. (Ans. B)

9. Each major division is $\frac{30}{10} = 3$ volts. Each minor division is $\frac{3}{5} = .6$ volts. 6 major + 2 minor divisions = $(6)(3) + (2)(.6) = 19.2$ volts. (Ans. D)

10. $33 \div 11 = 3$ columns by $27 \div 8$ rounded down to 3 rows. $(3)(3) = 9$. (Ans. B)

11. $\sqrt{5} = 2.236$ approx. Finding the absolute value of the difference between 2.236 and each of 2.1, 2.2, 2.125, and 2.5 yields .136, .036, .111, and .264, respectively. Thus, 2.2 (or $2\frac{1}{5}$) is closest to $\sqrt{5}$. (Ans. B)

12. Use a proportion: $\frac{1\frac{1}{2}}{x} = \frac{.3\%}{100\%} = \frac{.003}{1}$, where x = capacity of the tank. Solving, x = 500. (Ans. D)

13. Total number of permutations = (6)(6)(6) = 216. (Ans. B)

14. 2 kilometers = 1.24 miles, which would require a MINIMUM of over $4\frac{1}{2}$ minutes for a superior athlete. (Ans. C)

15. 32,000,000 = 3.2×10^7 and .000028 = 2.8×10^{-5}. Then, $(3.7\times10^7)(2.8\times10^{-5}) = 8.96 \times 10^2$. (Ans. C)

16. +1 and -1 are their own multiplicative inverses. The multiplicative inverse of 0 doesn't exist. The multiplicative inverse of +.1 is +10. (Ans. A)

17. There are 100,000 centimeters in a kilometer. Since 1 inch ≈ 2.5 centimeters, 1 yard ≈ (36)(2.5) = 90 centimeters. Thus, the number of yards in 100,000 centimeters = 100,000/90 = (100,000)/[(36)(2.5)]. (Ans. C)

18. His net worth after 1 year = ($120,000)(.625) = $75,000. His net worth after 2 years = (75,000)(1.40) = $105,000. Thus, $105,000/$120,000 = .875 = $87\frac{1}{2}$%. (Ans. C)

19. The sum of all fifty numbers = (50)(38) = 1900. By discarding the numbers 45 and 55, the new sum is 1800 for 48 numbers. The mean is then 1800/48 = 37.5. (Ans. D)

20. Any number ending in a 6 which is raised to a positive integral value will still have 6 as its last digit. Only choice B ends in a 6. (Ans. B)

TEST 4

DIRECTIONS: Each question or incomplete statement is followed by several suggested answers or completions. Select the one that BEST answers the question or completes the statement. *PRINT THE LETTER OF THE CORRECT ANSWER IN THE SPACE AT THE RIGHT.*

1. A dealer sold two calculators for $15 each, one at a profit of 25% of its cost, the second at a loss of 25% of its cost. 1.____
The COMBINED effect of the two transactions is
   A. no gain or loss B. a gain of $2
   C. a gain of $3 D. a loss of $2

2. One hundred dollars is invested at a rate of interest of 8% per annum compounded semi-annually. 2.____
The TOTAL value of the investment, in dollars, at the end of one year will be
   A. 116.64 B. 108.16 C. 108.08 D. 108.00

3. If the distance from the earth to the moon is approximately 380,000 kilometers, then this distance, in meters, is 3.____
   A. 3.8×10^8 B. 3.8×10^7 C. 3.8×10^5 D. 3.8×10^2

4. If 14_{five} is subtracted from 123_{four}, the result, in base ten, is 4.____
   A. 18 B. 63 C. 109 D. 1299

5. Two junior high school classes took the same test. The first class of 20 students attained an average grade of 80%. The second class of 30 students attained an average grade of 70%. 5.____
The AVERAGE grade for all students in both classes is
   A. 75% B. 74% C. 73% D. 72%

6. In a class studying the relationship between the metric system and the English system, the following statements were made by students: a 6.____
   I. meter is a little more than a yard
   II. liter is a little more than a quart
   III. kilometer is more than a mile
   IV. kilogram is more than a pound

   Which of these statements if FALSE?
   A. I B. II C. III D. IV

7. A pupil adds his test scores and divides the sum by the number of scores. 7.____
The result of this procedure would be the
   A. arithmetic mean B. median
   C. mode D. standard deviation

8. If the product of two positive integers is divisible by 6, which of the following must be TRUE? 8.____
   A. One integer must be divisible by 2, and the other integer must be divisible by 3.
   B. At least one of the integers must be divisible by 6.
   C. At least one of the integers must be an even number.
   D. Neither of the integers can be a prime number.

9. A gas tank with a capacity of 15 gallons is $\frac{5}{16}$ full. 9.____

   How many gallons of fuel must be added to the tank for it to be $\frac{5}{8}$ full?
   A. $4\frac{11}{16}$ B. $5\frac{5}{8}$ C. $9\frac{3}{8}$ D. $10\frac{5}{16}$

10. Mr. Jones bought a house for $50,000. He sold the house at a profit of 20% of his original cost. The house was resold by the new purchaser at a profit of 20% of his cost. 10.____
    What percent of Mr. Jones' original purchase price is the final selling price of the house?
    A. 44% B. 122% C. 140% D. 144%

11. A man invested $1000 at 12% per year, compounded quarterly, for a period of 5 years. 11.____
    Which of the following represents the total of his investment at the end of that time?
    A. $1000\ (1.03)^{20}$ B. $1000\ (1.05)^{12}$
    C. $1000\ (1.12)^{5}$ D. $1000\ (1.12)^{20}$

12. The number designated by 2021_{three} can be denoted in the binary system by 12.____
    A. 111101_{two} B. 101011_{two}
    C. 110111_{two} D. 101111_{two}

13. A representation for the number .00792 in scientific notation is 13.____
    A. 7.92×10^{-3} B. 7.92×10^{-4}
    C. 7.92×10^{2} D. 7.92×10^{3}

14. An eleventh year mathematics class studying positive and negative exponents examined a number of relationships in the metric system. 14.____
    Which of the following is NOT a correct relationship?
    A. $1\ mm = 10^{-2}\ cm$ B. $1\ cm^3 = 10^{-3} L$
    C. $1\ kg = 10^{6}\ mg$ D. $1\ cm = 10^{-5} km$

15. The last digit of 7^{253} is 15.____
    A. 1 B. 5 C. 7 D. 9

16. Of the following, the property that the set {-1,0,1} does NOT possess is 16.____
   A. closure under addition
   B. closure under multiplication
   C. an identity element for multiplication
   D. inverse elements for addition

17. A pupil is informed that his percentile rank on a test given to a certain group is 70. 17.____
This means that
   A. his score is in the upper 30% of the test scores of the group
   B. his score is in the lower 30% of the test scores of the group
   C. he answered 70 of the items correctly
   D. he answered 70% of the items correctly

18. A number written in base 7 is 1231_{seven}. 18.____

This number written in base 5 is
   A. 3323_{five} B. 3233_{five} C. 1321_{five} D. 463_{five}

19. A television console is listed in a catalog for $1000. If the set is sold with successive discounts of 20% and 10%, the ACTUAL selling price will be 19.____
   A. $700   B. $720   C. $780   D. $850

20. At a certain college, 1/3 of all applications sent to prospective students were never returned. Of those returned, 2/5 were rejected and 1/6 of those accepted decided not to attend. 20.____
How many applications were sent out if 1,000 freshmen were admitted?
   A. 6000   B. 2000   C. 3000   D. 4500

KEY (CORRECT ANSWERS)

1.	D	11.	A
2.	B	12.	A
3.	A	13.	A
4.	A	14.	A
5.	B	15.	C
6.	C	16.	A
7.	A	17.	A
8.	C	18.	A
9.	A	19.	B
10.	D	20.	C

SOLUTIONS TO PROBLEMS

1. The first calculator's cost to the dealer = \$15 ÷ 1.25 = \$12. The second calculator's cost to the dealer = \$15 ÷ .75 = \$20. The combined effect for the dealer was (\$15+\$15) - (\$12+\$20) = -\$2; thus a loss of \$2. (Ans. D)

2. Total value at the end of one year = $\$100(1.04)^2 = \$108.16$. (Ans. B)

3. Since 1 kilometer = 1000 meters, 380,000 km = (380,000)(1000) = 380,000,000 or 3.8×10^8 m. (Ans. A)

4. $14_{five} = (1)(5) + 4 = 9_{ten}$. $123_{four} = (1)(16) + (2)(4) + 3 = 27_{ten}$. The difference is 18, base 10. (Ans. A)

5. Average = $\dfrac{(20)(.80) + (30)(.70)}{50}$ = .74 or 74%. (Ans. B)

6. A kilometer is about $\frac{5}{8}$ of a mile. (Ans. C)

7. The arithmetic mean = sum of numbers divided by the number of numbers. (Ans. A)

8. If (A)(B)/6 is a whole number, we can conclude that either A or B or both A,B is(are) even. Furthermore, at least one of A,B must be divisible by 3. (Ans. C)

9. The required amount of fuel = $15(\frac{5}{8} - \frac{5}{16}) = 4\frac{11}{16}$. (Ans. A)

10. Mr. Jones sold his house for (\$50,000)(1.20) = \$60,000. The new buyer sold the house for (\$60,000)(1.20) = \$72,000. Now, \$72,000 is (72,000/50,000) × 100 = 144% of \$50,000. (Ans. D)

11. $T = P(1 + \frac{R}{n})^{nt}$, where T = total, P = principal (investment), R = annual compounded rate, n = number of times per year being compounded, t = number of years. Thus, $T = 1000(1.03)^{20}$. (Ans. A)

12. $2021_{three} = 2(27) + 0(9) + 2(3) + 1 = 61$ in base 10. This is equivalent to 111101_{two}. (Ans. A)

13. $.00792 = 7.92 \times .001 = 7.92 \times 10^{-3}$. (Ans. A)

14. The CORRECT statement for A is 1 mm = 10^{-1} cm. (Ans. A)

15. 7^1 ends in 7, 7^2 ends in 9, 7^3 ends in 3, 7^4 ends in 1. This cycle is repeated, so that in order to find the last digit of 7^{253}, divide 253 by 4. The remainder of this division is 1, and thus corresponds to 7^1 which ends in 7. (Note that if there were no remainder, this would have been equivalent to a remainder of 4, corresponding to 7^4 which ends in 1.) (Ans. C)

16. Use the example 1 + 1 = 2, and 2 is not an element of {-1,0,1}. (Ans. A)

17. A percentile rank indicates the *relative* position of a score when the scores are arranged from LOWEST to HIGHEST. 70, as a percentile, means that *approximately* 70% of all the scores are LOWER and 30% of all the scores are HIGHER. (Ans. A)

18. 1231_{seven} = (1)(343) + (2)(49) + (3)(7) + 1 = 463.

With base 5, the rightmost column is ones, next column is fives, next column is twenty-fives, fourth column is 125's. Now, 463 = (3)(125) + (3)(25) + (2)(5) + 3(1), so the answer is 3323_{five}. (Ans. A)

19. Discount of 20% = ($1000)(.80) + $800, followed by a Discount of 10%= ($800)(.90) = $720 = answer. (Ans. B)

20. Let x = number of applications sent out. Then, 2/3x = number of applications returned; (3/5)(2/3x) = 2/5x = number of applicants accepted; (5/6)(3/5x) = 1/3x decided to attend. Thus, 1/3x = 1000 and so x = 3000. (Ans. C)

TEST 5

DIRECTIONS: Each question or incomplete statement is followed by several suggested answers or completions. Select the one that BEST answers the question or completes the statement. *PRINT THE LETTER OF THE CORRECT ANSWER IN THE SPACE AT THE RIGHT.*

1. In a three digit number, the units digit is two more than the tens digit. The sum of the digits is 12. The number with the digits reversed is 198 less than the original number. 1.___
The original number must be between
   A. 100 and 200
   B. 200 and 300
   C. 400 and 500
   D. 600 and 700

2. If the tenth term of an arithmetic sequence is 15 and the twentieth term is 35, then the thirtieth term is 2.___
   A. 525
   B. 50
   C. 55
   D. 61

3. The expressions a+bc and (a+b)(a+c) are 3.___
   A. *never* equal
   B. equal when a+b+c = 1
   C. *always* equal
   D. equal when a+b+c = 0

4. Four pupils answered a question. Pupil A's answer was 37.5×10^{-6}, Pupil B's answer was $\frac{3}{8} \times 10^{-6}$, Pupil C's answer was $\frac{15}{4} \times 10^{-5}$, and Pupil D's answer was $.000037\frac{1}{2}$. 4.___
The answer that was NOT equivalent to the others was that of Pupil
   A. A
   B. B
   C. C
   D. D

5. If the original selling price of a certain article, including a profit of 40% of the cost, were \$18.20, and if the profit were to be reduced to 30% of the cost, the selling price would become 5.___
   A. \$13.39
   B. \$13.65
   C. \$16.38
   D. \$16.90

6. If a 4% stock whose par value is \$60.00 is purchased at a price that will make the investment yield a return of 5%, the purchase price is 6.___
   A. \$30
   B. \$48
   C. \$75
   D. \$82

7. If a piece of property was sold for \$5,780 at a loss of 15% of the cost, the cost of the property was 7.___
   A. \$4,913
   B. \$6,647
   C. \$6,800
   D. \$7,200

8. If the single discount equivalent to three successive discounts is 38.8% and the first two discounts are 20% and 10%, then the third discount, in percent, is 8.___
   A. 8.8
   B. 15
   C. 17
   D. 30

9. The SMALLEST integral value of k ($k \neq 0$) that will make 8820k the cube of a positive integer is 9.____

A. 100 B. 150 C. 1000 D. 1050

10. A wholesaler sells a certain article to the retailer at a profit of 60% of the cost. The retailer then sells this article to the consumer at a profit of 25% of his cost. 10.____
The consumer pays $14.40.
The cost to the wholesaler was

A. $7.20 B. $7.78 C. $10.80 D. $12.24

11. Two bicycles start traveling from the same point at the same time. One heads due west at 8 mph and the other heads due south at 15 mph. 11.____
They will be 51 miles apart in _____ hours.

A. 2 B. approximately $2\frac{1}{4}$
C. 3 D. 9

12. At the end of the first two years of school, a pupil attains an average of 83% in eight majors. 12.____
The average required in five majors in the third year at school in order to achieve an overall average of 85% is

A. 86.5% B. 87% C. 88.2% D. 89%

13. To win an election, a candidate needs 3/4 of the votes cast. 13.____
If after 2/3 of the votes have been counted, a candidate has 5/6 of what he needs, what part of the remaining votes does he still need?

A. 1/8 B. 1/4 C. 3/8 D. 1/2

14. A sells an article for D dollars, less 20% and 10%. B sells the same article for D dollars less 25%. 14.____
What additional discount should B allow in order to match A's selling price?

A. 1.8% B. 2% C. 4% D. 5%

15. A radioactive isotope loses 1/3 of its strength during the first minute of its existence, 1/3 of its remaining strength during the second minute, 1/3 of its remaining strength during the third minute, etc. 15.____
How long, to the nearest minute, will it be before the isotope will have lost 87% of its original activity?
_____ minutes.

A. 2 B. 3 C. 4 D. 5

16. A refrigerator was originally marked to sell at a profit of 66 2/3% of the cost. It was finally sold at a profit of 33 1/3% of the cost. 16.____
What percent discount did the purchaser receive on the marked price?

A. 15 B. 20 C. 25 D. 33 1/3

17. A store offers a discount of 30%. An additional discount, in percent, to make the combined discount equivalent to a single discount of 37% would be 17.____

A. 7 B. 10 C. 23 D. 67

18. A sample of brass contained $1\frac{3}{4}$ pounds of copper, $1\frac{1}{4}$ pounds of zinc, and 2 ounces of impurities. 18.____
The number of pounds of copper in one ton of this type of brass is

A. 560 B. 800 C. 1080 D. 1120

19. When the temperature drops from 37°F to -8°F, the number of degrees the temperature on the Centigrade scale will fall during the same period is 19.____

A. $7\frac{2}{9}$ B. 25 C. 49 D. 57

20. As part of its aircraft officer training program, the Navy sends sailors to radio school. Of those who are sent to radio school, 1/3 drop out during the course. Of those who graduate, 4/5 are assigned to aircraft carriers. 20.____
If 3/4 of these become officers, how many sailors should the Navy send to radio school if it needs 60 aircraft officers?

A. 120 B. 150 C. 180 D. 300

KEY (CORRECT ANSWERS)

1. D	11. C
2. C	12. C
3. C	13. C
4. B	14. C
5. D	15. D
6. B	16. B
7. C	17. B
8. B	18. D
9. D	19. B
10. A	20. B

SOLUTIONS TO PROBLEMS

1. Any three digit number can be represented as $100h + 10t + u$. From the conditions of the problem, we get three equations:
   1) $u - t = 2$
   2) $u + t + h = 12$
   3) $100h + 10t + u = 100u + 10t + h + 198$ which reduces to $-u + h = 2$

   Solving, $u = 4$, $t = 2$, $h = 6$; so the answer is 624. (Ans. D)

2. The nth term of an arithmetic progression with first term x and difference d is $x + (n-1)d$. Thus, $x + 9d = 15$ and $x + 19d = 35$. Solving, $x = -3$ and $d = 2$. The thirtieth term is $-3 + (29)(2) = 55$. (Ans. C)

3. $(a+b)(a+c) = a^2 + ab + ac + bc$. In order for this expression to equal $a+bc$, we need $a^2 + ab + ac = a$, which implies $a(a+b+c-1) = 0$. Now, either $a = 0$ or $a+b+c-1 = 0$; i.e., $a+b+c = 1$. Note that choice C does NOT give the FULL answer but is the BEST choice. (Ans. C)

4. Pupils A, C, and D have answers equivalent to .0000375, whereas Pupil B's answer is .000000375. (Ans. B)

5. Let C = cost. $18.20 = (1.40)(C), so C = $13.00. Now, the new profit = (13)(1.30) = $16.90. (Ans. D)

6. Let x = purchase price. Then, $(60)(.04) = (x)(.05)$. Solving, x = $48. (Ans. B)

7. Let x = cost. $5780 = .85x$. Thus, x = $6800. (Ans. C)

8. Let the original price = 1 (for simplicity). A single discount of 38.8% means the final sale price = .612. Two successive discounts of 20% and 10% would amount to a price of $(.8)(.9) = .72$. Letting x be the third discount, the final price $= .72(1 - \frac{x}{100})$. Thus, $.612 = .72(1 - \frac{x}{100})$.

   Solving, $x = 15$. (Ans. B)

9. $8820 = 2^2 \cdot 3^2 \cdot 5 \cdot 7^2$. In order to multiply this product by some factor so that the new number will be a perfect cube (and smallest non-zero perfect cube), the factor would be $2 \cdot 3 \cdot 5^2 \cdot 7 = 1050$. Note that $(8820)(1050) = 9,261,000$, which is $(210)^3$. (Ans. D)

10. Let c = wholesaler cost. The cost to the retailer = 1.6c and so the cost to the consumer becomes $(1.6c)(1.25) = 2c$. If 2c = $14.40, c = 7.20. (Ans. A)

11. Let h = number of hours. Then, $(8h)^2 + (15h)^2 = 51^2$, since the Pythagorean Theorem can be used. Solving, $h = 3$. (Ans. C)

12. An average of 83% for eight subjects means a total of 664 percentage points. Let x = average for the next five subjects, so that 5x = the total percentage points for these 5 subjects. To average 85% for all 13 subjects, 85% = (664+5x)/13. Solving, x = 88.2%. (Ans. C)

13. Let V = number of votes to be cast. After $\frac{2}{3}V$ have been tallied, the candidate has $\frac{5}{6}$ of the $\frac{3}{4}V$ he needs to win. $(\frac{5}{6})(\frac{3}{4}V) = \frac{5}{8}V$. From the remaining $\frac{1}{3V}$ votes he needs to be nominated, $\frac{3}{4}V - \frac{5}{8}V = \frac{1}{8}V$ times. Finally, $\frac{1}{8}V/\frac{1}{3}V = \frac{3}{8}$. (Ans. C)

14. Two consecutive discounts of 20% and 10% on D dollars means .90(.80D)= .72D is the selling price. If the first discount is 25%, the selling price is then .75D (B's first discount). In order to match .72D as the final selling price, a second discount of x% means (100-x)(.75D) = .72D. Then, x = 4%. (Ans. C)

15. Let x = number of minutes required. After x minutes, the isotope will retain $(\frac{2}{3})^x \cdot S$ of its strength, where S = original strength. We seek x such that the retention will be $\frac{13}{100}$ - S. Solving, $(\frac{2}{3})^x = \frac{13}{100}$ by Logs yields x = 5.03 or about 5 minutes. (Ans. D)

16. Let C = cost. Then, $1\frac{2}{3}C$ = original marked price. The item was finally sold at $1\frac{1}{3}C$. The percent discount on the marked price is $[(1\frac{2}{3} - 1\frac{1}{3})/1\frac{2}{3}][100] = 20\%$. (Ans. B)

17. Let P = original price. After one discount of 30%, the price is .708. If the second discount is x%, then the new price is $(\frac{100-x}{100})(.70P)$. Since the combined discount is equivalent to one 37% discount, $(\frac{100-x}{100})(.70P) = .63P$. Solving, x = 10. (Ans. B)

18. This sample contains $1\frac{3}{4} + 1\frac{1}{4} + \frac{1}{8} = 3\frac{1}{8}$ lbs. Let x = number of pounds of copper in 1 ton of this brass sample. $\frac{x}{2000} = \frac{1.75}{3.125}$. Solving by cross-multiplication, x = 1120. (Ans. D)

19. Use $C = \frac{5}{9}(F-32)$. 37°F converts to $2\frac{7}{9}$°C and -8°F converts to $-22\frac{1}{9}$°C. The drop is $24\frac{8}{9}$° or approx. 25°. (Ans. B)

20. Let x = number of sailors sent to school. Then, $\frac{2}{3}x$ graduate. Subsequently, $(\frac{4}{5})(\frac{2}{3}x) = \frac{8}{15}x$ are assigned to aircraft carriers. Finally, $(\frac{3}{4})(\frac{8}{15}x) = \frac{2}{5}x$ = number of officers = 60. Thus, x = 150. (Ans. B)

EXAMINATION SECTION

DIRECTIONS: Each question or incomplete statement is followed by several suggested answers or completions. Select the one that BEST answers the question or completes the statement. *PRINT THE LETTER OF THE CORRECT ANSWER IN THE SPACE AT THE RIGHT.*

1. Each edge of a cube is increased by 50%. The percent of increase in the surface area of the cube is 1.____
   A. 50 B. 125 C. 150 D. 300 E. 750

2. Through a point P inside the triangle ABC, a line is drawn parallel to the base AB, dividing the triangle into two equal areas. 2.____
   If the altitude to AB has a length of 1, then the distance from P to AB is
   A. 1/2 B. 1/4 C. $2 - \sqrt{2}$ D. $\frac{2 - \sqrt{2}}{2}$ E. $\frac{2 + \sqrt{2}}{8}$

3. If the diagonals of a quadrilateral are perpendicular to each other, the figure would always be included under the general classification 3.____
   A. rhombus
   B. rectangle
   C. square
   D. isosceles trapezoid
   E. none of the above

4. If 78 is divided into three parts which are proportional to 1, 1/3, 1/6, the middle part is 4.____
   A. 9 1/3 B. 13 C. 17 1/3 D. 18 1/3 E. 26

5. The value of $(256)^{.16} \cdot (256)^{.09}$ is 5.____
   A. 4 B. 16 C. 64 D. 256.25 E. -16

6. Given the true statement: If a quadrilateral is a square, then it is a rectangle. It follows that, of the converse and the inverse of this true statement, 6.____
   A. only the converse is true
   B. only the inverse is true
   C. both are true
   D. neither is true
   E. the inverse is true, but the converse is sometimes true

7. The sides of a right triangle are a, a + d, and a + 2d, with <u>a</u> and <u>d</u> both positive. 7.____
   The ratio of <u>a</u> to <u>d</u> is
   A. 1:3 B. 1:4 C. 2:1 D. 3:1 E. 3:4

8. The value of $x^2 - 6x + 13$ can never be less than 8.____
   A. 4 B. 4.5 C. 5 D. 7 E. 13

9. A farmer divides his herd of <u>n</u> cows among his four sons so that one son gets one-half the herd, a second son gets one-fourth, a third son gets one-fifth, and the fourth son gets 7 cows. Then, <u>n</u> is 9.____
   A. 80 B. 100 C. 140 D. 180 E. 240

10. In triangle ABC, with AB = AC = 3.6, a point D is taken on AB at a distance 1.2 from A. Point D is joined to point E in the prolongation of AC so that triangle AED is equal in area to triangle ABC. Then, AE equals 10.____
   A. 4.8 B. 5.4 C. 7.2 D. 10.8 E. 12.6

11. The logarithm of .0625 to the base 2 is 11.____
   A. .025 B. .25 C. 5 D. -4 E. -2

12. By adding the same constant to each of 20, 50, 100, a geometric progression results. The common ratio is 12.____
   A. 5/3 B. 4/3 C. 3/2 D. 1/2 E. 1/3

13. The arithmetic mean (average) of a set of 50 numbers is 38. If two numbers, namely 45 and 55, are discarded, the mean of the remaining set of numbers is 13.____
   A. 36.5 B. 37 C. 37.2 D. 37.5 E. 37.52

14. Given the set S whose elements are zero and the even integers, positive and negative. Of the five operations applied to any pair of element: (1) addition, (2) subtraction, (3) multiplication, (4) division, (5) finding the arithmetic mean (average), those operations that yield only elements of S are 14.____
   A. all B. 1, 2, 3, 4 C. 1, 2, 3, 5
   D. 1, 2, 3 E. 1, 3, 5

15. In a right triangle, the square of the hypotenuse is equal to twice the product of the legs. One of the acute angles of the triangle is 15.____
   A. 15° B. 30° C. 45° D. 60° E. 75°

16. The expression $\dfrac{x^2 - 3x + 2}{x^2 - 5x + 6} \div \dfrac{x^2 - 5x + 4}{x^2 - 7x + 12}$, when simplified, is 16.____
   A. $\dfrac{(x-1)(x-6)}{(x-3)(x-4)}$ B. $\dfrac{x+3}{x-3}$ C. $\dfrac{x+1}{x-1}$
   D. 1 E. 2

17. If $y = a + \dfrac{b}{x}$, where <u>a</u> and <u>b</u> are constants, and if y = 1 when x + -1, and y = 5 when x = -5, then a + b equals 17.____
   A. -1 B. 0 C. 1 D. 10 E. 11

18. Let <u>r</u> and <u>s</u> be positive numbers with <u>r</u> greater than <u>s</u>. Let R = r + 1 and S = s + 1. The difference in percent by which r exceeds <u>s</u> and <u>R</u> exceeds <u>S</u> is 18.____

A. $\frac{100(r-s)}{r}$ B. $\frac{100(r-s)}{s}$ C. $\frac{100(r-s)}{r+1}$

D. $\frac{100(r-s)}{s+1}$ E. none of the above

19. With the use of three different weights, namely 1 lb., 3 lb., and 9 lb., how many objects of different weights can be weighed if the objects to be weighed and the given weights may be placed in either pan of the scale? 19.___
A. 15 B. 13 C. 11 D. 9 E. 7

20. It is given that x varies directly as y and inversely as the square of z, and that $x = 10$ when $y = 4$ and $z = 14$. Then, when $y = 16$ and $z = 7$, x equals 20.___
A. 180 B. 160 C. 154 D. 140 E. 120

21. If p is the perimeter of an equilateral triangle inscribed in a circle, the area of the circle is 21.___
A. $\frac{\pi p^2}{3}$ B. $\frac{\pi p^2}{9}$ C. $\frac{\pi p^2}{27}$ D. $\frac{\pi p^2}{81}$ E. $\frac{\pi p^2\sqrt{3}}{27}$

22. The line joining the midpoints of the diagonals of a trapezoid has length 3. If the longer base is 97, then the shorter base is 22.___
A. 94 B. 92 C. 91 D. 90 E. 89

23. The set of solutions for the equation $\log_{10}(a^2-15a) = 2$ consists of 23.___
A. two integers
B. one integer and one fraction
C. two irrational numbers
D. two non-real numbers
E. no numbers, that is, the set is empty

24. A chemist has m ounces of salt water that is m% salt. How many ounces of salt must he add to make a solution that is 2m% salt? 24.___
A. $\frac{m}{100+m}$ B. $\frac{2m}{100-2m}$ C. $\frac{m^2}{100-2m}$ D. $\frac{m^2}{100+2m}$ E. $\frac{2m}{100+m}$

25. The symbol $|a|$ means $+a$ if a is greater than or equal to zero, and $-a$ if a is less than or equal to zero; the symbol $<$ means *less than*; the symbol $>$ means *greater than*. The set of values x satisfying the inequality $|3-x| <$ consists of all x such that 25.___
A. $x^2 < 49$ B. $x^2 > 1$ C. $1 < x^2 < 49$
D. $-1 < x < 7$ E. $-7 < x < 1$

26. The base of an isosceles triangle is $\sqrt{2}$. The medians to the legs intersect each other at right angles. The area of the triangle is 26.___
A. 1.5 B. 2 C. 2.5 D. 3.5 E. 4

27. Which one of the following statements is NOT true for the equation $ix^2 - x + 2i = 0$ where $i \equiv \sqrt{-1}$? 27.____

A. The sum of the roots is 2.
B. The discriminant is 9.
C. The roots are imaginary.
D. The roots can be found by using the quadratic formula.
E. The roots can be found by factoring, using imaginary numbers

28. In triangle ABC, AL bisects angle A and CM bisects angle C. Points L and M are on BC and AB, respectively. The sides of triangle ABC are a, b, and C. Then, $\frac{AM}{MB} = k\frac{CL}{LB}$ where k is 28.____

A. 1 B. $\frac{bc}{a^2}$ C. $\frac{a^2}{bc}$ D. $\frac{c}{b}$ E. $\frac{c}{a}$

29. On an examination of $\underline{n}$ questions, a student answers correctly 15 of the first 20. Of the remaining questions, he answers one-third correctly. All the questions have the same credit. If the student's mark is 50%, how many different values of $\underline{n}$ can there be? 29.____

A. 4 B. 3 C. 2 D. 1
E. the problem cannot be solved

30. $\underline{A}$ can run around a circular track in 40 seconds; $\underline{B}$, running in the opposite direction, meets $\underline{A}$ every 15 seconds. What is $\underline{B}$'s time to run around the track, expressed in seconds? 30.____

A. $12\frac{1}{2}$ B. 24 C. 25 D. $27\frac{1}{2}$ E. 55

31. A square, with an area of 40, is inscribed in a semi-circle. The area of a square that could be inscribed in the entire circle with the same radius is 31.____

A. 80 B. 100 C. 120 D. 160 E. 200

32. The length $\underline{l}$ of a tangent, drawn from point A to a circle, is 4/3 of the radius $\underline{r}$. The (shortest) distance from A to the circle is 32.____

A. $\frac{1}{2}r$ B. r C. $\frac{1}{2}$ l D. 2/3 l
E. a value between $\underline{r}$ and $\underline{l}$

33. A harmonic progression is a sequence of numbers such that their reciprocals are in arithmetic progression. Let S_n represent the sum of the first $\underline{n}$ terms of the harmonic progression; for example, S_3 represents the sum of the first three terms. If the first three terms of a harmonic progression are 3, 4, 6, then 33.____

A. $S_4 = 20$ B. $S_4 = 25$ C. $S_5 = 49$ D. $S_6 = 49$ E. $S_2 = \frac{1}{2}S_4$

34. Let the roots of $x^2 - 3x + 1 = 0$ be $\underline{r}$ and $\underline{s}$. Then, the expression $r^2 + s^2$ is 34.____

A. a positive integer
B. a positive fraction greater than 1
C. a positive fraction less than 1
D. an irrational number
E. an imaginary number

35. The symbol $\geq$ means *greater than or equal to*; the symbol $\leq$ means *less than or equal to*. 35.___

In the equation $(x-m)^2 - (x-n)^2 = (m-n)^2$, m is a fixed positive number, and n is a fixed negative number. The set of values x satisfying the equation is

A. $x \geq 0$
B. $x \leq n$
C. $x = 0$
D. the set of all real numbers
E. none of these

36. The base of a triangle is 80, and one of the base angles is 60°. The sum of the other two sides is 90. The shortest side of the triangle is 36.___

A. 45 B. 40 C. 36 D. 17 E. 12

37. When simplified, the product $(1-1/3)(1-1/4)(1-1/5)\ldots(1-1/n)$ becomes 37.___

A. $1/n$ B. $2/n$ C. $\frac{2(n-1)}{n}$

D. $\frac{2}{n(n+1)}$ E. $\frac{3}{n(n+1)}$

38. If $4x + \sqrt{2x} = 1$, then x 38.___

A. is an integer
B. is fractional
C. is irrational
D. is imaginary
E. may have two different values

39. Let S be the sum of the first nine terms of the sequence, $x + a, x^2 + 2a, x^3 + 3a, \ldots.$ Then, S equals 39.___

A. $\frac{50a + x + x^8}{x + 1}$ B. $50a - \frac{x + x^{10}}{x-1}$

C. $\frac{x^9 - 1}{x + 1} + 45a$ D. $\frac{x^{10} - x}{x-1} + 45a$

E. $\frac{x^{11} - x}{x - 1} + 45a$

40. In triangle ABC, BD is a median. CF intersects BD at E so that BE = ED. Point F is on AB. Then, if BF = 5, BA equals 40.___

A. 10 B. 12 C. 15 D. 20
E. none of these

41. On the same side of a straight line, three circles are drawn as follows: a circle with a radius of 4 inches is tangent to the line, the other two circles are equal, and each is tangent to the line and to the other two circles. The radius of the equal circles is 41.___

A. 24 B. 20 C. 18 D. 16 E. 12

42. Given three positive integers a, b, and c. Their greatest common divisor is D; their least common multiple is M. Then, which two of the following statements are TRUE? 42.____

I. The product MD cannot be less than abc.
II. The product MD cannot be greater than abc.
III. MD equals abc if and only if a, b, c are each prime.
IV. MD equals abc if and only if a, b, c are relatively prime in pairs. (This means: no two have a common factor greater than 1.)

The CORRECT answer is:
A. I, II B. I, III C. I, IV D. II, III E. II, IV

43. The sides of a triangle are 25, 39, and 40. The diameter of the circumscribed circle is 43.____
A. 133/3 B. 125/3 C. 42 D. 41 E. 40

44. The roots of $x^2 + bx + c = 0$ are both real and greater than 1. Let $s = b + c + 1$. Then, s 44.____
A. may be less than zero
B. may be equal to zero
C. must be greater than zero
D. must be less than zero
E. must be between -1 and +1

45. If $(\log_3 x)(\log_x 2x)(\log_{2x} y) = \log_x x^2$, then y equals 45.____

A. 9/2 B. 9 C. 18 D. 27 E. 81

46. A student on vacation for d days observed that 46.____
I. it rained 7 times, morning or afternoon
II. when it rained in the afternoon, it was clear in the morning
III. there were five clear afternoons
IV. there were six clear mornings
Then, d equals
A. 7 B. 9 C. 10 D. 11 E. 12

47. Assume that the following three statements are true: 47.____
1. All freshmen are human.
2. All students are human.
3. Some students think.
Given the following four statements:
I. All freshmen are students.
II. Some humans think.
III. No freshmen think.
IV. Some humans who think are not students.

Those which are logical consequences of 1, 2, and 3 are
A. II B. IV C. II, III D. II, IV E. I, II

48. Given the polynomial $a_0x^n + a_1x^{n-1} + \ldots + a_{n-1}x + a_n$, where n is a positive integer or zero, and a_0 is a positive integer. The remaining a's are integers or zero. Set $h = n + a_0 + |a_1| + |a_2| + \ldots + |a_n|$. [See example 25 for the meaing of $|x|$.] The number of polynomials with h = 3 is 48.____
A. 3 B. 5 C. 6 D. 7 E. 9

49. For the infinite series 1 - 1/2 - 1/4 + 1/8 - 1/16 - 1/32 + 1/64 - 1/128 - ... let S be the (limiting sum). Then, S equals 49.____

A. 0 B. 2/7 C. 6/7 D. 9/32 E. 27/32

50. A club with <u>x</u> members is organized into four committees in accordance with these two rules: 50.____

I. Each member belongs to two and only two committees.
II. Each pair of committees has one and only one member in common.

Then, <u>x</u>

A. cannot be determined
B. has a single value between 8 and 16
C. has two values between 8 and 16
D. has a single value between 4 and 8
E. has two values between 4 and 8

KEY (CORRECT ANSWERS)

1. B	11. D	21. C	31. B	41. D
2. D	12. A	22. C	32. C	42. E
3. E	13. D	23. A	33. B	43. B
4. C	14. D	24. C	34. A	44. C
5. A	15. C	25. D	35. E	45. B
6. D	16. D	26. A	36. D	46. B
7. D	17. E	27. A	37. B	47. A
8. A	18. E	28. E	38. B	48. B
9. C	19. B	29. D	39. D	49. B
10. D	20. B	30. B	40. C	50. D

SOLUTIONS TO PROBLEMS

1. S(old) = $6x^2$. S(new) = $6(1.5x)^2 = 13.50x^2$.
Increase = $7.5x^2 = \frac{5}{4}(6x^2)$

Increase (%) = 125
(Ans. B)

2. Let x be the distance from P to AB. By similar triangles,
$\frac{1}{2} = \frac{(1-x)^2}{1^2}$ ... $1 - x = \pm\frac{1}{\sqrt{2}}$ $\therefore$ $x = \frac{2 - \sqrt{2}}{2}$ (negative sq. root rejected)
(Ans. D)

3. There are a variety of figures satisfying the given conditions and not falling within the classifications (A), (B), (C), (D); for example, the *kite*. (Ans. E)

4. $x + \frac{1}{3}x + \frac{1}{6}x = 78$. $9x = 468$. $\frac{1}{3}x = 17\ 1/3$. (Ans. C)

5. $(256)^{.16}(256)^{.09} = (256)^{.25} = (256)^{1/4} = 4$. (Ans. A)

6. The converse is: If a quadrilateral is a rectangle, then it is a square.
The inverse is: If a quadrilateral is not a square, then it is not a rectangle.
Both statements are false.

or

Use Venn diagram to picture the sets mentioned. (Ans. D)

7. $a^2 + (a+d)^2 = (a+2d)^2$ $\therefore$ $a = 3d$ $\therefore$ $\frac{a}{d} = \frac{3}{1}$. (Ans. D)

8. $x^2 - 6x + 13 = (x-3)^2 + 4$. The smallest value for this expression, 4, is obtained when x = 3.

or

Graph $y = x^2 - 6x + 3$. The turning point, whose ordinate is 4, is a minimum point. (Ans. A)

9. $n = \frac{1}{2}n + \frac{1}{4}n + \frac{1}{5}n + 7$. n = 140. (Ans. C)

10. Let the altitude from B to AC be <u>h</u>. Then, the altitude from D to AE is 1/3<u>h</u>. Let AE = x. Then,
$\frac{1}{2} \cdot \frac{1}{3}hx = \frac{1}{2}h(3.6)$ $\therefore$ $x = 10.8$. (Ans. D)

11. Let $\log_2 .0625 = x$ $\therefore$ $2^x = .0625 = \frac{1}{2^4}$ $\therefore$ $x = -4$. (Ans. D)

12. Let a = the constant.

$$\frac{20 + a}{50 + a} = \frac{50 + a}{100 + a} \quad \therefore a = 25 \quad \therefore r = \frac{5}{3}$$ (Ans. A)

13. Arith. mean = $\frac{\text{sum of numbers}}{\text{number of numbers}}$

$\therefore S = 50 \times 38 = 1900 \quad \therefore x = \frac{1900 - 45 - 55}{48} = 37.5$ (Ans. D)

14. Addition, subtraction, and multiplication with even integers always yield even integers.
(Note: This is a good opportunity to underscore operational restrictions imposed by the available domain.)
(Ans. D)

15. $c^2 = 2ab \therefore a^2 + b^2 = 2ab \therefore (a-b)^2 = 0 \therefore a = b.$
Since the right triangle is isosceles, one of the acute angles is 45°. (Ans. C)

16. $\frac{(x-2)(x-1)}{(x-3)(x-2)} \cdot \frac{(x-3)(x-4)}{(x-4)(x-1)} = 1$ (Ans. D)

17. $y = a + \frac{b}{x}$ $\quad 1 = a - b$

$5 = a - \frac{1}{5}b \quad \therefore b = 5 \text{ and } a = 6$

(Ans. E)

18. $\left(\frac{r - s}{s} - \frac{(r+1) - (s+1)}{s + 1}\right) 100 = \frac{100(r-s)}{s(s+1)}$
(Ans. E)

19.

Weights used	No. of Weighings Possible
1. Singly	3
2. Two at a time (same pan)	3
3. Three at a time (same pan)	1
4. Two at a time (diff. pans)	3
5. Three at a time (diff. pans)	3
Total	13

or

$111_3 = 1 \cdot 3^2 + 1 \cdot 3 + 1 = 13_{10}$, so that the number of weighings equals the sum of the weights, when the weights are related in this manner. (Ans. B)

20. $x = \frac{Ky}{Z^2} \quad 10 = \frac{K(4)}{14^2} \quad \therefore K = \frac{10 \cdot 14^2}{4} \quad \therefore x = \frac{\frac{10 \cdot 14^2 \cdot 16}{4}}{7^2} = 160$
(Ans.B)

21. $R = \frac{2}{3}\text{ altitude} = \frac{2}{3} \cdot \frac{1}{2} \cdot \frac{p}{3}\sqrt{3} = \frac{p}{3\sqrt{3}} \quad \therefore A = \frac{\pi p^2}{27}$ (Ans. C)

22. The median of a trapezoid goes through the midpoints of the diagonals. Let x be the length of the shorter base.

$\therefore$ length of median $= \frac{x}{2} + 3 + \frac{x}{2}$

$\therefore \frac{1}{2}(x+97) = \frac{x}{2} + 3 + \frac{x}{2} \quad \therefore x = 91$

(Ans. C

23. $\log_{10}(a^2-15a) = 2 \therefore 10^2 = a^2 - 15a \therefore a = 20$ or $a = -5$

(Ans. A)

24. $\dfrac{\frac{m^2}{100} + x}{m + x} = \dfrac{2m}{100} \quad \therefore x = \dfrac{m^2}{100 - 2m}$ (Ans. C)

25. Let AB be a straight line segment with its midpoint at 3, and its right end at B. Each of the two intervals from A to 3 and from 3 to B is less than 4. Hence, B is to the left of 7 and A is to the right of -1.

or

$|3-x| < 4$

$\therefore 3 - x < 4 \quad \therefore -x < 1 \quad \therefore x > -1$

$-4 < 3 - x \quad \therefore -7 < -x \quad \therefore x < 7$

$\therefore -1 < x < 7$

(Ans. D)

26. $x^2 + x^2 = 2 \therefore x = 1 \therefore DF = \frac{\sqrt{2}}{2}$

But $\frac{AD}{AE} = \frac{2}{3} \therefore \frac{DF}{EG} = \frac{2}{3}$

$\therefore EG = \frac{3\sqrt{2}}{4} \quad \therefore$ altitude $CDF = \frac{3\sqrt{2}}{2}$

$\therefore A = \frac{1}{2} \cdot \sqrt{2} \cdot \frac{3\sqrt{2}}{2} = \frac{3}{2}$

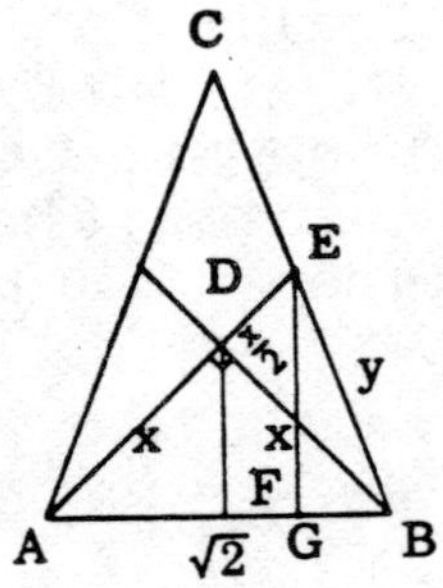

Fig. 1

or

$x^2 + x^2 = 2 \therefore x = 1$

$\therefore y^2 = 1 + \frac{1}{4} \therefore y = \frac{\sqrt{5}}{2} \therefore BC = \sqrt{5}$ etc. (Ans. A)

27. Sum of roots is $\frac{1}{i} = -i$. (Ans. A)

28. The bisector of an angle of a triangle divides the opposite sides into segments proportional to the other two sides

$\therefore \frac{AM}{MB} = \frac{b}{a}$ and $\frac{CL}{LB} = \frac{b}{c}$

Since $\frac{c}{a} \cdot \frac{b}{c} = \frac{b}{a}$, $k = \frac{c}{a}$ (Ans. E)

29. $\frac{15 + \frac{1}{3}(x-20)}{x} = \frac{1}{2}$ $x = 50$ (Ans. D)

30. Let x = B's time in seconds. Letting 1 represent the length of the track, we have $\frac{1}{40}(15) + \frac{1}{x}(15) = 1$ $\therefore x = 24$ (Ans. B)

31. Let 2s be the side of the smaller square.
Then $\frac{r-s}{2s} = \frac{2s}{r+s}$ $\therefore r = \sqrt{50}$
Let S be the side of the larger square
$S = r\sqrt{2} = 10$ $\therefore A = 100$
(Ans. B)

32. The point A, the point of tangency, and the center of the circle, determine a right triangle with one side $\underline{l}$, another side $\underline{r}$, and the hypotenuse x+r, where x is the shortest distance from A to the circle.

$(\frac{4}{3}r)^2 + r^2 = (x+r)^2$ $\therefore x = \frac{2}{3}f = \frac{1}{2}l$ (Ans. C)

33. $\frac{1}{3}, \frac{1}{4}, \frac{1}{6}, \frac{1}{12}$, 0 with $d = -\frac{1}{12}$ $\therefore$ the terms of the H.P. are

3, 4, 6, 12 only $\therefore S_4 = 25$. (Ans. B)

34. $x^2 - 3x + 1 = 0$ $\therefore rs = 1$ and $r + s = 3$
$\therefore (r + s)^2 = r^2 + 2rs + s^2 = 9$ $\therefore r^2 + s^2 = 7$.
(Ans. A)

35. $(x - m)^2 - (x - n)^2 = (m - n)^2$ $M > 0$ $n < 0$
Since $(m - n)^2 > 0$ $(x - m)^2 > (x-n)^2$
$\therefore |x-m| > |x-n|$

$x - m > x - n$
not usable

$2x < m + n$
$x < \frac{m + n}{2}$

or

Solving for x, we have $x(-m+n) = -mn + n^2$ $x = n$
(Ans. E)

36. Let the triangle be ABC, with AB = 80, BC = a, CA = b = 90 - a, $\angle B = 60°$. Let CD be the altitude to AB. Let x = BD.
$\therefore$ $CD = \sqrt{3}x$ $\quad a = 2x \quad b = 90 - 2x$

$\therefore$ $3x^2 + (80-x)^2 = (90-2x)^2$

$\therefore$ $x = \frac{17}{2}$ $\quad\therefore$ $a = 17 \quad b = 73$

(Ans. D)

37. $(1 - \frac{1}{3})(1 - \frac{1}{4})(1 - \frac{1}{5}) \dots (1 - \frac{1}{n})$
$= \frac{2}{3} \cdot \frac{3}{4} \cdot \frac{4}{5} \cdot \dots \frac{n-2}{n-1} \frac{n-1}{n} = \frac{2}{n}$
(Ans. B)

38. $4x + \sqrt{2x} = 1 \quad \therefore 4x - 1 = -\sqrt{2x}$

$16x^2 - 10x + 1 = 0 \quad \therefore x = \frac{1}{8}$

$x = \frac{1}{2}$ does not satisfy the original equation.

or

Let $y = \sqrt{x} \quad \therefore 4y^2 + \sqrt{2}y - 1 = 0$

$y = \frac{2\sqrt{2}}{8}, \quad \frac{-4\sqrt{2}}{8}, \quad x = y^2 = \frac{1}{8}, \frac{1}{2}$ reject

(Ans. B)

39. $x + x^2 + x^3 + \dots + x^9$

$S_1 = \frac{x(1-x^9)}{1-x} = \frac{x^{10} - x}{x - 1}$
$a + 2a + 3a + \dots + 9a$

$S_2 = \frac{9}{2}(a + 9a) = 45a \quad S = S_1 + S_2$ (Ans. D)

40. Let G be a point on EC so that FE = EG. Connect D with G. Then, FDGB is a parallelogram.
$\therefore$ DG = 5 $\quad$ AF = 10 $\quad$ AB = 15
(Ans. C)

41.

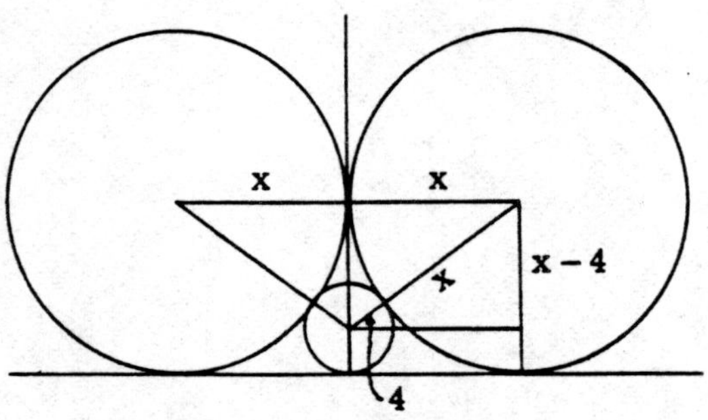

Fig. 2

$x^2 + (x-4)^2 = (x+4)^2 \quad x = 16, 0$ (Ans. D)

42. Represent a, b, c in terms of their prime factors. Then D is the product of all the common prime factors, each factor taken as often as it appears the least number of times in <u>a</u> or <u>b</u> or <u>c</u>. M is the product of all the non-common prime factors, each factor taken as often as it appears the greatest number of times in <u>a</u> or <u>b</u> or <u>c</u>.
Therefore, MD may be less than abc, but it cannot exceed abc. Obviously, MD equals abc when there are no common factors. (Ans. E)

43. Let h be the altitude to side 39. Then, $\frac{2R}{25} = \frac{40}{h}$.

But, $\frac{1}{2}h \quad 39 = \text{Area} = \sqrt{s(s-a)(s-b)(s-c)}$

$\therefore h = \frac{2}{39}\sqrt{52 \cdot 13 \cdot 12 \cdot 27} = 24 \qquad \therefore 2R = \frac{125}{3}$

(Ans. B)

44. Let the roots be $1 + m$ and $1 + n$ with <u>m</u> and <u>n</u> both positive. $\therefore 1 + m + 1 + n = -b$ and $(1+m)(1+n) = c$ $\therefore s = b + c + 1 = mn > 0$. (Ans. C)

45. Since $\log_a b = \frac{\log_c b}{\log_c a}$, we have, with base x,

$$\frac{\log x}{\log 3}\ \frac{\log 2x}{\log x}\ \frac{\log y}{\log 2x} = 2$$

$\log y = 2 \log 3 = \log 9 \quad \therefore y = 9.$ (Ans. B)

46.

	rainy mornings	non-rainy mornings
rainy afternoons	a	b
non-rainy afternoons	c	e

$d = a + b + c + e \qquad a + b + c = 7 \qquad a = 0$
$c + e = 5 \qquad b + e = 6 \qquad \therefore e = 2 \qquad \therefore d = 9$
(Ans. B)

47.

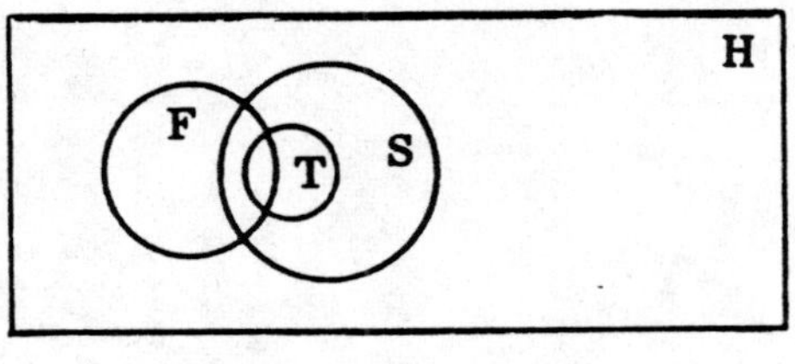

(Ans. A)

48. For h = 3, we can have $1x^2$, $1x^1 + 1$, $1x^1 - 1$, $2x^1$, $3x^0$ (Ans. B)

49. Combine the terms in threes, as follows,

$$\frac{1}{4} + \frac{1}{32} + \frac{1}{256}, \ldots \qquad \therefore S = \frac{\frac{1}{4}}{1 - \frac{1}{8}} = \frac{2}{7}$$

or

Since there is absolute convergence, the terms may be rearranged to yield the three series

$$1 + \frac{1}{8} + \frac{1}{64} + \ldots, \qquad -\frac{1}{2} - \frac{1}{16} - \frac{1}{128} - \ldots,$$

$$-\frac{1}{4} - \frac{1}{32} - \frac{1}{256} - \ldots$$

$$S_1 = \frac{1}{1 - \frac{1}{8}} = \frac{8}{7} \qquad S_2 = \frac{-\frac{1}{2}}{1 - \frac{1}{8}} = -\frac{4}{7}$$

$$S_3 = \frac{-\frac{1}{4}}{1 - \frac{1}{8}} = -\frac{2}{7} \qquad \therefore S = \frac{2}{7}$$

(Ans. B)

50. This problem may be interpreted as a miniature finite geometry of 4 lines and 6 points, so that each pair of lines has only 1 point in common, and each pair of points has only 1 line in common.

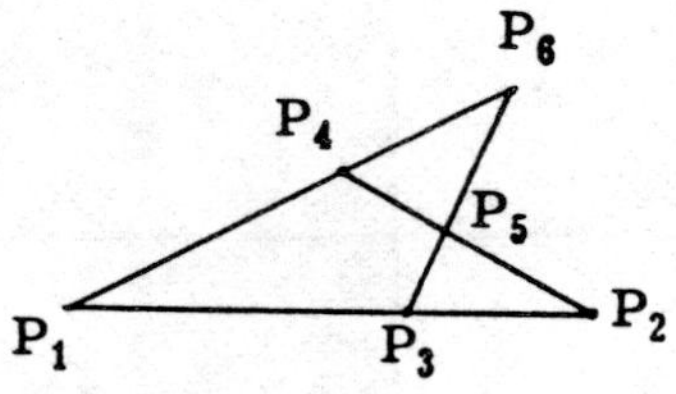

Fig. 3

$C(4,2) = \frac{4!}{2!2!} = 6$, displayed as follows

	Committees			
	A	B	C	D
Members	a	b	d	f
	c	e	a	e
	b	d	f	c

(Ans. D)

EXAMINATION SECTION

DIRECTIONS: Each question or incomplete statement is followed by several suggested answers or completions. Select the one that BEST answers the question or completes the statement. *PRINT THE LETTER OF THE CORRECT ANSWER IN THE SPACE AT THE RIGHT.*

1. All of the following secrete digestive enzymes EXCEPT the 1.___
   A. pancreas
   B. salivary glands
   C. stomach
   D. small intestine
   E. liver

2. Soon after fertilization, the dividing zygote of the amphibian forms a hollow ball of cells surrounding a central cavity. 2.___
   This stage in development is called the
   A. morula
   B. blastula
   C. gastrula
   D. primitive streak
   E. fetus

3. The two products of the *light reactions* of photosynthesis that are required for the synthetic *dark reactions* are ATP and 3.___
   A. carbon dioxide
   B. the reduced form of coenzyme NADP
   C. oxygen
   D. glucose
   E. ribulose-1, 5-bisphosphate (RuBP)

4. Vertebrate skeletal muscle is able to contact as a result of muscle membrane depolarization due to the action of 4.___
   A. neurotransmitters
   B. Ca^{2+} ions
   C. actin and myosin
   D. phosphocreatine
   E. myoglobin

5. Assuming that all are of the same size, which of the following fishes would you expect to produce the *greatest* volume of urine per unit time? 5.___
   A. Bony fish living in freshwater
   B. Bony fish living in an estuary
   C. Bony fish living in the ocean
   D. Shark living in the ocean
   E. All about the same

6. One of the functions of light in the process of photosynthesis is to 6.___
   A. raise the energy level of electrons
   B. cause the formation of water
   C. cause the formation of ribulose-diphosphate
   D. fix CO_2
   E. oxidize NADP (nicotinamide adenine dinucleotide phosphate)

7. In mammalian embryonic development, the embryo proper develops from the 7.____
   A. trophoblast
   B. amnion
   C. inner cell mass
   D. primary yolk sac
   E. placenta

8. Hydrogen bonds 8.____
   A. have bond energy about equal to covalent bonds
   B. have bond energy much larger than covalent bonds
   C. are important in maintaining protein conformations
   D. are too weak to be of importance in biological molecules
   E. are any bonds between hydrogen and another atom

9. The MAIN function of the nucleolus is to 9.____
   A. direct the transcriptive activities of the nucleus
   B. coordinate the replication of chromosomal DNA
   C. synthesize components of the nuclear membrane
   D. synthesize ribosomal RNA
   E. regulate the condensation of chromosomes as the cell approaches metaphase

10. Which of the following would tend to shift a population out of Hardy-Weinberg equilibrium? 10.____
   A. Barriers to migration
   B. Prevention of mutation
   C. Population size increase
   D. Prevention of genetic drift
   E. Preferential mating

11. In the modern understanding of the concept of natural selection, the fittest individuals are those who 11.____
   A. produce the largest number of progeny
   B. are adapted to the widest diversity of environments
   C. produce most highly variable offspring
   D. survive for the largest number of years
   E. have the largest number of fertile offspring

12. Recombinant DNA technology uses which of the following to cleave DNA molecules into polynucleotide fragments? 12.____
   A. Reverse transcriptases
   B. DNA topoisomerases
   C. Restriction enzymes
   D. Plasmids or episomes
   E. Recombinases

13. During the development of a typical vertebrate embryo, the mesoderm germ layer produces the following series of structures: 13.____
   A. Epidermis, nails, and hair
   B. Dermis, blood vessels, and vertebrae
   C. Neural tube, brain and cranial nerves
   D. Lining of the gut, liver, and pancreas
   E. All of the above

14. The stem length of pea plants is genetically determined by a pair of alleles, *T* for tall and *t* for short. *T* is completely dominant over *t*. If the gene frequency for *T* is 0.9 in a given population, what will be the frequency of short-stemmed pea plants in the population? 14.____
   A. 0.1 B. 0.01 C. 0.5 D. 0.05 E. 0.15

15. The pituitary gland is attached to and secretes its hormones in response to neurahormonal stimulation from the 15.____
   A. thalamus
   B. hypothalamus
   C. cerebrum
   D. medullaoblongata
   E. cerebellum

16. To say that the genetic code is *degenerate* means that 16.____
   A. a given codon may specify more than one amino acid
   B. a given amino acid may be specified by more than one codon
   C. some of the codons are nonsense codons
   D. the code is nonoverlapping
   E. nonsense suppressor mutations occur in tRNA genes

17. When mammalian eyes become accommodated for close vision, the 17.____
   A. ciliary muscles are contracted and the lens becomes more convex
   B. ciliary muscles are relaxed and the lens becomes more convex
   C. ciliary muscles are contracted and the lens becomes flattened
   D. ciliary muscles are relaxed and the lens becomes flattened
   E. eyeball undergoes auteroposterior shortening

18. The movement of materials across a cell membrane from a region of low concentration to a region of high concentration 18.____
   A. is termed free diffusion
   B. occurs only in osmosis
   C. requires the expenditure of energy
   D. is termed faciliated diffusion
   E. none of the above

19. The liver of the mammal has many important functions. One function is the synthesis of a nitrogen waste product in the form of 19.____
   A. ammonia
   B. urea
   C. nitrates
   D. nitric acid
   E. nitrous oxide

20. Which of the following organs plays a major role in the immune function? 20.____
   A. Thyroid
   B. Pituitary
   C. Pancreas
   D. Pineal
   E. Thymus

21. The phylum chordata is usually judged to be *most closely* related to the 21.____
   A. Arthropoda
   B. Annelida
   C. Echinodermata
   D. Mollusca
   E. Coelenterata

22. The organelle MOST involved in the energy-producing functions of the cell is the 22.____
   A. nucleus
   B. Golgi complex
   C. ER
   D. mitochondrion
   E. ribosome

23. A feature common to the chromosomes of both prokaryotic and eukaryotic cells is the 23.____
   A. presence of DNA and histones in about equal amounts
   B. circularity of the DNA molecules
   C. involvement of DNA polymerase in chromosomal replication
   D. presence of the pyrimidines uracil and cytosine
   E. location of the chromosomes within a cell

24. Which of the following is homeothermic? 24.____
   A. Pisces
   B. Amphibia
   C. Aves
   D. Reptilia
   E. Insects

25. Mammalian somatic motor neurons 25.____
   A. leave the spinal cord via the ventral root
   B. enter the spinal cord via the dorsal root
   C. innervate pressure receptors in muscle
   D. have their cell bodies outside the spinal cord
   E. innervate visceral organs

26. If a portion of a DNA base sequence is G-A-T, the complementary portion of a mRNA base sequence must be 26.____
   A. C-T-A
   B. C-T-U
   C. C-U-A
   D. G-A-T
   E. C-U-U

27. The amylase present in saliva is *most likely* to be involved in the digestion of which component of a bacon, lettuce and tomato sandwich? 27.____
   A. Bacon
   B. Lettuce
   C. Tomato
   D. Bun
   E. Butter

28. 28.____

INITIAL SOLUTION CONCENTRATIONS

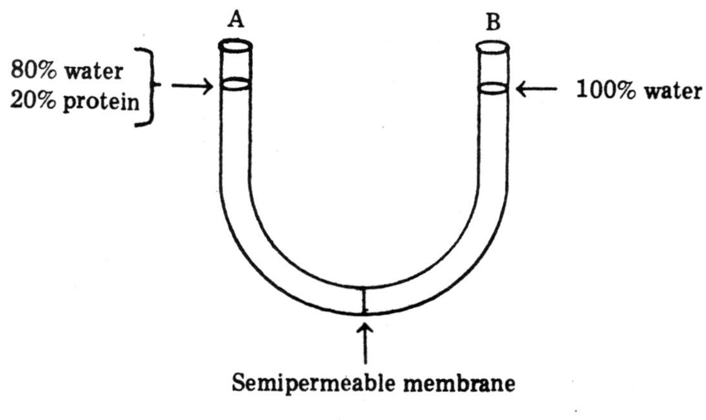

In the U-shaped tube with a semipermeable membrane separating Solution A from Solution B in the diagram on the preceding page, the water level will
- A. rise inside A, because water will pass from the area of greater concentration of water to the area of lesser concentration of water
- B. rise inside B, because water will pass from the area of lesser concentration of water to the area of greater concentration of water
- C. rise inside B as the protein concentration equalizes on both sides
- D. remain the same because atmospheric pressure is equal on both sides of the system
- E.

29. All of the solar energy that is converted by photosynthesis into the biomass of an ecosystem is ultimately lost from the ecosystem as 29.____
    - A. exports of biomass
    - B. organisms die
    - C. more biomass is produced
    - D. heat
    - E. decreased entropy

30. The majority of the known species of multicellular animals in the animal kingdom are characterized by 30.____
    - A. no skeleton
    - B. bony exoskeleton
    - C. chitinous endoskeleton
    - D. bony endoskeleton
    - E. chitinous exoskeleton

31. Which of the following is one of the morphogenetic movements that forms the gastrula of vertebrate embryos? 31.____
    - A. Differentiation
    - B. Cleavage
    - C. Metamorphosis
    - D. Induction
    - E. Invagination

32. In adult mammals, a blood vessel that carries deoxygenated blood is the 32.____
    - A. dorsal aorta
    - B. ventral aorta
    - C. pulmonary vein
    - D. pulmonary artery
    - E. coronary artery

33. Peptide linkages are found in 33.____
    - A. enzymes
    - B. nucleic acids
    - C. nucleosides
    - D. fatty acids
    - E. carbohydrates

34. ATP is a chemical compound classified as a 34.____
    - A. nucleoside
    - B. nucleotide
    - C. nucleic acid
    - D. deoxyriboside
    - E. nucleopeptide

35. When toxic nonbiodegradable fat-soluble organic chemicals, such as DDT, are introduced into an ecosystem, they become 35.____

A. diluted and dispersed as they pass through the food chain
B. harmless as organisms excrete them into the environment
C. less toxic in higher trophic levels
D. an energy source for tertiary consumers
E. more concentrated in successive levels of the food chain

36. During contraction of vertebrate striated muscle cells, 36.____

I. the thick filaments slide past the thin filaments in an energy-dependent process
II. calcium ions are pumped rapidly into the sarcoplasmic reticulum
III. the creatine phosphate concentration in the cell rises
IV. the actin molecules of the thin filament contract
V. the myosin molecules are replaced by tropomyosin

The CORRECT answer is:

A. I
B. I, III
C. I, IV
D. I, II, III, IV
E. IV *only*

37. A *basic* difference between all prokaryotic and all eukaryotic cells is that prokaryotic cells lack a 37.____

A. cell wall
B. plasma membrane
C. centriole
D. chlorophyll
E. nuclear envelope

38. All flowering plants are classified as 38.____

A. bryophytes
B. phytoplankton
C. gymnosperms
D. angiosperms
E. sea anemones

39. Escherichia coli is a common intestinal bacterium. One would expect a typical E. coli cell to be about the size of a(n) 39.____

A. human liver cell
B. polyribosome
C. amoeba
D. mitochondrion
E. microfilament

40. Hemophilia is a sex-linked disease characterized by the inability of blood to clot. Prince Frederick was a hemophiliac. 40.____
Which statement must be TRUE of Frederick's family? His

A. mother must have been a carrier
B. father must have been a hemophiliac
C. grandfather must have been a carrier
D. sister must have been a hemophiliac
E. uncle could have been a carrier

41. In the oxidation-reduction reaction 41.____

$$2MnO_4^- + 5C_2O_4^{2-} + 16H^+ \rightarrow 2Mn^{2+} + 10CO_2 + 8H_2O$$

the oxidation number of each carbon atom changes from
A. +2 to +4 B. +3 to +6 C. +3 to +4
D. +4 to +2 E. +3 to +2

42. Considering the nuclear reaction below, what is X? 42.____

$$X + \text{proton} \rightarrow {}^{22}Mg + \text{neutron}$$

A. ^{22}Na B. ^{23}Na C. ^{21}Mg D. ^{23}Mg E. ^{21}Ne

43. Which trend in the halogen family occurs with increasing atomic number? 43.____
A. *Decreasing* ionic radius
B. *Decreasing* melting points
C. *Increasing* covalent radius
D. *Increasing* electronegativity
E. *Increasing* first ionization potential

44. In which of the following species does phosphorus exhibit its *highest* oxidation number? 44.____
A. PCl_3 B. P_4 C. H_3PO_3 D. PH_3 E. P_2O_5

45. In which of the following solutions would CaF_2 be LEAST soluble? 45.____
A. 0.01M $CaCl_2$ B. 0.02M $CaCl_2$
C. 0.01M NaF D. 0.02M NaF
E. 0.02M NaCl

46. A mixture of gases containing CO_2 and SO_2 is allowed to effuse from one container through a pinhole into a second container which has been evacuated. 46.____
A. The rate of effusion for CO_2 is *faster* because the molecules of CO_2 are *lighter*.
B. The rate of effusion for SO_2 is *faster* because the molecules of SO_2 are *lighter*.
C. The rate of effusion for CO_2 is *slower* because the molecules of CO_2 are *lighter*.
D. The rate of effusion for SO_2 is *faster* because the molecules of SO_2 are *heavier*.
E. Both compounds will effuse at the same rate since they are both at the same temperature.

47. The numbers of protons and neutrons, respectively, in $^{17}_{8}O^{2-}$ are 47.____
A. 8, 17 B. 8, 10 C. 9, 8 D. 6, 17 E. 8, 9

48. The percent composition, by weight, of nitrogen in the compound $(NH_4)_2Cr_2O_7$ is (Atomic weights: H = 1, N = 14, O = 16, Cr = 52) 48.____

A. $$\frac{14}{14 + 4(1) + 2(52) + 7(16)} \times 100$$

B. $$\frac{2(14)}{2(14) + 8(1) + 2(52) + 7(16)} \times 100$$

C. $\frac{14}{14 + 1 + 52 + 16}$ x 100

D. $\frac{2(14)}{2(14) + 4(1) + 2(52) + 7(16)}$ x 100

E. $\frac{2(14)}{8(1) + 2(52) + 7(16)}$ x 100

49. How many unpaired electrons are in the ground state of a selenium atom (Z=34)? 49.____
A. One B. Two C. Three D. Four E. Zero

50. The PRINCIPAL attractive force contributing to lattice energy in an ionic solid is 50.____
A. coulombic repulsion
B. electrostatic attraction
C. London forces
D. Van der Waals forces
E. hydrogen bonding

51. Which gives the MOST basic solution when dissolved in water? 51.____
A. H_3PO_4
B. NaH_2PO_4
C. P_2O_5
D. $NaNO_3$
E. $P_2O_5Na_3PO_4$

52. How many liters of 5.0 molar ethyl alcohol (C_2H_5OH) can be prepared by dissolving 460 grams of ethyl alcohol in water? (C_2H_5OH M.W. = 46) 52.____
A. 0.5 B. 10 C. 2.0 D. 50 E. 5.0

53. What is the molarity of a solution resulting from the addition of 200 ml of 0.6M H_2SO_4 to 500 ml of 0.4M H_2SO_4 solution? 53.____

A. $\frac{(0.6)(0.2) + (0.4)(0.5)}{0.7}$

B. $\frac{0.6 + 0.4}{2}$

C. $\frac{200/0.6 + 500/0.4}{700}$

D. $\frac{(0.6)(200) + (0.4)(500)}{1000}$

E. (0.6)(200) + (0.4)(500)

54. What is the geometry of SO_2 and the hybridization of the central atom? 54.____
A. Linear, sp
B. Linear, sp^2
C. Bent, sp
D. Bent, sp^2
E. Triangular, sp^3

55. The data shown below were obtained for the reaction 55.____
$A + 2B \rightarrow 2C + D$

Experiment	Initial [A](M)	Initial [B](M)	Initial rate of appearance of D ($M\ min^{-1}$)
1	1.0×10^{-4}	1.0×10^{-2}	0.65×10^{-6}
2	2.0×10^{-4}	1.0×10^{-2}	1.30×10^{-6}
3	2.0×10^{-4}	0.50×10^{-2}	0.65×10^{-6}
4	0.50×10^{-4}	2.0×10^{-2}	0.65×10^{-6}

According to these data, the rate law for this system is rate =

A. $k\frac{[C]^2\ [D]}{[A]\ [B]^2}$ B. k[A][B] C. $k[A][B]^2$

D. $k[B]^2$ E. k[A]

56. The rate of most reactions tends to double with a 10°C increase in temperature. This is thought to be due to a(n) 56.____

A. *decrease* in the activation energy
B. *increase* in the activation energy
C. *increase* in the equilibrium constant
D. *increase* in the fraction of molecules possessing at least the activation energy
E. *decrease* in the fraction of molecules possessing at least the activation energy

57. Which reaction has the MOST positive value of ΔS? 57.____

A. $2NO_{2(g)} \rightarrow N_2O_{4(l)}$ B. $2NO_{2(g)} \rightarrow N_2O_{4(g)}$

C. $N_2O_{4(l)} \rightarrow 2NO_{2(g)}$ D. $N_2O_{4(g)} \rightarrow 2NO_{2(g)}$

E. $N_2O_{4(l)} \rightarrow 2NO_{2(l)}$

58. The trigonal planar BCl_3 molecule is nonpolar. What is the explanation for this? 58.____

A. Boron and chlorine have the same electro-negativity.
B. The net polarity is zero due to the symmetry of the molecule.
C. The polarity of each boron-chlorine bond is zero.
D. Boron and chlorine have the same electron affinity.
E. The electron density around the boron is the same as around the chlorine.

59. Which of the following will produce a change in the value of the equilibrium constant for a reaction? 59.____

A. *Increase* the concentration of reactant
B. *Decrease* the concentration of product
C. Addition of a suitable catalyst
D. *Increase* the temperature of the reaction
E. All of the above

60. When 1.00 g of liquid water (M.W. = 18.0) is produced from H_2 and O_2 at a constant temperature (25°C) and pressure (1 atm), 15.8 kilojoules are produced. What is the molar heat of formation of liquid water, in kilojoules? 60.____

A. -15.8 x 18.0 B. 15.8 x 18.0

C. $\frac{15.8}{18.0}$ D. $\frac{-15.8}{18.0}$

E. $\frac{-18.0}{15.8}$

61. Consider Crystalline solids made from the following types of particles. Which type of particles gives the solid with the LOWEST melting point? 61.____

A. Small non-polar molecules
B. Small polar molecules
C. Positive and negative ions
D. Positive ions and mobile electrons
E. Atoms covalently bonded in a continuous array

62. If the Group Numbers of elements x and z in the Periodic Table are VIA and VIIA, respectively, then what is the overall charge on the following Lewis dot formula? 62.____

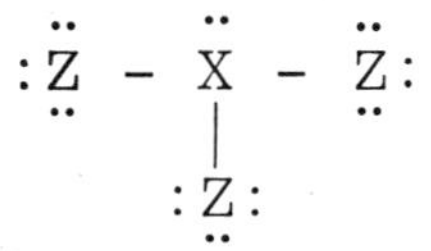

A. +1 B. -1 C. +2 D. -2 E. +3

63. The equation for the Haber process for production of ammonia is $N_2 + 3H_2 \rightarrow 2NH_3$. What is the MAXIMUM number of moles of NH_3 which can be produced on reaction of a mixture containing 5 moles of N_2 and 6 moles of H_2? 63.____

A. 9 B. 10 C. 6 D. 2 E. 4

64. A liter of solution contains 0.00001 moles of hydrochloric acid. What is the pH of this solution? 64.____

A. 1.0 B. 4.0 C. -4.0 D. -5.0 E. 5.0

65. When solid NaOH is added to water, it dissolves and the solution becomes warm (sometimes even hot!). The signs of ΔG, ΔH, and ΔS, respectively, are 65.____

A. +, +, + B. +, -, +
C. -, -, - D. -, +, +
E. -, -, +

66. The unbalanced equation for the oxidation of ammonia is: 66.____

$$NH_3 + O_2 \rightarrow NO + H_2O$$

After balancing the equation, which is the CORRECT set of coefficients for the substances from left to right?

A. 2, 3, 2, 3 B. 3, 2, 3, 2
C. 4, 5, 4, 6 D. 4, 6, 4, 6
E. 2, 2, 2, 3

67. Which substance is oxidized in this reaction? 67.___

$3Cu + 8H^+ + 2NO_3^- \rightarrow 3Cu^{2+} + 2NO + 4H_2O$

A. NO　　B. NO_3^-　　C. H^+　　D. Cu　　E. Cu^{2+}

68. Experimentally, it was found that 1.5×10^{-6} moles of $BaSO_4$ would dissolve in one liter of 0.001M Na_2SO_4 solution. 68.___
Assuming ideal solution behavior, what is the solubility product constant for $BaSO_4$?

A. $(1.5 \times 10^{-6})^2$　　B. $(1.5 \times 10^{-6})^2(10^{-3})$

C. $\frac{(1.5 \times 10^{-6})^2}{10^{-3}}$　　D. $(1.5 \times 10^{-6})(10^{-3})$

E. $\frac{10^3}{1.5 \times 10^{-6}}$

69. Which one of the following concentration terms is temperature dependent? 69.___

A. % by weight　　B. Molality
C. Molarity　　D. Mole fraction
E. None of the above

70. What is the molecular weight of an ideal gas if a 15.0 g sample occupies 25.5 liters at 100°C and 1 atmosphere of pressure? 70.___

A. $\frac{(15)(0.082)(100)}{(1)(25.5)}$　　B. $\frac{(15)(0.082)(373)}{(1)(25.5)}$

C. $\frac{(15)(82.0)(100)}{(1)(25.5)}$　　D. $\frac{(15)(82.0)(373)}{(760)(25.5)}$

E. $\frac{(15)(0.082)(373)}{(760)(25.5)}$

71. Which compound gives the BEST yield of a *single* alkene on treatment with ethanolic KOH? 71.___

A.
```
       CH3
        |
  CH3 — C — CH3
        |
        OH
```

B.
```
         Br
         |
  CH3 —CH—CH2—CH3
```

C. 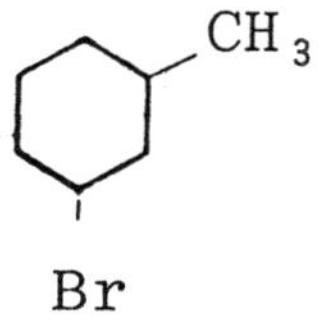

D. 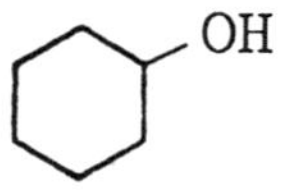

E.
```
               Br
               |
  CH3—CH2—CH—CH2—CH3
```

72. Which of the following reactions would give 72.____

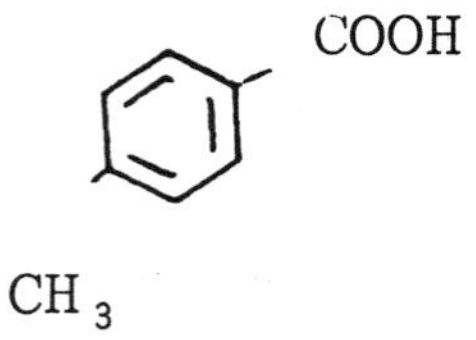

A. CH_3MgBr + 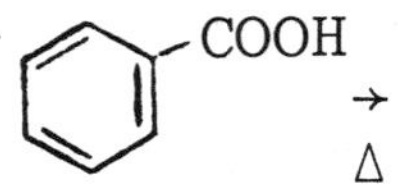

B. CH_3OH + 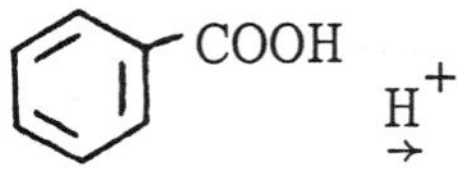

C. 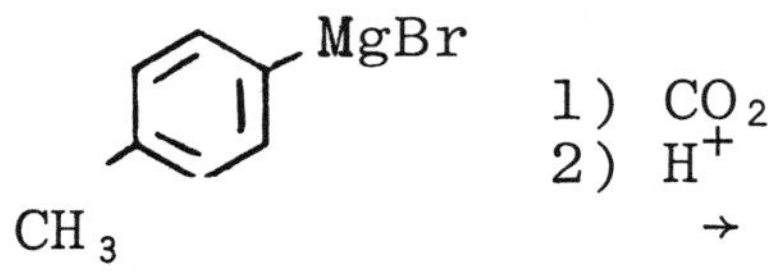

D. $NaHCO_3$ + 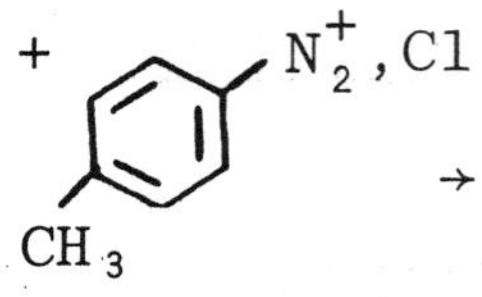

E. $LiAlH_4$ + 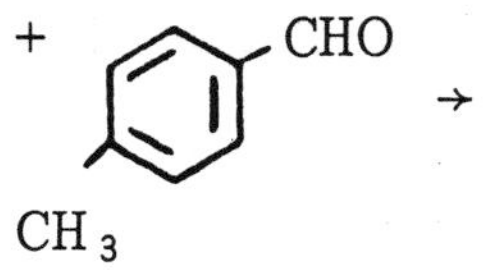

73. What is the product of the following reaction? 73.____

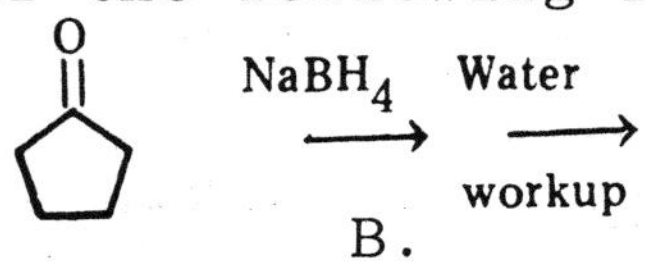

A. 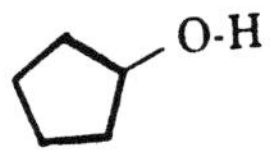

B. 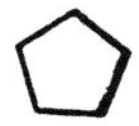

C. $HO_2C\text{-}CH_2CH_2CH_2CO_2H$

D. 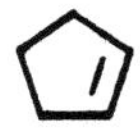

E. 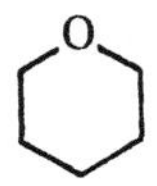

74. Which of the following is the STRONGEST acid? 74.____

A. $ClCH_2CH_2CO_2H$

B. Cl_2CHCO_2H

C. $CH_3CHClCO_2H$

D. $ClCH_2CHClCO_2H$

E. $CH_3CH_2CO_2H$

75. Which of the following reactions will proceed by an S_N2 reaction mechanism? 75.____

A. $CH_3CH_2OH + K_2Cr_2O_7 \rightarrow CH_3\text{-}\overset{O}{C}\text{-}OH$

B. $CH_4 + O_2 \xrightarrow[\text{heat}]{} CO_2 + H_2O$

C. $CH_3CH_2Br + NaNH_2 \rightarrow CH_2{=}CH_2 + NaBr + NH$

D. $CH_3CH_2Br + NaCN \rightarrow CH_3CH_2CN + NaBr$

E. $CH_3{-}CH{=}CH_2 + HBr \rightarrow CH_3{-}CH(Br){-}CH_3$

76. Which of the following statements is TRUE for the S_N2 reaction shown below? 76.____

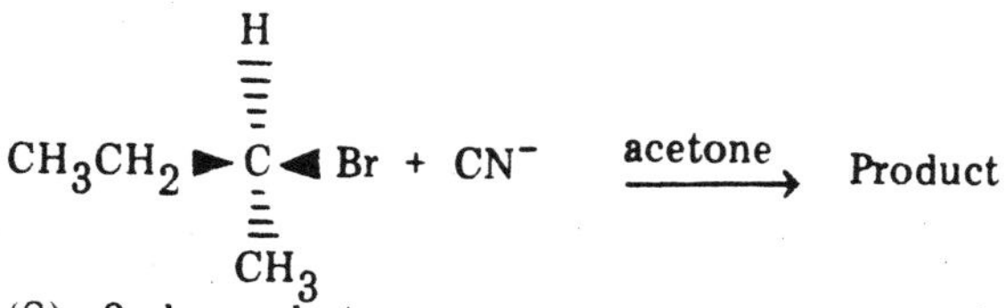

(S) - 2 - bromobutane

A. The product will be a racemate.
B. A change in the concentration of the cyanide ion will not alter the rate of reaction.
C. A carbocation intermediate will be formed.
D. The reaction will occur with inversion of configuration.
E. The reaction will occur with retention of configuration.

77. What is the reagent and reaction condition that will bring about the conversion of benzoic acid to benzoyl chloride? 77.____

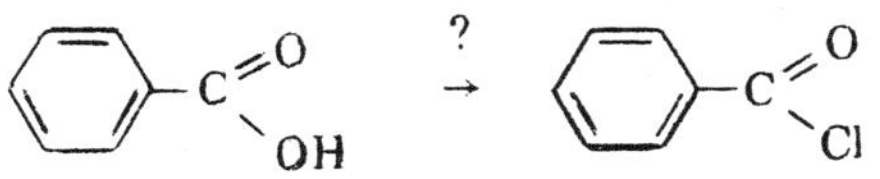

A. HCl (in CCl_4)
B. CH_3Cl (reflux)
C. Fe, Cl_2
D. $SOCl_2$ (reflux)
E. $AlCl_3$

78. Which alcohol undergoes acid-catalyzed dehydration MOST readily when heated with concentrated sulfuric acid? 78.____

A. $CH_3CH_2CH_2CH_2CH_2OH$

B. $CH_3CH(OH)CH_2CH_2CH_3$

C. 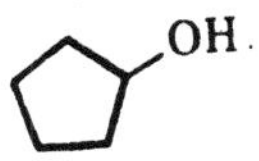

D. CH_3CH_2OH

E. $CH_3CH_2C(CH_3)_2OH$

79. D.(-)-Ribose shown below contains how many chiral centers? 79. ____

A. One

B. Two

C. Three

D. Four

E. None

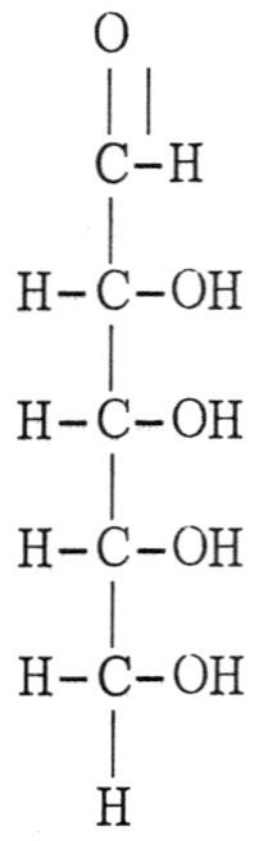

D-(-)-Ribose

80. Which of the following phenols is the STRONGEST acid? 80. ____

A. 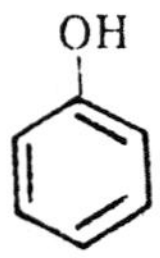

B. 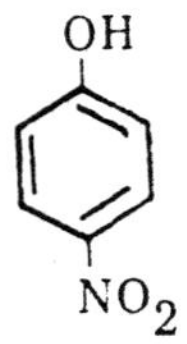

C. 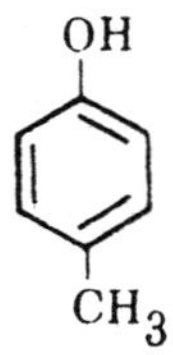

D. 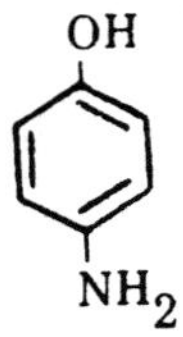

E. 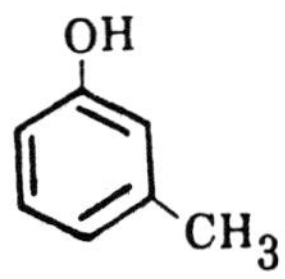

81. Reaction of 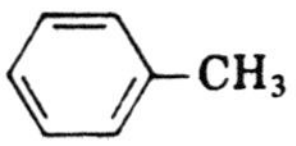 with a mixture of HNO_3 and H_2SO_4 would give predominately which of the following compounds? 81. ____

A. 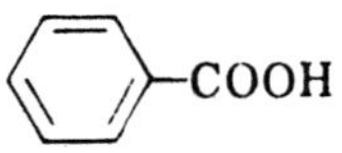

B. 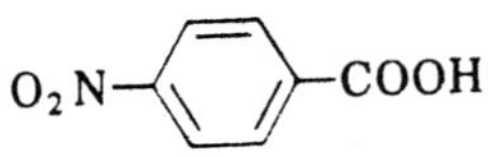

C. 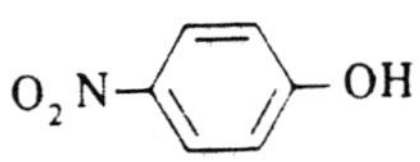

D. 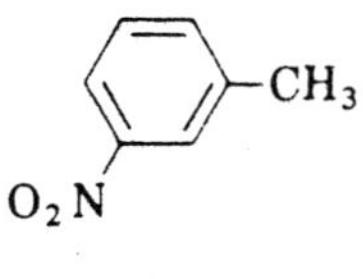

E. 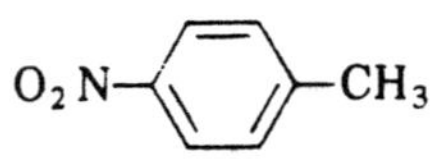

82. In the bromination of benzene ($Br_2/FeBr_3$), one of the reactive intermediates is: 82.____

A. 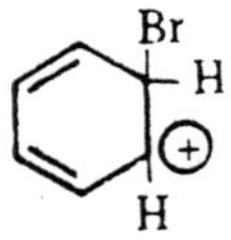

B. 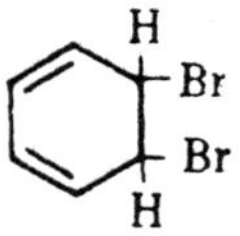

C. 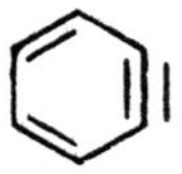

D. 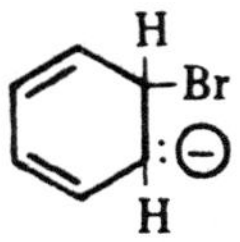

E. 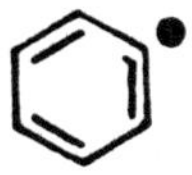

83. Which compound is *most likely* to have an infrared spectrum with a large peak between 1750-1700 cm^{-1} (5.77-5.88μ)? 83.____

A. CH_3-O-CH_3

B. $CH_3-\overset{O}{\overset{||}{C}}-CH_3$

C. $CH_3-CH_2-\overset{-H}{\overset{|}{N}}-CH_2-CH_3$

D. CH_3-CH_2-OH

E. CH_3-CH_2-I

84. How many hydrogens in the compound below are exchangeable with the deuterium in D_2O under basic catalysis? 84.____

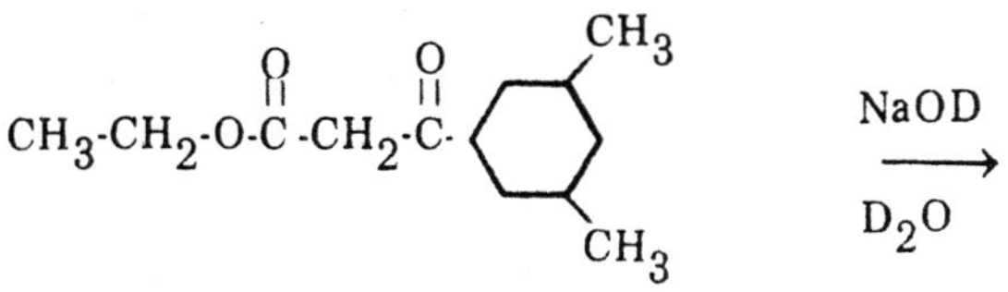

A. Two
B. Four
C. Five
D. Seven
E. Thirteen

85. Propionaldehyde, CH_3CH_2CHO, is allowed to react with ethyl magnesium bromide, CH_3CH_2MgBr. Upon hydrolysis, compound A is formed. Oxidation of A by potassium dichromate-sulfuric acid gives compound B. 85.____
What is B?

A. $CH_3CH_2\overset{O}{\overset{||}{C}}CH_3$

B. $CH_3CH_2\overset{O}{\overset{||}{C}}CH_2CH_3$

C. $CH_3CH_2\overset{OH}{\overset{||}{C}}HCH_2CH_3$

D. (CH_3CH_2) COH

E. $CH_3CH_2CH_2OCH_2CH_3$

86. What is the product of the following sequence of reactions? 86.____

$$CH_3\text{-}CH_2\text{-}CH_2\text{-}\overset{O}{\overset{\|}{C}}\text{-}OH \xrightarrow{SOCl_2} A \xrightarrow[\text{excess}]{NH_3} B$$

A. $CH_3\text{-}CH_2\text{-}\overset{NH_2}{\overset{|}{C}H}\text{-}\overset{O}{\overset{\|}{C}}\text{-}OH$

B. $CH_3\text{-}CH_2\text{-}CH_2\text{-}CH_2\text{-}NH_2$

C. $CH_3\text{-}CH_2\text{-}CH_2\text{-}CH_2\text{-}Cl$

D. $CH_3\text{-}CH_2\text{-}CH_2\text{-}\overset{O}{\overset{\|}{C}}\text{-}NH_2$

E. 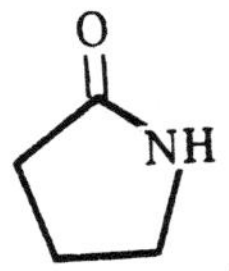

87. Which of the following is NOT an ester? 87.____

A. $CH_3\text{-}\overset{O}{\overset{\|}{C}}\text{-}O\text{-}CH_3$

B. $H\text{-}\overset{O}{\overset{\|}{C}}\text{-}O\text{-}CH_2\text{-}CH_3$

C. $CH_3\text{-}\underset{H}{\underset{|}{\overset{O\text{-}CH_3}{\overset{|}{C}}}}\text{-}O\text{-}CH_3$

D. $CH_3\text{-}O\text{-}\overset{O}{\overset{\|}{C}}\text{-}H$

E. 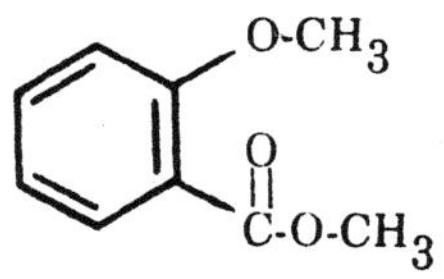

88. The correct hybridization state of the central carbon in neopentane, 88.____

$$CH_3\text{—}\underset{CH_3}{\underset{|}{\overset{CH_3}{\overset{|}{C}}}}\text{—}CH_3$$

and the approximate angles between the C-C bonds is

A. sp^2 and 120°

B. sp^3 and 90°

C. sp and 180°

D. sp^3 and 109°

E. sp and 109°

89. What is the product of the following reaction? 89.____

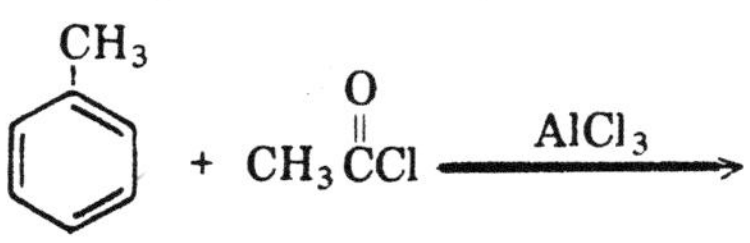

A. 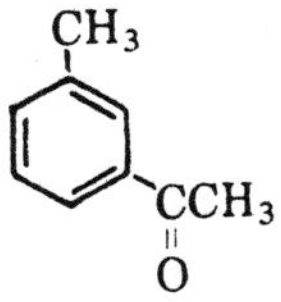

B. 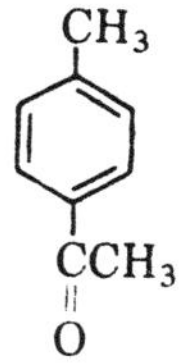

C. 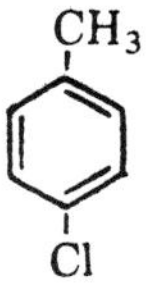

D. 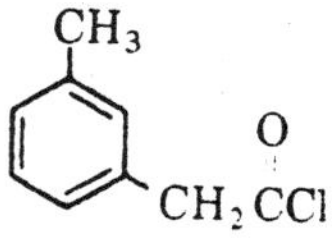

E. 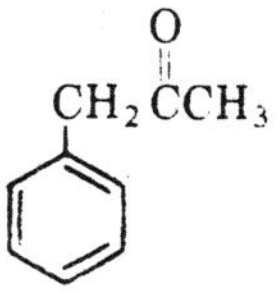

90. Aniline ($C_6H_5NH_2$) will react *most rapidly* with 90.____

A. 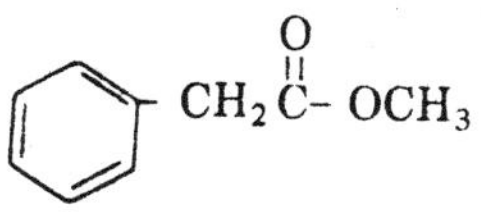

B. 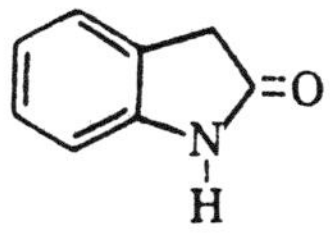

C. $(CH_3)_2CH\text{-}\overset{\overset{O}{\|}}{C}\text{-}Cl$

D. 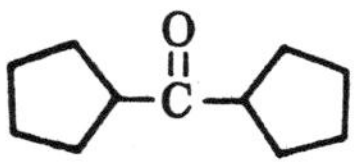

E. 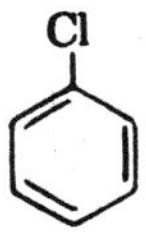

91. In the reaction sequence 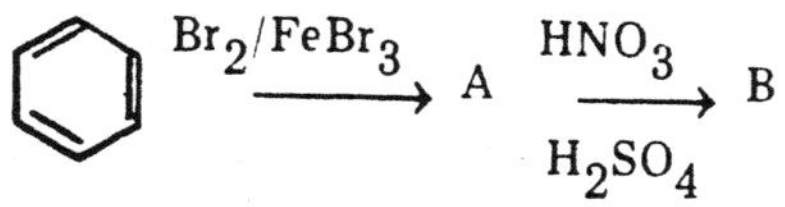 91.____

the MAJOR product is:

A. 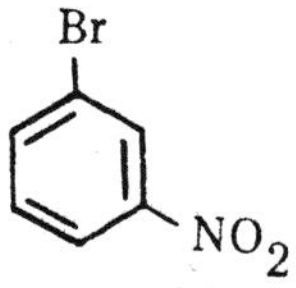

B. 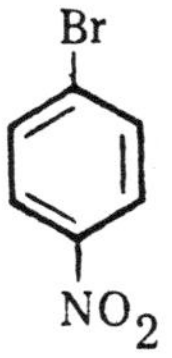

C. 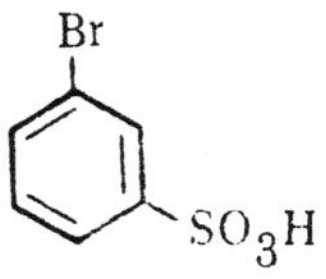

D. 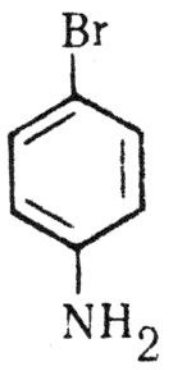

E. 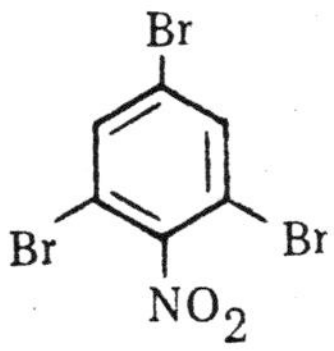

92. From the following compounds (which have similar molecular weights), select the one which has the *highest* boiling point. 92.____

A. $CH_3CH_2\underset{\underset{O}{\|}}{C}CH_3$ B. $CH_3CH_2OCH_2CH_3$

C. $CH_3CH_2CO_2H$

D. $CH_3CH_2CH_2CH_2OH$

E. $CH_3CH_2CH_2CH_2CH_3$

93. Which of the following is a product of 93.____

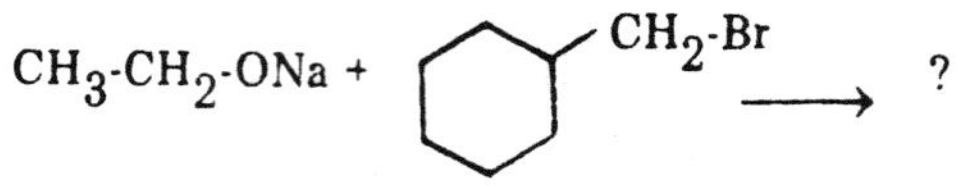

A. 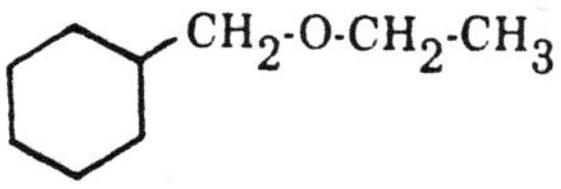

B. 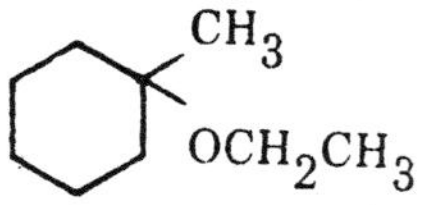

C. 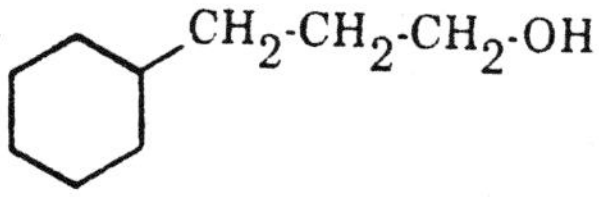

D. 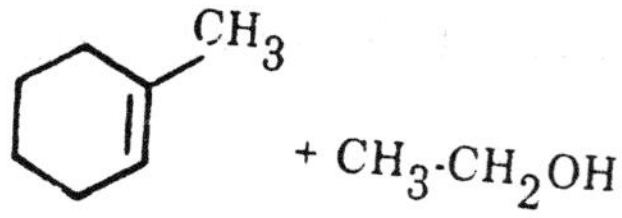

E. 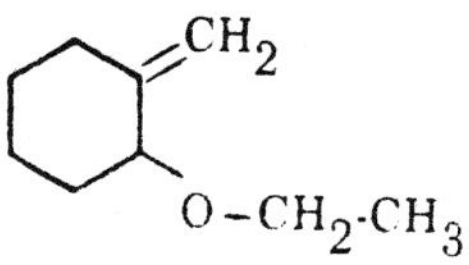

94. Which of the following reactions listed below would have the *lowest* energy of activation (E act.)? 94.____

A. $Cl{-}Cl \rightarrow Cl\cdot + Cl\cdot$

B. $Cl\cdot + CH_3{-}H \rightarrow HCl + \cdot CH_3$

C. $CH_3{-}CH_3 \rightarrow \cdot CH_3 + \cdot CH_3$

D. $\cdot CH_3 + Cl{-}Cl \rightarrow CH_3{-}Cl + Cl\cdot$

E. $\cdot CH_3 + \cdot CH_3 \rightarrow CH_3{-}CH_3$

95. Which of the following compounds will undergo nitration the *fastest* when treated with a mixture of concentrated H_2SO_4 and HNO_3? 95.____

A. 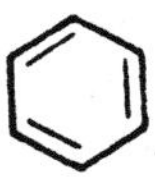

B. 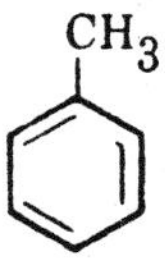

C. 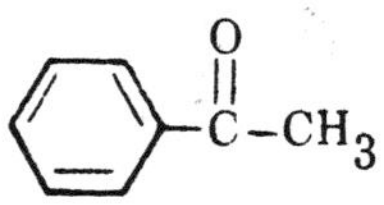

D. 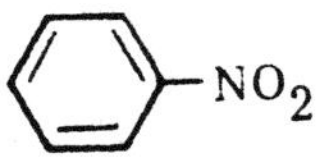

E. 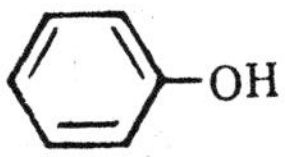

96. Which of the following compounds is capable of intramolecular (internal) hydrogen bonding? 96.____

A. 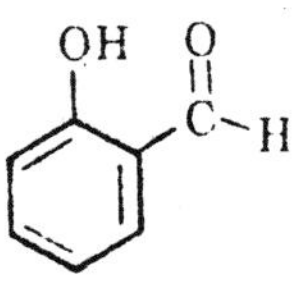

B. 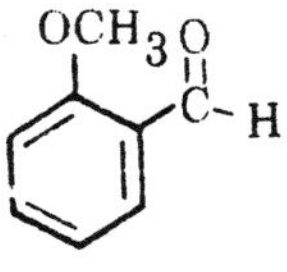

C. 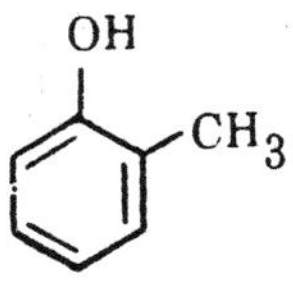

D. 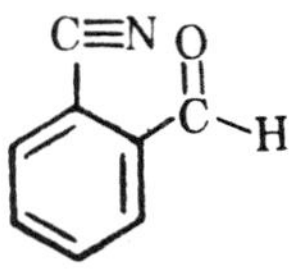

E. 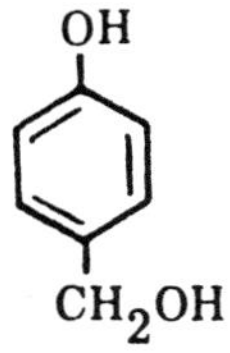

97. Select the IUPAC name for 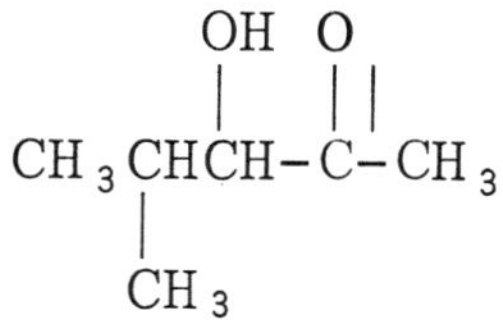 97.___

A. 3-hydroxy-2-hexanone
B. 3-hydroxy-4-hexanone
C. 3-hydroxy-2-methyl-4-pentanoate
D. 3-hydroxy-4-methyl-2-pentanal
E. 3-hydroxy-4-methyl-2-pentanone

98. Which of the following is achiral and, therefore, will NOT rotate plane polarized light? 98.___

A. 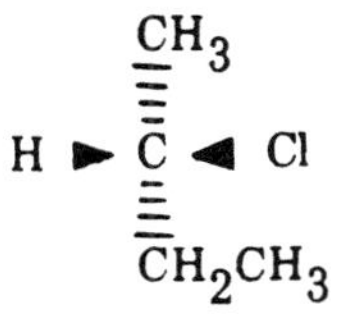

B. an equimolar mixture of

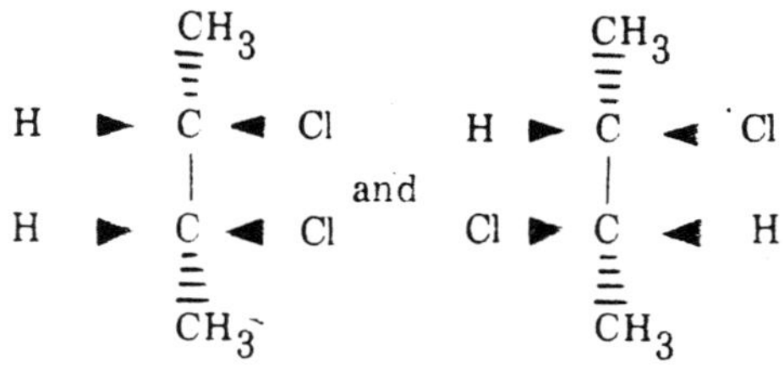

C. 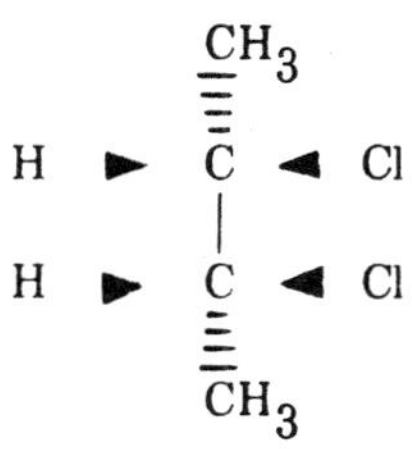

D. 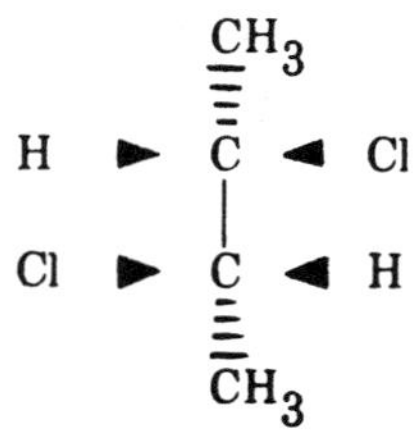

E. 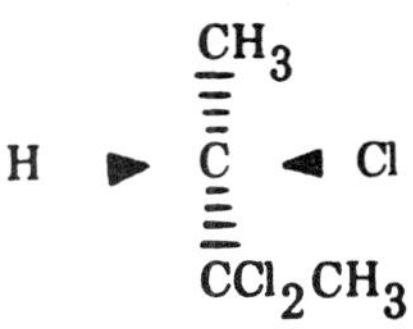

99. Which compound is chiral and, therefore, has a nonsuperimposable mirror image? 99.___

A. 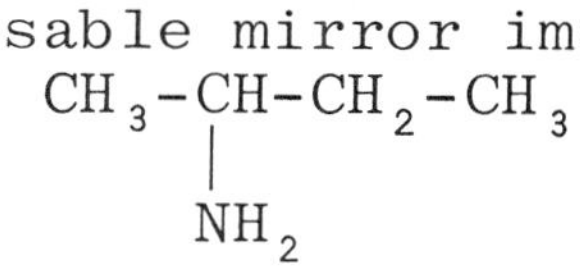

B. $CH_3-CH_2-CH_2-CH_2-NH_2$

C. $CH_3-\underset{\displaystyle CH_3}{\underset{|}{CH}}-CH_2-NH_2$

D. $CH_3-CH_2-\underset{\displaystyle NH_2}{\underset{|}{CH}}-CH_2-CH_3$

E.

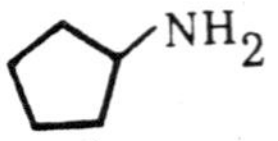

100. The fact that the allyl carbocation ($CH_2=CH-\overset{+}{C}H_2$) is more stable than primary carbocations such as $CH_3CH_2\overset{+}{C}H_2$ can BEST be accounted for on the basis of 100.___

A. lack of steric hindrance in the allyl carbocation
B. tautomerism in the allyl carbocation
C. the electron withdrawing characteristic of the double bond in the allyl carbocation
D. resonance stabilization of the allyl carbocation
E. hydrogen bonding in the allyl carbocation

KEY (CORRECT ANSWERS)

1. E	21. C	41. C	61. A	81. E
2. B	22. D	42. A	62. A	82. A
3. B	23. C	43. C	63. E	83. B
4. A	24. C	44. E	64. E	84. A
5. A	25. A	45. D	65. E	85. B
6. A	26. C	46. A	66. C	86. D
7. C	27. D	47. E	67. D	87. C
8. C	28. A	48. B	68. D	88. D
9. D	29. D	49. B	69. C	89. B
10. E	30. E	50. B	70. B	90. C
11. E	31. E	51. E	71. E	91. B
12. C	32. D	52. C	72. C	92. C
13. B	33. A	53. A	73. A	93. A
14. B	34. B	54. D	74. B	94. E
15. B	35. E	55. B	75. D	95. E
16. B	36. A	56. D	76. D	96. A
17. A	37. E	57. C	77. D	97. E
18. C	38. D	58. B	78. E	98. C
19. B	39. D	59. D	79. C	99. A
20. E	40. A	60. A	80. B	100. D

EXAMINATION SECTION

TEST 1

DIRECTIONS: Each question or incomplete statement is followed by several suggested answers or completions. Select the one that BEST answers the question or completes the statement. *PRINT THE LETTER OF THE CORRECT ANSWER IN THE SPACE AT THE RIGHT.*

1. In MOST carbohydrate molecules, the ratio of hydrogen atoms to oxygen atoms is 1.___
   A. 1:2 B. 2:1 C. 3:1 D. 1:3

2. Which compound is inorganic? 2.___
   A. Amino acid B. Protein
   C. Nucleic acid D. Water

3. An intern has a microscope with a 10x eyepiece and 10x and 40x objectives. He observed 40 onion epidermal cells across the diameter of his low-power field. 3.___
   The number of cells he would MOST probably observe under high power would be
   A. 1 B. 40 C. 10 D. 4

4. Which organelle is found inside the nucleus of an animal cell? 4.___
   A. Centriole B. Nucleolus
   C. Chloroplast D. Mitochondrion

5. In an Ameba, the process of engulfing organisms is MOST closely associated with the life function known as 5.___
   A. respiration B. excretion
   C. nutrition D. reproduction

6. All the chemical reactions that take place within a plant or animal cell are known as 6.___
   A. transport B. synthesis
   C. respiration D. metabolism

7. If the contractile fibers of a certain animal permit a limited amount of movement, but the animal remains in a fixed position much of the time, it is referred to as being 7.___
   A. phototropic B. motile
   C. autotrophic D. sessile

8. The BEST description of the nutritional pattern of a protozoan such as the Paramecium is 8.___
   A. heterotrophic and intracellular
   B. autotrophic and intracellular
   C. heterotrophic and extracellular
   D. autotrophic and extracellular

9. Which two organisms have a ventral nerve cord? 9.___
   A. Hydra and human
   B. Earthworm and human
   C. Earthworm and grasshopper
   D. Grasshopper and Hydra

10. An insect larva is about to undergo metamorphosis. Compared with a sample of fluid from this insect earlier in the larval stage, a sample of circulatory fluid from this insect at this time would NORMALLY show a(n) 10.___
   A. *decrease* in hemoglobin
   B. *decrease* in nitrogen content
   C. *increase* in blood cells
   D. *increase* in certain hormones

11. A similarity between enzymes and hormones is that both of these substances are 11.___
   A. chemical secretions of living things
   B. chemical excretions of living things
   C. substances used in treatment of bacterial infections
   D. substances used to promote mutations

12. Neurohumors are produced as the result of 12.___
   A. excretion in nephrons
   B. respiration in alveoli
   C. synthesis in nerve cells
   D. hydrolysis in muscle cells

13. Which environmental factor is DIRECTLY associated with the excretion of ammonia as the major nitrogenous waste from an organism? 13.___
   A. Intensity of sunlight
   B. Amount of water available
   C. Concentration of nitrogen in the soil
   D. Concentration of oxygen in the air

14. Which metabolic waste is produced as the result of the synthesis of maltose from two glucose molecules? 14.___
   A. Water
   B. Carbon dioxide
   C. Salt
   D. Urea

15. Compared to a cell that is carrying on anaerobic respiration, a cell that is carrying on aerobic respiration 15.___
   A. uses less oxygen
   B. uses less carbon dioxide
   C. produces more ATP
   D. produces more alcohol

16. In the grasshopper, the structure involved in respiratory gas exchange is the 16.___
   A. skin
   B. nephridium
   C. Malpighian tubule
   D. tracheal tubule

17. Molecules larger than the membrane pores of a cell could enter the cell by the process of 17.___
   A. diffusion
   B. osmosis
   C. pinocytosis
   D. cyclosis

18. In plants, the production of poisons, drugs, waxes, and fibers is a DIRECT result of 18.___
    A. respiration B. hydrolysis
    C. digestion D. synthesis

19. To be used by muscle cells, starch must be chemically converted to 19.___
    A. amino acids B. simple sugars
    C. fatty acids D. simple proteins

20. Organisms are classified as heterotrophs if they derive their metabolic energy from 20.___
    A. photosynthesis
    B. inorganic raw materials
    C. lightning
    D. preformed organic compounds

21. Which substance is produced as a result of the action of lipase? 21.___
    A. Fatty acid B. Protease
    C. Amino acid D. Glucose

22. By which process do carbon dioxide molecules leave a plant and enter the atmosphere? 22.___
    A. Digestion B. Osmosis
    C. Photosynthesis D. Diffusion

23. Growth responses in plants due to unequal auxin distribution are called 23.___
    A. tropisms B. mutations
    C. stimuli D. synapses

24. The diffusion of water molecules into and out of cells is called 24.___
    A. cyclosis B. pinocytosis
    C. osmosis D. homeostasis

25. The leaf structures closely associated with both transpiration and excretion are 25.___
    A. lenticels
    B. stomates
    C. waxy surfaces
    D. elongated epidermal cells

26. A functional difference between animals and green plants is that green plants are able to 26.___
    A. synthesize glucose
    B. break down carbohydrates
    C. carry on aerobic respiration
    D. carry on locomotion

27. The cells in the stem of a plant through which water is transported upward are known as _____ cells. 27.___
    A. epidermal B. guard
    C. phloem D. xylem

28. In a plant, starch molecules in the leaf cells are hydrolyzed 28.___
A. intracellularly B. extracellularly
C. by pinocytosis D. by osmosis

29. Autotrophic activity in green plant cells is MOST closely associated with organelles called 29.___
A. mitochondria B. ribosomes
C. vacuoles D. chloroplasts

30. Large numbers of motile aerobic bacteria accumulate along portions of a filament of green algae exposed to blue and red light. Few bacteria accumulate in areas exposed to green and yellow light. 30.___
The bacteria form this pattern because
A. bacteria need red and blue light for fermentation
B. more oxygen is released by algae cells in areas exposed to red and blue light
C. more glucose diffuses out of the algae cells exposed to green and yellow light
D. water is warmer in areas exposed to green and yellow light

---

KEY (CORRECT ANSWERS)

1. B	11. A	21. A
2. D	12. C	22. D
3. C	13. B	23. A
4. B	14. A	24. C
5. C	15. C	25. B
6. D	16. D	26. A
7. D	17. C	27. D
8. A	18. D	28. A
9. C	19. B	29. D
10. D	20. D	30. B

TEST 2

DIRECTIONS: Each question or incomplete statement is followed by several suggested answers or completions. Select the one that BEST answers the question or completes the statement. *PRINT THE LETTER OF THE CORRECT ANSWER IN THE SPACE AT THE RIGHT.*

1. The sperm cells produced by a male member of a species differ from the egg cells produced by a female member of the same species in that the sperm cells are 1.___
   A. smaller than the egg cells
   B. less numerous than the egg cells
   C. stationary, whereas egg cells are motile
   D. diploid, whereas egg cells are monoploid

2. Which statement is TRUE of budding? 2.___
   It
   A. produces zygotes by fertilization
   B. involves an equal division of cytoplasm
   C. produces gametes by meiosis
   D. is an asexual form of reproduction

3. Which occurs in the process of cleavage? 3.___
   A. Meiosis B. Regeneration
   C. Mitosis D. Synapsis

4. In Hydra, asexual reproduction differs from sexual reproduction in that asexual reproduction does NOT involve 4.___
   A. mitotic cell division B. cytoplasmic division
   C. fusion of nuclei D. division of the nucleus

5. External fertilization and external development are characteristic of 5.___
   A. bulldogs B. pigeons
   C. rattlesnakes D. trout

6. Which structure would be found in a plant cell during mitotic cell division but NOT in an animal cell? 6.___
   A. Centriole B. Centromere
   C. Cell plate D. Spindle apparatus

7. In normal human endocrine glands, mitotic cell division produces 7.___
   A. uncontrolled growth of cancerous tissue
   B. normal monoploid gametic tissue
   C. cells specialized for the secretion of hormones
   D. cells programmed for the production of hemoglobin

8. The cells in the petals of a particular flower each contain twenty-four chromosomes. 8.___
   A normal sperm nucleus produced in a pollen grain of this flower contains a MAXIMUM of _____ chromosomes.
   A. 6 B. 12 C. 18 D. 24

9. The development of a bee's egg without fertilization is known as 9.___
   A. meiosis B. replication
   C. metamorphosis D. parthenogenesis

10. Plant and animal breeders usually sell or destroy undesirable specimens and use only desirable ones for breeding. This practice is referred to as 10.___
   A. vegetative propagation B. artificial selection
   C. natural breeding D. random mating

11. Experimental evidence indicates that DNA is the genetic material. This evidence comes from studies involving 11.___
   A. bacterial transformations
   B. plant transpiration
   C. animal nutrition
   D. protozoan locomotion

12. Which diagram BEST illustrates the structure of a portion of a DNA molecule? 12.___

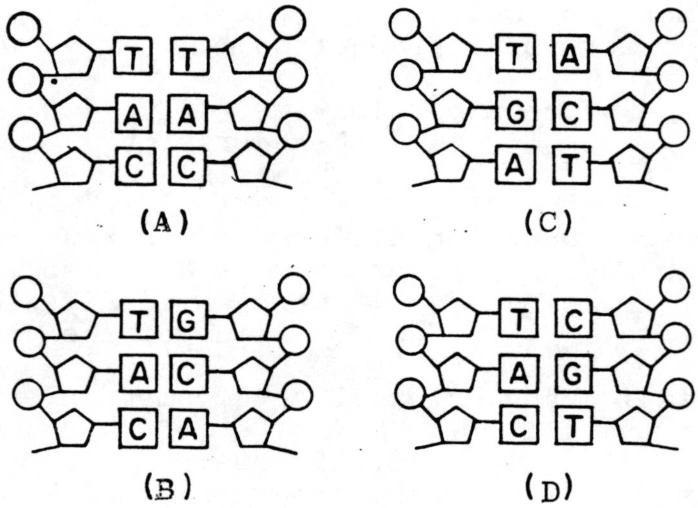

13. Changes in the genetic composition of a chromosome may be the result of 13.___
   A. nondisjunction B. crossing-over
   C. independent assortment D. replication

14. Two parents, both heterozygous for blood type A, produce a child. What are the chances that the child has blood type A? 14.___
   A. 1 out of 4 B. 1 out of 2
   C. 3 out of 4 D. 1 out of 1

15. When pure white and pure red four o'clocks are crossed, all the offspring are pink. 15.___
The phenotype of the offspring illustrates the pattern of inheritance known as
   A. dominance   B. segregation
   C. incomplete dominance   D. multiple alleles

16. In horses, black color is dominant over chestnut color. Two black horses produce both a black and a chestnut-colored offspring. 16.___
If coat color is controlled by a single pair of genes, it can BEST be assumed that
   A. in horses, genes for hair color frequently mutate
   B. one of the parent horses is homozygous dominant and the other is heterozygous for hair color
   C. both parent horses are homozygous for hair color
   D. both parent horses are heterozygous for hair color

17. When a strain of fruit flies homozygous for light body color is crossed with a strain of fruit flies homozygous for dark body color, all of the offspring have light body color. 17.___
This illustrates the principle of
   A. segregation   B. dominance
   C. incomplete dominance   D. independent assortment

18. A colorblind man marries a woman with normal vision. Her mother was colorblind. They have one child. 18.___
What is the chance that this child is colorblind?
   A. 0%   B. 25%   C. 50%   D. 100%

19. All of the following are kingdoms EXCEPT 19.___
   A. animal   B. protozoa   C. protist   D. plant

20. According to the heterotroph hypothesis, there was no free oxygen in the primitive atmosphere until the appearance of the early 20.___
   A. heterotrophs   B. saprophytes
   C. parasites   D. autotrophs

21. According to evolutionary theory, which group of organisms is believed to be among the EARLIEST to evolve on Earth? 21.___
   A. Birds   B. Algae   C. Mammals   D. Reptiles

22. Lamarck's theory involving the inheritance of acquired characteristics is based on the concept that 22.___
   A. the environment selects the adaptation of greatest survival value
   B. adaptations arise due to the needs of the organism
   C. cells are the unit of structure and function of living things
   D. more offspring are produced than can possibly survive

23. The forelegs of a frog and a horse are examples of structures that are 23.___
A. heterotrophic B. homozygous
C. hermaphroditic D. homologous

24. The similarity among the blood proteins of all the mammals may be taken as evidence for evolutionary relationships based upon 24.___
A. comparative anatomy B. geographic distribution
C. comparative embryology D. comparative biochemistry

25. 25.___

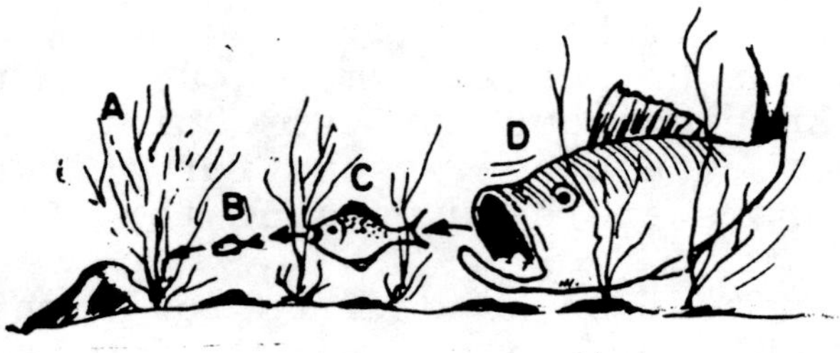

In the diagram of the food chain shown above, which organism represents the primary consumer?
A. A B. B C. C D. D

26. Different species of animals in a community would MOST likely be similar in 26.___
A. physical structure
B. size
C. abiotic requirements
D. number of offspring produced

27. When species of plants and animals are introduced into a new habitat, they often become pests in the new habitat, even though they were not pests in their native habitats. The MOST probable reason for this is that in the new habitat they 27.___
A. have fewer natural enemies
B. have a much lower mutation rate
C. develop better resistance to the new climate
D. learn to use different foods

28. In which form is nitrogen NORMALLY absorbed from the soil by grasses? 28.___
A. Nitrates B. Uric acid
C. Ammonia D. Molecular nitrogen

29. The organisms which prevent the Earth from becoming covered with the bodies of dead organisms are known as 29.___
A. herbivores B. parasites
C. producers D. saprophytes

30. Interactions between organisms which influence their development and survival are known as 30.___
A. biotic factors
B. inorganic substances
C. physical conditions
D. chemical factors

KEY (CORRECT ANSWERS)

1. A	11. A	21. B
2. D	12. C	22. B
3. C	13. B	23. D
4. C	14. C	24. D
5. D	15. C	25. B
6. C	16. D	26. C
7. C	17. B	27. A
8. B	18. C	28. A
9. D	19. B	29. D
10. B	20. D	30. A

TEST 3

DIRECTIONS: Each question or incomplete statement is followed by several suggested answers or completions. Select the one that BEST answers the question or completes the statement. *PRINT THE LETTER OF THE CORRECT ANSWER IN THE SPACE AT THE RIGHT.*

Questions 1-4.

DIRECTIONS: Questions 1 through 4 are to be answered on the basis of the diagram below, which represents reactants A and B and enzyme C, and on your knowledge of biology.

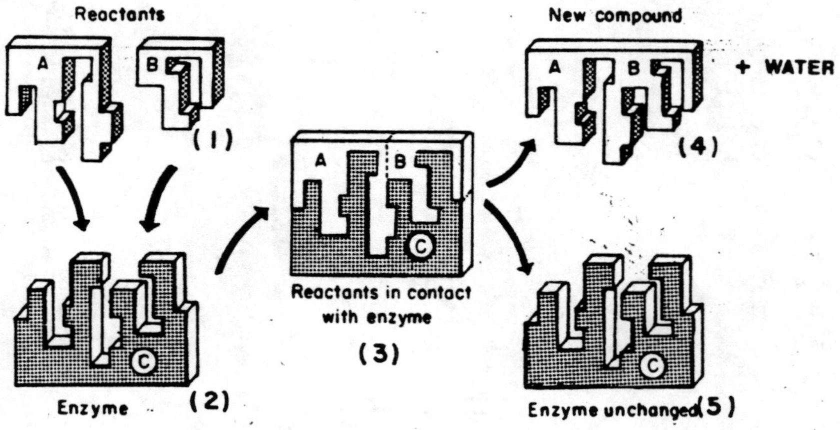

1. Enzyme C increases the rate at which molecules of A unite with molecules of B without itself being altered. Enzyme C is a 1.___
   A. vitamin B. substrate
   C. catalyst D. nucleotide

2. Enzyme C will work only with reactants A and B. This provides evidence for a characteristic of enzymes known as 2.___
   A. specificity B. hydrolysis
   C. deactivation D. synthesis

3. Molecules of the compound represented by figure 4 resulted from a process known as 3.___
   A. carbon fixation B. enzymatic hydrolysis
   C. intracellular digestion D. dehydration synthesis

4. Figure 3 BEST represents a(n) 4.___
   A. enzyme-coenzyme complex B. enzyme-substrate complex
   C. chemical replication D. bacterial transformation

Questions 5-9.

DIRECTIONS: Questions 5 through 9 are to be answered on the basis of the diagram below, which represents a cellular process in animals, and on your knowledge of biology.

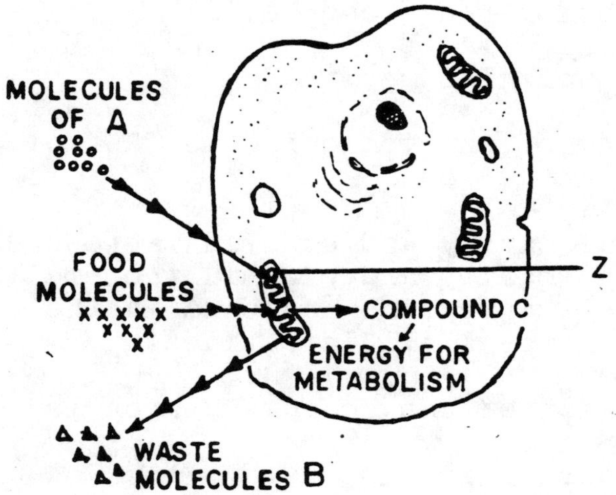

5. The substance labeled *food* is MOST likely molecules of 5.___
   A. starch B. glucose
   C. urea D. chlorophyll

6. Compound C MOST likely represents molecules of 6.___
   A. oxygen B. glucose C. ATP D. DNA

7. If this cell is carrying on aerobic respiration, B represents molecules of a waste product known as 7.___
   A. carbon dioxide B. ATP
   C. ethyl alcohol D. pyruvic acid

8. If this represents a kidney cell from the human body, the molecules of A are MOST probably 8.___
   A. carbon dioxide B. enzymes
   C. lipids D. oxygen

9. The cell organelle labeled Z is known as a 9.___
   A. chloroplast B. mitochondrion
   C. nucleolus D. vacuole

10. In which process is light energy converted to chemical energy? 10.___
    A. Photosynthesis B. Dehydration synthesis
    C. Aerobic respiration D. Hydrolysis

11. In humans, which gland regulates the level of calcium in the bloodstream? 11.___
    A. Ovary B. Pancreas
    C. Parathyroid D. Salivary

12. In humans, urine is eliminated from the bladder through the 12.___
A. urethra B. ureter
C. nephron D. collecting tubule

13. Which process in the liver will increase the level of sugar in the blood? 13.___
A. Formation of droplets of lipid
B. Destruction of red blood cells
C. Synthesis of bile
D. Hydrolysis of glycogen

14. In humans, which of the following is TRUE of carbohydrate digestion? 14.___
It begins
A. in the oral cavity and ends in the esophagus
B. in the oral cavity and ends in the small intestine
C. in the small intestine and ends in the large intestine
D. and ends in the small intestine

15. The CHIEF function of the sensory neuron is to transmit impulses 15.___
A. to the central nervous system
B. away from the effectors
C. away from the central nervous system
D. to the receptors

Questions 16-20.

DIRECTIONS: Questions 16 through 20 are to be answered on the basis of the diagram below, which represents the exchange of materials between capillaries and cells, and on your knowledge of biology.

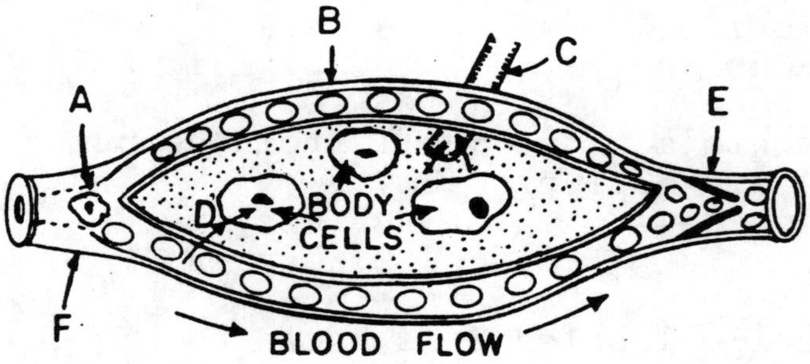

16. Blood vessel B has walls that are very thin. 16.___
This enables this type of vessel to
A. transport hemoglobin to body cells
B. transport red blood cells into the tissue spaces
C. withstand the pressure of the blood coming from veins
D. easily transport substances into and out of the blood

17. A function of cell A is to 17.___
   A. carry oxygen
   B. engulf disease-producing organisms
   C. transport digested food
   D. produce hemoglobin

18. A substance which diffuses in the direction indicated by D is MOST likely 18.___
   A. fibrin B. oxygen C. urea D. bile

19. Which vessel MOST likely contains the greatest amount of carbon dioxide? 19.___
   A. F B. B C. C D. E

20. Excess intercellular fluid (ICF) is constantly drained off by lymphatic vessels. 20.___
Which letter represents such a vessel?
   A. E B. B C. C D. F

21. The part of the plant embryo which develops into the roots and the lower portion of the stem is the 21.___
   A. cotyledon B. epicotyl C. hypocotyl D. seed coat

22. Which is the embryonic germ layer that gives rise to the tissue involved with impulse transmission? 22.___
   A. Endoderm B. Echinoderm
   C. Mesoderm D. Ectoderm

23. Which structure functions as a reservoir for waste products that accumulate during the embryological development of a bird such as a robin? 23.___
   A. Yolk B. Amnion C. Allantois D. Placenta

24. In humans, the cleavage of a zygote NORMALLY begins in the 24.___
   A. ovary B. oviduct C. testis D. vagina

Questions 25-27.

DIRECTIONS: Questions 25 through 27 are to be answered on the basis of the diagram below, which represents the major stages of the human menstrual cycle, and on your knowledge of biology.

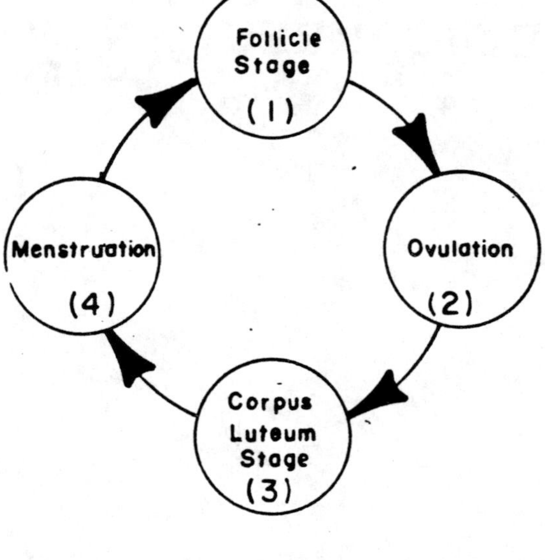

25. During which stage does an egg cell leave a follicle? 25.___
A. 1 B. 2 C. 3 D. 4

26. During which stage does the uterine tissue break down? 26.___
A. 1 B. 2 C. 3 D. 4

27. Stage 3 takes place within which structure? 27.___
A. Ovary B. Pituitary gland
C. Vagina D. Oviduct

Questions 28-30.

DIRECTIONS: Questions 28 through 30 are to be answered on the basis of the diagram below of a flower and on your knowledge of biology.

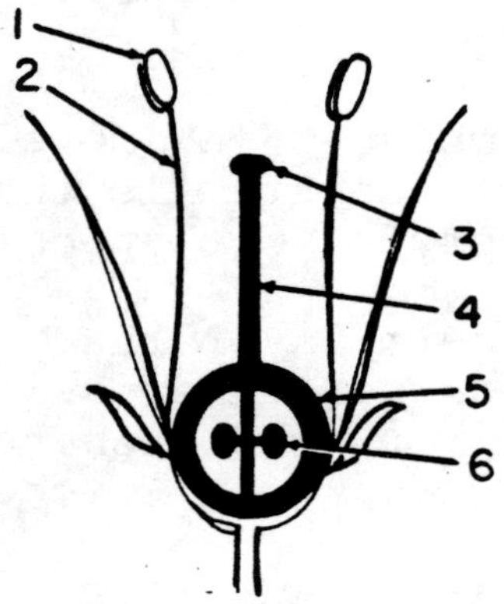

28. Which structure produces cells which form sperm nuclei? 28.___
A. 1 B. 2 C. 3 D. 4

29. In which structure do fertilization and development occur? 29.___
A. 1 B. 6 C. 3 D. 4

30. Which structures are collectively known as the pistil? 30.___
A. 1 and 2 B. 2, 4, and 6
C. 1 and 6 D. 3, 4, and 5

KEY (CORRECT ANSWERS)

1. C	11. C	21. C
2. A	12. A	22. D
3. D	13. D	23. C
4. B	14. B	24. B
5. B	15. A	25. B
6. C	16. D	26. D
7. A	17. B	27. A
8. D	18. B	28. A
9. B	19. D	29. B
10. A	20. C	30. D

TEST 4

DIRECTIONS: Each question or incomplete statement is followed by several suggested answers or completions. Select the one that BEST answers the question or completes the statement. *PRINT THE LETTER OF THE CORRECT ANSWER IN THE SPACE AT THE RIGHT.*

1. The PRINCIPAL function of genes is to 1.___
   A. maintain continuity from one generation to the next
   B. aid in the excretion of waste products from the organism
   C. cause mutations to occur
   D. aid in the maintenance of the water balance in the cell

2. A normal bacterial cell carries on the chemical reaction represented below. 2.___

$$\text{Substance A} \xrightarrow{\text{enzyme X}} \text{Substance B} \xrightarrow{\text{enzyme Y}} \text{Substance C}$$

   A certain mutant bacterial cell can produce substance B but not substance C.
   The mutation was MOST likely the result of a change in the gene that codes for
   A. enzyme X
   B. enzyme Y
   C. substrate A
   D. substrate C

3. RNA carries out the original instructions found in molecules of 3.___
   A. ATP
   B. DNA
   C. PTC
   D. ADP

4. Both DNA and RNA molecules contain 4.___
   A. uracil bases
   B. ribose sugars
   C. phosphate groups
   D. thymine bases

5. Any change that affects the base sequence in an organism's DNA is known as a 5.___
   A. chromosomal recombination
   B. chromosomal disjunction
   C. gene replication
   D. gene mutation

6. If a living algal cell has its chloroplasts removed, neither that organism nor its asexually produced offspring can regain chloroplasts, despite the presence of nuclear genes. 6.___
   This provides evidence for
   A. gene mutations
   B. the *one gene-one enzyme* hypothesis
   C. the individuality of organisms
   D. cytoplasmic inheritance

Questions 7-10.

DIRECTIONS: Questions 7 through 10 are to be answered on the basis of the diagram below, which represents some events associated with synthesis within a cell.

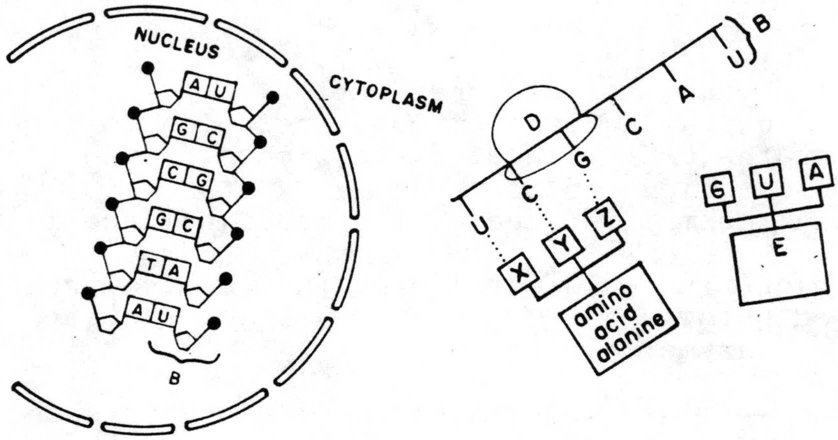

7. Letter B MOST likely represents 7.___
   A. nuclear DNA B. transfer RNA
   C. messenger RNA D. protein

8. Letter D represents a cytoplasmic organelle known as a 8.___
   A. ribosome B. chloroplast
   C. nucleolus D. mitochondrion

9. The sequence of nitrogenous bases that are represented by X, Y, and Z are 9.___
   A. T-U-C B. U-C-G C. A-G-C D. A-T-C

10. Letter E MOST likely represents a(n) 10.___
   A. amino acid other than alanine
   B. enzyme molecule
   C. ribose molecule
   D. nucleotide building block

11. In the relationship $p^2 + 2pq + q^2$, the letters p and q represent the 11.___
   A. homozygous dominant individuals in the population
   B. frequencies of the dominant and recessive alleles
   C. homozygous recessive individuals in the population
   D. frequency of the dominant and recessive phenotypes

12. When a white moth lands on a white birch tree, its color has a high adaptive value. 12.___
If the trees become covered with black soot, the moth's white trait in this environment would MOST probably
   A. still have the same adaptive value
   B. increase in adaptive value
   C. mutate to the black trait
   D. lose its adaptive value

13. The gene frequencies in a population would MOST likely change if 13.___
A. mating became random
B. the population was very large
C. mutation rates increased
D. migrations did not occur

14. Geographic isolation of one species of organisms into two populations would MOST likely result in 14.___
A. increasing the mutation frequency in one population
B. minimizing the differences in traits which occur between the populations
C. preventing a new species from forming one population
D. maintaining the differences in traits which occur between the populations

15. Asexual reproduction generally does NOT lead to changes in gene frequencies because in asexually reproducing species 15.___
A. large populations cannot be produced easily
B. mutations cannot occur
C. there is little opportunity for genetic recombination
D. there is no gene pool

Questions 16-18.

DIRECTIONS: Questions 16 through 18 are to be answered on the basis of the diagram below. Letters A through M represent species of organisms and the vertical distances between the dotted lines represent long periods of time in which major environmental changes have occurred.

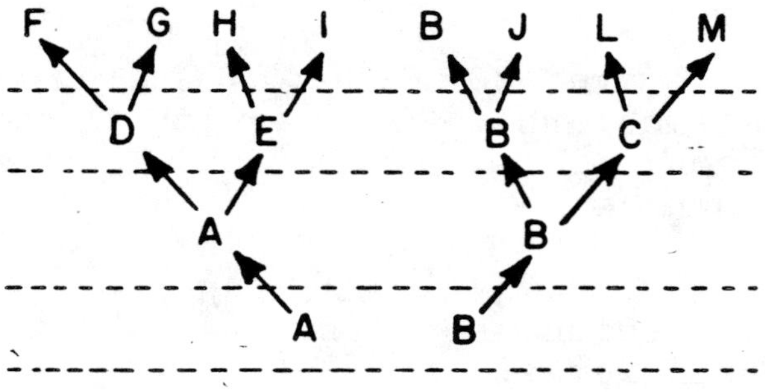

16. Which two organisms have the CLOSEST common ancestor? 16.___
A. F and G B. F and H C. J and M D. G and M

17. Which organism was the FIRST to become extinct? 17.___
A. A B. B C. C D. J

18. Which species appears to have been MOST successful in surviving changes in the environment over time? 18.___
A. A B. B C. E D. D

Questions 19-20.

DIRECTIONS: Questions 19 and 20 are to be answered on the basis of the information below and on your knowledge of biology.

A certain insect species is a pest that destroys hundreds of acres of forest by eating the leaves of trees. A new pesticide is used on the insect and successfully kills most of the species. The next year, however, the population of the insect is large again, and treatment with the pesticide has little effect on it.

19. The insects that survived the pesticide PROBABLY 19.___
 A. acquired the ability to resist the pesticide
 B. developed resistance through use and disuse
 C. learned how to avoid the pesticide in their habitat
 D. had genetic resistance to the pesticide

20. Initially, the presence of the pesticide in the environment MOST probably 20.___
 A. caused mutations to occur in the insects
 B. acted as a selecting agent for the insects
 C. killed only predators of the insect
 D. made the trees more resistant to insect attack

21. A particular species of fish has a very narrow range of tolerance for changes of water temperature and dissolved oxygen. 21.___
For the fish, the temperature and oxygen content represent
 A. autotrophic conditions B. a community
 C. abiotic factors D. symbiosis

22. In an aquatic biome, the original source of energy is 22.___
 A. fish B. algae C. sunlight D. water

23. In a certain area, over 80 inches of fairly evenly distributed rainfall occurs. As a result, there is no well-defined dry season. 23.___
This area is known as a
 A. tundra
 B. taiga
 C. temperature deciduous forest
 D. tropical rain forest

24. Which accomplishment by humans has made the MOST positive ecological impact on the environment? 24.___
The
 A. importation of organisms such as the starling and the Japanese beetle into the United States
 B. reforestation and soil-cover planting measures to prevent soil erosion
 C. extinction or near extinction of many predators to prevent the death of prey animals
 D. use of pesticides and other similar crop-improvement chemicals to regulate the insect population

25. Drastic changes in air temperature would be LEAST likely to affect which biome? 25.___
   A. Tundra
   B. Temperate deciduous forest
   C. Marine
   D. Taiga

Questions 26-28.

DIRECTIONS: Questions 26 through 28 are to be answered on the basis of the chart below and on your knowledge of biology.

Ecological Plant Survey

Number of Individual Organisms

Year	Assorted Grasses	Assorted Shrubs	Oak Trees	Hickory Trees	Beech Trees	Maple Trees
1860	6,000	2,000	100	150	40	20
1880	5,000	2,800	109	158	80	60
1900	4,500	2,500	125	170	128	130
1910	3,000	2,320	180	195	175	200
1920	1,200	2,142	150	170	190	250
1940	800	1,975	130	130	200	400
1960	785	1,860	120	135	226	407

26. The change in the number of plants in each category between 1860 and 1960 is an example of which ecological principle? 26.___
   A. Succession
   B. Adaptive radiation
   C. Evolution
   D. Mutation

27. Which is the dominant member of the climax community in this survey? 27.___
   A. Grasses
   B. Shrubs
   C. Hickory trees
   D. Maple trees

28. The climax community in this survey would be located in which environment? 28.___
   A. Tundra
   B. Temperate deciduous forest
   C. Taiga
   D. Tropical rain forest

29. When a garden became infested with a large population of aphids, ladybird beetles were introduced into the community as predators on the aphids. 29.___
The resultant decrease in the aphid population was due to
   A. biological control
   B. parthenogenesis
   C. vegetative propagation
   D. chemosynthesis

30\. Which sequence of land biomes is CORRECTLY arranged in order of increasing latitude? 30.___

A. Tundra, taiga, deciduous forest, tropical forest
B. Tropical forest, deciduous forest, taiga, tundra
C. Tundra, deciduous forest, tropical forest, taiga
D. Tropical forest, taiga, tundra, deciduous forest

KEY (CORRECT ANSWERS)

1. A	11. B	21. C
2. B	12. D	22. C
3. B	13. C	23. D
4. C	14. D	24. B
5. D	15. C	25. C
6. D	16. A	26. A
7. C	17. A	27. D
8. A	18. B	28. B
9. C	19. D	29. A
10. A	20. B	30. D

EXAMINATION SECTION

TEST 1

DIRECTIONS: Each question or incomplete statement is followed by several suggested answers or completions. Select the one that BEST answers the question or completes the statement. *PRINT THE LETTER OF THE CORRECT ANSWER IN THE SPACE AT THE RIGHT.*

1. In the normal human body, an increase in the amount of glucose in the blood stimulates the production of 1.___
   A. cortin B. insulin C. secretin
   D. iodine E. ptyalin

2. Exact similarity between chromosomes of the various cells within the same tissue of a plant or animal is LARGELY due to the mechanism of 2.___
   A. segregation B. meiosis C. mitosis
   D. fertilization E. maturation

3. Marriages of closely related persons are USUALLY inadvisable from a biological standpoint because 3.___
   A. undesirable recessive characters are more likely to appear in following generations
   B. such unions are likely to be sterile
   C. desirable characteristics, even when dominant, are less likely to be transmitted to future generations
   D. such unions generally produce physically weaker children
   E. at least one-fourth of the children are likely to be hemophiles

4. Much of the water entering an amoeba by osmosis is eliminated by the action of the 4.___
   A. contractile vacuole B. gastric vacuole
   C. ectoplasm D. cytoplasmic crystals
   E. pseudopodia

5. The rate of flow (quantity per second) of man's blood is GREATEST in the 5.___
   A. venae cavae B. radial artery
   C. portal vein D. capillaries
   E. aorta

6. MOST of the world's supply of sugar as a commercial product is obtained from _____ and _____. 6.___
   A. leaves; stems B. fruits; stems C. roots; stems
   D. seeds; stems E. seeds; roots

7. The essential cellular component divided and redistributed by the process of mitosis is the 7.___
   A. plasma membrane B. cytoplasm
   C. plastid D. chromatin
   E. central spindle

8. The discharge of adrenalin into the blood causes 8.____
   A. dilation of the blood vessels of the stomach
   B. increased absorption of sugar by the liver
   C. an increase in the speed and force of the heart beat
   D. constriction of the blood vessels of the muscles
   E. a slowing down of respiration

9. Synthesis of glucose from carbon dioxide and water in green plants occurs ONLY in the 9.____
   A. epidermis
   B. sieve tubes
   C. cambium
   D. chlorophyll-bearing cells
   E. root hairs

10. Identify the TRUE statement regarding syphilis. 10.____
   A. It is transmitted only by sexual contact.
   B. It attacks mainly the reproductive organs.
   C. Its treatment is the same as that for gonorrhea.
   D. Its transmission from one generation to the next follows Mendel's laws.
   E. It is possible to have a latent form of the disease without recognizable symptoms.

11. Similarities in the characteristics of identical twins are caused PRINCIPALLY by 11.____
   A. the presence of similar genes in all cells
   B. similar environmental conditions before birth
   C. similar environmental conditions after birth
   D. simultaneous fertilization of an ovum by two similar sperm cells
   E. identical genetic mutation

12. Gametes differ from spores in that gametes 12.____
   A. may unite and form zygotes
   B. are produced only by gametophytes
   C. are produced only by animals
   D. are capable of independent motion
   E. are always the larger in size

13. The poisonous effect on the human body of inhaled carbon monoxide is caused by its 13.____
   A. chemical action on lung tissue
   B. replacement of the oxygen in oxyhemoglobin
   C. insolubility in blood plasma
   D. forming insoluble precipitates in the blood
   E. paralyzing effect on the respiratory center of the brain

14. Tropisms of leaves are often produced DIRECTLY by 14.____
   A. turgor changes in certain cells
   B. contractions of wood fibers
   C. electrical conductivity of sieve tubes
   D. digestion of starch
   E. increase of sugar in the cells

15. A climax community is MOST likely to be found in regions where 15. ___
   A. man has greatly modified his surroundings
   B. there are no dominant organisms
   C. conditions have remained relatively constant for a period of many years
   D. distinct changes in climatic conditions have recently occurred
   E. plants are relatively uniform in size

16. An internal secretion of the mucosa of the upper part of the small intestine stimulates the 16. ___
   A. flow of ptyalin
   B. flow of pancreatic juices
   C. dilation of the cardiac sphincter
   D. production of thyroxin
   E. absorption of water in the large intestine

17. A hyperthyroid condition is characterized by 17. ___
   A. low blood pressure
   B. a tendency toward obesity
   C. low body temperature
   D. increased metabolism
   E. severely retarded mental activity

18. Which of the following types of cells in the human male contains one-half the ordinary number of chromosomes? 18. ___
   A. All of the somatic cells
   B. Somatic cells of the reproductive organs only
   C. Spermatozoa
   D. Primary spermatocytes
   E. T-cells

Questions 19-20.

DIRECTIONS: Questions 19 and 20 are to be answered on the basis of the following information.

S = short-haired (dominant)
s = long-haired (recessive)

19. The parents of a litter of long-haired cats are 19. ___
   A. SS + Ss   B. SS + ss   C. Ss + Ss
   D. Ss + ss   E. ss + ss

20. The parents of a litter of short-haired hybrid cats are MOST likely to be 20. ___
   A. SS + Ss   B. SS + ss   C. Ss + Ss
   D. Ss + ss   E. SS + SS

Questions 21-23.

DIRECTIONS: Questions 21 through 23 are to be answered on the basis of the following diagram.

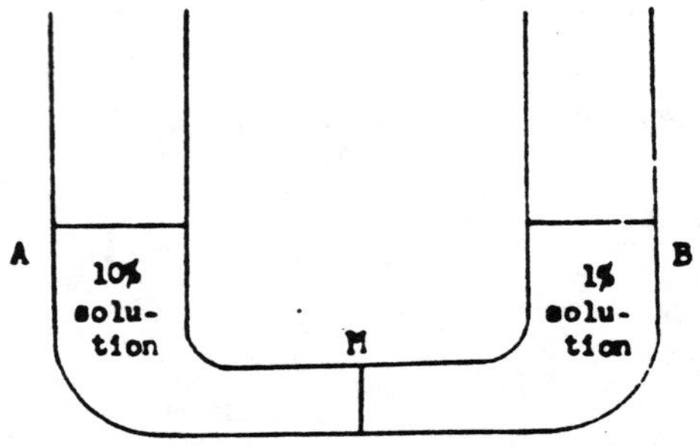

A 10% solution of cane sugar in water (A) is separated from a 1% solution of cane sugar in water (B) by a membrane (M) permeable to water but NOT to cane sugar. The levels of the two liquids are the same.

21. Molecules of water will pass through the membrane 21.____
   A. in one direction only
   B. in both directions at all times
   C. until the total number of molecules is the same on both sides
   D. only until the solution on one side is saturated
   E. only until a final constant difference in level is attained; then their passage will cease

22. When equilibrium between the two solutions is attained, 22.____
   A. the levels of the two solutions will be equal
   B. there will be an equal number of sugar molecules in each solution
   C. there will be an equal number of water molecules in each solution
   D. no molecules will pass through the membrane in either direction
   E. equal numbers of water molecules will be passing through the membrane in each direction

23. If the membrane were equally permeable to water and to sugar, 23.____
   A. the concentration in A and B would remain unchanged, even after a long period of time
   B. the concentration of sugar would ultimately become equal in A and B
   C. no diffusion would take place through the membrane
   D. the level in B would become ten times as high as in A
   E. there would be excessive pressure on the membrane

24. Some insects carry disease germs on their bodies and transmit diseases to man merely by contact. Other insects' bodies act as *culture tubes* in which the disease organisms pass a part of their life cycle.
Which one of these insects is a *culture tube* type of carrier for the disease named after it? 24.___
   A. Housefly - tuberculosis
   B. Mosquito - malaria
   C. Cockroach - typhoid fever
   D. Housefly - common cold
   E. Body louse - typhus fever

25. 25.___

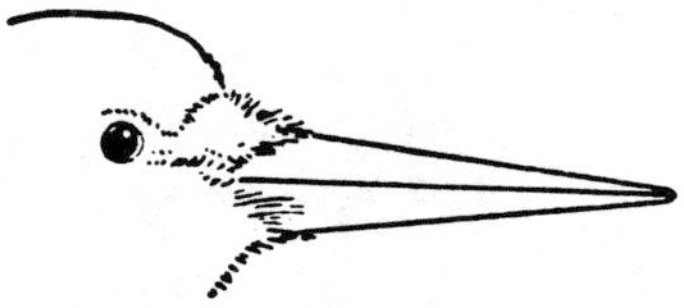

The bird beak shown above is of MOST value to its possessor for
   A. crushing seeds
   B. drilling for and extracting insects
   C. catching fish
   D. tearing flesh from bones
   E. capturing insects in flight

26. One of the MOST important functions of root hairs is to 26.___
   A. increase the plant's sensitivity to stimuli
   B. enable roots to penetrate deeper into the soil
   C. increase the root's total absorbing surface
   D. protect the delicate parts of the root from injury
   E. increase the total food storage capacity of the root

27. The presence of certain useless structures in man's body, such as the appendix and the muscles in the outer ears, may be an indication that 27.___
   A. man had a remote ancestor who used these organs
   B. man has always been as he is today
   C. man can regenerate organs at will
   D. these structures have helped man to survive
   E. man has undoubtedly descended from the monkey

28. Food is digested in the alimentary tract because 28.___
   A. the body needs energy
   B. food is required for building new cells
   C. oxidation would not take place unless the foods were digested
   D. man cannot live unless his nutrition requirements are met
   E. there are enzymes present which change the food into soluble form

29. Which one of the following traits distinguishes all birds from all reptiles? 29.____
   A. Birds lay eggs.
   B. Birds have internal body skeletons.
   C. Birds are warm-blooded.
   D. In birds the nerve cord is dorsally located in the body.
   E. Birds have legs.

30. Each secretes hormones EXCEPT the 30.____
   A. pituitary gland
   B. lymph nodes
   C. parathyroid glands
   D. adrenal glands
   E. islets of the pancreas

31. Which is an example of sexual reproduction? 31.____
   A. Mature yeast plants develop outgrowths which, when shed, are the young yeast plants.
   B. A mature paramecium divides into two offspring.
   C. A fish hatchery worker pours some salmon milt into a jar of salmon eggs which later hatch into young salmon.
   D. A gardener plants pieces of potatoes containing *eyes* and later harvests a crop of potatoes.
   E. A fern plant produces many brown spores on the undersides of the leaves. These spores give rise to young plants.

32. It is sometimes desirable to mix a small amount of white clover seed with the grass seed when seeding a new lawn because the clover 32.____
   A. furnishes shade to the young grass plants when they first come up
   B. tends to crowd out weeds
   C. produces carbon dioxide
   D. protects the young grass plants from injury until the sod is well established
   E. has root structures which harbor nitrogen-fixing bacteria

33. A _____ is *cold-blooded*. 33.____
   A. frog
   B. goose
   C. bat
   D. whale
   E. polar bear

34. One of the MOST marked differences between animal cells and plant cells is that 34.____
   A. plant cells have chromosomes
   B. animal cells ordinarily have a nucleus
   C. animal cells contain protoplasm
   D. animal cells have a variety of shapes
   E. plant cells usually have thick, rigid walls

35. Blood flowing through the pulmonary veins is distinguished from blood flowing through the large jugular vein in the neck region in that the blood in the pulmonary veins 35.____
   A. carries disease-resisting substances known as antibodies

B. contains nutrient substances, such as sugar, fats, and amino acids
C. has more white blood cells
D. carries a fresh supply of oxygen
E. has a higher concentration of carbon dioxide

36. A group of organisms protected by a *suit of armor* is 36.___
A. sponges B. arthropods C. amphibians
D. roundworms E. primates

37. All EXCEPT _____ constitute real homes for living things. 37.___
A. the oceans
B. inland ponds and lakes
C. the air over the earth
D. swiftly flowing fresh-water streams
E. the land mass of the earth

38. Why can a green plant continue to carry on photosynthesis after the oxygen surrounding it has been removed by a chemical absorbing agent? 38.___
A. Green plants do not use oxygen.
B. Green plants use carbon dioxide in respiration.
C. Transpiration serves the same function in green plants as respiration does in animals.
D. Green plants use nitrogen instead of oxygen.
E. Green plants release free oxygen as a by-product in food manufacturing.

39. Four of the following offer evidence that living things have gone through long ages of gradual development on the earth. 39.___
Which one does NOT offer evidence supporting this theory?
A. Many fossils of animals and plants show series of changes from simple to complex forms.
B. The whale has bones, which suggest that its ancestors may have had legs.
C. A very young human embryo is hardly distinguishable from a very young fish embryo.
D. The hand and arm of a man are similar, bone for bone, to the forefoot and foreleg of a horse.
E. There is only one species of mankind living upon the earth at the present time.

40. 40.___

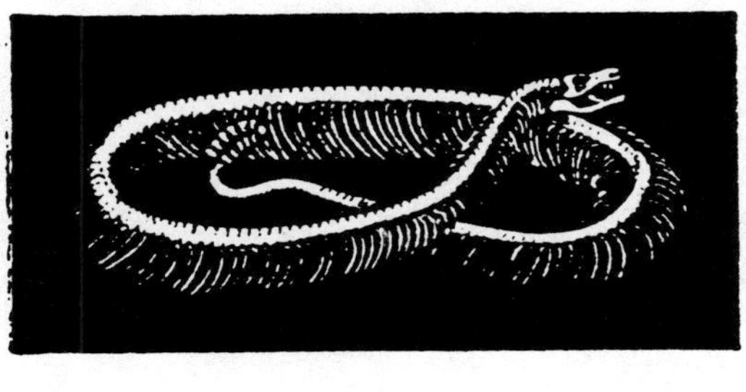

The above skeleton indicates that the animal belonged to the _____ group.
A. roundworm B. arthropod C. echinoderm
D. chordate E. mollusk

41. The GREATEST disturbers of the balance of nature have been 41.____
   A. the carnivorous animals
   B. the insects
   C. civilized people
   D. volcanoes and earthquakes
   E. bacteria and fungi

42. The Mediterranean fruit fly has eight chromosomes in each of its body cells. 42.____
The normal number of chromosomes in one of its sperm cells or egg cells would, therefore, be
   A. two B. four C. eight
   D. sixteen E. thirty-two

43. A characteristic of the offspring of asexual reproduction is that they 43.____
   A. are apt to resemble each other and the parent more closely than is true of the offspring of sexual reproduction
   B. differ markedly from each other in hereditary traits
   C. are likely to show many mutations
   D. can adapt themselves better to changing environmental conditions than the offspring of sexual reproduction
   E. are very unpredictable as to the physical and genetic traits they will possess

44. Bone tissue is hard because 44.____
   A. the body needs a strong, rigid supporting framework
   B. the possession of an internal skeleton distinguishes the chordates from all other phyla of animals
   C. the muscles require places for attachment in order to function properly
   D. it is needed to protect delicate parts of the body from injury
   E. calcium compounds are deposited in the spaces between and around the cells

45. *So we may doubt whether, in cheese and timber, worms are generated or if beetles and wasps in cow dung, or if butterflies, shellfish, eels, and such life be procreated of putrefied matter. To question this is to question reason, sense, and experience. If he doubts this, let him go to Egypt, and there he will find the fields swarming with mice begot of the mud of the Nile, to the great calamity of the inhabitants.* 45.____
In the above paragraph, the theory under question is that of
   A. sexual reproduction B. special creation
   C. spontaneous generation D. vegetative reproduction
   E. regeneration

46. The wings of India's *dead leaf* butterfly are shaped like a leaf and the undersides are colored like a dead leaf. 46.____
This butterfly is an example of
   A. symbiosis B. protective resemblance
   C. warning coloration D. metamorphosis
   E. None of these

47. If you are about the right weight, the BEST way for you to stay that way is to 47.____
   A. exercise every day
   B. eat meals that contain enough vitamins and minerals
   C. cut out all desserts and snacks
   D. adjust your calorie intake to your calorie needs
   E. None of the above

48. It has been observed that increasing the amount of x-irradiation increases the number of mutations per thousand irradiated organisms. 48.____
Which graph indicates this process?

A.
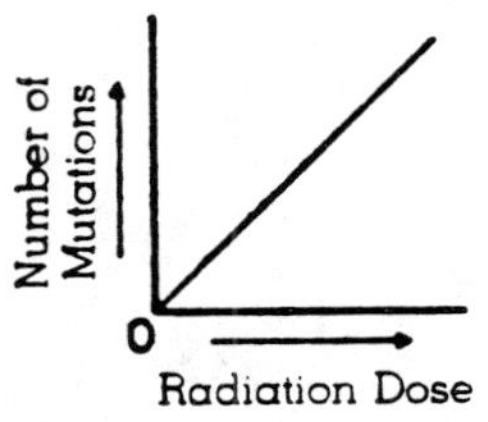

B.
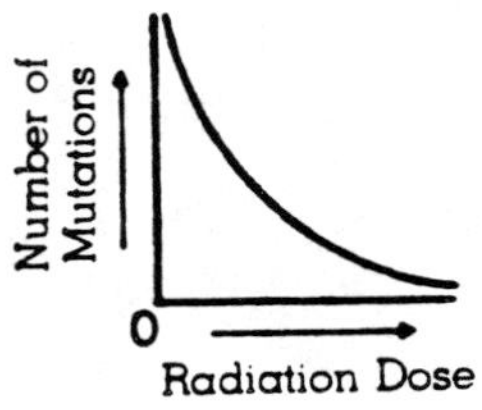

C.
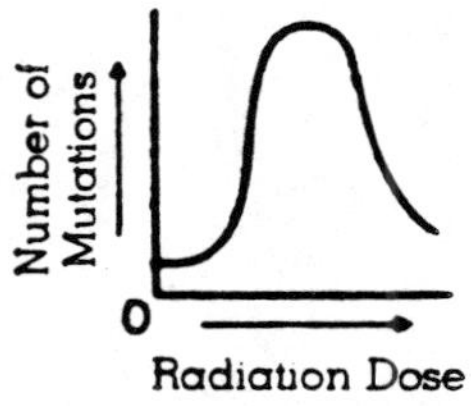

D.
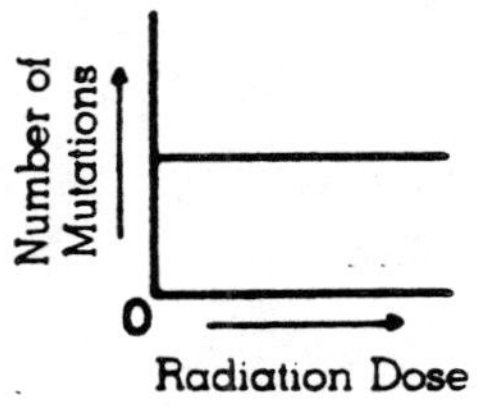

E. None of the above

49. Beans were growing in one garden patch and asparagus was growing in another adjacent patch. Equal amounts of salt were added to the soil in both patches. All of the beans died, and all of the asparagus lived. 49.____
Which is the MOST acceptable explanation for these observations?
   A. Asparagus plants can tolerate larger amounts of salt than beans can.
   B. Asparagus plants use the salt to build tissue.
   C. Some substance other than salt killed the beans.
   D. Bean plants do not need as much water as asparagus plants do.
   E. None of the above

50. 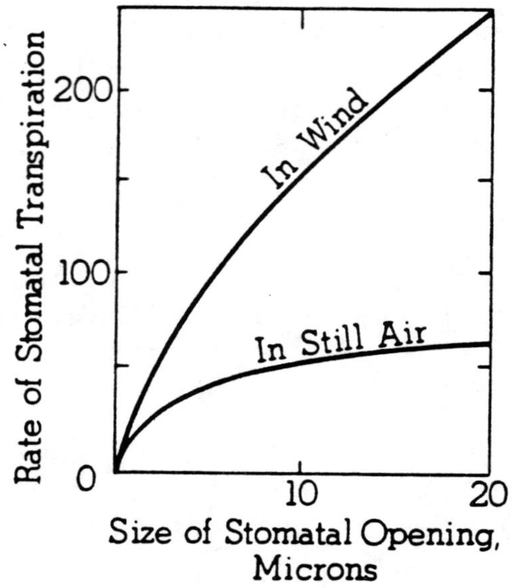

50.____

The above graph describes corn plants with equal areas of leaf surface.
A plant in _____ would PROBABLY lose water fastest.

A. wind, stomatal openings 10 microns
B. wind, stomatal openings 15 microns
C. still air, stomatal openings 10 microns
D. still air, stomatal openings 20 microns
E. None of the above

KEY (CORRECT ANSWERS)

1. B	11. A	21. B	31. C	41. C
2. C	12. A	22. E	32. E	42. B
3. A	13. B	23. B	33. A	43. A
4. A	14. A	24. B	34. E	44. E
5. E	15. C	25. B	35. D	45. C
6. C	16. B	26. C	36. B	46. B
7. D	17. D	27. A	37. C	47. D
8. C	18. C	28. E	38. E	48. A
9. D	19. E	29. C	39. E	49. A
10. E	20. B	30. B	40. D	50. B

TEST 2

DIRECTIONS: Each question or incomplete statement is followed by several suggested answers or completions. Select the one that BEST answers the question or completes the statement. *PRINT THE LETTER OF THE CORRECT ANSWER IN THE SPACE AT THE RIGHT.*

1. Which one of the following statements regarding the endocrine glands is TRUE? 1.___
   A. The removal of any endocrine gland will cause death.
   B. Overactivity of a gland produces effects similar to those produced by underactivity.
   C. Large numbers of different kinds of hormones may be found in the alimentary canal.
   D. Overactivity of a gland may always be corrected by the administration of a synthetic hormone.
   E. The activity of one gland is often affected by the products of others.

2. Differences in genetic composition in similar-appearing individuals may be discovered experimentally by 2.___
   A. the use of x-rays
   B. the use of hormones
   C. a back-cross
   D. crossing-over
   E. regeneration

3. The variety of present day forms of animals and plants may be reasonably explained on the basis that 3.___
   A. each form has been specially created
   B. present forms have resulted from effort on the part of individual organisms to adapt themselves to changing environments
   C. any environmental change always produces structural changes that are hereditary
   D. all new forms are better fitted for survival than their predecessors
   E. all present forms have developed as results of variations that have occurred in previous generations

4. The parathyroid glands in man are important because certain processes in them influence the 4.___
   A. concentration of calcium in the blood
   B. metabolism of carbohydrates
   C. rate of growth
   D. sodium and potassium balance in the blood
   E. oxidative metabolism

5. Enzymes differ from inorganic catalysts in that enzymes 5.___
   A. are more resistant to extremes of temperature
   B. must be present in greater concentration to be effective
   C. are most effective at temperatures of about 212°F
   D. catalyze only specific reactions
   E. cannot be obtained in crystalline form

6. Chemical compounds in dead organisms are transformed into compounds usable by plants CHIEFLY by the action of 6.____
   A. inorganic elements in soil
   B. saprophytic bacteria and fungi
   C. parasitic fungi
   D. unicellular animals
   E. pathogenic microorganisms

7. Exchange of material between two homologous chromosomes in synapsis is known as 7.____
   A. fertilization B. linkage
   C. crossing-over D. hybridization
   E. cleavage

8. A person born with an underactive anterior lobe of the pituitary gland is LIKELY to be 8.____
   A. a cretin B. a giant
   C. a midget D. feeble-minded
   E. diabetic

9. The GREATEST amount of heat energy will be furnished to the body by complete oxidation of one gram of 9.____
   A. glucose B. sucrose C. starch
   D. fat E. protein

10. Inactivation of the vagus nerve results in 10.____
   A. an acceleration of the heart beat
   B. blindness
   C. loss of sensation of pain
   D. an increase in the flow of saliva
   E. impairment of the sense of taste

11. An animal's intelligence is correlated CHIEFLY with 11.____
   A. its ability to form conditioned reflexes
   B. the complexity of its pattern of instinctive behavior
   C. the sum of all its simple reflex actions
   D. the usefulness to the animal of its instinctive behavior
   E. the keenness of its sense organs

12. One difference between the nutrition of higher animals and plants is the relatively larger proportion of the animal's food 12.____
   A. used in the synthesis of carbohydrates
   B. used in the synthesis of organic components of protoplasm
   C. used in the synthesis of supporting tissue
   D. stored within the organism
   E. oxidized

13. During the development of a fruit from a flower, an ovule becomes the 13.____
   A. entire fruit B. fleshy part of the fruit
   C. endosperm D. embryo
   E. seed

14. The GREATEST degree of precipitation will be obtained when rabbit blood serum which has been immunized against human blood serum is mixed with diluted blood serum of 14.___
   A. non-immunized rabbits B. squirrels
   C. monkeys D. man-like apes
   E. man

15. A disease which might be contracted from some food that an individual has eaten is 15.___
   A. typhus fever B. anemia C. diabetes
   D. trichinosis E. ringworm

16. *The evidence seems to show beyond question that our present species of plants have descended...from simpler and fewer species which formerly existed - back, to a single kind which throve in remotest antiquity.* 16.___
   On the basis of this statement alone, it might follow that
   A. the number of species of plants is decreasing
   B. generally speaking, plants are becoming simpler
   C. an organism could become so complex that its very complexity would lead to its extinction
   D. the number of species of plants is increasing
   E. ancient plants were more successful than modern plants

17. An example of a flowering plant is a(n) 17.___
   A. fern B. mushroom C. moss
   D. arbor vitae E. corn

18. An individual could continue to live a fairly normal life after the removal or destruction of any EXCEPT one 18.___
   A. adrenal gland B. kidney
   C. lung D. cerebral hemisphere
   E. parathyroid gland

19. Two well-watered geranium plants, in sealed pots, were placed under two dry bell jars, X and Y. The leaves of the plant under Jar X were coated with vaseline on both upper and lower surfaces, while those of the plant under Jar Y were not coated. The two bell jars were then placed in bright sunlight for 8 hours. 19.___
   At the end of this time, what was the condition of the inside surface of the bell jars?
   A. Jar X showed less moisture than Jar Y.
   B. Jar X showed more moisture than Jar Y.
   C. Each jar was perfectly dry,
   D. Each jar was very moist with no noticeable difference in amount.
   E. Jar X was covered with many fine droplets of vaseline.

20. A man is able to maintain his balance when he sits, stands, or walks PRIMARILY because of the functioning of the 20.___
   A. medulla oblongata connecting the brain and the spinal cord
   B. adrenal glands secreting adrenalin into the blood stream

C. spinal cord
D. solar plexus or nerve center in the stomach region of the abdomen
E. semicircular canals in the ears

21. What is the MOST important reason for cutting many branches off a deciduous tree that is to be transplanted? It 21.___
A. prevents too great a water loss until the roots are reestablished
B. tends to reduce the rate of photosynthesis
C. increases the rate of water absorption
D. increases the efficiency of food production
E. exposes more surface to the atmosphere

22. When a sip of water goes *down the wrong way*, there is improper functioning of the 22.___
A. larynx B. trachea C. pharynx
D. epiglottis E. Eustachian tubes

23. Wheat is planted three years in succession in Field X, while soybeans are planted three years in succession in Field Y. 23.___
The soil nitrogen will PROBABLY
A. increase in Field X
B. increase in Field Y
C. decrease in Field Y
D. decrease equally in both fields
E. be unaffected in either field

Questions 24-26.

DIRECTIONS: For each of Questions 24 through 26, select the organism that belongs to a different phylum from the other four.

24. A. Sunfish B. Starfish C. Trout 24.___
D. Bass E. Codfish

25. A. Pine B. Sunflower C. Oak 25.___
D. Fern E. Dandelion

26. A. Ameba B. Paramecium C. Euglena 26.___
D. Malarial parasite E. Hydra

27. On the basis of photosynthesis and conditions necessary for this process to occur, it should be possible to produce a marked increase in plant growth in a closed greenhouse room by 27.___
A. slowly releasing a continuous supply of carbon dioxide into the room from a carbon dioxide tank
B. drying the air in the room with a calcium chloride apparatus
C. providing electric light during the day in addition to the usual sunlight
D. uncapping a bottle containing a chlorophyll solution and allowing its vapors to pass into the air in the room

E. slowly releasing a continuous supply of pure oxygen into the room from an oxygen tank

28. External fertilization in animals is MOST often associated with 28.___
A. a land habitat
B. small size
C. parental care of the young
D. asexual reproduction
E. living in water

29. Which statement might BEST account for the fact that the trout, which is a very active fish, is most frequently found in the swift, well-churned type of stream? 29.___
A. Swiftly flowing water contains less decaying organic matter.
B. The trout escapes most of its natural enemies by living in the rapids.
C. Water in the rapids is more highly oxygenated than relatively still water.
D. Food is more easily caught in a swiftly flowing stream.
E. The trout gets considerable satisfaction from skirting danger.

30. When blood passes through the pancreas, the amount of _____ in the blood _____. 30.___
A. digestive enzyme; increases
B. insulin; increases
C. sugar; increases
D. adrenalin; increases
E. hormone; decreases

31. The scientific name of the leopard frog is *Rana pipiens* and that of the bullfrog is *Rana catesbiana*. These scientific names indicate that both frogs belong to the same 31.___
A. genus B. species C. class D. order E. family

32. Wheat rust can be eliminated BEST by 32.___
A. dusting wheat fields with insect poisons
B. encouraging ladybird beetles to multiply rapidly
C. spreading lime on the fields before plowing
D. getting rid of all common barberry bushes in the vicinity
E. draining the swamps and wet lands in that region

Questions 33-39.

DIRECTIONS: Questions 33 through 39 are on the MOST effective measures for preventing certain diseases. For each disease named, select from the following KEY the best preventive.

KEY
A. Water treatment and milk pasteurization
B. Eradication of insect carriers
C. An addition to or a subtraction from one's diet
D. Immunization, such as vaccination or inoculation
E. Eugenics

33. Yellow fever 33.___

34. Anemia 34.___

35. Diphtheria 35.___

36. Rabies 36.___

37. Rickets 37.___

38. Night blindness 38.___

39. Undulant fever 39.___

Questions 40-43.

DIRECTIONS: For Questions 40 through 43, select from the following KEY the scientific classification which might be applied to each statement.

KEY
A. Generalization
B. Problem
C. Fact by definition
D. Hypothesis
E. Fact by demonstration

40. Would an orchardist who raises cherries for the market consider the robin a harmful or a beneficial bird? 40.___

41. The robin may have developed in antiquity from reptile ancestors. 41.___

42. Why do robins migrate to southern latitudes in the winter? 42.___

43. All members of the thrush family of birds have spotted breasts, either in the young or in the adult stage. 43.___

44. According to current theories, what is the order in which the following plants appeared on Earth, the earliest listed FIRST? 44.___

I. Ferns II. Angiosperms III. Algae

The CORRECT answer is:
A. I, II, III B. I, III, II C. II, I, III
D. III, I, II E. II,III, I

45. In a kidney transplant, a person would have the BEST chance for the organ to be accepted by his body if the kidney came from his 45.___
A. brother B. fraternal twin C. mother
D. identical twin E. father

46. 46.___

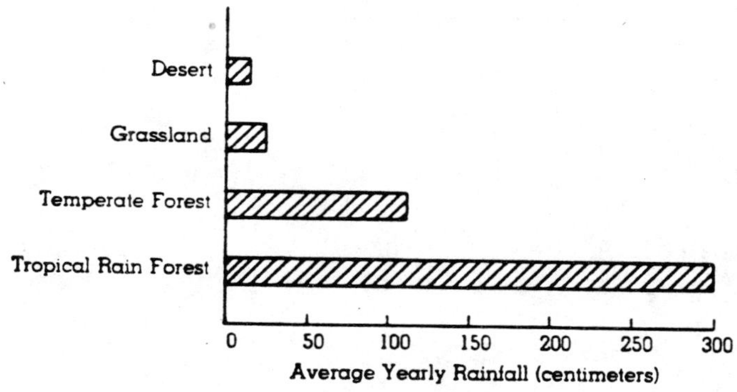

Identify the conclusion MOST closely related to the information presented in the above graph.
A. There is a relationship between temperature and the types of plants existing in an ecosystem.
B. The amount of available water is a factor that determines the types of plants growing in a region.
C. Areas of limited rainfall have the widest variety of plants.
D. There is a relationship between latitude and the types of plants existing in an ecosystem.
E. None of the above.

Questions 47-48.

DIRECTIONS: Questions 47 and 48 are to be answered on the basis of the following graph.

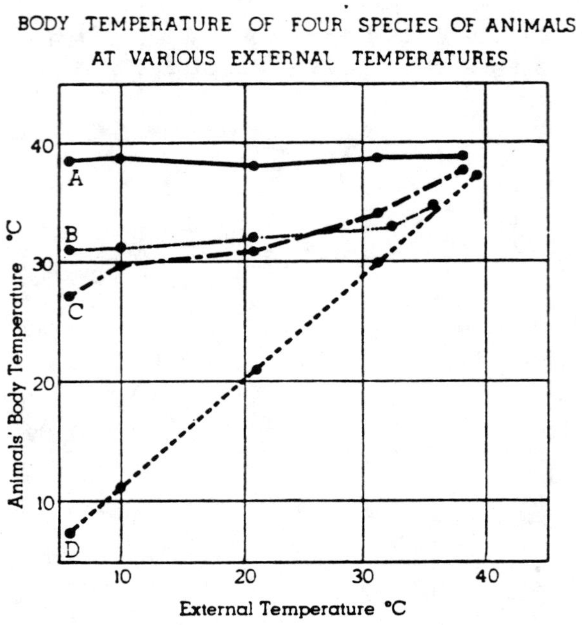

47. Which curve represents a cold-blooded animal? 47.___
A. A B. B C. C D. D E. None of these

48. Which curve represents an animal that is warm-blooded and whose temperature is LEAST affected by changes in external temperature? 48.___
A. A B. B C. C D. D E. None of the abo

Questions 49-50.

DIRECTIONS: Questions 49 and 50 are to be answered on the basis of the following illustration.

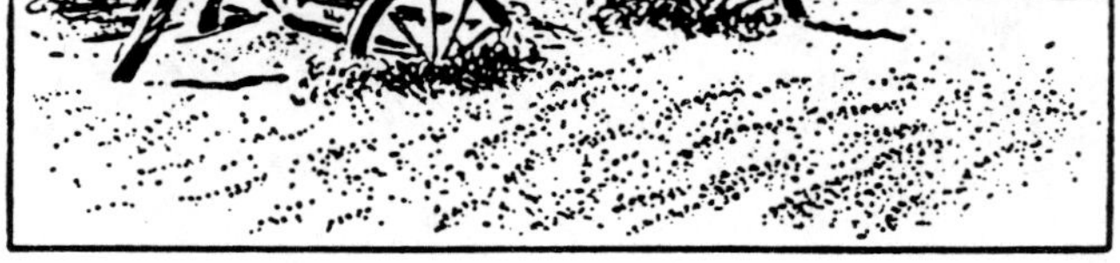

49. In the scene above, _____ has occurred. 49.___
A. a dust storm
B. sheet erosion
C. gullying
D. a snowstorm
E. a flood

50. The MOST probable cause of this occurrence was 50.___
A. overgrazing range land followed by floods
B. forest removal followed by heavy rains
C. a sudden drop in temperature followed by high winds
D. a forest fire
E. wheat farming on dry plains followed by high winds

KEY (CORRECT ANSWERS)

1. E	11. A	21. A	31. A	41. D
2. C	12. E	22. D	32. D	42. B
3. E	13. E	23. B	33. B	43. A
4. A	14. E	24. B	34. C	44. D
5. D	15. D	25. D	35. D	45. D
6. B	16. D	26. E	36. D	46. B
7. C	17. E	27. A	37. C	47. D
8. C	18. D	28. E	38. C	48. A
9. D	19. A	29. C	39. A	49. A
10. A	20. E	30. B	40. B	50. E

TEST 3

DIRECTIONS: Each question or incomplete statement is followed by several suggested answers or completions. Select the one that BEST answers the question or completes the statement. *PRINT THE LETTER OF THE CORRECT ANSWER IN THE SPACE AT THE RIGHT.*

1. Three groups of tadpoles of the same age were placed in a bowl containing pond water. The pituitary glands of the tadpoles in Group I were removed; the thyroid glands of the tadpoles in Group II were removed; and the tadpoles of Group II were left intact. In two weeks, only the tadpoles of Group III began to change into frogs. These observations are evidence that in frogs, the 1.____
   A. thyroid gland controls metamorphosis
   B. pituitary gland controls metamorphosis
   C. pituitary gland controls the thyroid gland
   D. thyroid and pituitary glands are both necessary for metamorphosis
   E. none of the above

2. John said that bean seeds sprout faster in the dark than in the light. 2.____
   Of the following, the BEST way for him to test this idea would be to moisten the seeds and then place
   A. some of the seeds in a dark refrigerator and the rest in sunlight
   B. all of the seeds in the sunlight for short periods of time and then move them into the dark
   C. some of the seeds in the dark and the rest in the light at the same temperature
   D. some of the seeds in the ground and the rest under a sunlamp
   E. none of the above

3. Which of the following would account for a fossil oyster found in your backyard? 3.____
   A. The oyster was probably fossilized by a volcanic eruption.
   B. Your backyard was probably once under water for a long time.
   C. The earth in your backyard is acid.
   D. The oyster evolved from a water animal to a land form.
   E. None of the above

4. As two students watched two squirrels in a park, the students made specific comments. 4.____
   Which of these comments was an assumption rather than an observation?
   A. The squirrels are getting ready to fight.
   B. One of the squirrels is moving faster than the other.
   C. The squirrels are not the same color.
   D. One of the squirrels dropped his nut.
   E. None of the above

5. The usual biological classification of plants and animals is based PRIMARILY on 5.___
   A. age
   B. structure
   C. geographical distribution
   D. size
   E. color

6. The CHIEF reason it is harder to breathe at high altitudes than at low ones is that at high altitudes 6.___
   A. the temperatures are lower
   B. there are fewer plants
   C. there is more CO_2
   D. the air pressure is lower
   E. None of the above

7. An animal is surely a bird if it 7.___
   A. flies
   B. lays eggs that hatch
   C. has feathers
   D. is warm-blooded
   E. has webbed feet

8. The featherlike gills of most species of fish PRIMARILY provide a 8.___
   A. large amount of surface area for the exchange of gases
   B. pump for the rapid flow of blood through the gill filaments
   C. filter for obtaining small particles of food from the water
   D. means for breaking down water into hydrogen and oxygen
   E. None of the above

Questions 9-26.

DIRECTIONS: In each of the following groups of items, there are several statements, phrases, or terms, each of which characterizes or suggests one of the five words or phrases listed above the questions. For each question, select that word or phrase from the above list to which it applies, or with which it is MOST significantly associated, and put the letter of your choice in the space at the right.

Questions 9-11.

A. Conjugation
B. Hybridization
C. Maturation
D. Inbreeding
E. Dominance

9. The breeding of parents CLOSELY related to each other. 9.___

10. Crossbreeding of parents differing in one or more hereditary characteristics. 10.___

11. The appearance of ONLY one of two contrasting characters when the potentialities of both are present in an individual. 11.___

Questions 12-14.

A. Ovum
B. Uterus
C. Vagina
D. Ovary
E. Oviduct

12. An egg; the female reproductive cell which, after fertilization, develops into a new member of the same species. 12.___

13. An organ in which the eggs or young of animals are retained during embryonic development. 13.___

14. An organ in which animal egg cells are produced. 14.___

Questions 15-17.

A. Dihybrid
B. Genotype
C. Mutant
D. Phenotype
E. Homozygote

15. An individual described or recognized by its visible characters WITHOUT reference to its hereditary factors. 15.___

16. An individual whose parents differ with respect to two pairs of hereditary characters. 16.___

17. An individual possessing an abrupt and heritable variation differing from any of its ancestors. 17.___

Questions 18-20.

A. Taxonomy
B. Paleontology
C. Cytology
D. Anatomy
E. Ecology

18. The scientific study of organisms of past geological periods, based on fossil remains. 18.___

19. The study of the structures and physiology of cells. 19.___

20. The study of the relations of organisms to each other and to their environment. 20.___

Questions 21-23.

A. Diastole
B. Peristalsis
C. Flexion
D. Tonus
E. Extension

21. A wave-like series of muscular contractions, progressing along the walls of various tubes of the body, propelling their contents. 21.___

22. A movement that bends one part upon another. 22.___

23. The stage of dilation of the heart or relaxation of the heart muscle. 23.___

Questions 24-26.

A. Blood
B. Neurilemma
C. Biceps
D. Neuron
E. Retina of the eye

24. Epithelial tissue 24.___

25. Vascular tissue 25.___

26. Muscular tissue 26.___

27. Identify the TRUE statement regarding the preservation of animal and plant remains. 27.___
   A. The most perfect fossils have been found in metamorphosed rock.
   B. Petrifaction preserves the organism without chemical change.
   C. Most ancient plants and animals ultimately were fossilized.
   D. Complete bodies of large animals have been preserved for thousands of years by low temperatures.
   E. Proterozoic rock is an abundant source of fossils.

28. Injection of pure water into the blood of an animal may indirectly cause its death by 28.___
   A. chemical reaction with hemoglobin
   B. plasmolysis of the corpuscles
   C. increasing external pressure upon the corpuscles
   D. swelling and bursting of the corpuscles
   E. destroying the permeability of the plasma membrane of the corpuscles

29. It is probable that the earliest organisms on the earth were MOST similar to present day 29.____
   A. saprophytic bacteria or fungi
   B. parasitic bacteria
   C. autophytic (autotrophic) bacteria or simple algae
   D. amoeba-like protozoans
   E. lichens

30. Mitotic cell division takes place 30.____
   A. principally in germ cells
   B. more commonly than any other form of cell division in organisms other than the lowest forms
   C. mainly in one-celled organisms
   D. mainly in vertebrates
   E. only under the influence of unfavorable conditions

31. The division of the Class Insecta into orders is made CHIEFLY on the basis of 31.____
   A. geographical distribution
   B. complexity of structures
   C. wing structure and mouth parts
   D. size and color
   E. egg-laying habits

32. The diploid number of chromosomes would be found in cells taken from what part of a moss plant? 32.____
   A. Archegonium   B. Antheridium   C. Protonema
   D. Calyptra   E. Capsule

33. The existence of cellulose-digesting protozoa in the intestines of termites is an example of 33.____
   A. a symbiotic relationship
   B. pathogenic parasitism
   C. saprophytism
   D. ecological succession
   E. a predatory relationship

34. Evidence of man's possible existence in the Pliocene Period is the discovery in sedimentary strata of that period of 34.____
   A. crude stone implements or eoliths
   B. crude metallic ornaments
   C. pottery
   D. complete skeletons of man-like creatures
   E. fossil remains of domesticated animals

35. Which one of the following is thought to have borne the GREATEST physical resemblance to man of today? 35.____
   A. Pithecanthropus erectus   B. Cro-Magnon man
   C. Neanderthal man   D. Piltdown man
   E. Peking man

36. The evolution of land plants from the Thallophytes to the Spermatophytes has been GENERALLY characterized by a(n) 36.___
A. *decrease* in structural size of the sexual generation
B. *increase* in the structural size and importance of the sexual generation
C. *decrease* in the functional importance of the sexual generation
D. *decreased* dependence on other plants and animals
E. *decrease* in number of complex structures

37. Colorblindness in man is a recessive sex-linked character. How many of the children of a colorblind mother and a father with normal vision will be colorblind? 37.___
A. All of the children
B. One-half of the girls and one-half of the boys
C. All of the girls and none of the boys
D. All of the boys and none of the girls
E. None of the children

38. Asphyxiation or suffocation victims are sometimes given a mixture of oxygen and carbon dioxide rather than pure oxygen because the carbon dioxide 38.___
A. stimulates the respiratory center in the medulla
B. decreases the danger to the victim of a shock resulting from sudden administration of pure oxygen
C. increases the speed with which gases pass through the lung tissue
D. decreases the viscosity of the blood
E. directly stimulates the rib muscles

39. The organism which is LEAST dependent upon other organisms for the procurement of essential food substances is 39.___
A. an amoeba
B. an autophytic (autotrophic) bacterium
C. a mushroom
D. bread mold
E. man

40. Iodide is added to salt to keep people from developing goiters. 40.___
The reason for using the iodide is MOST similar to the reason for
A. applying antiseptic to a cut
B. taking aspirin for a fever
C. adding chlorine to water to kill bacteria
D. adding fluoride to drinking water to prevent tooth decay
E.

41. Which of the following is PROBABLY a drawing of plant cells? 41.___

A.
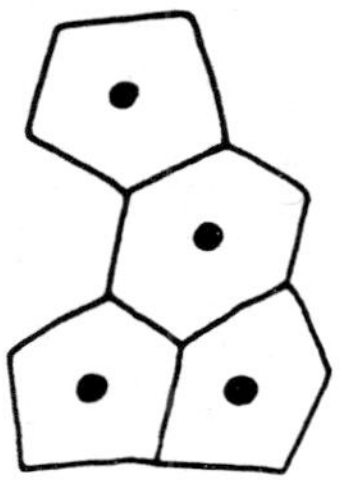

B.
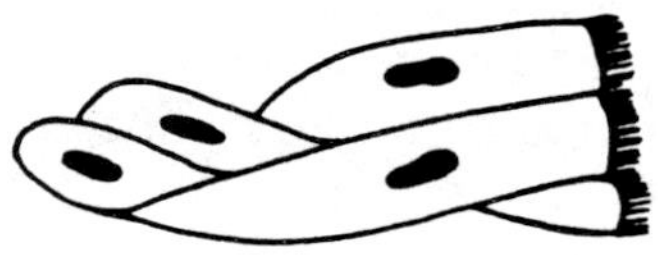

C. 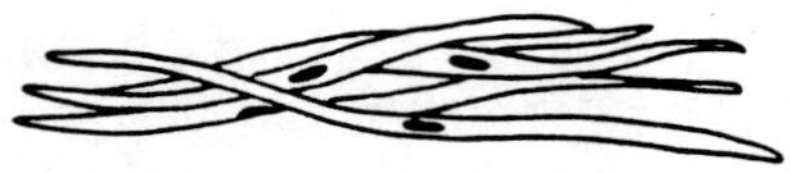

D. 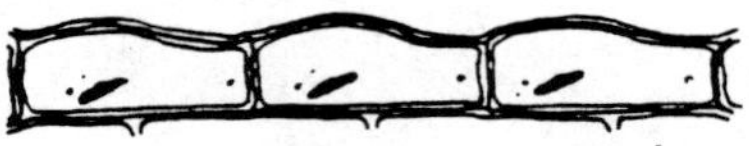

E. None of the above

42. The significance of meiosis for heredity lies in which statement? 42.___

A. The great variety of gene combinations that it makes possible
B. The doubling of the chromosome number in the sex cells of the offspring
C. The production of offspring identical with the parents
D. The potential for many offspring
E. None of the above

43. An experimenter wants to know whether a mouse is more likely to turn left or right in a maze. 43.___
Which experimental design is BEST for this purpose?

A. 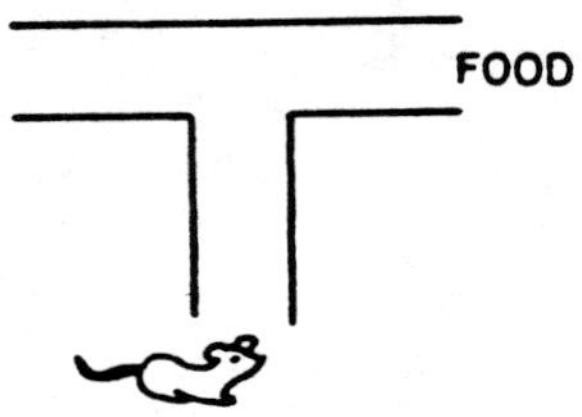

B. 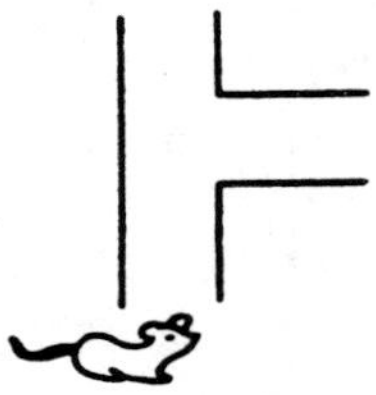

C. 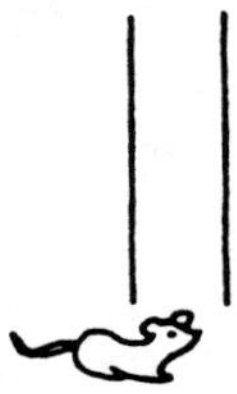

D. 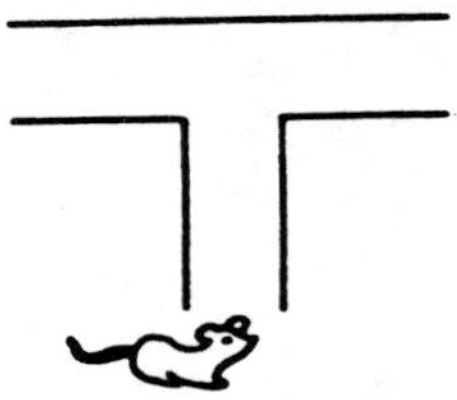

E. None of the above

44. Two plants with pink flowers were crossed, and the following results were obtained: 27 red, 31 white, and 63 pink-flowered plants. 44.___
These data indicate that the color of the pink flowers is due to

A. sex-linked recessiveness
B. sex-linked dominance
C. incomplete dominance
D. translocation
E. chromotropsin

45. What is the BEST reason why only consumer organisms and very few producer organisms are found at great ocean depths? 45.___
   A. In deep water, consumer organisms ingest any producer organisms at a rate that prevents reproduction of the producers.
   B. Photosynthesis requires the presence of light.
   C. Increased pressure favors the survival of heterotrophs and not of autotrophs.
   D. Autotrophs are independent of heterotrophs in deep water.
   E. The enormous pressure inhibits growth.

Questions 46-47.

DIRECTIONS: Questions 46 and 47 are to be answered on the basis of the following diagram of the food web.

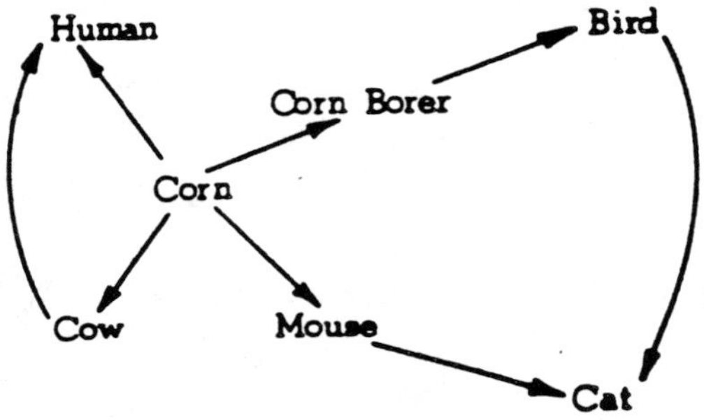

46. Which of these is a PRIMARY producer in this food web? 46.___
   A. Bird B. Cat C. Corn D. Human E. Mouse

47. The food web above includes _____ primary (first-order) consumers? 47.___
   A. One B. Two C. Three D. Four E. Five

Questions 48-50.

DIRECTIONS: Questions 48 through 50 are to be answered on the basis of the following table.

POPULATION RECORDS FOR 9 SPECIES OF BIRDS THAT APPEARED TO BE MOST SERIOUSLY AFFECTED BY APPLICATION OF DDT DUST ON A 40-ACRE PLOT

SPECIES	NO. OF BIRDS COUNTED BEFORE DUSTING	NUMBER OF BIRDS COUNTED DURING FIRST 6 DAYS AFTER DUSTING					
		1st Day	2nd Day	3rd Day	4th Day	5th Day	6th Day
Texas wren	3	2	2	1	0	0	0
Carolina wren	5	1	0	0	0	0	0
Kentucky warbler	1	0	0	0	0	0	0
Yellow-breasted chat	3	0	0	0	0	0	0
Cardinal	10	8	6	5	2	1	1
Blue grosbeak	2	0	0	0	0	0	0
Painted bunting	4	4	3	2	2	0	0
Lark sparrow	8	2	2	2	2	1	1
Field sparrow	5	4	4	4	3	3	1
Total	41	21	17	14	9	5	3

Study the above table and read each question carefully. Then, in the space at the right, mark the letter of your answer according to the KEY below.

KEY
A. The table tends to support the statement.
B. The table tends to contradict the statement.
C. The table furnishes no conclusive evidence, either supporting or contradicting the statement.

48. Within two days after application of DDT to the 40-acre plot, a decrease in numbers was noted in all nine species of birds listed. 48.___

49. Ground-nesting birds were MOST seriously affected by the spreading of DDT over the plot. 49.___

50. DDT MUST be used with extreme caution in areas occupied by birds. 50.___

KEY (CORRECT ANSWERS)

1. D	11. E	21. B	31. C	41. D
2. C	12. A	22. C	32. E	42. A
3. B	13. B	23. A	33. A	43. D
4. A	14. D	24. E	34. A	44. C
5. B	15. D	25. A	35. B	45. B
6. D	16. A	26. C	36. A	46. C
7. C	17. C	27. D	37. D	47. D
8. A	18. B	28. D	38. A	48. A
9. D	19. C	29. C	39. B	49. C
10. B	20. E	30. B	40. D	50. A

EXAMINATION SECTION

TEST 1

DIRECTIONS: Each question or incomplete statement is followed by several suggested answers or completions. Select the one that BEST answers the question or completes the statement. *PRINT THE LETTER OF THE CORRECT ANSWER IN THE SPACE AT THE RIGHT.*

1. If a protein contains 80 amino acids, its corresponding gene must contain AT LEAST how many nucleotides? 1.___
   A. 40 B. 120 C. 240 D. 360 E. 480

2. Which one of the following is characteristic ONLY of mitosis and NOT of meiosis? 2.___
   A. Synapsis occurs
   B. Cells with identical genotypes are produced
   C. Splitting of centromeres takes place
   D. Homologous chromosomes separate
   E. Spindle fibers are formed

3. The PRIMARY role of oxygen in respiration is to 3.___
   A. yield energy in the form of ATP as it is passed down the respiratory chain
   B. act as an acceptor for electrons and hydrogen ions to form water
   C. combine with carbon to form CO_2
   D. combine with lactic acid to form pyruvic acid
   E. catalyze the reactions of glycolysis

4. Fetal cells sloughed off into the amniotic fluid can be collected and cultured. 4.___
   The cultured cells CANNOT be used for prenatal diagnosis of
   A. identical twinning
   B. paternity
   C. genetic diseases whose metabolic basis is known
   D. the sex of the fetus
   E. aneuploidy

5. The function of the Loop of Henle is to 5.___
   A. rid the body of excess urea and ammonia
   B. rid the body of excess hydrogen ions
   C. return reusable nutrients to the blood
   D. produce a sugar gradient capable of concentrating urine
   E. produce a salt gradient capable of concentrating urine

6. The cells of the testis that are MOST like the follicle cells of the ovary in that they respond to the pituitary hormone LH by producing steroid hormones are 6.___
   A. spermatids B. endometrial cells
   C. stem cells D. interstitial cells
   E. germ cells

7. Bacteriophages are 7.____
   A. organelles
   B. organisms
   C. prokaryotes
   D. bacteria
   E. viruses

8. When an aerobic organism is temporarily deprived of O_2, it obtains its chemical energy from 8.____
   A. the substrate level of ATP synthesis in glycolysis
   B. the oxidation of pyruvic acid to acetyl-CoA
   C. the respiratory electron transport chain
   D. chemiosmotic coupling
   E. metabolism of succinic acid in the TCA cycle

9. Examination of the eukaryotic cell surface by the electron microscope reveals that the plasma membrane 9.____
   A. is composed of a single layer of molecules approximately 75 Angstrom units in thickness
   B. is composed exclusively of phospholipids
   C. invaginates into the cellular cytoplasm to form canals and vesicles
   D. invaginates to form cristae on which are arranged the electron transport systems
   E. is composed exclusively of proteins

10. In a research project, a chemical was introduced to developing embryos that selectively destroyed the mesoderm germ layer. 10.____
    Which of the following structures would be absent in the fetus?
    A. Brain
    B. Pectoralis muscle
    C. Epidermis
    D. Intestinal mucosa
    E. Adrenal medulla

11. A restriction endonuclease produces a break in 11.____
    A. DNA at a specific base sequence
    B. tRNA at a specific base sequence
    C. any nucleic acid at the end of the molecule
    D. proteins at a specific amino acid sequence
    E. DNA at the 3' terminal end *only*

12. All chemosynthetic autotrophic prokaryotes belong to the 12.____
    A. bacteria
    B. fungi
    C. protozoa
    D. viruses
    E. tracheophytes

13. The carbon dioxide carried in the blood from the tissues to the lungs is MOST commonly found in the form of 13.____
    A. carbaminohemoglobin
    B. free carbon dioxide
    C. carbonic acid
    D. bicarbonate ions
    E. membrane-bound carbon dioxide

14. The regulation of body temperature, water balance, and appetite are a function of the 14.____
    A. thalamus
    B. hypothalamus
    C. medulla oblongata
    D. anterior lobe of pituitary
    E. cerebrum

15. In sex-linkage 15.___
   A. the recessive autosomal characters of the father are expressed in the sons
   B. X-linked characters of the mother must be expressed in the daughters
   C. the X-linked characters of the mother are never expressed in the daughters
   D. the primary sexual characteristics are determined by the sex hormones
   E. normal male fruitflies and humans always have a Y-chromosome

16. Assuming Hardy-Weinberg conditions, when 16 percent of a population is homozygous recessive for a trait, the percent that is heterozygous is 16.___
   A. 30 B. 25 C. 48 D. 24 E. 36

17. One of the evolutionary adaptations of reptiles for a terrestrial environment was 17.___
   A. a thin, pliable skin
   B. a four-chambered heart
   C. air breathing lung
   D. a shelled egg with extraembryonic membranes
   E. legs for rapid locomotion

18. According to the theory of natural selection, the environment *selects* ONLY those characteristics which 18.___
   A. fit the organism to future environmental change
   B. *increase* the life span of the individual
   C. *increase* the number of offspring which reach reproductive age
   D. result in stronger individuals
   E. affect social behavior

19. If acetylcholine were released at a synapse and acetylcholinesterase was inhibited, the 19.___
   A. postsynaptic neuron would not respond to the acetylcholine
   B. postsynaptic neuron would produce a single nerve impulse
   C. postsynaptic neuron would produce an abnormally long series of nerve impulses
   D. acetylcholine would not diffuse across the synapse
   E. acetylcholine would spontaneously decompose

20. Cystic fibrosis is inherited as a simple autosomal recessive. Suppose a woman who is heterozygous for this trait marries a man who is also heterozygous for it. What is the probability that they will have a child who is heterozygous for the trait? 20.___
   A. 0 B. 1/4 C. 1/2 D. 2/3 E. 3/4

KEY (CORRECT ANSWERS)

1.	C	11.	A
2.	B	12.	A
3.	B	13.	D
4.	A	14.	B
5.	E	15.	E
6.	D	16.	C
7.	E	17.	D
8.	A	18.	C
9.	C	19.	C
10.	B	20.	C

TEST 2

DIRECTIONS: Each question or incomplete statement is followed by several suggested answers or completions. Select the one that BEST answers the question or completes the statement. *PRINT THE LETTER OF THE CORRECT ANSWER IN THE SPACE AT THE RIGHT.*

1. Which of the following statements is TRUE of the archenteron? 1.____
   A. The cavity of the archenteron is called the blastocoel.
   B. The cavity of the archenteron represents the beginning of the primitive gut.
   C. The archenteron is formed during blastula formation.
   D. The cavity of the archenteron represents the first cavity of the developing heart.
   E. The archenteron is formed by a closing of the neural tube.

2. Which part of the cell is involved MOST directly with the synthesis of ribosomal subunits? 2.____
   A. Nucleolus
   B. Microtubules
   C. Endoplasmic reticulum
   D. Golgi apparatus
   E. Nuclear envelope

3. Which of the following substances is a nucleotide? 3.____
   A. Estrogen
   B. Growth hormone (somatotropin)
   C. Insulin
   D. Adenosine triphosphate (ATP)
   E. Amylose

4. Which of the following is NOT a function of microtubules? 4.____
   A. Maintaining or controlling the shape of the cell
   B. Movement of chromosomes during anaphase
   C. Temporary storage of proteins prior to secretion
   D. Forming the structural elements of the centrioles
   E. Activity of cells and flagella

5. The thymus gland is involved in 5.____
   A. the regulation of calcium metabolism
   B. the development of the immune response
   C. regulation of the activity of the thyroid gland
   D. endocrine and exocrine functions
   E. reproductive physiology

6. At different stages during the normal sequence of events in the menstrual cycle, there is an increase in progesterone, FSH, and estrogen. 6.____
   Which one of the following is the CORRECT sequence of *initial* increases in each substance, beginning with menstruation?
   A. Estrogen, FSH, progesterone
   B. FSH, estrogen, progesterone

C. Estrogen, progesterone, FSH
D. FSH, progesterone, estrogen
E. Progesterone, estrogen, FSH

7. Suppose an individual is heterozygous for ten different independently assorting genes. 7.____
How many genetically different gametes will be possible from this individual?
A. 10 B. 20 C. 10^2 D. 200 E. 2^{10}

8. Viruses may not be considered true living organisms because they 8.____
A. are too small
B. can only reproduce in the cells of another living organism
C. are not eukaryotes
D. are extremely primitive organisms
E. can only replicate in an anaerobic environment

9. One of the MAJOR advantages in using scanning electron microscopy as opposed to transmission electron microscopy is that 9.____
A. greater magnification can be obtained
B. greater resolving power can be obtained
C. the specimen does not have to be treated with chemicals
D. a three-dimensional image can be obtained
E. there is no advantage

10. The following gland is both endocrine and exocrine in function. 10.____
A. Thyroid B. Liver C. Adrenal
D. Pancreas E. Pituitary

11. Sucrose is 11.____
A. a disaccharide of glucose and fructose
B. a trisaccharide of galactose, glucose, and fructose
C. the technical term for blood sugar
D. the major subunit of cellulose
E. the major subunit of starch

12. The intracellular ion that is PRIMARILY responsible for triggering muscle contraction is 12.____
A. sodium B. potassium C. phosphorus
D. calcium E. magnesium

13. In which two of the following phyla do most biologists place the MOST primitive bilaterally symmetrical animals? 13.____
A. Chordata and Hemichordata
B. Coelenterata (Cnidaria) and Ctenophora
C. Onycophora and Arthropoda
D. Echinodermata and Chaetognatha
E. Platyhelminthes and Nemertina

14. A classic example of primary embryonic induction is the induction by the vertebrate chordamesoderm of the 14.___
A. vertebrae
B. axial musculature
C. neural tube
D. heart
E. liver primordium

15. In which of the following organelles is water synthesized from oxygen and hydrogen? 15.___
A. Nucleus
B. Mitochrondria
C. Ribosomes
D. Lysosomes
E. Golgi apparatus

16. The biological significance of the evolution of fleshy fruits such as the apple and the peach is that such fruits are 16.___
A. necessary for seed transpiration
B. to protect the seeds from being eaten by animals
C. exposed to rigorous natural selection because the matured ovary wall is triploid
D. important sources of vitamin C for the plant
E. adaptations to securing seed dispersal by animals

17. In a simple food chain, animals with the SMALLEST population *probably* 17.___
A. are least likely to be an endangered species
B. have a very high biotic potential
C. are physically smaller than the others in the food chain
D. are herbivorous
E. are carnivorous

18. Which of the following enzymes acts on carbohydrates? 18.___
A. Carboxypeptidase
B. Trypsin
C. Chymotrypsin
D. Lipase
E. Amylase

19. All of the following processes require energy input EXCEPT 19.___
A. active transport
B. muscle contraction
C. DNA synthesis
D. maintenance of the resting potential of neurons
E. osmosis

20. The movement of fluid from the arteriole end of a mammalian capillary bed into the interstitial spaces is PRIMARILY due to 20.___
A. hydrostatic pressure
B. osmotic pressure
C. active transport by the capillary walls
D. contraction of skeletal muscles
E. contraction of smooth muscle of the capillary walls

KEY (CORRECT ANSWERS)

1. B	11. A
2. A	12. D
3. D	13. E
4. C	14. C
5. B	15. B
6. B	16. E
7. E	17. E
8. B	18. E
9. D	19. E
10. D	20. A

EXAMINATION SECTION

DIRECTIONS: Each question or incomplete statement is followed by several suggested answers or completions. Select the one that BEST answers the question or completes the statement. *PRINT THE LETTER OF THE CORRECT ANSWER IN THE SPACE AT THE RIGHT.*

1. According to the Second Law of Thermodynamics, 1.___
   A. energy can neither be created nor destroyed
   B. energy can be created or destroyed
   C. any system isolated from an energy source tends to decrease in entropy
   D. organisms could not evolve
   E. any system isolated from an energy source tends toward its least ordered state

2. The distinction between the anaerobic metabolism of glucose in muscle cells and in yeast cells is the 2.___
   A. formation of lactic acid (lactate) in muscle cells and the formation of ethanol in yeast cells
   B. formation of acetate in yeast cells and lactate in muscle cells
   C. synthesis of more ATP per glucose molecule in muscle than in yeast cells
   D. formation of carbon dioxide in muscle but not in yeast cells
   E. synthesis of less ATP per glucose molecule in muscle cells

3. Organisms that obtain their energy from light can be termed 3.___
   A. autotrophic B. holotrophic C. chemotrophic
   D. heterotrophic E. heliotrophic

4. An investigator isolated small particles from cancer cells which hydrolyzed protein and concluded that these were 4.___
   A. ribosomes B. lipid vacuoles
   C. lysosomes D. food vacuoles
   E. mitochondria

5. The first enzyme-catalyzed reaction in the glycolysis of glucose is 5.___
   A. deamination B. lipolysis C. phosphorylation
   D. hydrolysis E. carboxylation

6. The generation of ATP (adenosine triphosphate) by the electron transport system (respiratory chain) occurs 6.___
   A. on the inner membrane of mitochondria
   B. on the outer surface of the nuclear envelope
   C. in the cytoplasm
   D. in the Golgi apparatus
   E. on the endoplasmic reticulum

7. Messenger ribonucleic acid (mRNA) differs from deoxyribonucleic acid (DNA) in that RNA 7.____
   I. contains thymine instead of uracil
   II. contains a ribose sugar
   III. is single-stranded

   The CORRECT answer is:
   A. I *only* B. II *only* C. III *only*
   D. I and III E. II and III

8. The so-called dark reactions (light-independent reactions) of photosynthesis 8.____
   A. do not occur during the daytime
   B. use the direct energy of light quanta
   C. occur in all plants cells
   D. do not require the products of the light reactions
   E. result in the assimilation (fixation) of carbon dioxide

9. If animal muscle cells are deprived of oxygen, anaerobic glycolysis will result and pyruvic acid will then be converted to 9.____
   A. alcohol B. glucose
   C. lactic acid D. phosphoric acid
   E. acetyl CoA

10. A sample of blood is added to a test tube containing a 1.6% salt solution. A short while later, the red blood cells are observed to be smaller and wrinkled in shape due to water loss. 10.____
    This indicates that
    A. red blood cells are isotonic to the 1.6% salt solution
    B. red blood cells are hypertonic to the 1.6% salt solution
    C. red blood cells are hypotonic to the 1.6% salt solution
    D. the 1.6% salt solution is hypotonic to the red blood cells
    E. the 1.6% salt solution is isotonic to the red blood cells

11. Which of the following is the key intermediate compound linking glycolysis to the Krebs cycle? 11.____
    A. NADH B. ATP C. Cytochrome b
    D. Succinic acid E. Acetyl Co A

12. A plant kept in the dark will not be able to produce glucose because light is necessary 12.____
    A. for the oxidation of glucose
    B. to excite electrons in the CO_2 molecules
    C. for activating enzymes necessary for converting CO_2 to glucose
    D. for sufficient ATP and reduced NADP to be available to synthesize glucose from CO_2
    E. for glucose phosphorylation

13. The First Law of Thermodynamics implies that living organisms cannot create their own energy but can only convert one form of energy into another. What, then, is the ULTIMATE source of energy for most living organisms? 13.___
   A. Chemical energy from the glucose molecule made by plants during photosynthesis
   B. The chemical energy released by the numerous hydrolytic reactions in a cell
   C. Heat energy from the sun
   D. Light energy from the sun
   E. ATP made in the mitochondria of both plants and animals

14. Which of the following is NOT a function of any hormone? 14.___
   A. Affects membrane transport of substances
   B. Regulates water balance in the body
   C. Changes the amount of activity of enzymes
   D. Promotes transcription of messenger RNA
   E. Acts as a source of energy

15. Which of the following pairs of structures have similarity of function? 15.___
_____ nervous system.
   A. Thyroid gland and sympathetic
   B. Adrenal cortex and sympathetic
   C. Adrenal cortex and parasympathetic
   D. Adrenal medulla and parasympathetic
   E. Adrenal medulla and sympathetic

16. In the nephron of the kidney, filtration occurs between 16.___
   A. Bowman's capsule and Henle's loop
   B. the glomerulus and Bowman's capsule
   C. the proximal tubule and Henle's loop
   D. Henle's loop and the vasa recta
   E. the peritubular network and the convoluted tubules

17. The stimulation of parasympathetic nerves would produce a(n) 17.___
   A. increase in peristaltic activity
   B. increase in perspiration
   C. decrease in salivary gland activity
   D. increase in blood pressure
   E. none of the above

18. Clotting of human blood 18.___
   A. requires that hemoglobin be present
   B. results from fibrin joining globulin
   C. is a result of platelets releasing fibrinogen
   D. depends on the formation of fibrin from fibrinogen
   E. is accelerated when Ca^{++} is removed

19. The muscle cells of the human heart are PRIMARILY nourished by 19.___
   A. blood within the four chambers of the heart
   B. fluid in the pericardial cavity
   C. the lymphatic system
   D. blood delivered by the coronary arteries
   E. blood delivered by the ductus arteriosus

20. Carbon dioxide passes from tissues to blood to lungs by 20.___
   A. diffusing from a region of high concentration to an area of lesser concentration
   B. diffusing from a region of lower to one of higher concentration
   C. active transport
   D. irreversibly binding to hemoglobin
   E. chemiosmosis

21. Products of digestion absorbed in the mammalian small intestine 21.___
   A. are carried directly to the heart by the posterior vena cava
   B. are carried to the spleen for processing
   C. must be further digested in the blood before they can be absorbed by the cells
   D. are processed by the cells of the small intestine, which then secrete ATP into the blood
   E. are carried to the liver by the hepatic portal vein

22. Which of the following are typically autotrophic? 22.___
   A. Protozoa B. Plants C. Animals
   D. Fungi E. Bacteria

23. Of the following phyla, the one that contains more species than the others combined is 23.___
   A. Annelida B. Arthropoda C. Mollusca
   D. Echinodermata E. Chordata

24. All chordates 24.___
   A. possess backbones
   B. possess a dorsal, tubular nerve cord at some stage of life
   C. lack larval forms
   D. have endoskeletons composed of cartilage
   E. have a water vascular system

25. In which of these kingdoms are the organisms entirely heterotrophic? 25.___
   A. Protista and Fungi B. Plantae and Fungi
   C. Animalia and Fungi D. Protista and Animalia
   E. Monera and Protista

26. Mendel's law of segregation reflects the fact that 26.___
   A. linkage never occurs in peas
   B. alleles segregate differently in males and females
   C. each member of an allelic pair of genes enters a separate cell during meiosis
   D. during the course of development, DNA becomes segregated in the nucleus, RNA in the cytoplasm
   E. increasing specialization in the course of evolution is characterized by a segregation of tissue types

27. A diploid cell (2N = 20) has how many tetrads at metaphase I? 27.___
   A. 0 B. 10 C. 20 D. 40 E. 80

28. For the human ABO blood typing system, which of the following is ALWAYS determined by a homozygous genotype? Type 28.___
   A. A
   B. B
   C. AB
   D. O
   E. all of the above

29. During the synthesis of a polypeptide at the ribosome site, the completed polypeptide is released when the 29.___
   A. ribosome reaches a termination codon
   B. ribosome reaches a termination anticodon
   C. tRNAs are depleted
   D. amino acids are depleted
   E. ribosome reaches the 5' end of the mRNA

30. A particular double-stranded DNA molecule was found to have 24% of its bases consist of adenine (A). What percentage of its bases would be expected to consist of guanine (G)? 30.___
   A. 24 B. 26 C. 48 D. 52 E. 76

31. In humans, a phenotype resulting from a homozygous autosomal recessive pair of genes would be expected to appear 31.___
   A. in unequal numbers in the two sexes
   B. phenotypically in every generation as long as one of the original parents manifested the trait
   C. only in those individuals who had at least one parent with the gene
   D. in approximately one-fourth of the children produced by two heterozygotes
   E. none of the above

32. One form of colorblindness is caused by a gene c carried on the X chromosome in humans. The gene is recessive to its normal allele C. Far more men are colorblind than women. 32.___
Geneticists explain this by pointing out that
   A. women possess no X chromosomes in their cells
   B. men carry no genes for color vision on their Y chromosomes
   C. men carry more genes for colorblindness than women do

D. colorblindness is inhibited by female sex hormones
E. colorblindness is promoted by male sex hormones

33. Sexual reproduction as compared with asexual reproduction ordinarily results in 33.___
A. more offspring
B. a greater inducement to reproduce
C. greater genetic diversity in the offspring
D. a higher frequency of well-adapted individual offspring
E. fewer individuals carrying recessive alleles

34. Gastrulation involves the 34.___
A. formation of the blastocoel
B. formation of germ layers
C. loss of the blastopore
D. formation of the blastula
E. final differentiation of the stomach

35. Of the germ layers comprising the early human embryo, which one forms MOST of the central nervous system? 35.___
A. Ectoderm B. Mesoderm C. Endoderm
D. Notochord E. Dermis

36. Embryonic induction is a process in which 36.___
A. embryonic tissues influence adjacent tissues to differentiate
B. an unfertilized egg is induced to develop
C. genes are transferred from one developing tissue to another
D. resting potentials are induced in neurons of embryos
E. the maternal parent induces expression of recessive genes in embryos

37. One of the loveliest sounds in nature is bird song. Such song is commonly associated with 37.___
A. hunger B. pugnacity C. territoriality
D. orientation E. happiness

38. A deciduous forest biome differs from that of the grassland biome in that the forest biome receives more 38.___
A. sunlight
B. CO_2 for photosynthesis
C. fixed nitrogen from the soil
D. moisture
E. ultraviolet light

39. Which of the following situations is MOST likely to result in genetic drift? 39.___
A. An increase in population size
B. A lack of gene mutation
C. A prevention of emigration
D. Random mating
E. Isolation of a small population from a larger one

40. Under Hardy-Weinberg conditions, 40.___
   A. dominant alleles eventually replace recessive alleles
   B. evolution occurs at a rapid rate
   C. the frequency of dominant alleles slowly increases
   D. gene frequencies remain constant
   E. a 50%-50% equilibrium is reached between dominant and recessive alleles

---

KEY (CORRECT ANSWERS)

1. E	11. E	21. E	31. D
2. A	12. D	22. B	32. B
3. A	13. D	23. B	33. C
4. C	14. E	24. B	34. B
5. C	15. E	25. C	35. A
6. A	16. B	26. C	36. A
7. E	17. A	27. B	37. C
8. E	18. D	28. D	38. D
9. C	19. D	29. A	39. E
10. C	20. A	30. B	40. D

EXAMINATION SECTION

DIRECTIONS: Each question or incomplete statement is followed by several suggested answers or completions. Select the one that BEST answers the question or completes the statement. *PRINT THE LETTER OF THE CORRECT ANSWER IN THE SPACE AT THE RIGHT.*

1. Vaporization is an example of a process for which _____ at all temperatures. 1.___
   A. ΔH and ΔG are positive
   B. ΔH and ΔS are positive
   C. ΔS and ΔG are positive
   D. ΔH and ΔS are negative
   E. ΔH and ΔG are negative

2. Which of the following elements is MOST electronegative? 2.___
   A. Li B. K C. C D. Ge E. N

3. What is the percentage of oxygen by weight in $Ba(HCO_3)_2$ (259g/mol)?
   A. 9.6% B. 18.5% C. 24.2% D. 37.1% E. 49.0%

4. What species is missing in the following nuclear equation? 4.___

$$^{235}_{92}U + ^{1}_{0}n \rightarrow ^{103}_{42}Mo + 2^{1}_{0}n + ?$$

   A. $^{131}_{50}Sn$ B. $^{132}_{50}Sn$ C. $^{131}_{52}Te$ D. $^{132}_{52}Te$ E. $^{132}_{51}Sb$

5. Two tanks of gas with identical volumes are filled at one atmosphere pressure and at the same temperature. If one tank contains H_2 and the other contains O_2, then 5.___
   A. both tanks contain the same mass of gas
   B. both tanks contain the same number of gas molecules
   C. both gases have the same density
   D. the molecules in both tanks are traveling at the same average speed
   E. the average kinetic energy in the H_2 tank is greater than in the O_2 tank

6. A solution of potassium acetate ($KC_2H_3O_2$) in water is 6.___
   A. basic because acetic acid molecules are formed
   B. basic because KOH molecules are formed
   C. acidic because acetic acid molecules are formed
   D. acidic because KOH molecules are formed
   E. neutral because potassium acetate is a salt

7. In an aqueous solution, the following equilibrium reactions are present: 7.___

$$Ag(NH_3)_2^+ \rightleftarrows Ag^+ + 2NH_3$$

$$NH_3 + H_2O \rightleftarrows NH_4^+ + OH^-$$

If the soluble salt, AgNO , is added to the solution, the following changes in concentration take place:

A. $[NH_3]$, $[NH_4^+]$, and $[OH^-]$ decrease

B. $[NH_3]$ increases; $[NH_4^+]$ and $[OH^-]$ decrease

C. $[NH_4^+]$ increases; $[NH_3]$ and $[OH^-]$ decrease

D. $[NH_4^+]$ and $[OH^-]$ increase; $[NH_3]$ decreases

E. $[NH_3]$ and $[OH^-]$ increase; $[NH_4^+]$ decreases

8. If an isotope of an element has an atomic number of 45 and a mass number of 103, another isotope of the element could have 8.____

A. 58 neutrons
B. fewer than 45 protons
C. more than 45 protons
D. 57 neutrons
E.

9. The conjugate acid of HPO_4^{2-} in water solution is 9.____

A. H^+ B. H_3PO_4 C. $H_4PO_4^+$ D. PO_4^{3-} E. $H_2PO_4^-$

10. Calculate the heat of reaction, $\Delta H°$, for the reaction 10.____

$$C_3H_8(g) + 5O_2(g) \rightarrow 3CO_2(g) + 4H_2O(l)$$

The necessary values for ΔH_f°, in Kcal/mole, are

$$H_2O(l) = -68.3,\ CO_2(g) = -94.0,\ C_3H_8(g) = -24.8$$

A. $1(-24.8) - 3(-94.0) - 4(-68.3)$
B. $-94.0 - 68.3 + 24.8$
C. $-24.8 - 94.0 - 68.3$
D. $3(-94.0) + 4(-68.3) - 1(-24.8)$
E. $3(-94.0) + 4(-68.3) + 1(-24.8)$

11. If a solution which is initially 1.00M in compound X undergoes a decomposition reaction for 20.0 sec at an average rate of 0.020 mol/l. sec, the new concentration of X will be ____ M. 11.____

A. 0.10 B. 0.40 C. 0.60 D. 1.0 E. 1.4

12. A gaseous mixture of 10 mole % nitrous oxide (N_2O), 20 mole % oxygen (O_2), and 70 mole % nitrogen (N_2) has a total pressure of 800 mm. 12.____
What is the partial pressure, in mm, of the nitrous oxide?

A. 800×0.10 B. $\frac{800}{0.10}$ C. $\frac{0.10}{800}$

D. 800×0.90 E. $\frac{800}{0.90}$

13. The simplest empirical formula for a compound was determined to be CH_2O, and its molecular weight was found to be 60g/mol. 13.___
How many atoms of hydrogen are in a molecule of this compound?
A. 2 B. 3 C. 4 D. 5 E. 6

14. In the following reaction, identify the oxidizing agent and the reducing agent: 14.___

$$4\,Zn + NO_3^- + 7\,OH^- \rightarrow NH_3 + 4ZnO_2^{2-} + 2H_2O$$

The oxidizing agent is ____; the reducing agent is ____.
A. Zn; NO_3^- B. NO_3^-; Zn C. OH^-; Zn^-
D. Zn; OH^- E. NO_3^-; OH^-

15. What is the ionization constant of a weak acid whose hydronium ion concentration is 3.0×10^{-5} in an 0.02M solution? 15.___
A. 1.8×10^{-11} B. 3.0×10^{-10} C. 3.0×10^{-3}
D. 4.5×10^{-12} E. 4.5×10^{-8}

16. Which one of the following 0.15m aqueous solutions has the LOWEST freezing point? 16.___
A. KCL B. $Al_2(SO_4)_3$ C. CH_3OH
D. C_2H_5OH E. NaOH

17. The boiling point of any liquid is 17.___
A. 100°C
B. the temperature at which as many molecules leave the liquid as return to it
C. the temperature at which the vapor pressure is equal to the external pressure
D. the temperature at which no molecules can return to the bulk of the liquid
E. the temperature at which the intermolecular forces are at their maximum

18. A gaseous sample contains 0.02000 moles of N_2. 18.___
How many atoms of nitrogen are in this sample?
A. 0.02000 B. 0.04000 C. 6.02×10^{23}
D. 12.04×10^{25} E. 24.08×10^{21}

19. In which of the following compounds does sulfur have an oxidation number of +2? 19.___
A. Na_2S B. Na_2S_2 C. $Na_2S_2O_3$
D. Na_2SO_3 E. Na_2SO_4

20. In which solvent should NaCl be MOST soluble? 20.___
A. CH_3OH (methyl alcohol)
B. C_8H_{18} (octane)
C. $(C_2H_5)_2O$ (diethyl ether)
D. CCl_4 (carbon tetrachloride)
E. C_6H_6 (benzene)

21. A common oxidation number of +2 exists for most period four transition metals because 21.___
   A. the elements are filling in the d orbitals
   B. of a d orbital screening effect
   C. the +2 oxidation state is always the most stable
   D. the 4s orbital fills before the 3d orbitals in these elements
   E. the 4s electrons are more easily removed than 3d electrons during ionization

22. If the rate of a reaction is second order with respect to component A, how will the rate change if the concentration of A is tripled? 22.___
It will
   A. double
   B. triple
   C. be six times as great
   D. be nine times as great
   E. be reduced to one-third its original value

23. An element has the electron configuration as follows: 23.___
$1s^2 2s^2 2p^6 3s^2 3p^6 3d^{10} 4s^2 4p^3$
This element
   A. is a transition element
   B. belongs to the halogen family
   C. has 33 neutrons
   D. belongs to Group V
   E. is an alkaline earth metal

24. When the following oxidation-reduction reaction is balanced, what is the correct stoichiometric coefficient for Sn^+ ? $Sn^{2+} + H^+ + Cr_2O_7^{2-} \rightarrow Sn^{4+} + Cr^{3+} + H_2O$ 24.___

A. 1 B. 2 C. 3 D. 4 E. 6

25. Which one of the following is the CORRECT chemical symbol for a particle containing 6 protons, 8 neutrons, and 7 electrons? 25.___
A. N B. C^+ C. C^- D. O^+ E. O^-

26. Select the one element below with a partially filled d-orbital subshell. 26.___
A. Pb B. Mg C. Se D. Cr E. Al

27. What mass of NaOH (40.0g/mol) should be weighted out to make 2.50 liters of 1.50M NaOH? 27.___
A. 40g B. 60g C. 100g D. 120g E. 150g

28. The solubility of Ag_2CrO_4 in water is x mol/L. Its solubility product constant, Ksp., is 28.___
A. $4x^3$ B. $4x^2$ C. $2x^2$ D. $2x^3$ E. x^2

29. The amount of heat it takes to raise the temperature of 1 gram of any substance by 1 degree celsius is ALWAYS 29.___
   A. the entropy of the substance
   B. the exothermic capacity of the substance
   C. the free energy of the substance
   D. the specific heat of the substance
   E. one (1) calorie

30. If 200 mL of 1.60M NaOH are diluted with water to a volume of 350 mL, the new concentration of the solution is 30.___

   A. $(\frac{200}{350})(\frac{1}{1.60})$ B. $(\frac{200}{350})(\frac{1.60}{1})$ C. $(\frac{1.60}{1})(\frac{200}{550})$

   D. $(\frac{350}{200})(\frac{1.60}{1})$ E. $(\frac{350}{200})(\frac{1}{1.60})$

KEY (CORRECT ANSWERS)

1. B	11. C	21. E
2. E	12. A	22. D
3. D	13. C	23. D
4. A	14. B	24. C
5. B	15. E	25. C
6. A	16. B	26. D
7. A	17. C	27. E
8. D	18. E	28. A
9. E	19. C	29. D
10. D	20. A	30. B

EXAMINATION SECTION

DIRECTIONS: Each question or incomplete statement is followed by several suggested answers or completions. Select the one that BEST answers the question or completes the statement. *PRINT THE LETTER OF THE CORRECT ANSWER IN THE SPACE AT THE RIGHT.*

1. The density of graphite (carbon) is 2.2 g/cm^3. Accordingly, which of the following graphite samples is the LARGEST? 1.___
   A. 12 g
   B. 12 cm^3
   C. 12 moles
   D. 12 atoms
   E. All are the same size

2. How many grams of copper are produced when 1.5 g of aluminum are reacted with excess $Cu(NO_3)_2$ according to the following equation: 2.___
   $2Al + 3Cu(NO_3)_2 \rightarrow 2Al(NO_3)_3 + 3Cu$.
   (The atomic masses of copper and aluminum are 63.5 and 27.0 a.m.u., respectively.)
   1.5 ×
   A. (2/3) × (27.0/63.5)
   B. (3/2 × (27.0/63.5)
   C. (2/3) × (63.5/27.0)
   D. (3/2) × (63.5/27.0)
   E. (63.5/27.0)

3. For the reaction between A and B to form C, it is found that when one combines 0.6 moles of A with 0.6 moles of B, all of the B reacts, 0.2 moles of A remain unreacted, and 0.4 moles of C are produced. 3.___
   What is the balanced equation for this reaction?
   A. A + 2B → C
   B. A + 3B → 2C
   C. 3A + 3B → 2C
   D. 3A + 2B → 3C
   E. 2A + 3B → 2C

4. If 3.00 g of a nitrogen-oxygen compound is found to contain 2.22 g of oxygen, what is the percentage of nitrogen in the compound? 4.___
   A. (3.00/2.22)(100/1)
   B. ((3.00 + 2.22)/3.00)(100/1)
   C. ((3.00 - 2.22)/2.22)(100/1)
   D. ((3.00 - 2.22)/3.00)(100/1)

5. A 10.0 liter sample of oxygen at 100°C and 1 atm is cooled to 27°C and expanded until the pressure is 0.5 atm. Find the final volume of the oxygen. 5.___
   A. (10.0)(1/5)(27/100)
   B. (10.0)(1/.5)(373/300)
   C. (10.0)(.5/1)(373/300)
   D. (10.0)(1/.5)(300/373)
   E. (10.0)(.5/1)(300/373)

6. When the volume of a gas is decreased at constant temperature, the pressure increases because the molecules 6.___
   A. move faster
   B. move slower
   C. become heavier
   D. become lighter
   E. strike a unit area of the container more often

7. Which of the following types of bonding is found in diamond? 7.___
   A. Covalent
   B. Hydrogen
   C. Van der Waal's
   D. Metallic
   E. Ionic

8. The molar volume of copper (63.5 g/mole) at 25°C is 7.09 cm^3 $mole^{-1}$. 8.___
   Which of the following is the density of copper at 25°C in g cm^{-3}?
   A. (63.5)/(7.09)
   B. (63.5)(7.09)
   C. (7.09)/(63.5)
   D. 7.09
   E. ((63.5)/(7.09))(25)

9. A strong acid can be distinguished from a weak acid of the same concentration by the fact that the strong acid 9.___
   A. neutralizes a base
   B. is a better conductor of electricity
   C. turns blue litmus paper red
   D. reacts with a metal to liberate hydrogen
   E. none of the above

10. Which of the following is NOT a colligative property (a property based on the number of particles present)? 10.___
   A. Boiling point elevation
   B. Sublimation energy
   C. Vapor pressure lowering
   D. Freezing point depression
   E. Osmotic pressure

11. Which of the following will be the final volume in mL when 400 mL of 0.6 M HCl is diluted to 0.5 M HCl? 11.___
   A. (400/1)(0.5/0.6)
   B. (400/1)(0.6/0.5)
   C. ((0.6 - 0.5)/1)(400/1)
   D. ((1,000 - 400)/1)(0.5/0.6)
   E. (0.6/0.5)((1,000 - 400)/1)

12. Chlorine bleaches are solutions that contain approximately 5% NaClO. 12.___
   These solutions are
   A. slightly acidic
   B. strongly acidic
   C. neutral
   D. slightly basic
   E. strongly basic

13. What is the hydroxide ion concentration $[OH^-]$ of a solution having a pH of 5.0? 13.___

A. 5×10^{-5} M B. 5×10 M
C. 1×10^{-5} M D. 1×10^{-9} M
E. 5×10^{-9} M

14. The solubility product of CuI is 5.1×10^{-12}. How many moles of Cu^+ will be in equilibrium with CuI in 1.0 liter of a 0.01 M KI solution? 14.___

A. 5.1×10^{-6} B. 2.3×10^{-6} C. 5.1×10^{-12}
D. 2.3×10^{-5} E. 5.1×10^{-10}

15. For the reaction: 15.___

$AgCl_{(s)} + 2NH_{3(aq)} \rightleftarrows Ag(NH_3)_2^+ + Cl^-$,

the equilibrium constant $K = 4 \times 10^{-3}$, which of the following statements is TRUE? [K_{sp} for AgCl is 1.0×10^{-10}]

A. The addition of NH_3 decreases the solubility of AgCl.
B. AgCl is more soluble in aqueous NH_3 than in water.
C. AgCl is more soluble in an aqueous solution containing Cl^- than in water.
D. AgCl is less soluble in aqueous NH_3 than in water.
E. None of the above

16. What is the equilibrium constant expression, K, for the gaseous reaction: $O_2 + 4HCl \rightleftarrows 2H_2O + 2Cl_2$? 16.___
K =

A. $\frac{[H_2O]^2[Cl_2]^2}{[O_2][HCl]^4}$ B. $\frac{[H_2O][Cl_2]}{[O_2][HCl]}$

C. $\frac{[O_2][HCl]^4}{[H_2O]^2[Cl_2]^2}$ D. $\frac{2[H_2O]2[Cl_2]}{[O_2]4[HCl]}$

E. $\frac{2[H_2O]^2 2[Cl_2]^2}{[O_2]4[HCl]^4}$

17. What would be the heat of formation, ΔH_f, for NO_2 gas if one considers the equations for the following reactions where all substances are gases? 17.___

$\frac{1}{2}N_2 + \frac{1}{2}O_2 \rightarrow NO$ $\Delta H^\circ_f = +21.6$ kcal

$NO_2 \rightarrow NO + \frac{1}{2}O_2$ $\Delta H^\circ = +13.5$ kcal

A. -28.7 kcal B. -8.1 kcal C. 35.1 kcal
D. 28.7 kcal E. 8.1 kcal

18. Which one of the following processes is accompanied by a decrease in entropy? 18.___

A. Freezing of water
B. Evaporation of water
C. Sublimation of carbon dioxide
D. Shuffling a deck of cards
E. Heating a balloon filled with a gas

19. Rates of reactions are USUALLY studied by 19.____
A. measuring the concentration of the reactants or products as a function of time
B. calculating the free energy change for the reaction
C. measuring the heat evolved under different conditions
D. measuring the amount of each reactant in the reaction
E. calculating the entropy change for the reaction

20. Suppose a solution, which is initially 0.60 M in compound X, undergoes a decomposition reaction. After 10 seconds, the concentration of X is 0.40 M. 20.____
Which of the following is the average rate of decomposition of X in mol/L sec?
A. 0.020 B. 0.040 C. 0.10 D. 0.20 E. 0.50

21. Which of the following is the number of hydrogen ions in the balanced reaction: $H_2SO_3(aq) + IO^-_3(aq) \rightarrow SO_4^{2-}(aq) + I^-(aq) + H^+(aq)$? 21.____
A. 2 B. 4 C. 6 D. 8 E. 10

22. Given the following half-cell reactions: 22.____
$Cl_2(g) + 2e^- \rightarrow 2Cl^-(aq)$ E° = +1.36v
$Cu^{2+}(aq) + 2e^- \rightarrow Cu(s)$ E° = +.34v
what is the value of E° for the following reaction:
$Cu^{2+}(aq) + 2Cl^-(aq) \rightarrow Cu(s) + Cl_2(g)$?

A. -2.38v B. -1.70v C. -1.02v D. +1.02v E. +1.70v

23. Which of the following represents the change in oxidation state of nitrogen during the chemical reaction: 23.____
$2NO + 3S + 4H_2O \rightarrow 2HNO_3 + 3H_2S$?
A. 1 B. 2 C. 3 D. 4 E. 5

24. The ion $^{9}_{4}Be^{2+}$ has _____ protons, _____ neutrons, and _____ electrons. 24.____
A. 4; 5; 4 B. 4; 5; 2
C. 5; 4; 2 D. 5; 4; 4
E. none of the above

25. The correct Lewis formula for a nitrate ion (NO_3^-) is 25.____

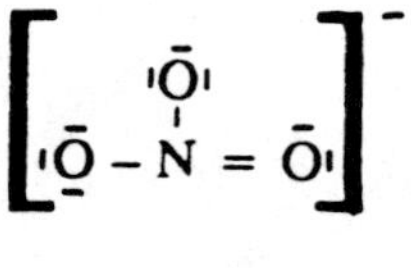

Which of the following are the oxygen-nitrogen-oxygen bond angles in this ion closest to?
A. 90° B. 109° C. 120° D. 150° E. 180°

26. Which of the following is the ground state electron configuration for $^{24}_{12}Mg^{2+}$? 26.____
A. $1s^2 2s^2 2p^6 3s^2$ B. $1s^2 2s^2 2p^6$
C. $1s^2 2s^2 2p^6 3s^2 3p^2$ D. $1s^2 2s^2 2p^4 3s$
E. $1s^2 2s^2 2p^6 3s^2 3p^6 3d^4 4s^2$

27. Antimony (Sb) has a smaller atomic radius than strontium (Sr) because of 27.___
   A. increased electron shielding
   B. the lanthanide contraction
   C. increased metallic character
   D. increased nuclear to electron attraction
   E. the difference in number of neutrons in their nucleus

28. Which of the following compounds would have the MOST polar bonds? 28.___
   A. BH_3 B. CH_4 C. NH_3 D. H_2O E. PH_3

29. The LEAST electronegative element can be found in the _____ corner of the periodic table. 29.___
   A. upper left B. upper right
   C. lower left D. lower right
   E.

30. In the nuclear reaction: ${}^{14}_{7}N + {}^{4}_{2}He \rightarrow {}^{17}_{8}O + X$, the symbol X represents which of the following? 30.___
   A. ${}^{4}_{2}He$ B. ${}^{1}_{0}n$ C. ${}^{0}{-1}e$ D. ${}^{0}{+1}e$ E. ${}^{1}_{1}H$

KEY (CORRECT ANSWERS)

1. C	11. B	21. C
2. D	12. D	22. C
3. E	13. D	23. C
4. E	14. E	24. B
5. D	15. B	25. C
6. E	16. A	26. B
7. A	17. E	27. D
8. A	18. A	28. D
9. B	19. A	29. C
10. B	20. A	30. E

EXAMINATION SECTION

TEST 1

DIRECTIONS: Each question or incomplete statement is followed by several suggested answers or completions. Select the one that BEST answers the question or completes the statement. *PRINT THE LETTER OF THE CORRECT ANSWER IN THE SPACE AT THE RIGHT.*

1. The equivalent weight of $CaCl_2$ (M.W. = 110) is 1.___
   A. 37 B. 55.5 C. 110 D. 220

2. 40.8 gm of mercury is used for the calibration of a pipette (Density = 13.6). What is the volume? 2.___
   A. 1 B. 2 C. 3 D. 4

3. In gas-liquid chromatography, it is necessary for the sample to be 3.___
   A. precipitated B. pulverized
   C. soluble in water D. volatilized

4. In flame photometry, the color of sodium in the flame is 4.___
   A. green B. purple C. red D. yellow

5. Thin layer chromatography has a distinct ADVANTAGE over paper chromatography in that it 5.___
   A. can be used with aqueous solutions
   B. is cheaper
   C. is faster
   D. uses less sample

6. Of the following, the one that the halogen ions do NOT include is 6.___
   A. chloride B. fluoride C. iodide D. sulfide

7. Beer's Law relates to 7.___
   A. calorimetry B. colorimetry
   C. gas volumes D. oxidation-reduction

8. The sulfides of lead and mercury are 8.___
   A. colloidal B. insoluble
   C. red in color D. soluble

9. The inert gases include all EXCEPT 9.___
   A. argon B. krypton C. methane D. neon

10. Of the following metals, the one which is in a different group from the others in the periodic table is 10.___
    A. lithium B. sodium C. magnesium D. cesium

11. The reaction of equimolar concentrations of NaOH and HCl is 11.___
   A. amphoteric titration B. coulemetric titration
   C. neutralization D. oxidation-reduction

12. 10.0 ml of a 0.1 normal solution contains 12.___
   A. 1 equivalent B. 1 microequivalent
   C. 1 milliequivalent D. 1 milligram

13. The assay of a compound that has maximum absorbency at 300 mu requires a spectrophotometer sensitive in which one of the following spectral regions? 13.___
   A. Infra-red B. Red
   C. Ultraviolet D. Visible

14. Which of the following is NOT an oxidizing agent? 14.___
   A. Ceric sulfate B. Citrate
   C. Ferricyanide D. Permanganate

15. A buffer solution contains 15.___
   A. a strong acid B. a weak acid or base
   C. an oxidizing agent D. sodium chloride

16. When a procedure calls for the d- or l-isomer of a substance, it may be possible to 16.___
   A. substitute the d- or l-isomer of a related substance
   B. use ½ the weight of a racemic mixture of the substance
   C. use twice the weight of the racemic mixture of the substance
   D. use the meso form of the substance

17. Hercuric ion will combine with which one of the following to form an undissociated salt? 17.___
   A. Carbonate B. Chloride C. Fluoride D. Sulfate

18. pH is defined as 18.___
   A. $[H^+]$ B. $[H^+]+[OH^+]$
   C. $-\log[H^+]$ D. $2-\log[H^+]$

19. Which of the following can be used to prepare a pH standard? 19.___
   A. Acetate B. Phosphate
   C. Potassium acid phthalate D. Veronal

20. The PREFERRED indicator to observe a pH change at 9.0 is 20.___
   A. bromthymol blue B. methyl orange
   C. methyl red D. phenolphthalein

21. The MOST effective buffer at pH of 6.8 is 21.___
   A. acetate B. barbiturate
   C. borate D. phosphate

22. The reaction involved in the titration of sodium oxalate by potassium permanganate is 22.____
   A. amphoteric titration   B. coulemetric titration
   C. neutralization   D. oxidation-reduction

23. Density is expressed BEST as 23.____
   A. mass/unit volume
   B. solubility per 100 ml
   C. specific gravity/unit volume
   D. volume/unit mass

24. 60°C converted to Fahrenheit is 24.____
   A. 110°F   B. 120°F   C. 130°F   D. 140°F

25. A substance with a melting point of +28°C at room temperature (25°C) will be a 25.____
   A. gas   B. liquid   C. mixture   D. solid

26. Which of the following has the HIGHEST boiling point? 26.____
   A. Acetic acid   B. Ethyl alcohol
   C. Methyl alcohol   D. Water

27. At constant pressure, which of the following will have the LOWEST freezing point? 27.____
   A. 0.1M NaCl   B. 0.2M NaCl
   C. 0.1M Na_2HPO_4 D. 0.2M NaH_2PO_4

28. In one liter, a 5% solution contains _____ gm. 28.____
   A. 5   B. 25   C. 50   D. 100

29. Which one of the following compounds, in aqueous solution, absorbs ultraviolet light? 29.____
   A. Fumaric acid   B. Glutamic acid
   C. Malic acid   D. Succinic acid

30. Which of the following statements is LEAST likely to be correct? 30.____
   Automated procedures
   A. are less costly than manual ones
   B. speed the rate of performance
   C. conserve laboratory space
   D. can be performed by less skilled personnel

31. The principle of the AutoAnalyzer is based on _____ analysis. 31.____
   A. sequential   B. discrete
   C. single   D. multiple

32. Atomic absorption is used to determine 32.____
   A. anions   B. atomic numbers
   C. cations   D. methyl groups

33. A nanogram of material is 33.____
A. 1×10^{-3} g
B. 1×10^{-6} g
C. 1×10^{-9} g
D. 1×10^{12} g

34. The Henderson-Hasselbalch equation is pH = 34.____
A. - log[H]
B. log[H]
C. $pK_a + \log \frac{[Acid]}{[Salt]}$
D. $pK_a + \log \frac{[Salt]}{[Acid]}$

35. In gas chromatography, the sample must be 35.____
A. liquid
B. inorganic
C. solid
D. volatilized

36. Atomic absorption spectroscopy requires 36.____
A. an extremely hot flame
B. a hollow cathode lamp
C. nuclear energy
D. vigorous mixing

37. Absolute temperature is _____ °C. 37.____
A. -100
B. -273
C. +100
D. +273

38. Gravimetric analysis PRIMARILY involves 38.____
A. amperometric voltages
B. colorimetry
C. titration
D. weighing

39. A gram molecular weight of a gas at standard conditions of temperature and pressure occupies _____ ml. 39.____
A. 1,000
B. 10,000
C. 22,400
D. 44,800

40. Infra-red analysis is MOST often used in 40.____
A. analytical chemistry
B. electrochemistry
C. organic chemistry
D. physical chemistry

41. Enzymes are 41.____
A. complex collagens
B. complex lipids
C. polysaccharides
D. protein catalysts

42. Vitamin A is 42.____
A. a nitrogenous compound
B. a protein catalyst
C. water insoluble
D. water soluble

43. Which of the following is destroyed in pasteurization? 43.____
A. Alkaline phosphatase
B. Calcium
C. Iron binding protein
D. Lactose

44. In the human cell, energy is stored as 44.____
A. adenosine monophosphate
B. adenosine triphosphate
C. creatine phosphokinase
D. nicotine adenine dinucleotide

45. The acid found in normal gastric juice is 45.____
A. citric
B. HCl
C. H_2SO_4
D. lactic

46. Albumin can be precipitated by addition of 46.____
A. blood serum
B. sodium chloride
C. sodium sulfate
D. water

47. Which of the following is NOT a reducing carbohydrate? 47.____
A. Fructose
B. Galactose
C. Glucose
D. Sucrose

48. The kinetic theory of matter explains that 48.____
A. the space between molecules of a gas is greater than the space occupied by the molecule itself
B. molecules of matter do not move unless agitated
C. molecules of matter are the ultimate particles of individual elements
D. molecules of matter are always in motion

49. Of the following, the PRIMARY purpose of standards and controls is to obtain 49.____
A. accuracy
B. priorities
C. replicates
D. reproducibility

50. Of the following, the BEST definition for accuracy in laboratory practice is 50.____
A. nearness to truth
B. reproducibility of replicates
C. within biological variation
D. within 2 standard deviations of the mean

KEY (CORRECT ANSWERS)

1. B	11. C	21. D	31. A	41. D
2. C	12. C	22. D	32. C	42. C
3. D	13. C	23. A	33. C	43. A
4. D	14. B	24. D	34. D	44. B
5. C	15. B	25. D	35. D	45. B
6. D	16. C	26. A	36. B	46. C
7. B	17. B	27. D	37. B	47. D
8. B	18. C	28. C	38. D	48. D
9. C	19. C	29. A	39. C	49. A
10. C	20. D	30. D	40. C	50. A

TEST 2

DIRECTIONS: Each question or incomplete statement is followed by several suggested answers or completions. Select the one that BEST answers the question or completes the statement. *PRINT THE LETTER OF THE CORRECT ANSWER IN THE SPACE AT THE RIGHT.*

1. Which of the following formulas does NOT correspond to a known substance? 1.___
   A. $NaClO_2$ B. $NaPO_3$ C. $NaSO_2$ D. $Na_2S_2O_3$

2. In the reaction between zinc and concentrated nitric acid, shown UNBALANCED as 2.___
   ___Zn + ___HNO_3 = ___$Zn(NO_3)_2$ + ___NO + ___H_2O ,

   the number which should appear in front of the formula for nitric acid after the equation has been balanced is
   A. 3 B. 4 C. 6 D. 8

3. The element whose valence electrons have the quantum designation $4s^2$, $4p^5$ is No. 3.___
   A. 7 B. 25 C. 28 D. 35

4. In the case of the following equilibrium reaction, $2NO + O_2 \rightleftarrows 2NO_2$ + heat, which of the following actions will result in a CHANGE in the numerical value of the equilibrium constant? 4.___
   A. Addition of NO_2
   B. Increase in the temperature
   C. Increase in the total pressure
   D. Introduction of a catalyst

5. Of the following, the STRONGEST oxidizing agent is 5.___
   A. Br_2 B. F_2 C. Na D. O_2

6. The ionization constant of acetic acid is 1.8×10^{-5}. What is the pH of a liter of a solution containing 0.5 moles of acetic acid and 0.25 moles of sodium acetate? 6.___
   A. 1.8 B. 3.2 C. 4.44 D. 5.05

7. The volume of 0.42 M H_2SO_4 solution which will be EXACTLY neutralized by 230 ml of 0.70 M NaOH is 7.___
   A. 138 B. 192 C. 276 D. 384

8. Of the following, the substance which will NOT react with 1 M NaOH is 8.___
   A. Al B. $AL(OH)_3$ C. Fe D. SO_2

9. Of the following precipitates, the one which will NOT dissolve in 0.3 M HCl is 9.___
   A. As_2S_3 B. CuS C. $MnNH_4PO_4$ D. ZnS

10. The ionization constant, K_B, of ammonium hydroxide is 1.8×10^{-5}. 10.___
What is the USEFUL range of pH's of the buffer solutions that can be made up from various mixtures of ammonium hydroxide and ammonium chloride?
A. 8.5 to 10.5 B. 7 to 13
C. 5.5 to 7.5 D. 2 to 6

11. The atomic number of an element is equal to the 11.___
A. number of neutrons in the nucleus
B. number of protons in the nucleus
C. sum of the protons and the electrons
D. sum of the protons and the neutrons

12. What will be the APPROXIMATE increase in the reaction rate for every 10°C rise in temperature? 12.___
_____ fold.
A. 1.5 B. 2.0 C. 2.5 D. 3.0

13. At standard temperature and pressure, one liter of hydrogen gas contains APPROXIMATELY the same number of molecules as 13.___
A. 0.5 liter of oxygen
B. 1.0 liter of sulfur dioxide
C. 1.5 liters of ozone
D. 2.0 liters of helium

14. The amount of $CuSO_4 \cdot 5H_2O$ that must be dissolved in 100 ml of water to produce a solution containing 1 mg Cu^{++} per ml is _____ g. 14.___
A. 0.100 B. 0.252 C. 0.393 D. 0.635

15. Of the following techniques, the one which would be the BEST to use in order to obtain absolute ethanol from the standard commercial product (95% ethanol, 5% water) is 15.___
A. fractional distillation
B. reaction with sodium, followed by distillation
C. reaction with zinc, followed by filtration
D. solvent extraction

16. Based upon mutual solubility considerations, which of the following would you expect to be the BEST solvent for a heavy machine oil? 16.___
A. Acetone B. Benzene C. Dioxane D. Ethanol

17. The specific gravity of concentrated hydrochloric acid reagent is 1.19. The solution contains 37% HCl. The molarity of the reagent is 17.___
A. 2 B. 6 C. 8 D. 12

18. The purpose of a magnetic damper is to 18.___
A. activate balance pans
B. eliminate counting of swings
C. keep the humidity down
D. remove static electricity

19. Quantities of waste flammable organic liquids should be destroyed by 19.___
   A. burning under controlled conditions
   B. dumping in a secluded area
   C. evaporating on a water bath in a hood
   D. flushing down the sink

20. Of the following determinations, which would be BEST for routine use in the quality control (i.e., testing of purity) of a solid benzene derivative? 20.___
   A. Diffusion coefficient   B. Melting range
   C. Solubility in toluene   D. Vapor pressure

21. The MEDIAN value in a column of figures is the ____ value. 21.___
   A. highest   B. lowest   C. mean   D. middle

22. The R_F in paper chromatography designates the 22.___
   A. distance between two solutes
   B. rate at which the fastest component migrates
   C. rate at which the slowest component migrates
   D. rate of solute migration compared to the solvent

23. An internal standard is used in flame photometry because it 23.___
   A. corrects for gas fluctuations
   B. forms a binary mixture
   C. increases the excitation
   D. simplifies calculations

24. In calcium analysis by atomic absorption, lanthanum is added to 24.___
   A. intensify the absorption
   B. intensify the emission
   C. prevent PO_4 interference
   D. reduce iron

25. The pressure of a mixture of three gases will be 25.___
   A. the product of the individual partial pressures
   B. the average of the partial pressures
   C. the sum of the partial pressures
   D. the partial pressure of the most volatile gas

26. Which of the following guides to the chemical literature deals EXCLUSIVELY with organic compounds? 26.___
   A. Abegg   B. Gmelin   C. Beilstein   D. Mellor

27. Of the following, the reagent which is employed in the separation and purification of ketones is 27.___
   A. Na_2CO_3 B. $NaHSO_3$ C. Cu_2Cl_2 D. $Ag(NH_3)_2Ol$

28. Of the following, the compound which exists as two geometrical isomers is 28.___
   A. $HOOCCH{=}CH_2$ B. $HOOCCH_2CH_2COOH$
   C. $HOOCCH{=}CHCOOH$ D. $HOOCC{=}CH$

29. The monomer from which Teflon plastic is produced is 29.___
A. $CF_2=CF_2$ B. CF_3COOH C. $CH_2=CH_2$ D. CHF=CHF

30. Of the following, the substance to start with in order to obtain the BEST yield of m-phenylenediamine is 30.___
A. aniline
B. benzenediazonium chloride
C. m-dichlorophenol
D. m-dinitrobenzene

31. What is the MOST likely reason for a blood glucose to be exceedingly high (above 1000 mg per 100 ml)? 31.___
The
A. patient ingested large amounts of carbohydrates
B. patient ingested reducing substances
C. patient was not fasting
D. specimen was contaminated from an infusion

32. If the pH of blood plasma is 7.1 and the dissolved CO_2 is 2.0 mmoles, then the HCO_3 is _____ mmoles. 32.___
A. 10 B. 20 C. 30 D. 40

33. A triglyceride is a compound of three 33.___
A. fatty acids
B. fatty acids and one glycerol
C. glycerols and one fatty acid
D. glycerol molecules

34. Starch can be determined by measuring the intensity of the blue color when it reacts with 34.___
A. alkaline copper
B. amylase
C. iodine
D. silver

35. After the complete hydrolysis of lecithin, which of the following is NOT present? 35.___
A. Choline
B. Ethanolamine
C. Glycerol
D. Phosphoric acid

36. Fehling's Solution is used in the analysis of 36.___
A. fat
B. protein
C. reducing sugar
D. starch

37. An antimetabolite that inhibits an enzyme reaction is 37.___
A. a heavy metal
B. a substance that chelates with the substrate
C. structurally related to the enzyme
D. structurally related to the substrate

38. Of the following enzymes, the one that is NOT present in the carbohydrate citric acid cycle is 38.___
A. fumarase
B. isocitric dehydrogenase
C. succinic dehydrogenase
D. triose phosphate isomerase

39. The xylose test, as performed in the clinical laboratory, is a test for 39.___
A. glomerular filtration B. kidney function
C. liver function D. malabsorption

40. Serum acid phosphatase will be FALSELY elevated when the 40.___
A. patient has urinary retention
B. patient was not fasting
C. serum alkaline phosphatase is elevated
D. serum is hemolyzed

41. The *diurnal* variation of a blood substance infers that it varies with the 41.___
A. age of the patient B. procedure used
C. sex of the patient D. time of day

42. A single peak in the Tiselius electrophoresis indicates that the 42.___
A. substance is a pure protein
B. substance is not a protein
C. solution contains mucopolysaccharides
D. solution is a mixture of proteins

43. 68 ml. of gastric juice were titrated to pH 7.0 and found to contain 138 mmoles per liter of acid. 43.___
What is the acidity in mmoles of the total volume of gastric juice?
A. 20.3 B. 14.4 C. 9.4 D. 4.9

44. The glucose oxidase method for blood glucose is PREFERRED over any other blood glucose test because 44.___
A. it is the fastest procedure
B. it requires the least expensive reagents
C. the reagents are readily stable
D. there is no interference from other reducing substances

45. Fluoride is used as a blood anticoagulant for glucose determinations because it 45.___
A. inhibits bacterial growth
B. inhibits glycolytic enzymes
C. precipitates calcium
D. prevents hemolysis

46. Deoxyribonucleoproteins form viscous solutions because they 46.___
A. are elongated
B. are spherical
C. contain protein
D. have a high molecular weight

47. Bromsulphonphthalein (BSP) is used as a liver function test because the dye is 47.___
A. excreted by the kidney B. excreted by the liver
C. not adsorbed to proteins D. stored in the liver

48. Proteins will NOT migrate in an electric field at ____ pH. 48.___
A. a neutral
B. an acid
C. an alkaline
D. an isoelectric

49. A pooled serum may be used as a 49.___
A. daily control
B. gas analysis control
C. primary standard
D. secondary standard

50. Which of the following is NOT a hormone? 50.___
A. Carotene
B. Estriol
C. Epinephrine
D. Secretin

KEY (CORRECT ANSWERS)

1. C	11. B	21. D	31. B	41. D
2. D	12. B	22. D	32. D	42. A
3. D	13. B	23. A	33. A	43. C
4. B	14. C	24. C	34. A	44. D
5. B	15. B	25. C	35. C	45. C
6. C	16. B	26. C	36. C	46. D
7. B	17. D	27. B	37. C	47. C
8. C	18. B	28. C	38. B	48. D
9. B	19. C	29. A	39. B	49. B
10. A	20. B	30. D	40. C	50. A

TEST 3

DIRECTIONS: Each question or incomplete statement is followed by several suggested answers or completions. Select the one that BEST answers the question or completes the statement. *PRINT THE LETTER OF THE CORRECT ANSWER IN THE SPACE AT THE RIGHT.*

1. One liter is APPROXIMATELY one 1.____
   A. pint B. quart
   C. half-gallon D. gallon

2. The temperature on the Kelvin (absolute) scale which corresponds to -60°C is 2.____
   A. -333 B. +213 C. +273 D. +333

3. How many liters of H_2 at STP would be displaced from 500 ml of 4M HCl by excess zinc? 3.____
   A. 11.2 B. 22.4 C. 44.8 D. 89.6

4. Metallic sodium should be stored in 4.____
   A. alcohol B. kerosene C. sawdust D. water

5. The reaction, 5.____
   $MnO_2 + H^+ + H_2C_2O_4 \rightarrow CO_2 + H_2O + MN^{++}$,

   is not balanced.
   After balancing it, select, of the following, the CORRECT number of moles of $H_2C_2O_4$ required to react with one mole of MnO_2.
   A. ½ B. 1 C. 2 D. 4

6. The pH of .01M HCl is 6.____
   A. 10^{-2} B. 1 C. 2 D. 3

7. The ionization constant of acetic acid is 1.8×10^{-5}. The hydrogen ion concentration in a solution of 0.5M acetic acid and 0.5M sodium acetate is 7.____
   A. $.9 \times 10^{-5}$M B. 1.8×10^{-5}M
   C. 3×10^{-3}M D. 3.3×10^{-12}M

8. A 50.0 ml sample of NaOH solution requires exactly 27.8 ml of 0.100M acid in titration. 8.____
   What is the normality of the NaOH?
   A. 0.0278 B. 0.0556 C. 0.112 D. 0.556

9. The solubility of $Pb(IO_3)_2$ in water is 4.0×10^{-5} moles/liter. 9.____
   What is the K_{sp} (solubility product) for $Pb(IO_3)_2$?

   A. 1.6×10^{-9} B. 2.4×10^{-13}
   C. 4.0×10^{-5} D. 12×10^{-5}

10. Light of 5000 Å (500 mμ) wave length 10.___
  A. is in the ultraviolet region
  B. is in the visible region
  C. contains twice as much energy as light of 2500 Å wave length
  D. is in the infra-red region

11. The compound Na_2S contains what percentage S? 11.___
  A. 33% B. 41% C. 59% D. 69%

12. A compound that has the power to neutralize an acid and form a salt is called a(n) 12.___
  A. buffer B. hetone C. anhydride D. alkali

13. Which of the following isotopes is NOT radioactive? 13.___
  A. C^{12} B. C^{14} C. Co^{60} D. H^3

14. The organic compound C_4H_{10} 14.___
  A. is a unique compound with no isomers
  B. exists in two isomeric forms
  C. exists in three isomeric forms
  D. exists in many (more than three) isomeric forms

15. Of the following, the STRONGEST reducing agent is ____ acid. 15.___
  A. acetic B. nitric C. oxalic D. phosphoric

16. Which of the following solutions has the LOWEST freezing point? 16.___
1M
  A. calcium sulfate B. calcium chloride
  C. sodium chloride D. sugar

17. The general formula for an organic aldehyde is 17.___
  A. RCHO B. RCOOH C. RCOR D. ROR

Questions 18-19.

DIRECTIONS: Questions 18 and 19 are to be answered on the basis of the following reversible reaction.

N_2O_4 (gas) $\rightleftarrows$ 2 NO_2 (gas)

18. Which expression CORRECTLY describes the equilibrium constant? (P stands for pressure) 18.___

  A. $P_{N_2O_4} / P^2_{NO_2}$ B. $P^2_{NO_2} / P_{N_2O_4}$

  C. $P_{NO_2} / P_{N_2O_4}$ D. $2 (P_{NO_2}) / P_{N_2O_4}$

19. If the total pressure on the reaction at equilibrium is suddenly increased at constant temperature, 19.____
   A. nothing would happen
   B. the equilibrium constant would change
   C. the reaction would shift toward NO_2 (gas)
   D. the reaction would shift toward N_2O_4 (gas)

20. A reaction requires 1 hour to run to completion at 30°C. The same reaction will run to completion in 15 minutes at APPROXIMATELY _____ °C. 20.____
   A. 20   B. 40   C. 50   D. 120

21. A quality control chart is used to 21.____
   A. check day-to-day variability
   B. define the laboratory accuracy
   C. define the laboratory workload
   D. find normal values

22. A primary standard is prepared by 22.____
   A. dilution of a solution
   B. always using oxidizing agents
   C. weighing on a gross balance
   D. weighing on an analytical balance

23. What part of a population will be included within ±2 standard deviation in a normal distribution curve? _____ percent. 23.____
   A. 65   B. 75   C. 85   D. 95

24. When a frozen control material is thawing and a portion is taken before complete melting and mixing, the obtained values are LIKELY to be 24.____
   A. high   B. low   C. unchanged   D. variable

25. The PROPER use of a volumetric pipette requires 25.____
   A. allowing it to drain   B. blowing it out
   C. washing it out   D. weighing the contents

26. When the skin is splashed with acid, it should 26.____
   A. immediately be covered with oil
   B. immediately be flushed with water
   C. immediately be flushed with weak acid
   D. not be touched

27. Fume hoods are used in laboratories to 27.____
   A. allow the use of a flame
   B. exhaust noxious fumes
   C. provide a well-lit work area
   D. provide storage space

28. How many milligrams of nitrogen are there in 40 milligrams of urea? 28.____
   A. 16.8   B. 18.5   C. 21.6   D. 24.6

29. The presence of barbiturates in a blood sample can BEST be determined by 29.___
   A. cellulose acetate electrophoresis
   B. fractional distillation
   C. paper electrophoresis
   D. thin layer chromatography

30. Urease is a(n) 30.___
   A. major constituent of urine
   B. nucleic acid metabolite
   C. protein metabolite
   D. enzyme

31. The MAJOR urinary excretory product of steroid metabolism is 31.___
   A. cholesterol
   B. estrogen
   C. 17-ketosteroids
   D. lanosteroid

32. The MAJOR polysaccharide involved in human metabolism is 32.___
   A. a-amylopectin
   B. amylose
   C. glycogen
   D. starch

33. The chemical identification of glucose can be made by the formation of a 33.___
   A. boron bead
   B. complex with bathophenanthrolene
   C. phenylhydrazine
   D. polymer

34. Which of the following has an asymmetric carbon atom? ____ acid. 34.___
   A. Acetic B. Lactic C. Oleic D. Succinic

35. Nitrogen is NOT present in 35.___
   A. glucuronic acid
   B. glutathione
   C. glycolic acid
   D. glycine

36. The MAJOR intracellular ion is 36.___
   A. calcium B. carbonate C. potassium D. sodium

37. The blood volume in a normal adult approximates ____ ml. 37.___
   A. 1000 B. 3000 C. 5000 D. 8000

38. The pH of normal blood is 38.___
   A. 6.40 B. 6.90 C. 7.40 D. 7.90

39. The serum protein involved in the clotting of blood is 39.___
   A. fibrinogen
   B. 1-globulin
   C. 2-globulin
   D. haptoglobin

40. Which one of the following tests can NOT be done on oxalated blood plasma? 40.___
   A. Calcium B. Creatinine C. Glucose D. Urine

41. The nitrogen content of proteins is MOST NEARLY ____ percent. 41.____
   A. 16.5 B. 18.5 C. 20.5 D. 22.5

42. Protein-bound iodine is a measure of _____ function. 42.____
   A. adrenal B. cardiac C. liver D. thyroid

43. Which of the following is NOT a liver function test? 43.____
   A. Cephalin flocculation B. Glucose tolerance
   C. Serum bilirubin D. Thymol turbidity

44. Heparin is often used as a(n) 44.____
   A. anticoagulant
   B. chelating agent in Ca^{++} analysis
   C. colored complex
   D. primary standard

45. Amino acids are bound together to form a protein through 45.____
   A. alcohol acid esters B. glycosidic linkages
   C. peptide bonds D. 3'5' phosphate bonds

46. Inulin is a polysaccharide of 46.____
   A. fructose B. galactose C. glucose D. lactose

47. A characteristic of isoenzymes is that 47.____
   A. the enzymes have identical activities at a given pH
   B. the protein moieties have the same charge densities
   C. the protein moieties have the same molecular weight
   D. a substrate is common to all the enzymes

48. The MOST likely journal to contain articles about elemental analysis is 48.____
   A. Analytical Chemistry
   B. Clinical Chemistry
   C. Journal of Chromatography
   D. Journal of Organic Chemistry

49. The Index Medicus contains 49.____
   A. abstracts of journal articles
   B. information about disease
   C. information about drugs
   D. references to journal articles by subject and author

50. When it is necessary to refer to published articles in the field of chemistry when only the subject is known, the BEST source of reference is 50.____
   A. CHEMICAL ABSTRACTS
   B. INDEX OF AMERICAN CHEMICAL SOCIETY
   C. INDEX OF CLINICAL CHEMISTRY
   D. INDEX MEDICUS

KEY (CORRECT ANSWERS)

1. B	11. B	21. A	31. B	41. D
2. B	12. D	22. D	32. B	42. C
3. B	13. A	23. D	33. B	43. A
4. B	14. B	24. D	34. C	44. A
5. B	15. C	25. A	35. B	45. C
6. C	16. B	26. B	36. C	46. D
7. B	17. A	27. B	37. D	47. C
8. B	18. B	28. C	38. C	48. A
9. B	19. D	29. A	39. A	49. D
10. B	20. C	30. D	40. B	50. A

EXAMINATION SECTION

TEST 1

DIRECTIONS: Each question or incomplete statement is followed by several suggested answers or completions. Select the one that BEST answers the question or completes the statement. *PRINT THE LETTER OF THE CORRECT ANSWER IN THE SPACE AT THE RIGHT.*

1. The degree of unsaturation in an organic compound may be found by shaking a specific weight of the substance with a standard solution of which one of the following? 1.___
   A. Sulfuric acid B. Potassium hydroxide
   C. Acetone D. Iodine

2. The structural formula for ∂ -amino propionic acid is 2.___
   A. 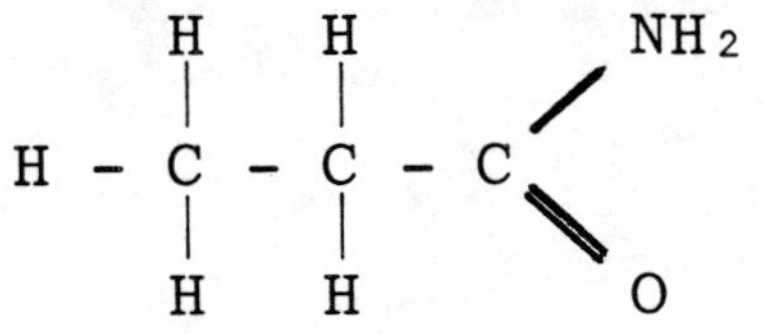
   B. 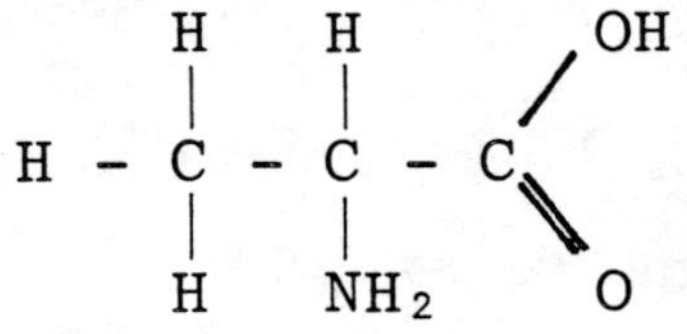
   C. 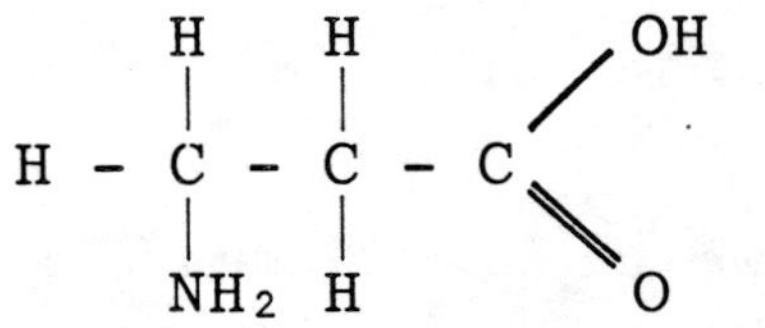
   D. 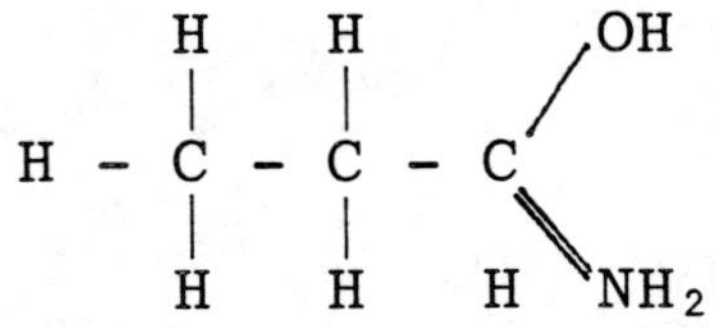

3. Of the following, the tertiary alcohol is 3.___
   A. $CH_3 \cdot CH_2 \cdot CH_2OH$
   B. $(CH_3)_3 \cdot COH$
   C. $(CH_3)_3C \cdot CH_2OH$
   D. $CH_3 \cdot CHOH \cdot CH_3$

4. Which one of the following is the empirical formula for ethyl cyclo pentane? 4.___
   A. C_7H_{13} B. C_7H_9 C. C_7H_{14} D. C_7H_{11}

5. The formula for xylene is 5.___
   A. $C_6H_5CH_3$
   B. $C_6H_3(CH_3)_3$
   C. $C_6H_4(CH_3)_2$
   D. $C_6(CH_3)_6$

6. A solution of the compound D (-) glucose in water will rotate the plane of polarized light to which one of the following? 6.___
   A. The right B. The left
   C. Either side D. Neither side

7. Of the following substances, the one which could NOT be represented by the empirical formula C_3H_6O is 7.___
   A. acetone B. propanol
   C. vinyl methyl ether D. ethinyl alcohol

8. An acidified solution of sucrose on standing is converted into a mixture of which one of the following pairs? 8.___
   A. Mannose and talose B. Glucose and fructose
   C. Idose and gulose D. Altose and sorbose

9. Which of the following are the CHIEF products in the Fischer-Tropsch synthesis? 9.___
   A. Acids B. Alcohols C. Aldehydes D. Detones

10. The name of the substance $(NH_2)_2$ CO is 10.___
   A. acetamide B. methylamide
   C. carbamide D. urea

11. Which one of the following molecules contains the GREATEST number of benzene rings? 11.___
   A. Quinone B. Naphthalene
   C. Phthalic anhydride D. Anthracene

12. The reagent phthalic anhydride is obtained CHIEFLY from the oxidation of 12.___
   A. phthalic acid B. turpentine
   C. anthracene D. naphthalene

13. Of the following forms of sulfur, which one is MOST readily soluble in carbon disulfide? 13.___
   A. Amorphous B. Prismatic C. Rhombic D. Plastic

14. Assume that solution *X* has a pH of 6.0. 14.___
   If solution *Y* has a hydronium ion concentration twice that of solution *X*, its pH will be APPROXIMATELY
   A. 3.0 B. 5.7 C. 6.0 D. 12.8

15. The triple point for CO_2 is -57°C and 5.2 atmospheres. 15.___
   In order to obtain liquid CO_2, the
   A. pressure must be below 5.2 atmospheres
   B. temperature must be below -57°C
   C. pressure must be below 5.2 atmospheres and temperature must be greater than -57°C
   D. pressure must be above 5.2 atmospheres and temperature must be greater than -57°C

16. The one of the following which is NOT an oxidation-reduction reaction is the 16.___
   A. replacement of iodine by chlorine in sodium iodide
   B. Haber process
   C. softening of hard water
   D. reaction of iron and copper sulfate

17. The nickel ion is USUALLY identified by 17.___
   A. cupferron
   B. dimethylglyoxime
   C. p-nitrobenzene azo resorcinol
   D. diphenyl benzidine

18. A mixture of $Al(OH)_3$ and $Fe(OH)_3$ can be separated easily by treatment with which one of the following? 18.___
   A. Sodium hydroxide solution
   B. Hydrochloric acid
   C. Sulfuric acid
   D. Ammonium hydroxide solution

19. A saturated solution of H_2S gas in water at atmospheric pressure and normal room temperature is APPROXIMATELY 19.___
   A. 0.001M B. 0.1M C. 0.5M D. 1.0M

20. By the addition of which one of the following can the blood-red color be produced in a confirmatory test for the Fe^{+++} ion? 20.___
A
   A. cyanate B. thiosulfate
   C. sulfide D. thiocyanate

21. Of the following, the element which in solution will form a white precipitate with chloride ion which will turn black on the addition of aqueous ammonia is 21.___
   A. lead B. silver C. tin D. mercury

22. When 27 grams of Al are added to one liter of 3N $CuSO_4$, the number of grams of Cu that will be displaced is (atomic weights: Cu = 64, Al = 27) 22.___
   A. 32 B. 64 C. 96 D. 128

23. The Fahrenheit and Centigrade scales of temperature have the same numerical reading at a temperature of 23.___
   A. -40° B. 0° C. 32° D. 212°

24. When a gas expands adiabatically, 24.___
   A. the temperature remains constant
   B. energy is liberated
   C. the pressure increases
   D. the environment remains unchanged

25. Of the following situations, the one in which no single electronic formula conforms both to the observed properties and to the octet rule is described as 25.___
   A. isomerism B. allotropism
   C. enantiomorphism D. resonance

KEY (CORRECT ANSWERS)

1. D
2. B
3. B
4. C
5. C

6. B
7. D
8. B
9. B
10. D

11. D
12. D
13. C
14. B
15. D

16. C
17. B
18. A
19. B
20. D

21. D
22. C
23. A
24. D
25. D

TEST 2

DIRECTIONS: Each question or incomplete statement is followed by several suggested answers or completions. Select the one that BEST answers the question or completes the statement. *PRINT THE LETTER OF THE CORRECT ANSWER IN THE SPACE AT THE RIGHT.*

1. Assuming that 100 ml of a 0.1 M solution of H_2SO_4 is needed to neutralize 200 ml of a $Ba(OH)_2$ solution, the normality of the $Ba(OH)_2$ solution is 1.___
   A. 0.05 B. 0.10 C. 0.20 D. 0.50

2. If 22.5 ml of HCl are needed to neutralize 25 ml of 0.1 N Na_2CO_3 solution, the normality of the acid is 2.___
   A. 0.037 B. 0.056 C. 0.111 D. 0.167

3. When a 0.1N solution of an acid of 25°C has a degree of ionization of 1%, the concentration of hydroxyl ions present is 3.___
   A. 10^{-3} B. 10^{-11} C. 10^{-12} D. 10^{-13}

4. If a compound has a negative heat of solution, at high temperatures it dissolves _____ rapidly and is _____ soluble. 4.___
   A. more; more
   B. more; less
   C. less; less
   D. less; more

5. In general, a 1 molar solution is any substance, when converted into molalities at a fixed temperature, will be 5.___
   A. less than 1 molal
   B. 1 molal
   C. more than 1 molal
   D. indeterminate

6. Eight liters of 0.86 N HBr solution contain _____ of HBr. 6.___
   A. 6800 millimoles
   B. 0.688 moles
   C. 6.88 moles
   D. 8000 millimoles

7. A solution of 4.5g of a pure nonelectrolyte in 100.0g of water was found to freeze at -0.465°C. The molecular weight of the solute is CLOSEST to which one of the following? 7.___
   A. 180 B. 172.4 C. 90 D. 86.2

8. A saturated solution of Ag_2SO_4 is 2.5×10^{-2} M. The value of its solubility product is 8.___
   A. 6.25×10^{-7}
   B. 1.6×10^{-5}
   C. 6.25×10^{-5}
   D. 1.25×10^{-3}

9. The concentration of hydronium ions in pure water, expressed in moles per liter, is 9.___

A. 10^{-7} B. 7 C. $1/10^{-7}$ D. 10^{-14}

10. If solid sodium acetate is added to a dilute solution of acetic acid, the pH will 10.___

A. increase
B. be unaffected
C. decrease
D. first decrease, then increase

11. The molality of a glucose solution containing 22.5 grams of glucose (atomic weights: C = 12; O = 16, H = 1) in 500 grams of water is CLOSEST to which one of the following? 11.___

A. 0.13 B. 0.25 C. 0.38 D. 0.50

12. Silver chloride was precipitated by adding HCl to a solution of a silver salt until the concentration of chloride ions is 0.20 mole/liter. 12.___
Ideally, the concentration of silver ions in this case should be ($K_{sp_{AgCl}} = 1.56 \times 10^{-10}$)

A. $\sqrt{1.56} \times 10^{-5}$ B. $\sqrt{7.8} \times 10^{-10}$

C. 7.8×10^{-10} D. 1.56×10^{-10}

13. Of the following, the solvent which is LEAST effective in dissolving fats is 13.___

A. alcohol B. chloroform
C. ether D. carbon tetrachloride

14. Of the following, the compound in which oxygen exhibits an oxidation state of +2 is 14.___

A. Cl_2O_6 B. BrO_2 C. $HClO_2$ D. F_2O

15. If 1.25 grams of a solid acid neutralize 25 ml of a 0.25M $Ba(OH)_2$ solution, the equivalent weight of the acid will be _____ grams. 15.___

A. 25 B. 50 C. 100 D. 200

16. When an element forms an oxide wherein the oxygen is 20% of the oxide by weight, the equivalent weight of the given element will be 16.___

A. 32 B. 40 C. 64 D. 128

17. In the reaction given below, the equivalent weight of HNO_3 (atomic weights: H = 1; N = 14; O = 16) is CLOSEST to which one of the following? 17.___

$$8HNO_3 + 3PhS \rightarrow 8NO + 3PbSO_4 + 4H_2O$$

A. 11.6 B. 21.0 C. 31.5 D. 63.0

18. The oxidation number of nickel in the compound $K_4[Ni(CN)_4]$ is 18.___
A. 0 B. +2 C. -2 D. +3

19. Of the following, the compound whose color is INCORRECTLY given is 19.___
A. $CrSO_4$ - red
B. $Cr_2(SO_4)_3$ - purple
C. K_2CrO_4 - yellow
D. $K_2Cr_2O_7$ - orange

20. According to the Bronsted Theory, which one of the following substances is classified as a base? 20.___
A. Cl^- B. H_3O^+ C. CH_3COOH D. NH_4^+

21. Of the following, the acid that is MOST closely related chemically to P_4O_6 is 21.___
A. HPO_3 B. H_3PO_3 C. H_3PO_4 D. $H_4P_2O_7$

22. According to the Lewis Theory of acids and bases, stannic chloride is 22.___
A. a base
B. neutral
C. an acid
D. amphoteric

23. Of the following pair of reagents which can be used to separate cupric and aluminum ions from manganous ions is NaOH and 23.___
A. Na_2O_2
B. tartrate ions
C. sodium bismuthate
D. NH_4OH

24. Compounds of manganese that do NOT exhibit para-magnetism are those in which the oxidation state is which one of the following? 24.___
A. +2 B. +4 C. +6 D. +7

25. An investigation of the energy sublevels of the electron shells in an atom discloses that the energy of the 3d subshell is GREATER than that of the _____ subshell. 25.___
A. 4f B. 4d C. 4p D. 4s

KEY (CORRECT ANSWERS)

1. B	6. C	11. B	16. A	21. B
2. C	7. A	12. C	17. B	22. C
3. B	8. C	13. A	18. A	23. B
4. A	9. A	14. D	19. A	24. D
5. D	10. A	15. C	20. A	25. D

TEST 3

DIRECTIONS: Each question or incomplete statement is followed by several suggested answers or completions. Select the one that BEST answers the question or completes the statement. *PRINT THE LETTER OF THE CORRECT ANSWER IN THE SPACE AT THE RIGHT.*

1. All of the following statements about the group of elements called the transitional elements are true EXCEPT that 1.___
   A. all of the transitional elements are predominantly metallic
   B. in aqueous solution many of their simple ions are colored
   C. most of the transitional elements show pronounced catalytic activity
   D. most of the transitional elements show only one valence state

2. When the specific heat of a metallic element is 0.214 calories/gram, the atomic weight will be CLOSEST to which one of the following? 2.___
   A. 6.6 B. 12 C. 30 D. 66

3. The MOST probable valence number for the atom with the total electron configuration, $1S^2 2S^2 2p^6 3S^2 3p^6 3d^{10} 4S^2 4p^5$, is 3.___
   A. -1 B. -3 C. +1 D. +3

4. Which one of the following groups of elements is analogous to the lanthanides? 4.___
   A. Halides B. Carbides C. Actinides D. Borides

5. Heating ammonia with air in the presence of a platinum catalyst will produce 5.___
   A. oxygen and nitrogen
   B. hydrogen and nitrogen dioxide
   C. water and nitric oxide
   D. ammonium hydroxide and nitrous oxide

6. Lavoisier's experiment to demonstrate the true nature of burning was made possible by the availability of which one of the following? 6.___
   A. The metal tin
   B. A lens for focusing sun's rays
   C. A glass retort
   D. A sensitive balance

7. Hydrogen that is used commercially is FREQUENTLY obtained from which one of the following? 7.___
   _____ gas.
   A. Marsh B. Coal C. Producer D. Water

8. In general, a plastic shows greater strength and rigidity as the polymer molecules show more 8.___
   A. crystallinity B. amorphous nature
   C. random arrangement D. atactic nature

9. An experiment designed to show the presence of water vapor in the air would PROBABLY employ which one of the following? 9.___
   A. Phosphorus B. Ammonium hydroxide
   C. Hydrated copper sulfate D. Sodium hydroxide

10. The type of electronic bonding found in potassium hydride is 10.___
    A. covalent B. coordinate covalent
    C. metallic D. ionic

11. Concentrated sulfuric acid is stored in 11.___
    A. wax bottles B. glass-stoppered bottles
    C. rubber-stoppered bottles D. copper containers

12. For BEST results when demonstrating the electrolysis of water, the laboratory assistant should make available an electric current of approximately 12.___
    A. 110 volts AC B. 20 volts AC
    C. 1.5 volts DC D. 18 volts DC

13. Hematite is an important ore of the metal 13.___
    A. iron B. boron C. magnesium D. plutonium

14. For the study of the action of metals on acids, students may be supplied safely with 14.___
    A. sodium B. zinc C. lithium D. potassium

15. Metallic potassium should be stored under 15.___
    A. water B. dilute hydrochloric acid
    C. fluorspar D. kerosene

16. Of the following, the substance with the LOWEST kindling temperature is 16.___
    A. white phosphorus B. sulfur
    C. magnesium D. calcium

17. A salt which will hydrolyze in water to form a basic solution is 17.___
    A. $CuSO_4$ B. NaCl C. KNO_3 D. Na_2CO_3

18. To keep blue litmus paper in a satisfactory condition in the laboratory, store it in a rubber-stoppered bottle and add one or two drops of 18.___
    A. HCl B. NH_4OH C. NaCl D. $Al_2(SO_4)_3$

19. Of the following salts, the one that is LEAST soluble in water is 19.___
    A. $MgCl_2$ B. $FeCl_2$ C. AgCl D. $CaCl_2$

20. A rapid chemical reaction will result if we treat ____ with ____. 20.___
   A. Al; Conc. HNO_3 B. Mg; dilute HCl
   C. Fe; cold Conc. H_2SO_4 D. Cu; cold dilute HCl

21. In order to show the dehydrating action of concentrated sulfuric acid in the laboratory, pour the acid on 21.___
   A. $NaHCO_3$ solution B. sucrose
   C. ethyl alcohol D. washing soda

22. To produce oil of wintergreen in the laboratory, add concentrated sulfuric acid to a mixture of ____ alcohol and ____ acid. 22.___
   A. ethyl; acetic B. methyl; formic
   C. methyl; salicylic D. ethyl; citric

23. One product that results when red hot iron is treated with steam is 23.___
   A. FeO B. H_2 C. $Fe(OH)_2$ D. Fe_2O_3

24. Antimony will burn in chlorine gas to produce the compound 24.___
   A. $SbCl_3$ B. SbCl C. $SbCl_2$ D. Sb_2Cl_5

25. When heated, carbon will readily reduce the compound 25.___
   A. Na_2O B. K_2O C. Al_2O_3 D. Pb_3O_4

KEY (CORRECT ANSWERS)

1. D
2. C
3. A
4. C
5. C

6. D
7. D
8. A
9. D
10. D

11. B
12. D
13. A
14. B
15. D

16. A
17. D
18. B
19. C
20. B

21. B
22. C
23. B
24. A
25. D

TEST 4

DIRECTIONS: Each question or incomplete statement is followed by several suggested answers or completions. Select the one that BEST answers the question or completes the statement. *PRINT THE LETTER OF THE CORRECT ANSWER IN THE SPACE AT THE RIGHT.*

1. During the electrolysis of brine in the laboratory, one observes that at the anode 1.___
   A. blue litmus is bleached
   B. litmus remains unchanged
   C. blue litmus turns red
   D. red litmus turns blue

2. To prepare a solution of calcium bicarbonate in the laboratory, one should 2.___
   A. dissolve the salt in hot water
   B. bubble excess CO_2 into $Ca(OH)_2$ solution
   C. add concentrated H_2SO_4 to $CaCO_3$
   D. treat washing soda with lime

3. A white salt will be formed if a bottle of concentrated NH_4OH is opened near exposed concentrated solutions of 3.___
   A. $Na(OH)$ B. H_2SO_4 C. $Ca(OH)_2$ D. HCl

4. Of the following gases, the formula of the one that is denser than air is 4.___
   A. CO_2 B. CH_4 C. NH_3 D. C_2H_4

5. To etch glass, the chemist employs the acid known as 5.___
   A. hydrofluoric B. hydrobromic
   C. hydrochloric D. hydriodic

6. A salt which will turn dark on exposure to sunlight has the formula 6.___
   A. $K_2C_2O_4$ B. $Fe_4[Fe(CN)_6]_3$ C. AgCl D. $CaCl_2$

7. A substance that will deliquesce in the normal laboratory atmosphere is 7.___
   A. copper sulphate B. sodium hydroxide
   C. silicon dioxide D. sucrose

8. A crystalline substance often used in laboratory experiments to demonstrate the presence of water of crystallization is 8.___
   A. calcium oxide B. copper sulfate
   C. sodium chloride D. sugar

9. The chemical formula of lodestone is 9.___
   A. FeO B. Fe_2O_3 C. Fe_3O_4 D. FeS

10. A substance commonly used in the chemistry laboratory as a desiccating agent is 10.___
A. $BaCl_2$ B. $CaCl_2$ C. KCl D. NaCl

11. Rhombic crystals of sulfur are USUALLY prepared from a solution of sulfur in 11.___
A. sulfurous acid B. alcohol
C. ether D. carbon disulfide

12. The electrolyte in the Edison storage cell is 12.___
A. KOH B. H_2SO_4 C. $FeCl_3$ D. NaCl

13. Chlorine may be prepared in the laboratory by the reaction between hydrochloric acid and 13.___
A. Al_3PO_4 B. MnO_2 C. KCl D. $FeSO_4$

14. A corrosive constituent of Fehling's Solution is 14.___
A. $AgNO_3$ B. Cl_2 C. H_2SO_4 D. NaOH

15. A gas commonly used as a refrigerant in home refrigerators is 15.___
A. argon B. chlorine C. freon D. neon

16. A salt frequently used to demonstrate crystallization from a supersaturated solution is 16.___
A. calcium chloride B. sodium thiosulfate
C. potassium permanganate D. magnesium sulfate

17. Commercial *10 volume* H_2O_2 is a solution with a strength of APPROXIMATELY 17.___
A. 30% B. 3% C. 1% D. 10%

18. Aqua regia is a mixture of concentrated ____ acids. 18.___
A. nitric and hydrofluoric
B. sulphuric and hydrochloric
C. sulphuric and nitric
D. nitric and hydrochloric

19. Rubber stoppers are GENERALLY used in reagent bottles containing 19.___
A. CS_2 B. C_2H_5OH C. HCl D. NaOH

20. The abrasive known as carborundum is the chemical compound ____ carbide. 20.___
A. aluminum B. tungsten C. silicon D. iron

21. A mineral which effervesces when treated with cold dilute hydrochloric acid is 21.___
A. calcite B. fluorite
C. chalcopyrite D. chalcocite

22. White phosphorus dissolves MOST readily in 22.___
A. carbon disulfide B. benzene
C. alcohol D. water

23. A reducing agent commonly employed in the silvering of glass is 23.___
A. sulfurous acid B. ferrous chloride
C. formaldehyde D. mercurous chloride

24. Zeolites are used GENERALLY for 24.___
A. catalysts in manufacturing sulfuric acid by the contact process
B. softening water
C. flux in soldering
D. cleaning chemical glassware

25. The mineral composed CHIEFLY of aluminum silicate is 25.___
A. feldspar B. amethyst C. quartz D. siderite

KEY (CORRECT ANSWERS)

1. A
2. B
3. D
4. A
5. A

6. C
7. B
8. B
9. C
10. B

11. D
12. A
13. B
14. D
15. C

16. B
17. B
18. D
19. D
20. C

21. A
22. A
23. C
24. B
25. A

TEST 5

DIRECTIONS: Each question or incomplete statement is followed by several suggested answers or completions. Select the one that BEST answers the question or completes the statement. *PRINT THE LETTER OF THE CORRECT ANSWER IN THE SPACE AT THE RIGHT.*

1. A liter of chlorine and a liter of oxygen measured under the same conditions of temperature and pressure will contain a(n) 1.___
   A. different number of atoms
   B. number of molecules depending upon the size of the molecules
   C. number of molecules depending upon the atomic weight
   D. equal number of molecules

2. Assuming that the same conditions of temperature and pressure prevail throughout the experiment, when 10 ml of hydrogen and 20 ml of oxygen are ignited, the number of ml of uncombined oxygen gas remaining will be 2.___
   A. 0.00 B. 7.50 C. 15.00 D. 18.75

3. A Leyden jar is used to 3.___
   A. hold corrosive liquids B. store an electric charge
   C. demonstrate interference D. store hot liquids

4. In the study of metallic sulfides, the following materials were furnished to the students: powdered sulfur, zinc dust, copper foil, iron filings, and lead shot. 4.___
   The GREATEST hazard in handling these materials would exist in the reaction between sulfur and
   A. zinc dust B. copper foil
   C. iron filings D. lead shot

5. Safety precautions require that we substitute, when possible, ____ for ____. 5.___
   A. HCl; H_2SO_4 B. H_2SO_4; HNO_3
   C. HNO_3; $HC_2H_3O_2$ D. $HC_2H_3O_2$; H_2CO_3

6. Temporary hardness in water is FREQUENTLY caused by the fact that the water contains 6.___
   A. $MgCO_3$ B. $Ca(HCO_3)_2$ C. $FeCl_3$ D. Na_2SO_4

7. With forceps (or a knife) make a small depression in a charcoal block. Place some zinc sulfate crystals into this depression and add a drop of water to make the crystals hold together. Using a blowpipe, heat the zinc sulfate for about one minute. Allow the residue to cool and add a drop of a particular reagent solution. Again heat the material using a blowpipe. 7.___
   The preceding directions refer to a demonstration on
   A. reduction with carbon

B. conversion of zinc sulfate to zinc sulfide
C. formation of microcosmic salt
D. the cobalt nitrate test for zinc

8. When steel wool burns in a bottle of oxygen, one should be instructed to 8.___
A. wrap the bottle in wire gauze
B. put a little water in the bottom of the bottle
C. hold the steel wool against the side of the bottle
D. add a catalyst to the steel wool

9. The CORRECT formula for chloric acid is 9.___
A. HCl B. HClO C. $HClO_2$ D. $HClO_3$

10. To demonstrate the thermite process, there should be included in the setup _____ oxide. 10.___
A. iron and aluminum B. lead and iron
C. aluminum and iron D. magnesium and aluminum

11. Of the following elements, the one that is USUALLY collected in the laboratory by the process of sublimation is 11.___
A. carbon B. iodine C. hydrogen D. nitrogen

12. When hydrogen sulfide is passed into a certain solution, it reacts to form a white precipitate. The solution referred to contains ions of 12.___
A. antimony B. zinc C. lead D. copper

13. When determining the presence of potassium in a mixture of potassium and sodium compounds by means of the flame test, one should 13.___
A. cut down the supply of air in the Bunsen burner
B. use a borax bead
C. use a very low flame
D. use blue cobalt glass

14. An example of a nuclear reaction is 14.___

$${}_7N^{14} + {}_2He^4 \rightarrow {}_1H^1 + x$$

The term x in this reaction represents
A. ${}_7N^{15}$ B. ${}_8O^{16}$ C. ${}_8O^{17}$ D. ${}_8O^{18}$

15. The law of multiple proportions is illustrated by the pair of compounds 15.___
A. KCl and $KClO_3$ B. $MnSO_4$ and $BaSO_4$
C. H_2O and H_2O_2 D. NaBr and NaCl

16. An alpha particle contains 16.___
A. 2 protons and 2 neutrons
B. 1 proton and 3 neutrons
C. 3 protons and 1 neutron
D. 2 electrons

17. The number of elements depicted on an up-to-date periodic chart of the atoms is 17.___
A. 96 B. 100 C. 102 D. 104

18. Sodium acetate is a salt of a ____ base and a ____ acid. 18.___
A. strong; strong B. strong; weak
C. weak; strong D. weak; weak

19. Destructive distillation of soft coal yields 19.___
A. coal gas and acetic acid
B. ammonia and coke
C. coal tar and charcoal
D. methamol and benzene

20. Of the two processes, oxidation and reduction, the reaction between hydrochloric acid and manganese dioxide involves 20.___
A. reduction *only*
B. oxidation *only*
C. neither oxidation nor reduction
D. oxidation and reduction

21. A brown ring appears in the test for a 21.___
A. chloride B. nitrate C. hydroxide D. sulfate

22. When cutting yellow phosphorus, one should 22.___
A. first dry the stick of phosphorus and then cut it on an asbestos pad
B. gently warm the phosphorus to drive off moisture
C. use a paper cutter so as to obtain even slices
D. cut the phosporus under water

23. In the laboratory experiment employing molasses, yeast, kerosene, and calcium hydroxide solution, the purpose of the calcium hydroxide is to 23.___
A. purify the products obtained from the molasses
B. test for carbon dioxide gas
C. prevent the kerosene from evaporating
D. neutralize unwanted by-product acids

24. A chemist orders the following materials and equipment: test tubes, Bunsen burner, magnifying glass, bar magnet, test tube holder, platform balance, iron powder, and powdered sulfur. 24.___
The planned experiment MOST likely would be a study of
A. allotropic forms of sulfur
B. magnetic lines of force
C. elements, compounds, and mixtures
D. crystallization

25. If a bottle of acid is dropped on the laboratory floor without injury to anyone, the FIRST act should be to 25.___
A. neutralize the area with sodium bicarbonate
B. discover who was responsible for the accident
C. pour concentrated ammonia water on area
D. spray area with a foam extinguisher

KEY (CORRECT ANSWERS)

1. D
2. C
3. B
4. A
5. A
6. C
7. D
8. B
9. D
10. C
11. B
12. B
13. D
14. C
15. C
16. A
17. C
18. B
19. B
20. B
21. B
22. D
23. B
24. C
25. A

EXAMINATION SECTION
TEST 1

DIRECTIONS: Each question or incomplete statement is followed by several suggested answers or completions. Select the one that BEST answers the question or completes the statement. *PRINT THE LETTER OF THE CORRECT ANSWER IN THE SPACE AT THE RIGHT.*

1. A property of ionic substances in the solid state is 1.____
   A. electrical conductivity B. a high melting point
   C. malleability D. high vapor pressure

2. In which noble gas are van der Waals forces the GREATEST? 2.____
   A. Ne B. Xe C. Kr D. Ar

3. The abnormally high boiling point of HF as compared to HCl is PRIMARILY due to intermolecular forces of attraction called 3.____
   A. network bonds B. electrovalent forces
   C. van der Waals forces D. hydrogen bonds

4. Hydrogen forms a negative ion when it combines with sodium to form NaH. 4.____
   This is PRIMARILY because hydrogen
   A. loses an electron to sodium
   B. has a greater attraction for electrons than sodium has
   C. is a larger atom than sodium
   D. has a smaller ionization energy than sodium

5. A molecule of iodine contains a _____ bond. 5.____
   A. ionic B. polar covalent
   C. nonpolar covalent D. metallic

6. Which represents the CORRECT order of activity for the Group VIIA elements? (> means greater than.) 6.____
   A. Bromine > iodine > fluorine > chlorine
   B. Fluorine > chlorine > bromine > iodine
   C. Iodine > bromine > chlorine > fluorine
   D. Fluorine > bromine > chlorine > iodine

7. Which group contains two metalloids? 7.____
   A. IIA B. IIB C. VA D. VB

8. A metallic element whose aqueous ions produce colorless solutions would be found in Period 4 and Group 8.____
   A. IA B. VIIA C. VIII D. O

9. Considered in succession, the elements in Period 2 of the Periodic Table show a decrease in atomic radius with increasing atomic number. 9.____
   This may BEST be explained by the fact that the
   A. nuclear charge increases
   B. number of principal energy levels increases

C. number of neutrons decreases
D. number of protons decreases

10. When the atoms of the elements of Group 0 are compared in order from top to bottom, the attractions between the atoms of each successive element _____ and the boiling point _____. 10.____
A. increase; decreases B. decrease; increases
C. increase; increases D. decrease; decreases

11. In the reaction $N_2 + 3H_2 \rightarrow 2NH_3$, how many grams of ammonia are produced when 1.0 mole of nitrogen reacts? 11.____
A. 8.5 B. 17 C. 34 D. 68

12. How many moles of KNO_3 are required to make 0.50 liter of a 2.0 M solution of KNO_3? 12.____
A. 1.0 B. 2.0 C. 0.50 D. 4.0

13. Eleven grams of a gas occupies 5.6 liters at STP. The molecular mass of this gas is 13.____
A. 11 B. 22 C. 44 D. 88

14. A compound which contains 75% carbon and 25% hydrogen by mass has the formula 14.____
A. CH_4 B. C_2H_2 C. C_2H_6 D. C_3H_8

15. According to the chart at the right, a solution containing 100 grams of KNO_3 per 100 grams of H_2O at 50°C is considered to be 15.____
A. dilute and unsaturated
B. dilute and supersaturated
C. concentrated and unsaturated
D. concentrated and supersaturated

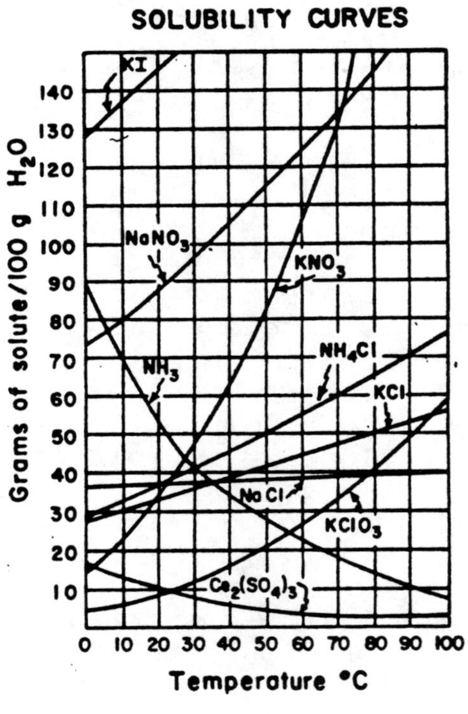

16. Given the equilibrium reaction: A + B $\rightleftarrows$ C + D + heat. What change in the reaction system will change the value of the equilibrium constant? 16.____

An increase in
- A. the concentration of A and B
- B. the concentration of C and D
- C. temperature
- D. pressure

17. Given the potential energy diagram shown at the right. With reference to energy, the reaction A + B $\rightarrow$ AB can BEST be described as 17.____
- A. endothermic, having a $+\Delta H$
- B. endothermic, having a $-\Delta H$
- C. exothermic, having a $+\Delta H$
- D. exothermic, having a $-\Delta H$

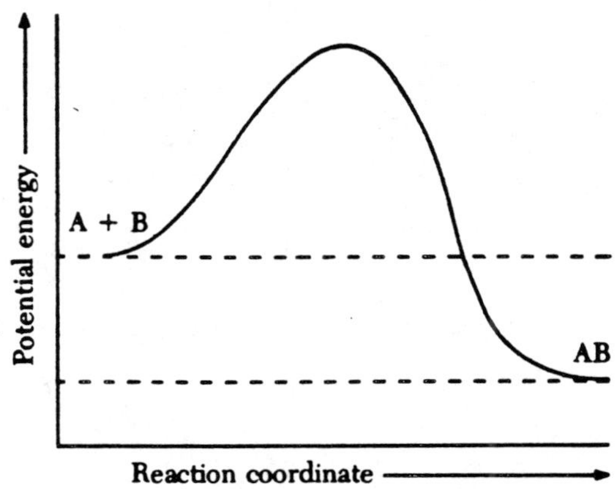

18. Which phrase BEST describes the following reaction: 18.____

$C(s) + \frac{1}{2}O_2(g) \rightarrow CO(g) + 26.4$ kcal?
- A. Exothermic with an increase in entropy
- B. Exothermic with a decrease in entropy
- C. Endothermic with an increase in entropy
- D. Endothermic with a decrease in entropy

19. Given the system at equilibrium: 19.____

$H_3PO_4 + 3H_2O \rightleftarrows 3H_3O^+ + PO_4^{-3}$

If $Na_3PO_4(s)$ is added, there will be a decrease in the concentration of

A. Na^+ B. PO_4^{-3} C. H_3O^+ D. H_2O

20. A chemical reaction is MOST likely to occur spontaneously if the 20.____
- A. free energy change (ΔG) is negative
- B. entropy change (ΔS) is negative
- C. activation energy (E) is positive
- D. heat of reaction (ΔH) is positive

21. When hydrochloric acid is neutralized by sodium hydroxide, the salt formed is sodium 21.____
- A. hydrochlorate
- B. chlorate
- C. chloride
- D. perchloride

22. The ionization constant of a weak acid is 1.8×10^{-5}. A reasonable pH for a 0.1 M solution of this acid would be 22.____

A. 1 B. 9 C. 3 D. 14

23. Which reaction illustrates amphoterism? 23.____

A. $H_2O + H_2O \rightarrow H_3O^+ + OH^-$ B. $HCl + H_2O \rightarrow H_3O^+ + Cl^-$
C. $NaCl \rightarrow Na^+ + Cl^-$ D. $NaOH \rightarrow Na^+ + OH^-$

24. A 1 molal solution of $MgCl_2$ has a HIGHER boiling point than a 1 molal solution of 24.____

A. $FeCl_3$ B. $CaCl_2$ C. $BaCl_2$ D. NaCl

25. A water solution of which gas contains more OH^- ions than H_3O^+ ions? 25.____

A. HCl B. NH_3 C. CO_2 D. SO_2

26. According to the table at the right, which metal will react with 1 molar HCl? 26.____

A. Au
B. Ag
C. Cu
D. Zn

STANDARD ELECTRODE POTENTIALS	
Ionic Concentrations 1 M Water at 298 K, 1 atm	
Half-Reaction	$E°$ *(volts)*
$F_2(g) + 2e^- \rightarrow 2F^-$	+2.87
$MnO_4^- + 8H^+ + 5e^- \rightarrow Mn^{2+} + 4H_2O$	+1.52
$Au^{3+} + 3e^- \rightarrow Au(s)$	+1.50
$Cl_2(g) + 2e^- \rightarrow 2Cl^-$	+1.36
$Cr_2O_7^{2-} + 14H^+ + 6e^- \rightarrow 2Cr^{3+} + 7H_2O$	+1.33
$MnO_2(s) + 4H^+ + 2e^- \rightarrow Mn^{2+} + 2H_2O$	+1.28
$\frac{1}{2}O_2(g) + 2H^+ + 2e^- \rightarrow H_2O$	+1.23
$Br_2(\ell) + 2e^- \rightarrow 2Br^-$	+1.06
$NO_3^- + 4H^+ + 3e^- \rightarrow NO(g) + 2H_2O$	+0.96
$\frac{1}{2}O_2(g) + 2H^+(10^{-7}M) + 2e^- \rightarrow H_2O$	+0.82
$Ag^+ + e^- \rightarrow Ag(s)$	+0.80
$\frac{1}{2}Hg_2^{2+} + e^- \rightarrow Hg(\ell)$	+0.79
$Hg^{2+} + 2e^- \rightarrow Hg(\ell)$	+0.78
$NO_3^- + 2H^+ + e^- \rightarrow NO_2(g) + H_2O$	+0.78
$Fe^{3+} + e^- \rightarrow Fe^{2+}$	+0.77
$I_2(s) + 2e^- \rightarrow 2I^-$	+0.53
$Cu^+ + e^- \rightarrow Cu(s)$	+0.52
$Cu^{2+} + 2e^- \rightarrow Cu(s)$	+0.34
$SO_4^{2-} + 4H^+ + 2e^- \rightarrow SO_2(g) + 2H_2O$	+0.17
$Sn^{4+} + 2e^- \rightarrow Sn^{2+}$	+0.15
$2H^+ + 2e^- \rightarrow H_2(g)$	0.00
$Pb^{2+} + 2e^- \rightarrow Pb(s)$	−0.13
$Sn^{2+} + 2e^- \rightarrow Sn(s)$	−0.14
$Ni^{2+} + 2e^- \rightarrow Ni(s)$	−0.25
$Co^{2+} + 2e^- \rightarrow Co(s)$	−0.28
$2H^+(10^{-7}M) + 2e^- \rightarrow H_2(g)$	−0.41
$Fe^{2+} + 2e^- \rightarrow Fe(s)$	−0.44
$Cr^{3+} + 3e^- \rightarrow Cr(s)$	−0.74
$Zn^{2+} + 2e^- \rightarrow Zn(s)$	−0.76
$2H_2O + 2e^- \rightarrow 2OH^- + H_2(g)$	−0.83
$Mn^{2+} + 2e^- \rightarrow Mn(s)$	−1.18
$Al^{3+} + 3e^- \rightarrow Al(s)$	−1.66
$Mg^{2+} + 2e^- \rightarrow Mg(s)$	−2.37
$Na^+ + e^- \rightarrow Na(s)$	−2.71
$Ca^{2+} + 2e^- \rightarrow Ca(s)$	−2.87
$Sr^{2+} + 2e^- \rightarrow Sr(s)$	−2.89
$Ba^{2+} + 2e^- \rightarrow Ba(s)$	−2.90
$Cs^+ + e^- \rightarrow Cs(s)$	−2.92
$K^+ + e^- \rightarrow K(s)$	−2.92
$Rb^+ + e^- \rightarrow Rb(s)$	−2.93
$Li^+ + e^- \rightarrow Li(s)$	−3.00

27. Which equation CORRECTLY represents reduction? 27.____

A. $Na^+ + 1e^- \rightarrow Na^0$ B. $Na^+ \rightarrow Na^0 + 1e^-$
C. $Cl^- + 1e^- \rightarrow Cl^0$ D. $Cl^- \rightarrow Cl^0 + 1e^-$

28. Which is the oxidizing agent in the following reaction: 28.____
$2Al + 3CuSO_4 \rightarrow Al_2(SO_4)_3 + 3Cu$?

A. Al^{+3} B. Cu^{+2} C. S^{+6} D. O^{-2}

29. Which is a redox reaction? 29.___
  A. $Ba^{+2} + SO_4^{-2} \rightarrow BaSO_4$
  B. $H^+ + OH^- \rightarrow H_2O$
  C. $Sn^0 + Sn^{+4} \rightarrow 2Sn^{+2}$
  D. $N^+ + NH_3 \rightarrow NH_4^+$

30. A reducing agent is a substance that 30.___
  A. gains protons
  B. loses protons
  C. gains electrons
  D. loses electrons

31. The reaction $C_3H_6 + H_2 \rightarrow C_3H_8$ is an example of 31.___
  A. substitution
  B. addition
  C. polymerization
  D. esterification

32. A triple covalent bond is contained in the molecule 32.___
  A. C_2H_2 B. C_2H_4 C. C_3H_6 D. C_3H_8

33. Which structural formula represents propene? 33.___

A. 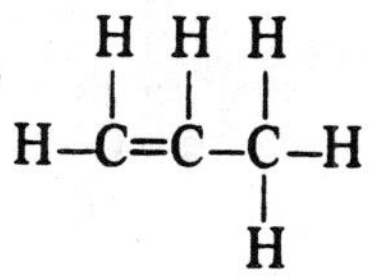

B. 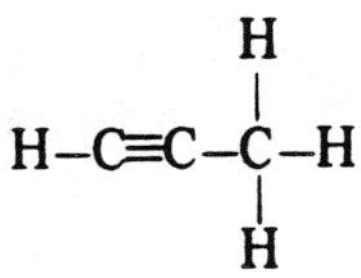

C. 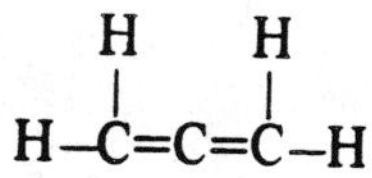

D. 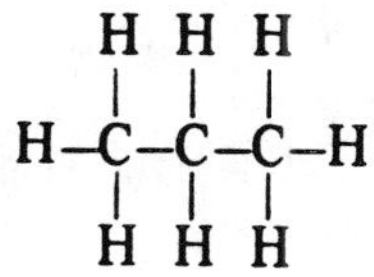

34. What is the I.U.C. name for the following compound? 34.___
  A. Dibromoethyne
  B. Dibromoethane
  C. 1,2-dibromoethyne
  D. 1,2-dibromoethane

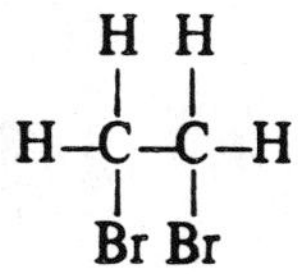

35. Which formula CORRECTLY represents an ester? 35.___
  A. $CH_3CH_2CH_2OH$
  B. CH_3COCH_3
  C. CH_3COOCH_3
  D. CH_3CH_2COOH

KEY (CORRECT ANSWERS)

1. B
2. B
3. D
4. B
5. C

6. B
7. C
8. A
9. A
10. C

11. C
12. A
13. C
14. A
15. D

16. C
17. D
18. A
19. C
20. A

21. C
22. C
23. A
24. D
25. B

26. D
27. A
28. B
29. C
30. D

31. B
32. A
33. A
34. D
35. C

TEST 2

DIRECTIONS: Each question or incomplete statement is followed by several suggested answers or completions. Select the one that BEST answers the question or completes the statement. *PRINT THE LETTER OF THE CORRECT ANSWER IN THE SPACE AT THE RIGHT.*

1. When one mole of a certain compound is formed from its elements under standard conditions, it absorbs 85 kilocalories of heat. A CORRECT conclusion from this statement is that the reaction has a _____ equal to _____ kcal/mole. 1.____
   A. ΔH_f^0; -85 B. ΔH_f^0; +85 C. ΔG_f^0; -85 D. ΔG_f^0; +85

2. When a catalyst is added to a reaction at equilibrium, the rate of the forward reaction _____ and the rate of the reverse reaction _____. 2.____
   A. decreases; decreases B. decreases; increases
   C. increases; decreases D. increases; increases

3. Equilibrium is reached in all reversible chemical reactions when the 3.____
   A. forward reaction stops
   B. reverse reaction stops
   C. concentrations of the reactants and the products become equal
   D. rates of the opposing reactions become equal

4. A solution at 25°C with a pH of 7 contains _____ OH^- ions. 4.____
   A. more H_3O^+ ions than
   B. fewer H_3O^+ ions than
   C. an equal number of H_3O^+ ions and
   D. no H_3O^+ ions or

5. Which acid is almost completely ionized in a dilute solution at 298K? 5.____
   A. CH_3COOH B. H_2S C. H_3PO_4 D. HNO_3

6. Which Brönsted acid has the WEAKEST conjugate base? 6.____
   A. HCl B. H_2SO_4 C. H_2S D. HNO_3

7. A solution of K_2CO_3 would have a pH CLOSEST to 7.____
   A. 1 B. 5 C. 3 D. 8

8. How many liters of 2.5 M HCl are required to EXACTLY neutralize 1.5 liters of 5.0 M NaOH? 8.____
   A. 1.0 B. 2.0 C. 3.0 D. 4.0

9. What are the Brönsted-Lowry bases in the reaction $H_2S + H_2O \rightleftarrows H_3O^+ + HS^-$? 9.____
   A. H_2S and H_2O B. H_2S and H_3O^+
   C. HS^- and H_2O D. HS^- and H_3O^+

10. How many moles of electrons are needed to reduce one mole of Fe^{3+} to Fe^{2+}? 10.____
A. One B. Two C. Three D. Five

11. Which change in oxidation number represents reduction? 11.____
A. -3 to 0 B. -2 to -3 C. 0 to +1 D. +1 to +2

12. Which pair will react spontaneously at 298K? 12.____
A. Cu + H_2O
B. Ag + H_2O
C. Ca + H_2O
D. Au + H_2O

13. When the equation _Al + $3NO_3^-$ + _H^+ → _Al^{3+} + $3H_2O$ + $3NO_2$ is completely balanced, the coefficient of Al will be 13.____
A. 1 B. 2 C. 3 D. 4

14. The oxidation number of sulfur in $Na_2S_2O_3$ is 14.____
A. -2 B. +2 C. +6 D. 0

15. In the reaction $Cl_2 + H_2O \rightarrow HClO + HCl$, the Cl_2 is 15.____
A. oxidized *only*
B. reduced *only*
C. both oxidized and reduced
D. neither oxidized nor reduced

16. Each member in the alkane series of hydrocarbons, when considered in successive order, has 1 more carbon atom and _____ more than the hydrocarbon preceding it. 16.____
A. one B. two C. three D. four

17. Which is an isomer of the compound propanoic acid CH_3CH_2COOH? 17.____
A. $CH_2 = CHCOOH$
B. $CH_3CH_2CH_2COOH$
C. $CH_3CH(OH)CH_2OH$
D. $HCOOCH_2CH_3$

18. Pentene is represented by the molecular formula 18.____
A. C_4H_8 B. C_4H_{10} C. C_5H_{10} D. C_5H_{12}

19. Which compound is a hydrocarbon? 19.____

(A) 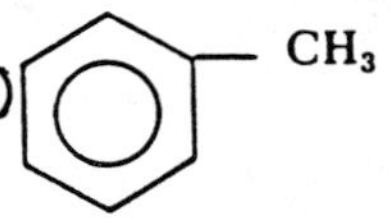

(C) 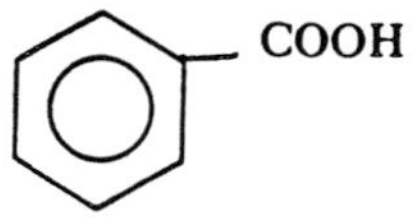

(B) 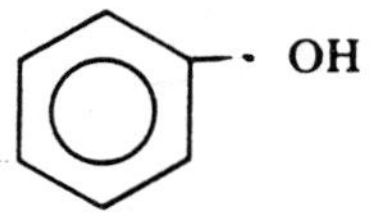

(D) 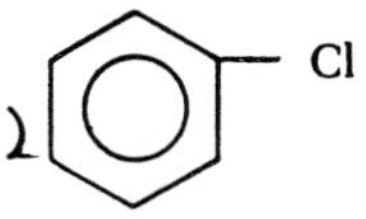

20. A molecule of _____ alcohol contains more than one hydroxyl group. 20.____
A. propanol B. butanol C. pentanol D. glycerol

21. As a sodium atom is oxidized, the number of protons in its nucleus 21.____
A. decreases
B. increases
C. remains the same
D. increases, then decreases

22. Given the reaction: $A(g) + B(g) \rightleftarrows AB(g)$. 22.___
As the pressure increases at a constant temperature, the rate of the forward reaction will
A. decrease B. increase
C. remain the same D. increase, then decrease

23. As the atmospheric pressure decreases, the temperature at which water will boil in an open container 23.___
A. decreases
B. increases
C. remains the same
D. cannot be determined from the information given

24. When an atom of bromine forms a bromide ion, the radius 24.___
A. decreases B. increases
C. remains the same D. decreases, then increases

25. When additional solid NaCl dissolves in a solution of NaCl in water, the pH of the solution 25.___
A. decreases B. increases
C. remains the same D. increases, then decreases

26. The MOST common property of all liquids is 26.___
A. definite shape B. definite volume
C. high compressibility D. high vapor pressure

27. A gas sample occupies 10. milliliters at one atmosphere of pressure. 27.___
If the volume changes to 20. milliliters and the temperature remains the same, the pressure will be ____ atm.
A. 1.0 B. 2.0 C. 0.25 D. 0.50

28. At constant pressure, which curve BEST shows the relationship between the volume of an ideal gas and its absolute temperature? 28.___
A. A
B. B
C. C
D. D

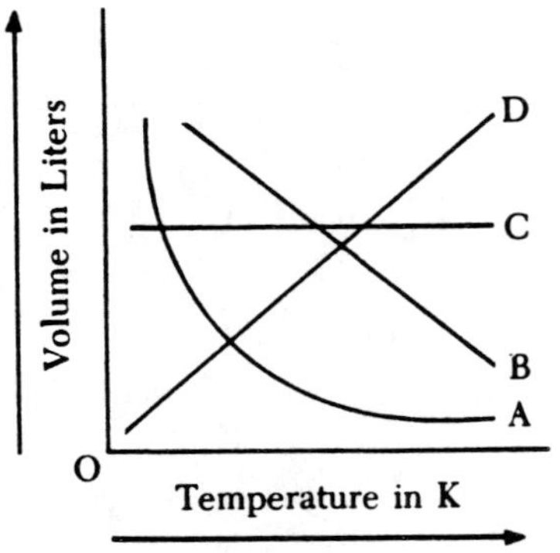

29. The average kinetic energies of the molecules in two gas samples could BEST be compared by measuring their 29.___
A. temperatures B. volumes
C. pressures D. densities

30. The volume of 1 mole of an ideal gas at 25°C and 1 atmosphere of pressure is 22.4 liters × 30.___

A. $\frac{1}{25}$ B. $\frac{25}{1}$ C. $\frac{298}{273}$ D. $\frac{273}{298}$

31. In the ground state, an atom of _____ contains electrons with a principal quantum number (n) of 4. 31.___
A. Kr B. Ar C. Ne D. He

32. In the equation ${}^{226}_{88}Ra \rightarrow {}^{222}_{86}Rn + X$, X represents a(n) 32.___
A. neutron B. proton
C. beta particle D. alpha particle

33. What is the TOTAL number of neutrons in an atom of ${}^{19}_{9}F$? 33.___
A. 9 B. 10 C. 19 D. 28

34. If the electron configuration of an atom of element X is $1s^2 2s^2 2p^4$, the electron dot symbol for the element is 34.___

A. X: B. $\cdot\dot{\underset{\cdot}{X}}\cdot$ C. $:\ddot{\underset{\cdot\cdot}{X}}:$ D. $\cdot\dot{\underset{\cdot\cdot}{X}}:$

35. A Mg^{+2} ion has the same electron configuration as 35.___
A. Na^0 B. Ar^0 C. F^- D. Ca^{2+}

KEY (CORRECT ANSWERS)

1. B
2. D
3. D
4. C
5. D

6. A
7. D
8. C
9. C
10. A

11. B
12. C
13. A
14. B
15. C

16. B
17. D
18. C
19. A
20. D

21. C
22. B
23. A
24. B
25. C

26. B
27. D
28. D
29. A
30. C

31. A
32. D
33. B
34. D
35. C

TEST 3

DIRECTIONS: Each question or incomplete statement is followed by several suggested answers or completions. Select the one that BEST answers the question or completes the statement. *PRINT THE LETTER OF THE CORRECT ANSWER IN THE SPACE AT THE RIGHT.*

1. Which equation represents sublimation? 1.____
   A. $H_2O(\ell) \rightarrow H_2O(g)$ B. $H_2O(s) \rightarrow H_2O(\ell)$
   C. $H_2O(s) \rightarrow H_2O(g)$ D. $H_2O(g) \rightarrow H_2O(\ell)$

2. All atoms of a given element MUST have the same 2.____
   A. atomic mass B. atomic weight
   C. mass number D. atomic number

3. According to the table at the right, heat is liberated during the formation of the compound 3.____
   A. nitrogen (II) oxide(g)
   B. ethyne(g)
   C. hydrogen fluoride(g)
   D. hydrogen iodide(g)

Standard Energies of Formation of Compounds at 1 atm and 298 K

Compound	*Heat (Enthalpy) of Formation kcal/mole* (ΔH_f°)	*Free Energy of Formation kcal/mole* (ΔG_f°)
Aluminum oxide Al_2O_3 (s)	—399.1	—376.8
Ammonia NH_3 (g)	—11.0	—4.0
Barium sulfate $BaSO_4$ (s)	—350.2	—323.4
Calcium hydroxide $Ca(OH)_2$ (s)	—235.8	—214.3
Carbon dioxide CO_2 (g)	—94.1	—94.3
Carbon monoxide CO (g)	—26.4	—32.8
Copper (II) sulfate $CuSO_4$ (s)	—184.0	—158.2
Ethane C_2H_6 (g)	—20.2	—7.9
Ethene C_2H_4 (g)	12.5	16.3
Ethyne (acetylene) C_2H_2 (g)	54.2	50.0
Hydrogen fluoride HF (g)	—64.2	—64.7
Hydrogen iodide HI (g)	6.2	0.3
Iodine chloride ICl (g)	4.2	—1.3
Lead (II) oxide PbO (s)	—52.4	—45.3
Magnesium oxide MgO (s)	—143.8	—136.1
Nitrogen (II) oxide NO (g)	21.6	20.7
Nitrogen (IV) oxide NO_2 (g)	8.1	12.4
Potassium chloride KCl (s)	—104.2	—97.6
Sodium chloride NaCl (s)	—98.2	—91.8
Sulfur dioxide SO_2 (g)	—71.0	—71.8
Water H_2O (g)	—57.8	—54.6
Water H_2O (ℓ)	—68.3	—56.7

Sample equation

$$2Al\ (s) + \tfrac{3}{2}O_2\ (g) \rightarrow Al_2O_3\ (s)$$

4. When 100 calories of heat energy is added to 10 grams of water at 20°C, the final temperature of the water will be ______°C. 4.____
   A. 10 B. 30 C. 40 D. 100

5. The vapor pressure of 25 milliliters of water at 25°C will be the same as 5.____
   A. 50. ml of water at 25°C
   B. 25 ml of water at 50°C
   C. 50. ml of alcohol at 25°C
   D. 25 ml of alcohol at 50°C

6. In what type of reaction do the products of the reaction ALWAYS possess more potential energy than the reactants? 6.___
   A. Endothermic B. Exothermic
   C. Spontaneous D. Redox

7. A neutral atom of $^{7}_{3}Li$ contains _____ electrons. 7.___
   A. seven B. ten C. three D. four

8. An atom with the electron configuration $1s^2 2s^2 2p^6 3s^2 3p^6 4s^2$ has an incomplete 8.___
   A. 2nd principal energy level
   B. 2s sublevel
   C. 3rd principal energy level
   D. 3s sublevel

9. Which of the following represents the CORRECT electron distribution of a transition element in the ground state? 9.___
   A. 2-8-8-1 B. 2-8-8-2 C. 2-8-18-2 D. 2-8-18-3

10. A 40.0 milligram sample of ^{33}P decays to 10.0 milligrams in 50.0 days. 10.___
    The half-life of ^{33}P is _____ days.
    A. 12.5 B. 25.0 C. 37.5 D. 75.0

11. The nucleus of a fluorine atom has a charge of 11.___
    A. 1+ B. 9+ C. 19+ D. 0

12. How many sublevels are completely occupied in the second principal energy level of a sodium atom in the ground state? 12.___
    A. One B. Two C. Three D. Four

13. The characteristic bright-line spectrum of an element is produced when electrons 13.___
    A. fall back to lower energy levels
    B. are gained by a neutral atom
    C. are emitted by the nucleus as beta particles
    D. move to higher energy levels

14. The CORRECT formula for aluminum sulfate is 14.___
    A. Al_2S_3 B. Al_3S_2 C. $Al_2(SO_4)_3$ D. $Al_3(SO_4)_2$

15. Which molecule is the MOST polar? 15.___
    A. H_2O B. H_2S C. H_2Se D. H_2Te

16. _____ bonding involves positive ions immersed in a sea of mobile electrons. 16.___
    A. Ionic B. Nonpolar covalent
    C. Polar covalent D. Metallic

17. Which sample of HCl MOST readily conducts electricity? 17.___
    A. HCl(s) B. HCl(ℓ) C. HCl(g) D. HCl(aq)

18. The forces of attraction which exist between hydrogen molecules in liquid hydrogen are due to 18.___
   A. ionic bonds   B. hydrogen bonds
   C. molecule-ion forces   D. van der Waals forces

19. Which compound is a network solid? 19.___
   A. SiO_2 B. Na_2O C. H_2O D. CO_2

20. The formula of a nonpolar molecule containing nonpolar bonds is 20.___
   A. CO_2 B. H_2 C. NH_3 D. H_2O

21. All elements in Period 3 have 21.___
   A. an atomic number of 3
   B. 3 valence electrons
   C. 3 occupied principal energy levels
   D. an oxidation number of +3

22. Which element has the HIGHEST ionization energy? 22.___
   A. Barium   B. Magnesium   C. Calcium   D. Strontium

23. Which group contains an element that is a liquid at room temperature? 23.___
   A. O   B. IIA   C. IB   D. IIB

24. Element X is a metal that forms an oxide with the formula X_2O. 24.___
   Element X is in group
   A. IA   B. IIA   C. VIA   D. VIIA

25. In which group do all the elements have the SAME number of electrons in the outermost principal energy level? 25.___
   A. VIB   B. VIII   C. O   D. IVA

26. Which is an alkaline earth metal? 26.___
   A. Na   B. Ca   C. Ga   D. Ta

27. The GREATEST percentage of oxygen by mass is contained by the compound 27.___
   A. BaO   B. CaO   C. MgO   D. SrO

28. Which gas is LESS dense than air at STP? 28.___
   A. CO_2 B. H_2S C. NH_3 D. SO_2

29. A compound contains 50% sulfur and 50% oxygen by mass. The empirical formula of this compound is 29.___
   A. SO   B. SO_2 C. SO_3 D. SO_4

30. Given the reaction: $C_3H_8(g) + 5O_2(g) \rightarrow 4H_2O(g) + 3CO_2(g)$. 30.___
   What is the TOTAL number of liters of CO_2 produced when 150 liters of O_2 reacts completely with C_3H_8?
   A. 90.   B. 150   C. 3.0   D. 250

31. What is the TOTAL volume, in liters, occupied by 56.0 grams of nitrogen gas at STP? 31.___

A. 11.2 B. 22.4 C. 33.6 D. 44.8

32. In a 30. gram sample of neon, the TOTAL number of atoms is _____ $\times 10^{23}$. 32.___

A. 12 B. 9.0 C. 3.0 D. 6.0

33. According to the table at the right, which compound released the GREATEST amount of energy per mole when it was formed from its elements? 33.___

A. Sulfur dioxide
B. Carbon dioxide
C. Magnesium oxide
D. Sodium chloride

Standard Energies of Formation of Compounds at 1 atm and 298 K

Compound	*Heat (Enthalpy) of Formation kcal/mole* (ΔH_f°)	*Free Energy of Formation kcal/mole* (ΔG_f°)
Aluminum oxide Al_2O_3 (s)	—399.1	—376.8
Ammonia NH_3 (g)	—11.0	—4.0
Barium sulfate $BaSO_4$ (s)	—350.2	—323.4
Calcium hydroxide $Ca(OH)_2$ (s)	—235.8	—214.3
Carbon dioxide CO_2 (g)	—94.1	—94.3
Carbon monoxide CO (g)	—26.4	—32.8
Copper (II) sulfate $CuSO_4$ (s)	—184.0	—158.2
Ethane C_2H_6 (g)	—20.2	—7.9
Ethene C_2H_4 (g)	12.5	16.3
Ethyne (acetylene) C_2H_2 (g)	54.2	50.0
Hydrogen fluoride HF (g)	—64.2	—64.7
Hydrogen iodide HI (g)	6.2	0.3
Iodine chloride ICl (g)	4.2	—1.3
Lead (II) oxide PbO (s)	—52.4	—45.3
Magnesium oxide MgO (s)	—143.8	—136.1
Nitrogen (II) oxide NO (g)	21.6	20.7
Nitrogen (IV) oxide NO_2 (g)	8.1	12.4
Potassium chloride KCl (s)	—104.2	—97.6
Sodium chloride NaCl (s)	—98.2	—91.8
Sulfur dioxide SO_2 (g)	—71.0	—71.8
Water H_2O (g)	—57.8	—54.6
Water H_2O (ℓ)	—68.3	—56.7

Sample equation

$2Al(s) + \frac{3}{2}O_2(g) \rightarrow Al_2O_3(s)$

34. Which saturated solution would have the HIGHEST S^{2-} ion concentration? 34.___

_____ (K_{sp} at 18°C = _____)

A. CdS; 3.6×10^{-29} B. CoS; 3.0×10^{-26}
C. PbS; 3.4×10^{-28} D. FeS; 3.7×10^{-19}

35. Which expression represents the solubility product constant, Ksp, of AgCl(s)? 35.___

K_{sp} =

A. $[Ag^+][Cl^-]$ B. $[Ag^+] + [Cl^-]$

C. $\frac{[Ag^+]}{[Cl^-]}$ D. $\frac{[Cl^-]}{[Ag^+]}$

KEY (CORRECT ANSWERS)

1. C	11. B	21. C	31. D
2. D	12. B	22. B	32. B
3. C	13. A	23. D	33. C
4. B	14. C	24. A	34. D
5. A	15. A	25. D	35. A
6. A	16. D	26. B	
7. C	17. D	27. C	
8. C	18. D	28. C	
9. C	19. A	29. B	
10. B	20. B	30. A	

EXAMINATION SECTION

DIRECTIONS: Each question or incomplete statement is followed by several suggested answers or completions. Select the one that BEST answers the question or completes the statement. *PRINT THE LETTER OF THE CORRECT ANSWER IN THE SPACE AT THE RIGHT.*

1. 1.____

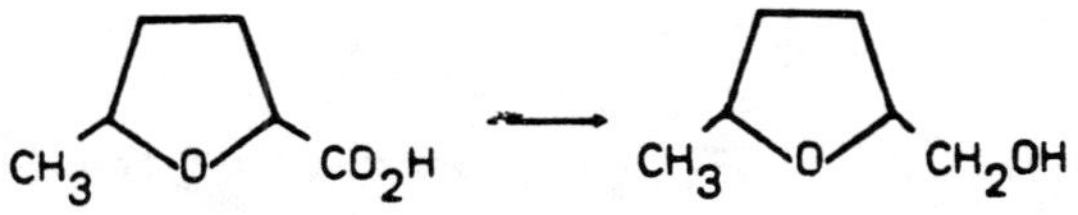

Which reagent could be used to accomplish the above conversion?

A. Aqueous $KMnO_4$
B. KOH in ethanol
C. H_2O_2 in aqueous acetone
D. CrO_3
E. $LiAlH_4$ followed by H_2O

2. Cyclopentadiene is an unusually acidic hydrocarbon and readily undergoes the following reaction: 2.____

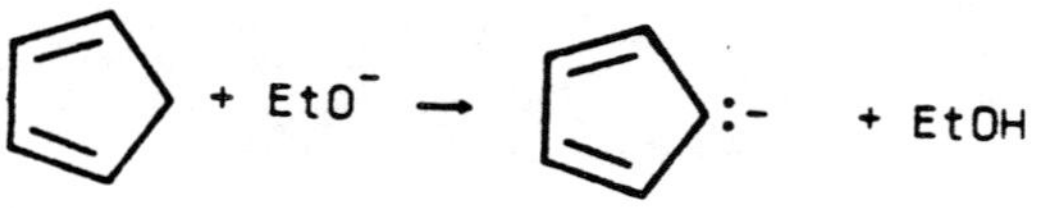

An explanation for this observation is:

A. Cyclopentadiene contains four sp^2 hybridized carbons
B. The ethoxide ion readily reacts with unsaturated hydrocarbons
C. Cyclopentadiene is an aromatic hydrocarbon
D. The reaction yields an aromatic carbocation
E. The reaction yields an aromatic carbanion

3. 3.____

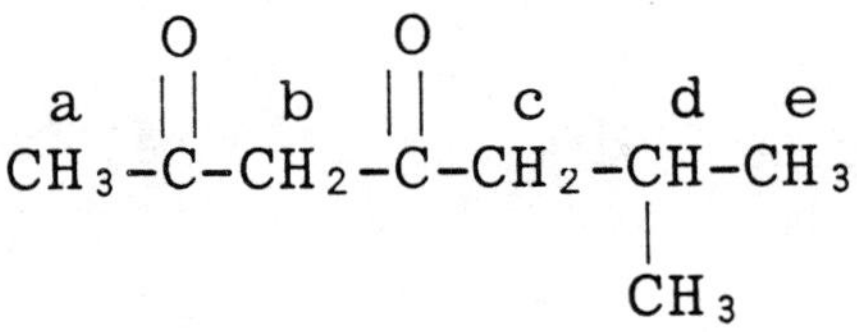

The hydrogen at which position in the above compound is MOST acidic?

A. a B. b C. c D. d E. e

4. Which of the following compounds will undergo elimination MOST readily by the E1 mechanism? 4.____

A. CH_3CH_2Br B. 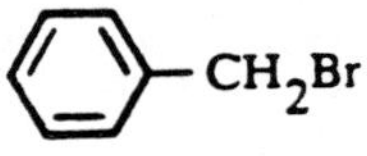

C. 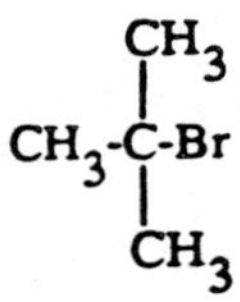

D. 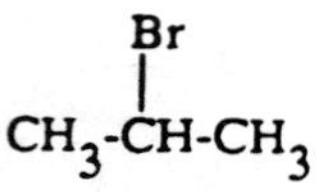

E. 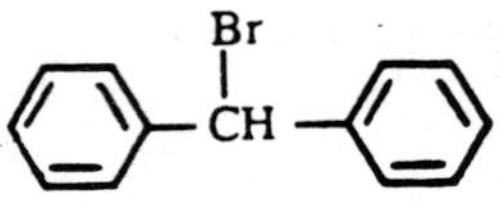

5. The benzyl carbanion 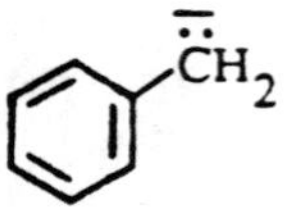 is an unusually stable carbanion. This stability arises from 5.____

A. the inductive effect of electron release by the phenyl group
B. resonance stabilization of the benzyl carbanion
C. steric hindrance by the large phenyl group
D. the conformation present in the benzyl carbanion
E. the hybridization of the charged carbon

6. How many PRIMARY hydrogens are present in the compound at the right? 6.____

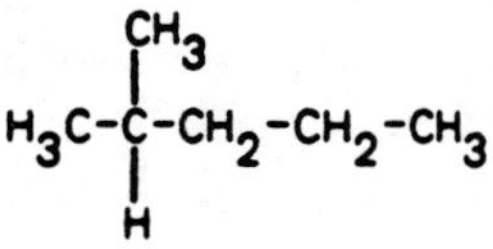

A. 1
B. 3
C. 4
D. 9
E. 14

7. Which of the structures below is an IMPORTANT resonance form of 7.____

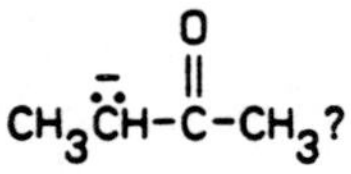?

A. 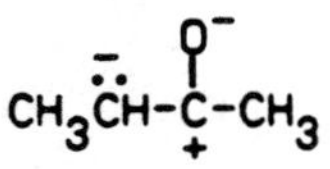

B. 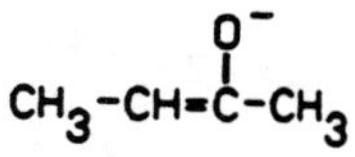

C. 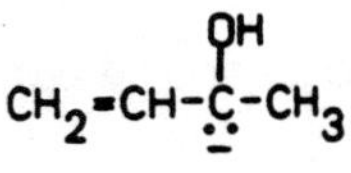

D. 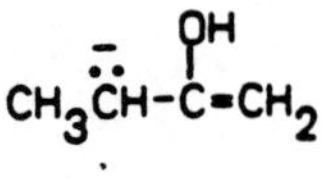

E. 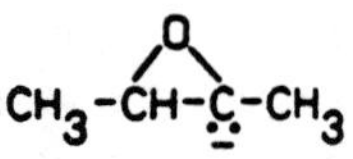

8. Identical molecules are capable of weakly bonding to one another through forces such as hydrogen bonding, dipolar interactions, and van der Waals forces. 8.____
From the following sets, select the molecules showing the WEAKEST self-association.

A. HF, HF
B. H_2O, H_2O
C. NH_3, NH_3
D. CH_4, CH_4
E. CH_3OH, CH_3OH

9. Which of the following combinations of reagents will yield the compound at the right after hydrolisis and work up? 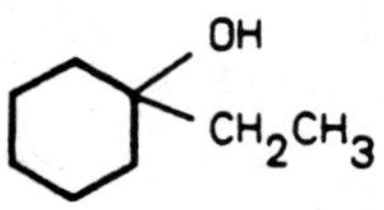 9.____

A. 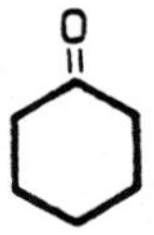 + $BrCH_2CH_3$

B. 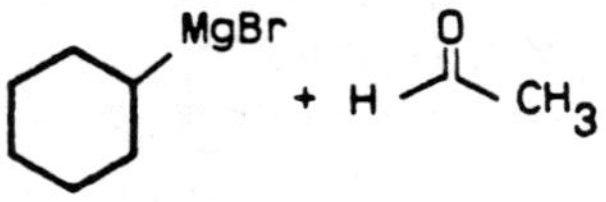

C. 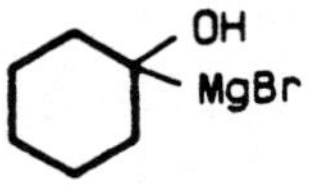 + $BrCH_2CH_3$

D. 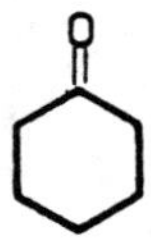 + $BrMgCH_2CH_3$

E. 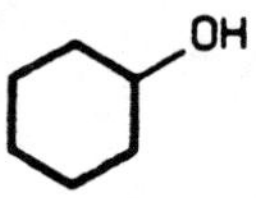 + $BrMgCH_2CH_3$

10. Which of the following is the MOST stable? 10.____

A. 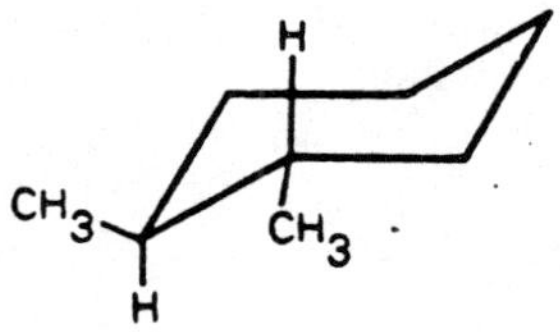

B. 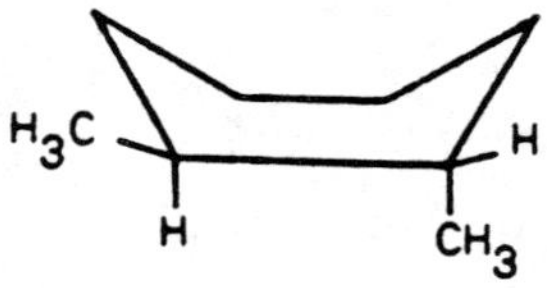

C. 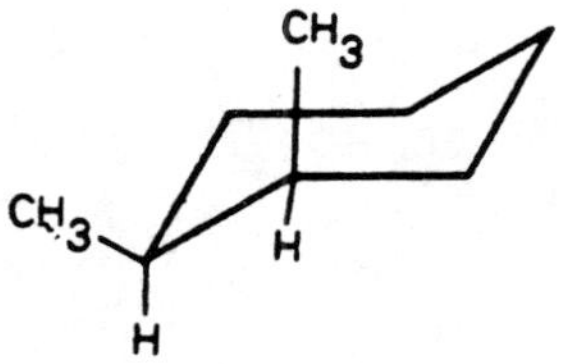

D. 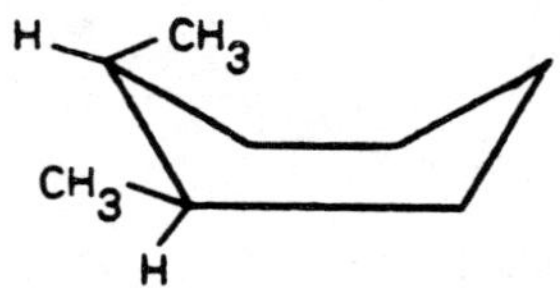

E. 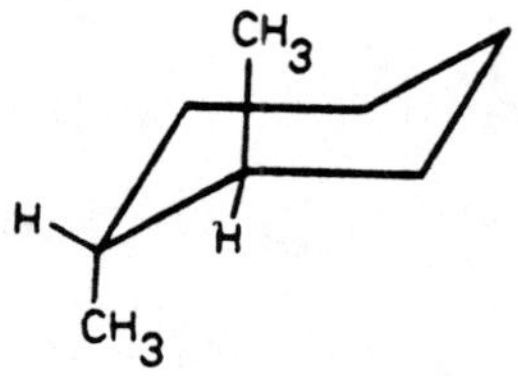

11. What is the product of the following reaction? 11.____

$$CH_3C \equiv CCO_2H + \text{excess } H_2 \xrightarrow{Pd}$$

A. 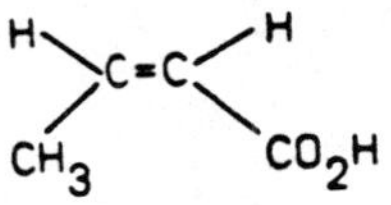

B. 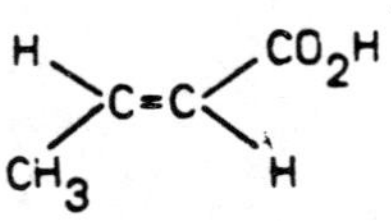

C. $CH_3C \equiv CCHO$

D. $CH_3C \equiv CH_2OH$

E. $CH_3CH_2CH_2CO_2H$

12. Which statement below is TRUE when comparing cis-2-hexene and trans-2-hexene? 12.____
These compounds
   A. have the same boiling point at atmospheric pressure
   B. liberate the same amount of heat when hydrogenated
   C. are nonsuperimposable mirror images
   D. will rotate the plane of polarized light
   E. produce the same alkane product upon catalytic hydrogenation

13. Although the molecular weights of acetic acid (60) and propionaldehyde (58) are quite similar, the former boils at a temperature of 69°C higher than the latter. 13.____
This phenomenon is due to
   A. effective hydrogen bonding in propionaldehyde
   B. effective hydrogen bonding in acetic acid
   C. ion-dipole interactions in propionaldehyde
   D. ion-dipole interactions in acetic acid
   E. dipole-dipole interactions in propionaldehyde

14. Which compound would NOT yield any $CH_3CH_2CH{=}O$ on ozonolysis? 14.____
   A. $CH_3CH_2CH{=}CHCH_2CH_3$
   B. $CH_3CH{=}CHCH_2CH_3$
   C. 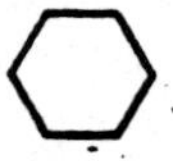 $=CHCH_2CH_3$
   D. $CH_2{=}CHCH_2CH{=}CH_2$
   E. $O{=}CHCH_2CH{=}CHCH_2CH_3$

15. Which of the following reactions MOST likely proceeds by the S_N2 mechanism? 15.____

A. $CH_3CH_2Cl + {}^-OH \rightarrow CH_3CH_2OH + Cl^-$

B. 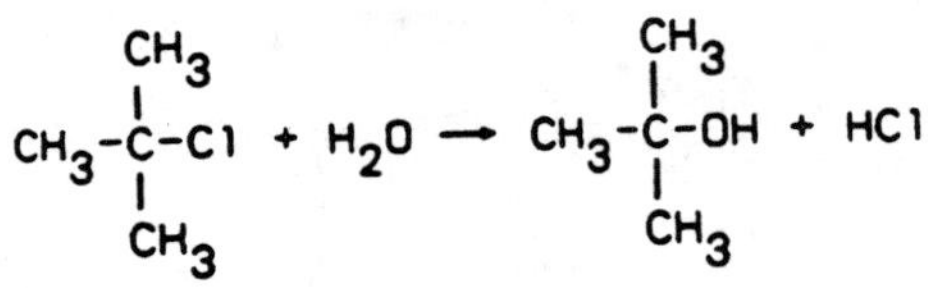

C. 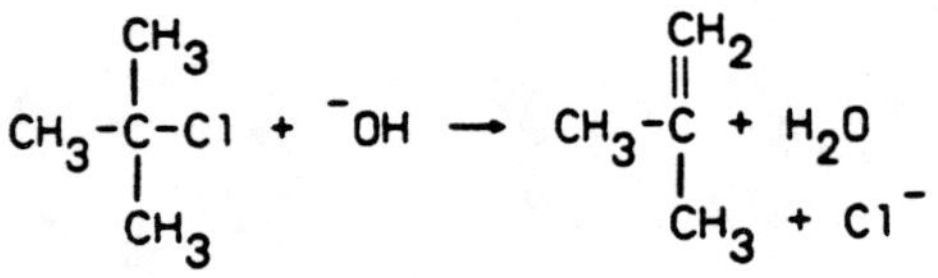

D. 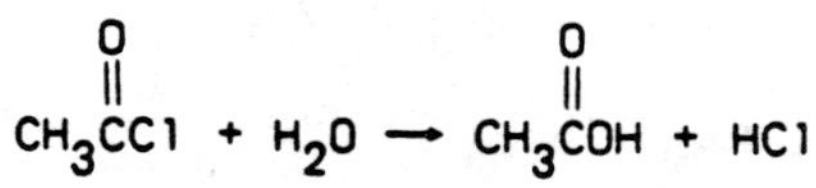

E. 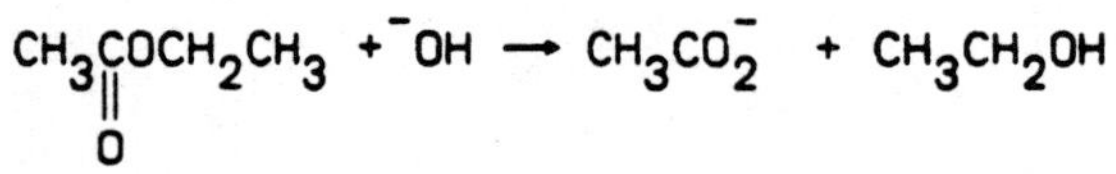

16. What is the PRINCIPAL organic product of this reaction sequence? 16.____

$$CH_3CH_2CH_2Br \xrightarrow[\text{Ether}]{Mg} \xrightarrow{D_2O}$$

   A. $CH_3CH_2CH_2D$
   B. $CH_3CH_2CH_2OD$
   C. $CH_3CD{=}CH_2$
   D. $CH_3CH_2CD{=}O$
   E. CH_3CH_2COOD

17. Which compound is soluble in aqueous HCl but separates from solution when excess aqueous NaOH is added? 17.____

A. 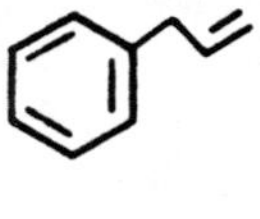

B. 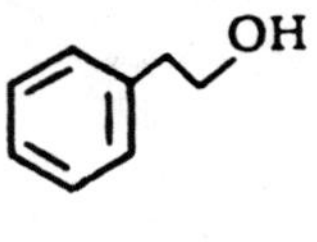

C. 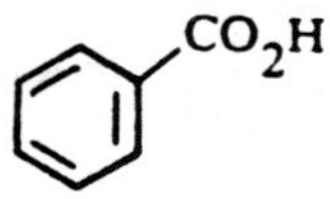

D. 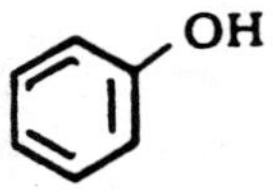

E. 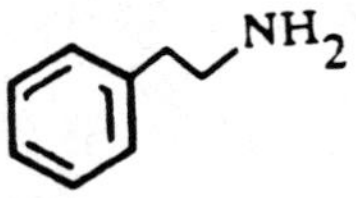

18. Which of the following would react MOST rapidly with aqueous NaOH? 18.____

A. $CH_3\overset{O}{\overset{\|}{C}}OCH_2CH_3$

B. $CH_3\overset{O}{\overset{\|}{C}}CH_3$

C. $CH_3CH_2OCH_2CH_3$

D. $CH_3\overset{O}{\overset{\|}{C}}Cl$

E. $CH_3\overset{O}{\overset{\|}{C}}NH_2$

19. The reaction of 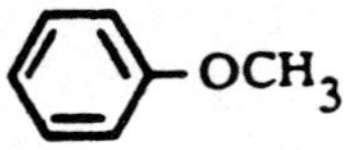 with HNO_3/H_2SO_4 will give ____ and will be ____ than nitration of benzene. 19.____

A. 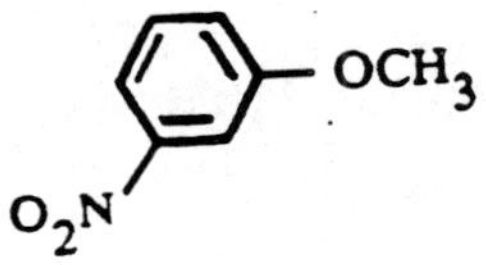 ; slower

B. 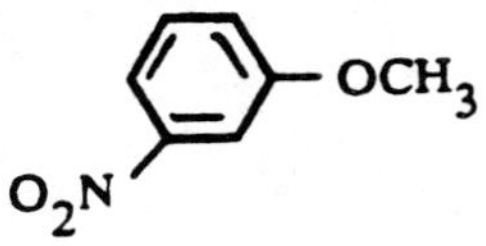 ; faster

C. 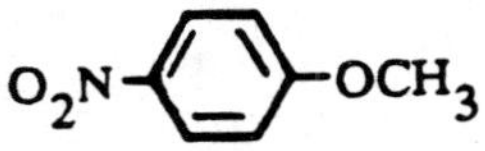 ; slower

D. 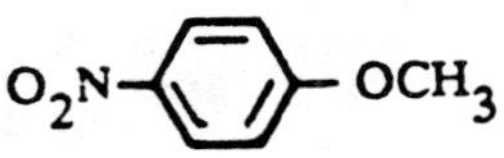 ; faster

E. 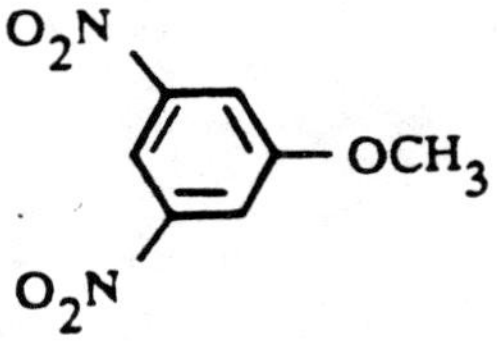 ; faster

20. Which of the following variations of experimental conditions has essentially no effect upon the position of the equilibrium of the hydrochloric acid catalyzed esterification of acetic acid, CH_3COOH, with ethyl alcohol, CH_3CH_2OH? 20.____

A. Addition of more hydrochloric acid
B. Removal of water as it is formed
C. Removal of ester as it is formed
D. Addition of excess ethyl alcohol
E. Addition of excess acetic acid

21. According to the Cahn-Ingold-Prelog convention, what is the CORRECT designation of the stereoisomer shown at the right? 21.____

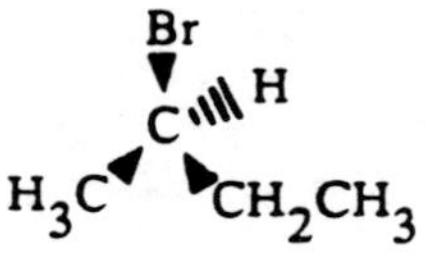

A. (S)
B. (R)
C. (R,S)
D. (Z)
E. Meso

22. The acid catalyzed addition of H_2O to 22.____

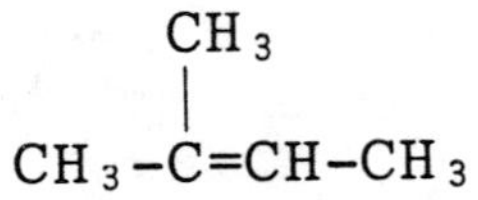

would yield predominantly

A. 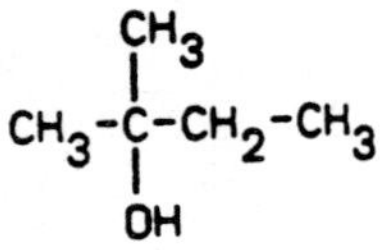

B. 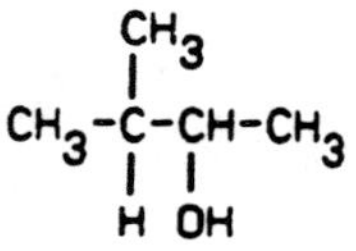

C. 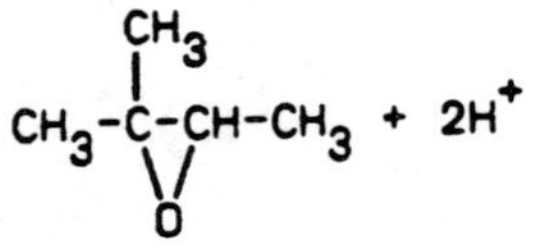

D. 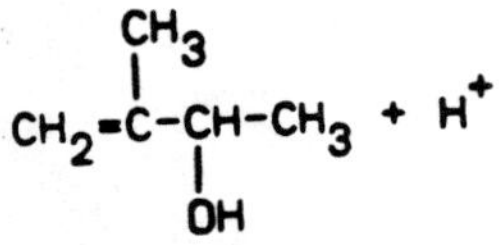

E. 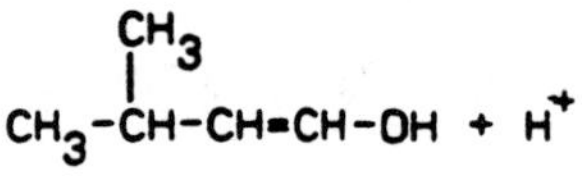

23. Which of the following is the MOST stable carbocation? 23.____

A. $H_3C-\overset{+}{C}H_2$

B. 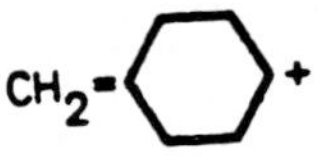

C. 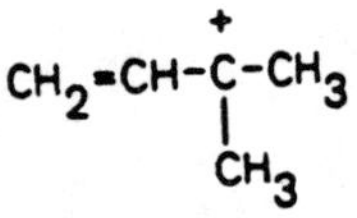

D. $CH_2=\overset{+}{C}H$

E. $H_3C-\overset{+}{C}H-CH_3$

24. Which of the structures below is a SECONDARY amine? 24.____

A. 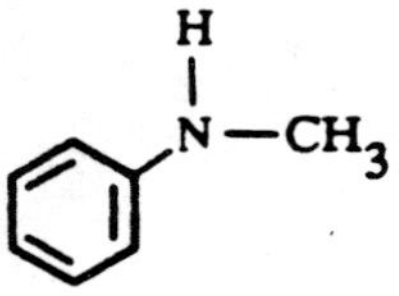

B. 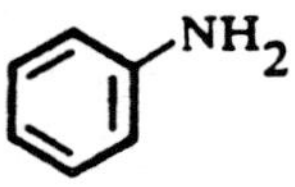

C. 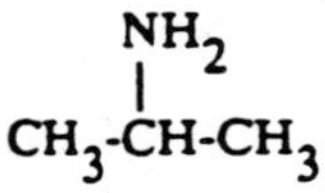

D. 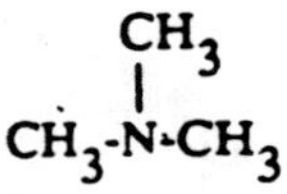

E. $H_2NCH_2CH_2NH_2$

25. Which of the following compounds is the STRONGEST acid? 25.____

A. 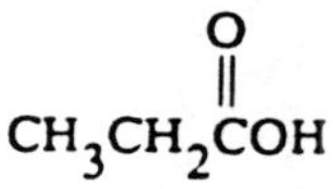

B. 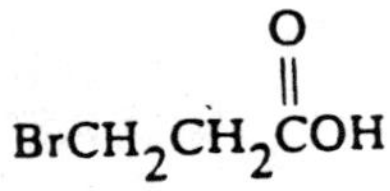

C. 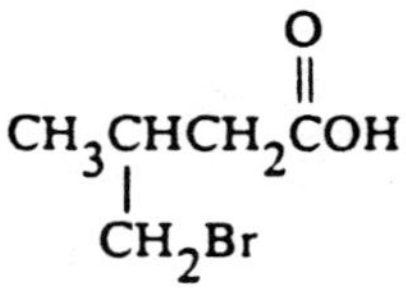

D. 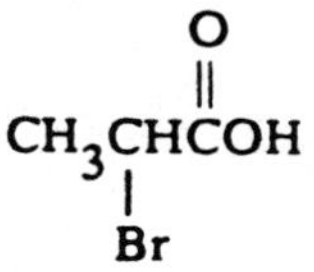

E. 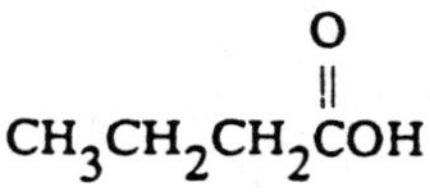

26. The transformation shown at the right is an example of 26.____
   A. dehydration
   B. reduction
   C. oxidation
   D. rearrangement
   E. mutarotation

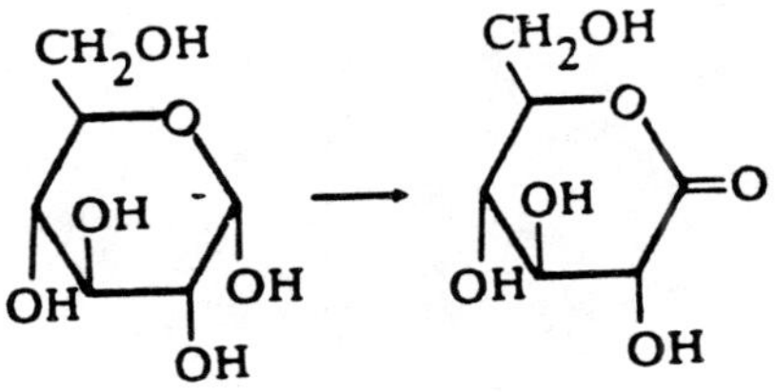

27. When ethyl benzene is brominated using iron as a catalyst, the predominant product is 27.____

A. 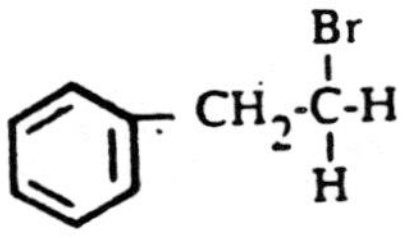

B. 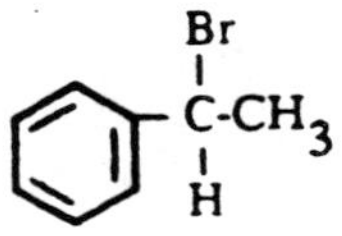

C. 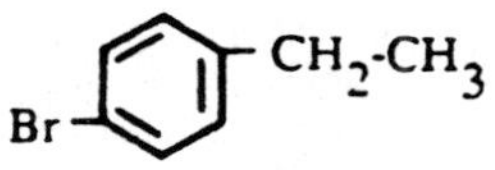

D. 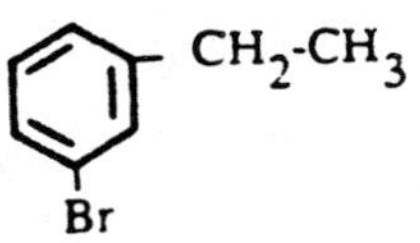

E. None of the above

28. Which molecule has a nonlinear structure, i.e., nuclei NOT in a straight line? 28.____
   A. H-C≡N
   B. O=C=O
   C. H-O-H
   D. H-Cl
   E. H-C≡C-H

29. Which Fischer projection represents a meso isomer? 29.____

A. 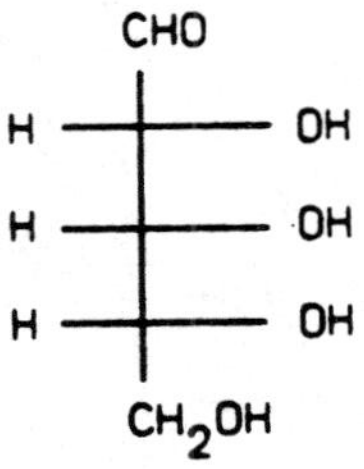

B. 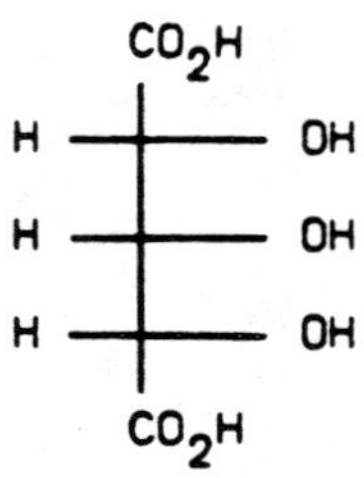

C. 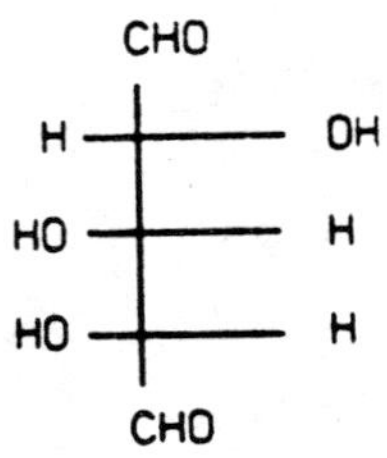

D. 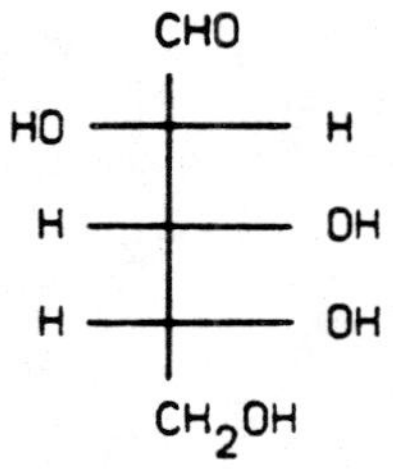

E. 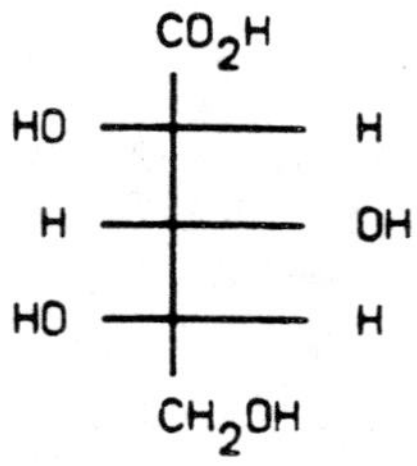

30. What would be the principal final product, C, of the reaction sequence below? 30.____

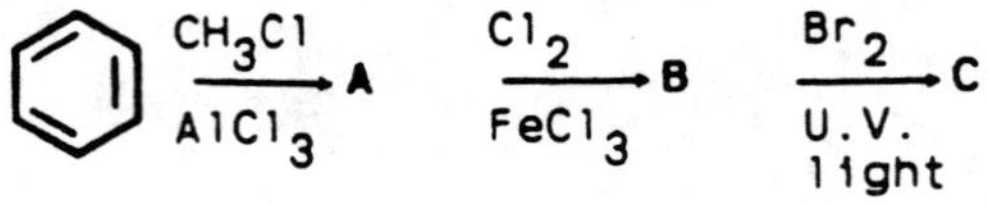

A. 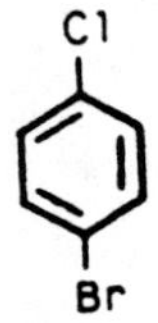

B. 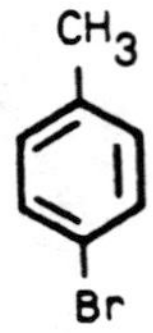

C. 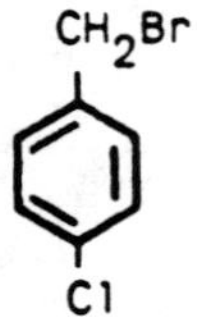

D. 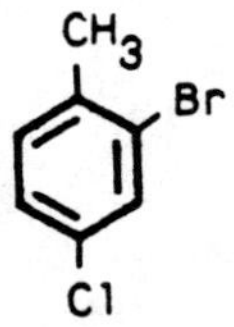

E. 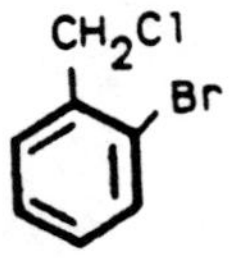

KEY (CORRECT ANSWERS)

1. E	11. E	21. B
2. E	12. E	22. A
3. B	13. B	23. C
4. C	14. D	24. A
5. B	15. A	25. D
6. D	16. A	26. C
7. B	17. E	27. C
8. D	18. D	28. C
9. D	19. D	29. B
10. A	20. A	30. C

EXAMINATION SECTION

DIRECTIONS: Each question or incomplete statement is followed by several suggested answers or completions. Select the one that BEST answers the question or completes the statement. *PRINT THE LETTER OF THE CORRECT ANSWER IN THE SPACE AT THE RIGHT.*

1. In the reaction A → E that has the following energy diagram, what is the intermediate? 1.___

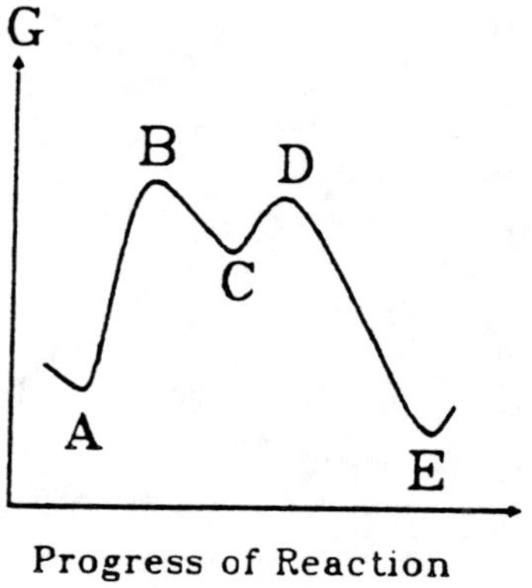

   A. A
   B. B
   C. C
   D. D
   E. E

2. A characteristic feature of the S_N2 reaction mechanism is that 2.___
   A. it follows first-order kinetics
   B. it produces stereochemical inversion of configuration
   C. there is no rate-determining step
   D. steric factors have little influence on the reaction rate constant
   E. collision of three or more particles is required

3. Which of the following alkyl bromides would react MOST rapidly by an S_N2 mechanism? 3.___

   A. $CH_3CH_2CH_2CH_2CH_2\text{-}Br$

   B. 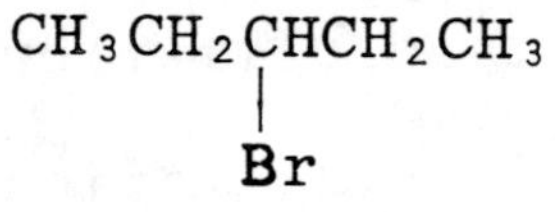

   C. 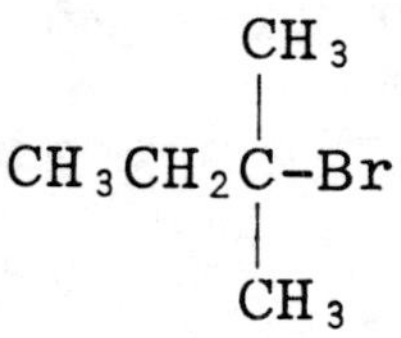

   D. 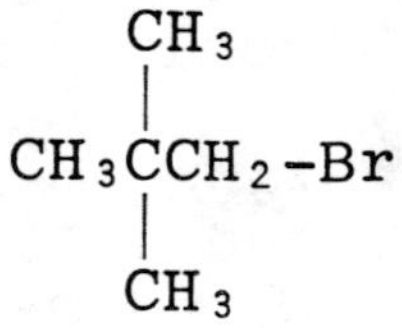

   E.

4. Which statement MOST correctly describes the rate determining step in the reaction below? 4.____

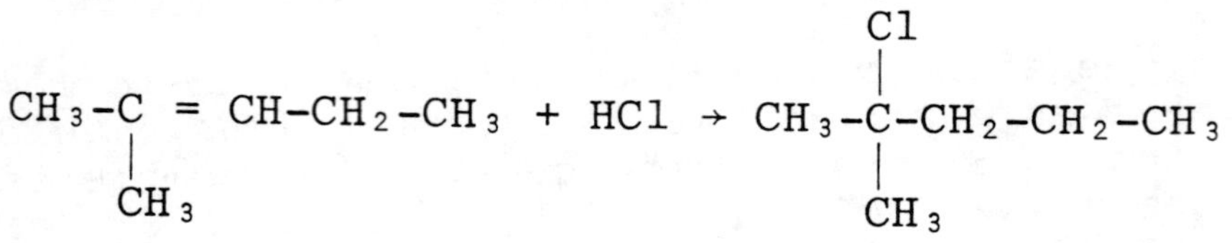

A. Formation of a 3° carbocation
B. Formation of a 2° carbocation
C. Formation of a 3° radical
D. Rearrangement of a 2° to 3° carbocation
E. Addition of Cl^- to a carbocation

5. Which of the following carbocations is the MOST stable? 5.____

A. $H_2C = \overset{+}{C}H$

B. $CH_3-\overset{+}{C}H_2$

C. 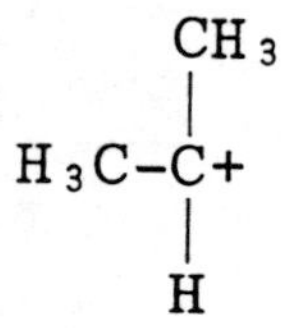

D. 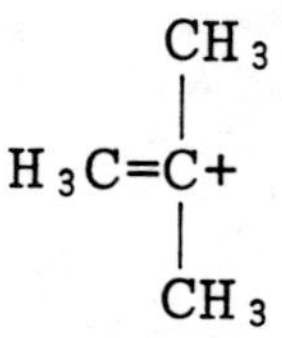

E. 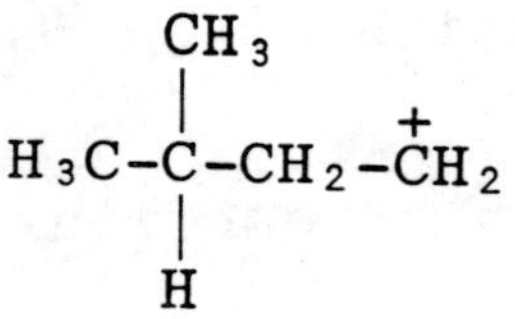

6. Nitration of toluene ($Ph-CH_3$) with HNO_3/H_2SO_4 occurs 6.____
A. faster than nitration of benzene and produces mostly ortho and para products
B. slower than nitration of benzene and produces mostly meta product
C. faster than nitration of benzene and produces mostly meta product
D. slower than nitration of benzene and produces mostly ortho and para products
E. at the same rate as nitration of benzene and produces mostly meta product

7. Which of the following does a strong infrared absorption band between 1750 and 1700 cm^{-1} (5.77 - 5.88μ) indicate the presence of? 7.____

A. $-NH_2$

B. 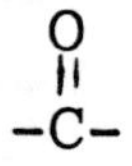

C. $-OH$

D. 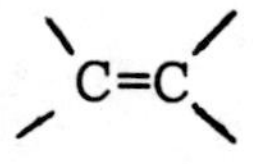

E. $-C{\equiv}C-$

8. Which of the compounds below would be MOST soluble in water? 8.___

A. $H_3C-CH_2-CH_2-CH_2-CH_3$

B. $Br-CH_2-Ch_2-CH_2-CH_3$

C. 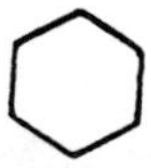

D. 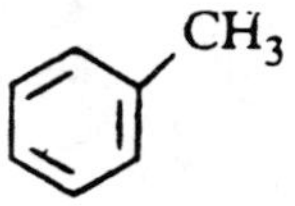

E.
```
      H
      |
H3C-C-CH3
      |
      OH
```

9. Which of the following pure liquids would be expected to show extensive intermolecular hydrogen bonding? 9.___

I. 2-butanol ($CH_3CH(OH)CH_2CH_3$)

II. Ethyl ether ($CH_3CH_2OCH_2CH_3$)

III. Acetone ($CH_3C(=O)CH_3$)

IV. Butyric acid ($CH_3CH_2CH_2CO_2H$)

The CORRECT answer is:

A. I *only* B. II *only* C. IV *only*
D. III *only* E. I and IV

10. Which of the following BEST describes the relationship between the two compounds shown below? 10.___

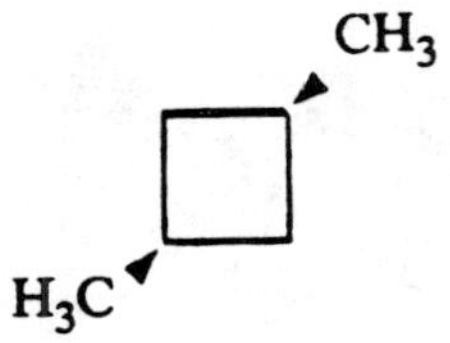

and

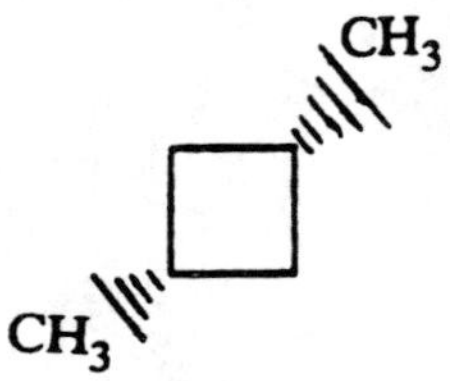

A. Structural isomers
B. Enantiomers
C. Diasteromers
D. Identical compounds
E. Meso compounds

11. Which of the conformations of 1,3-dimethylcyclohexane is the LEAST stable? 11.___

A. 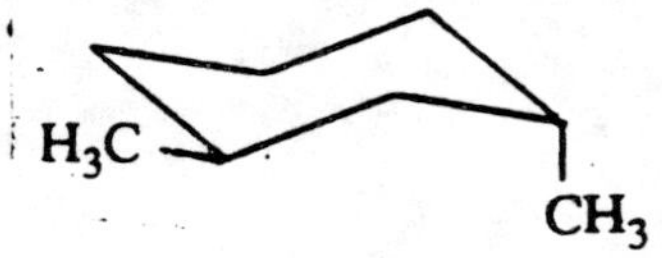

B. 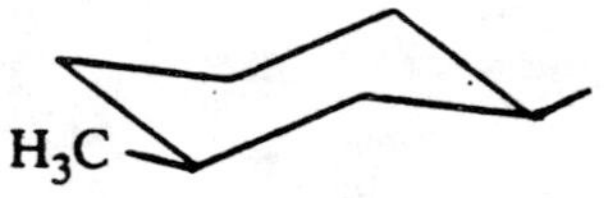

C. 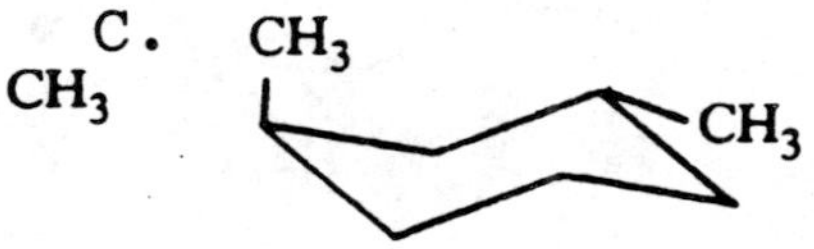

D. 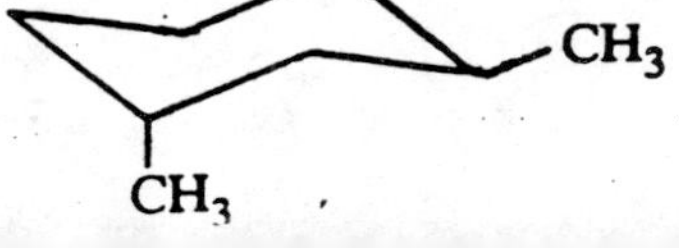

E. 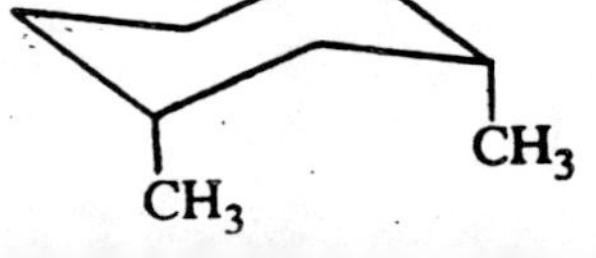

12. Which of the following compounds is NOT super-imposable on its mirror image? 12.___

A.
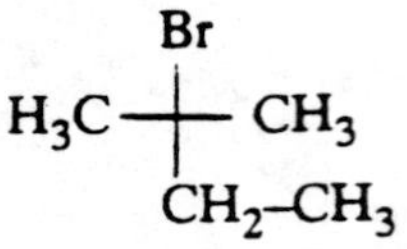

D.
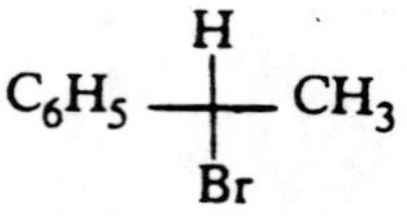

B.
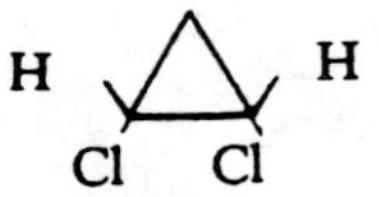

E.
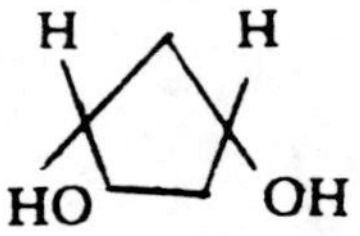

C.
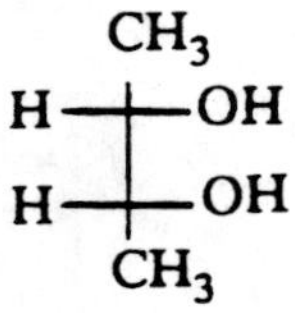

13. Which of the following compounds is a tertiary (3°) amine? 13.___

A.
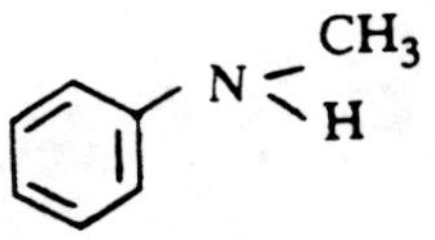

B.
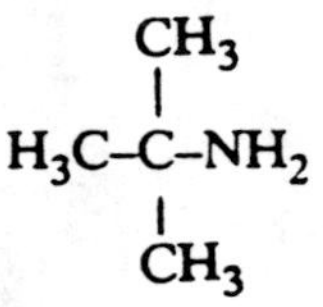

D.
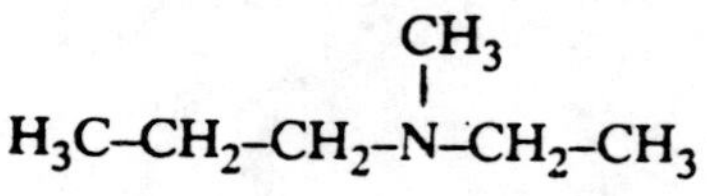

C.
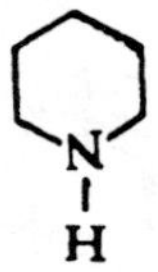

E.
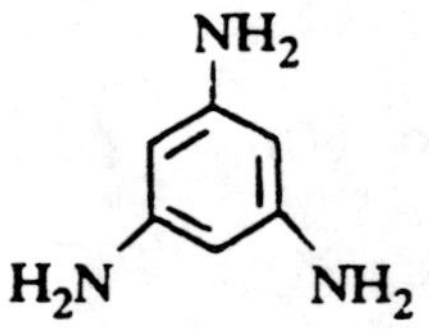

14. Which structure represents a trans (E) isomer? 14.___

A.
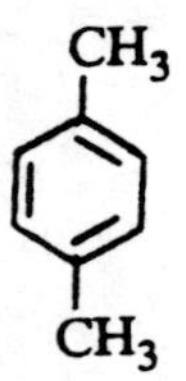

C.
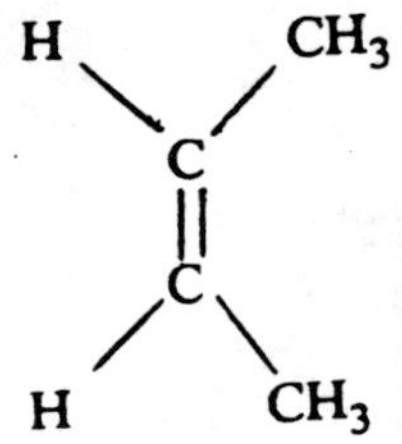

E.
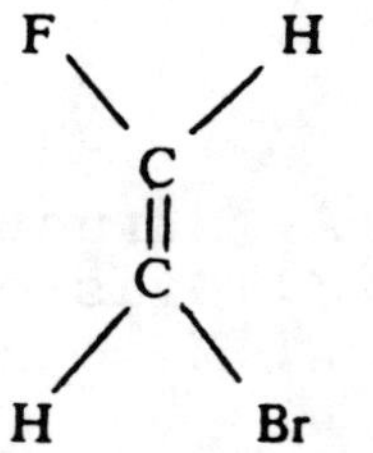

B.
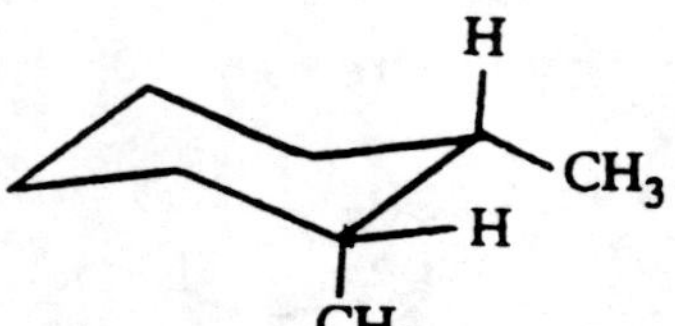

D.
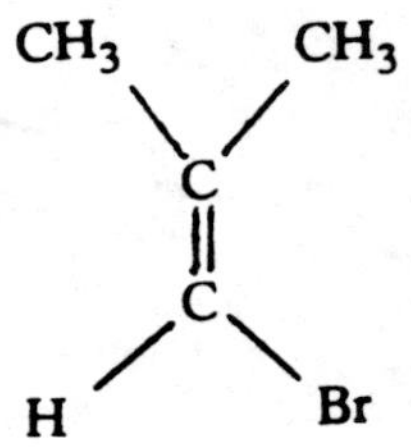

15. Which of the following will undergo a free radical bromination MOST rapidly? 15.___

A. $CH_3-CH-CH_3$
|
CH_3

B. CH_3
|
CH_3-C-CH_3
|
CH_3

C. CH_4

D. CH_3-CH_3

E. 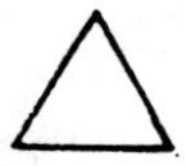

16. Which combination of reagents will produce 16.___

OH
|
$CH_3CH_2CCH_3$?
|
CN

A. $CH_3CH_2CH_2CH_3$ + KOH + KCN

B. O
||
$CH_3CH_2CCH_3$ + HCN + KCN

C. OH
|
$CH_3CH_2CHCH_3$ + KCN

D. Cl
|
$CH_3CH_2CHCH_3$ + KCN

E. CN
|
$CH_3CH_2CHCH_3$ + KOH

17. Which set of reactants could be used to prepare 17.___

OH
|
$CH_3CH_2CHCH_3$?

A. CH_3CH_2MgBr + 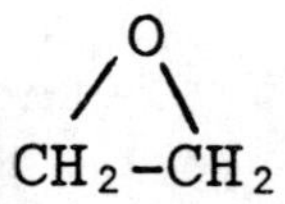

B. O
||
CH_3CH_2MgBr + CH_3CH

C. CH_3CH_2Br + CH_3CH_2ONa

D. O
||
$CH_3CH_2CH_2MgBr$ + HCH

E. O
||
CH_3MgI + $CH_3CH_2COCH_3$

18. What is the product of the following sequence of reactions? 18.___

$$CH_3\text{-}CH_2\text{-}Br \xrightarrow{Mg} \xrightarrow{CO_2} \xrightarrow{H_3O^+}$$

A. $CH_3\text{-}CH_2\text{-}OH$

B. $CH_3\text{-}CH_2\text{-}\overset{O}{\overset{\|}{C}}\text{-}H$

C. $CH_3CH_2\text{-}\overset{O}{\overset{\|}{C}}\text{-}OH$

D. $CH_3\text{-}CH_2\text{-}CH_3$

E. $CH_3CH_2\text{-}CH_2\text{-}Br$

19. What is the MAJOR product of the following reaction? 19.___

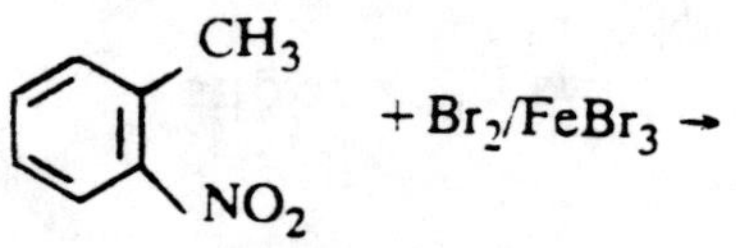

A. 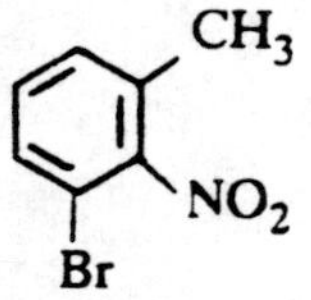

B. 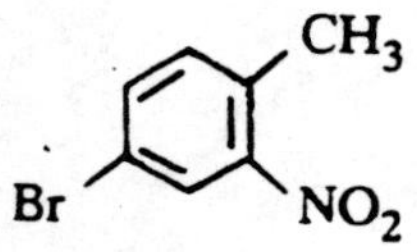

C. 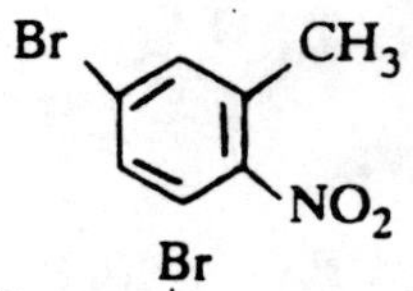

D. 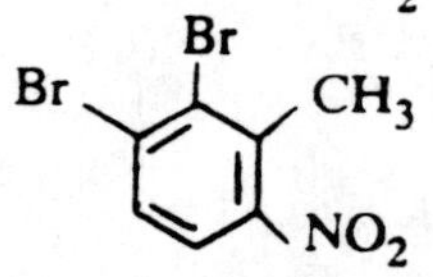

E. 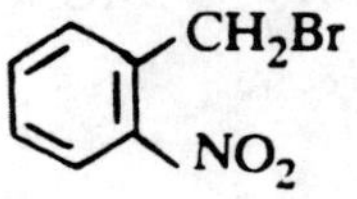

20. Which reagent, followed by the appropriate work-up procedure, could you use to effect the following conversion: 20.___

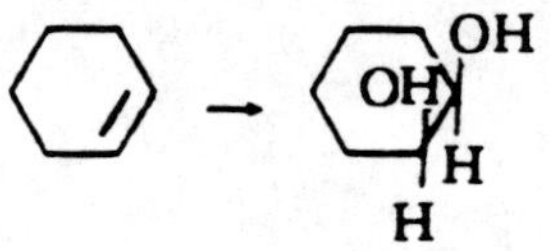 ?

A. $H_2O/^-OH$

B. H_2SO_4

C. $(BH_3)_2$

D. $CH_3\overset{O}{\overset{\|}{C}}OH$

E. $KMnO_4/OH^-$

21. Which compound would be the product of the reaction shown below? 21.___

$$\underset{\displaystyle CH_3}{CH_3\text{-}\underset{|}{C}H\text{-}CO_2H} \xrightarrow{LiAlH_4} \xrightarrow{H_3O^+}$$

A. $CH_3-CH_2-CH(CH_3)-OH$ (CH₃ on the CH)

B. $CH_3-C(CH_3)_2-OH$

C. $CH_3-CH(CH_3)-CH_3$

D. $CH_3-CH(CH_3)-CH_2-OH$

E. $CH_3-CH(CH_3)-O-CH_3$

22. What is the product of the following addition reaction? 22.___

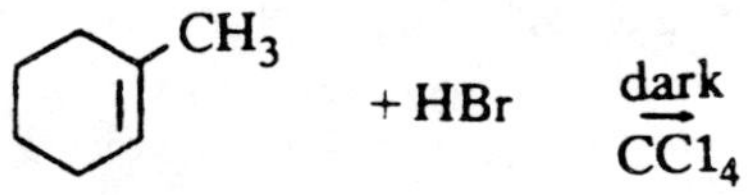

A. 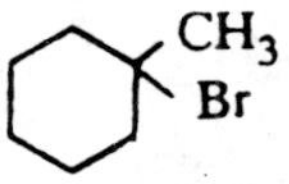

B. 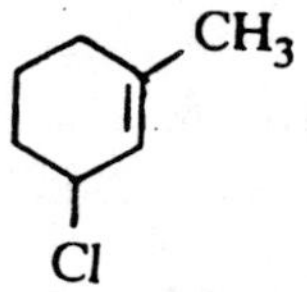

C. 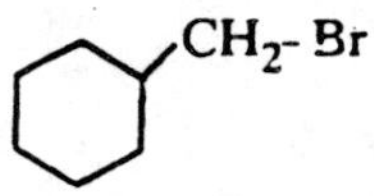

D. 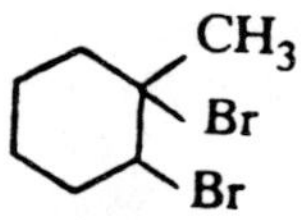

E. 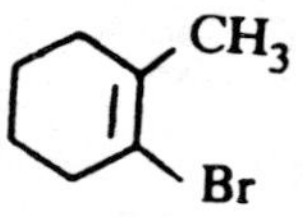

23. Which of the following are the two Brönsted-Lowry bases represented in the equilibrium below? 23.___
HOAc + NaCN ⇄ HCN + NaOAc

A. HOAc + NaCN B. HOAc + NaOAc C. NaCn + NaOAc
D. NaCn + HCN E. HOAc + HCN

24. Which of the compounds below would be MOST acidic? 24.___

A. 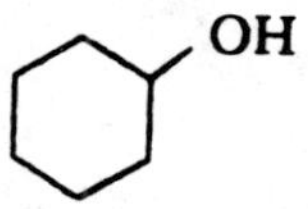

B. 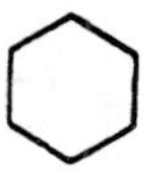

C. 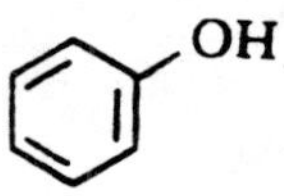

D. 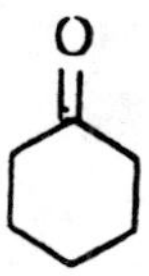

E. 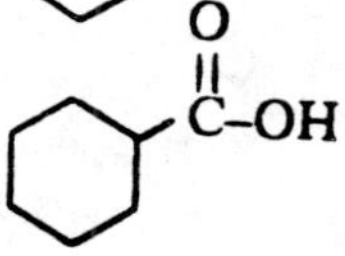

25. The MOST acidic hydrogen(s) in the following compound are attached to which of the following carbons? 25.___

```
                 O         O              O
                 ||        ||             ||
CH3-CH2-C-CH2-C-CH2-CH2-C-O-CH3
 ↑    ↑       ↑             ↑           ↑
 1    2       3             4           5
```

A. 1 B. 2 C. 3 D. 4 E. 5

26. Which of the following is a group that is both deactivating and ortho, para directing in the nitration reaction of substituted benzenes? 26.___

A. $-COOH$ B. $-CH_3$ C. $-Br$ D. $-NO_2$ E. $-OCH_3$

27. Which of the following ions is stabilized by resonance? 27.___

A.
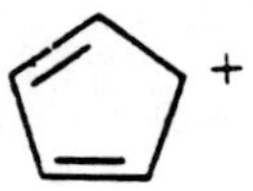

B.
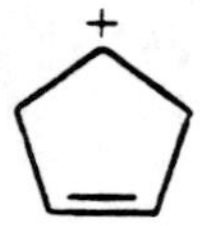

C.
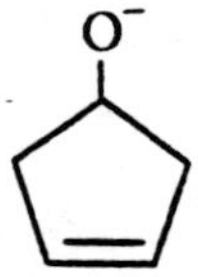

D.
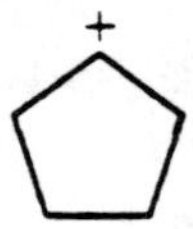

E.
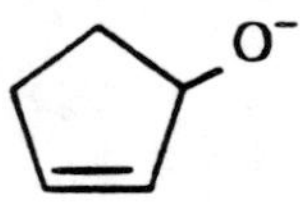

28. How does the hybridization of carbon change during the oxidation sequence: $CH_3-OH \rightarrow CH_2=O \rightarrow HCO_2H \rightarrow CO_2$? 28.___

A. sp^2, sp^2, sp^2, sp B. sp^3, sp^2, sp, sp
C. sp^2, sp^3, sp^3, sp^3 D. sp^3, sp^2, sp^2, sp
E. sp^3, sp^3, sp^3, sp^2

29. Treatment of benzoic acid with thionyl chloride followed by addition of ethanol gives which of the following as the MAJOR product? 29.___

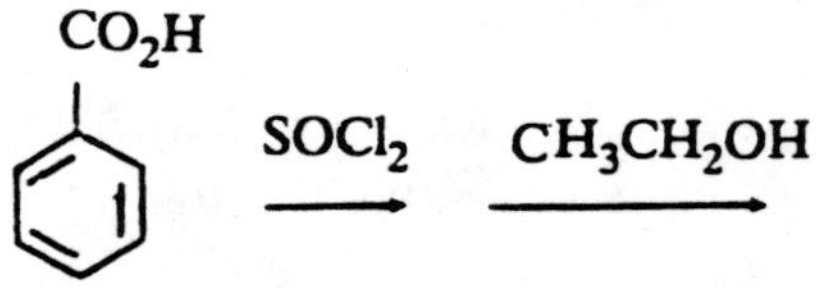

A.
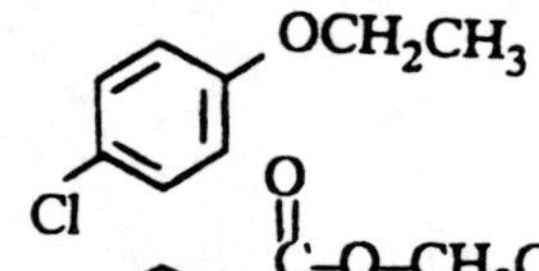

B.
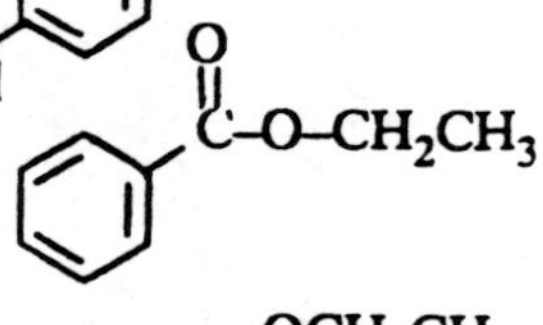

C.
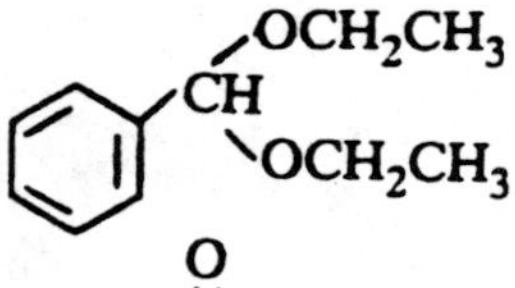

D.
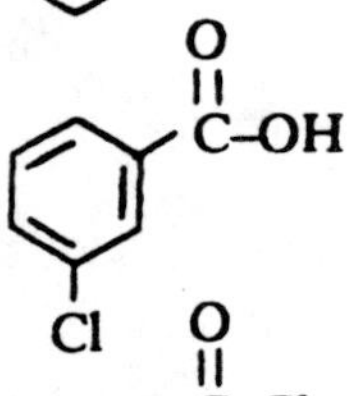

E.
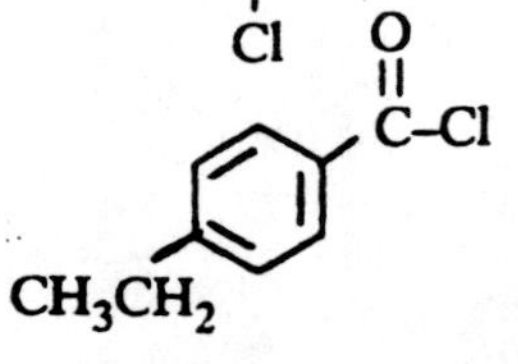

30. What is the MAJOR product (B) of the following reaction sequence? 30.___

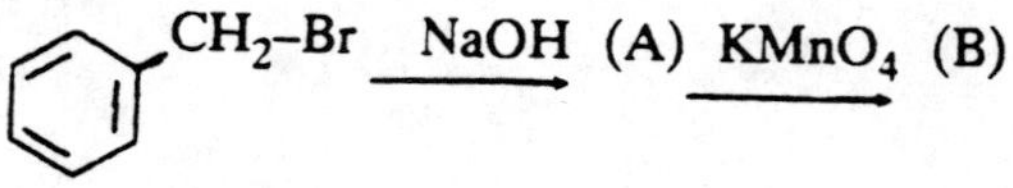

A. 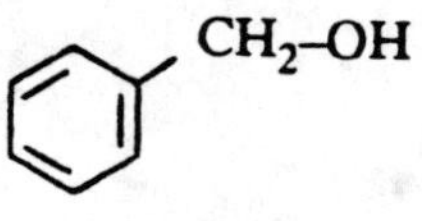

B. 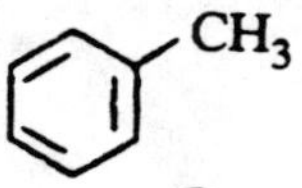

C. 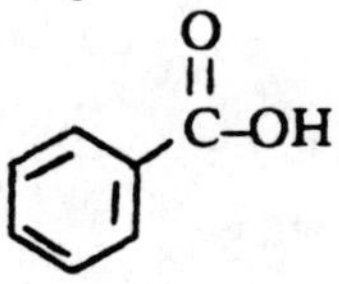

D. 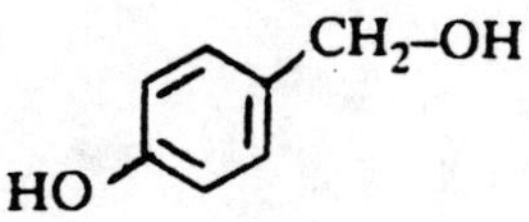

E. 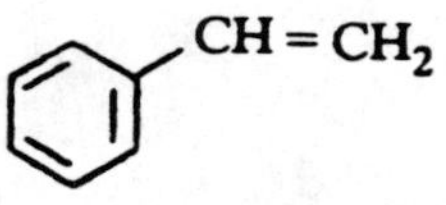

KEY (CORRECT ANSWERS)

1. C	11. E	21. D
2. B	12. D	22. A
3. A	13. D	23. C
4. A	14. E	24. E
5. D	15. A	25. C
6. A	16. B	26. C
7. B	17. B	27. A
8. E	18. C	28. D
9. E	19. B	29. B
10. D	20. E	30. C

SCIENCE READING COMPREHENSION

EXAMINATION SECTION

DIRECTIONS FOR THIS SECTION:
Each question or incomplete statement is followed by several suggested answers or completions. Select the one that BEST answers the question or completes the statement. *PRINT THE LETTER OF THE CORRECT ANSWER IN THE SPACE AT THE RIGHT.*

TEST 1

PASSAGE

Photosynthesis is a complex process with many intermediate steps. Ideas differ greatly as to the details of these steps, but the general nature of the process and its outcome are well established. Water, usually from the soil, is conducted through the xylem of root, stem and leaf to the chlorophyl-containing cells of a leaf. In consequence of the abundance of water within the latter cells, their walls are saturated with water. Carbon dioxide, diffusing from the air through the stomata and into the intercellular spaces of the leaf, comes into contact with the water in the walls of the cells which adjoin the intercellular spaces. The carbon dioxide becomes dissolved in the water of these walls, and in solution diffuses through the walls and the plasma membranes into the cells. By the agency of chlorophyl in the chloroplasts of the cells, the energy of light is transformed into chemical energy. This chemical energy is used to decompose the carbon dioxide and water, and the products of their decomposition are recombined into a new compound. The compound first formed is successively built up into more and more complex substances until finally a sugar is produced.

Questions 1-8.

1. The union of carbon dioxide and water to form starch results in an excess of 1. ...
   A. hydrogen B. carbon C. oxygen
   D. carbon monoxide E. hydrogen peroxide
2. Synthesis of carbohydrates takes place 2. ...
   A. in the stomata
   B. in the intercellular spaces of leaves
   C. in the walls of plant cells
   D. within the plasma membranes of plant cells
   E. within plant cells that contain chloroplasts
3. In the process of photosynthesis, chlorophyl acts as a 3. ...
   A. carbohydrate B. source of carbon dioxide
   C. catalyst D. source of chemical energy
   E. plasma membrane
4. In which of the following places are there the GREATEST number of hours in which photosynthesis can take place during the month of December? 4. ...
   A. Buenos Aires, Argentina B. Caracas, Venezuela
   C. Fairbanks, Alaska D. Quito, Ecuador
   E. Calcutta, India
5. During photosynthesis, molecules of carbon dioxide enter the stomata of leaves because 5. ...
   A. the molecules are already in motion
   B. they are forced through the stomata by the son's rays
   C. chlorophyl attracts them
   D. a chemical change takes place in the stomata
   E. oxygen passes out through the stomata

6. Besides food manufacture, another USEFUL result of photosynthesis is that it 6. ...
   A. aids in removing poisonous gases from the air
   B. helps to maintain the existing proportion of gases in the air
   C. changes complex compounds into simpler compounds
   D. changes certain waste products into hydrocarbons
   E. changes chlorophyl into useful substances
7. A process that is almost the exact reverse of photosynthesis is the 7. ...
   A. rusting of iron B. burning of wood
   C. digestion of starch D. ripening of fruit
   E. storage of food in seeds
8. The leaf of the tomato plant will be unable to carry on photosynthesis if the 8. ...
   A. upper surface of the leaf is coated with vaseline
   B. upper surface of the leaf is coated with lampblack
   C. lower surface of the leaf is coated with lard
   D. leaf is placed in an atmosphere of pure carbon dioxide
   E. entire leaf is coated with lime

TEST 2

PASSAGE

The only carbohydrate which the human body can absorb and oxidize is the simple sugar glucose. Therefore, all carbohydrates which are consumed must be changed to glucose by the body before they can be used. There are specific enzymes in the mouth, the stomach, and the small intestine which break down complex carbohydrates. All the monosaccharides are changed to glucose by enzymes secreted by the intestinal glands, and the glucose is absorbed by the capillaries of the villi.

The following simple test is used to determine the presence of a reducing sugar. If Benedict's solution is added to a solution containing glucose or one of the other reducing sugars and the resulting mixture is heated, a brick-red precipitate will be formed. This test was carried out on several substances and the information in the following table was obtained. "P" indicates that the precipitate was formed and "N" indicates that no reaction was observed.

Material Tested	Observation
Crushed grapes in water	P
Cane sugar in water	N
Fructose	P
Molasses	N

Questions 1-2.

1. From the results of the test made upon crushed grapes in water, one may say that grapes contain 1. ...
   A. glucose B. sucrose C. a reducing sugar
   D. no sucrose E. no glucose
2. Which one of the following foods probably undergoes the LEAST change during the process of carbohydrate digestion in the human body? 2. ...
   A. Cane sugar B. Fructose C. Molasses
   D. Bread E. Potato

TEST 3

PASSAGE

The British pressure suit was made in two pieces and joined around the middle in contrast to the other suits, which were one-piece suits with a removable helmet. Oxygen was supplied through a tube, and a container of soda lime absorbed carbon dioxide and water vapor. The pressure was adjusted to a maximum of 2 1/2 pounds per square inch (130 millimeters) higher than the surrounding air. Since pure oxygen was used, this produced a partial pressure of 130 millimeters, which is sufficient to sustain the flier at any altitude.

Using this pressure suit, the British established a world's altitude record of 49,944 feet in 1936 and succeeded in raising it to 53,937 feet the following year. The pressure suit is a compromise solution to the altitude problem. Full sea-level pressure can not be maintained, as the suit would be so rigid that the flier could not move arms or legs. Hence a pressure one third to one fifth that of sea level has been used. Because of these lower pressures, oxygen has been used to raise the partial pressure of alveolar oxygen to normal.

Questions 1-9.

1. The MAIN constituent of air not admitted to the pressure suit described was 1. ...
   A. oxygen B. nitrogen C. water vapor
   D. carbon dioxide E. hydrogen
2. The pressure within the suit exceeded that of the surrounding air by an amount equal to 130 millimeters of 2. ...
   A. mercury B. water C. air
   D. oxygen E. carbon dioxide
3. The normal atmospheric pressure at sea level is 3. ...
   A. 130 mm B. 250 mm C. 760 mm
   D. 1000 mm E. 1300 mm
4. The water vapor that was absorbed by the soda lime came from 4. ...
   A. condensation
   B. the union of oxygen with carbon dioxide
   C. body metabolism
   D. the air within the pressure suit
   E. water particles in the upper air
5. The HIGHEST altitude that has been reached with the British pressure suit is about 5. ...
   A. 130 miles B. 2 1/2 miles C. 6 miles
   D. 10 miles E. 5 miles
6. If the pressure suit should develop a leak, the 6. ...
   A. oxygen supply would be cut off
   B. suit would fill up with air instead of oxygen
   C. pressure within the suit would drop to zero
   D. pressure within the suit would drop to that of the surrounding air
   E. suit would become so rigid that the flier would be unable to move arms or legs
7. The reason why oxygen helmets are unsatisfactory for use in efforts to set higher altitude records is that 7. ...
   A. it is impossible to maintain a tight enough fit at the neck

B. oxygen helmets are too heavy
C. they do not conserve the heat of the body as pressure suits do
D. if a parachute jump becomes necessary, it can not be made while such a helmet is being worn
E. oxygen helmets are too rigid

8. The pressure suit is termed a compromise solution because 8. ...
A. it is not adequate for stratosphere flying
B. aviators can not stand sea-level pressure at high altitudes
C. some suits are made in two pieces, others in one
D. other factors than maintenance of pressure have to be accommodated
E. full atmospheric pressure can not be maintained at high altitudes

9. The passage implies that 9. ...
A. the air pressure at 49,944 feet is approximately the same as it is at 53,937 feet
B. pressure cabin planes are not practical at extremely high altitudes
C. a flier's oxygen requirement is approximately the same at high altitudes as it is at sea level
D. one-piece pressure suits with removable helmets are unsafe
E. a normal alveolar oxygen supply is maintained if the air pressure is between one third and one fifth that of sea level

TEST 4

PASSAGE

Chemical investigations show that during muscle contraction the store of organic phosphates in the muscle fibers is altered as energy is released. In doing so, the organic phosphates (chiefly adenoisine triphosphate and phospho-creatine) are transformed anaerobically to organic compounds plus phosphates. As soon as the organic phosphates begin to break down in muscle contraction, the glycogen in the muscle fibers also transforms into lactic acid plus free energy; this energy the muscle fiber uses to return the organic compounds plus phosphates into high-energy organic phosphates ready for another contraction. In the presence of oxygen, the lactic acid from the glycogen decomposition is changed also. About one-fifth of it is oxidized to form water and carbon dioxide and to yield another supply of energy. This time the energy is used to transform the remaining four-fifths of the lactic acid into glycogen again.

Questions 1-5.

1. The energy for muscle contraction comes directly from the 1. ...
A. breakdown of lactic acid into glycogen
B. resynthesis of adenosine triphosphate
C. breakdown of glycogen into lactic acid
D. oxidation of lactic acid
E. breakdown of the organic phosphates

2. Lactic acid does NOT accumulate in a muscle that 2. ...
   A. is in a state of lacking oxygen
   B. has an ample supply of oxygen
   C. is in a state of fatigue
   D. is repeatedly being stimulated
   E. has an ample supply of glycogen
3. The energy for the resynthesis of adenosine triphosphate and phospho-creatine comes from the 3. ...
   A. oxidation of lactic acid
   B. synthesis of organic phosphates
   C. change from glycogen to lactic acid
   D. resynthesis of glycogen
   E. change from lactic acid to glycogen
4. The energy for the resynthesis of glycogen comes from the 4. ...
   A. breakdown of organic phosphates
   B. resynthesis of organic phosphates
   C. change occurring in one-fifth of the lactic acid
   D. change occurring in four-fifths of the lactic acid
   E. change occurring in four-fifths of glycogen
5. The breakdown of the organic phosphates into organic compounds plus phosphates is an 5. ...
   A. anobolic reaction
   B. aerobic reaction
   C. endothermic reaction
   D. exothermic reaction
   E. anaerobic reaction

TEST 5

PASSAGE

And with respect to that theory of the origin of the forms of life peopling our globe, with which Darwin's name is bound up as closely as that of Newton with the theory of gravitation, nothing seems to be further from the mind of the present generation than any attempt to smother it with ridicule or to crush it by vehemence of denunciation. "The struggle for existence," and "natural selection," have become household words and every-day conceptions. The reality and the importance of the natural processes on which Darwin founds his deductions are no more doubted than those of growth and multiplication; and, whether the full potency attributed to them is admitted or not, no one is unmindful of or at all doubts their vast and far-reaching significance. Wherever the biological sciences are studied, the "Origin of Species" lights the path of the investigator; wherever they are taught it permeates the course of instruction. Nor has the influence of Darwinian ideas been less profound beyond the realms of biology. The oldest of all philosophies, that of evolution, was bound hand and foot and cast into utter darkness during the millennium of theological scholasticism. But Darwin poured new life-blood into the ancient frame, the bonds burst, and the revivified thought of ancient Greece has proved itself to be a more adequate expression of the universal order of things than any of the schemes which have been accepted by the credulity and welcomed by the superstition of seventy later generations of men.

Questions 1-7.

1. Darwin's theory of the origin of the species is based on 1. ...
   A. theological deductions B. the theory of gravitation
   C. Greek mythology
   D. natural processes evident in the universe
   E. extensive reading in the biological sciences
2. The passage implies that 2. ...
   A. thought in ancient Greece was dead
   B. the theory of evolution is now universally accepted
   C. the "Origin of Species" was seized by the Church
   D. Darwin was influenced by Newton
   E. the theories of "the struggle for existence" and "natural selection" are too evident to be scientific
3. The idea of evolution 3. ...
   A. was suppressed for 1,000 years
   B. is falsely claimed by Darwin
   C. has swept aside all superstition
   D. was outworn even in ancient Greece
   E. has revolutionized the universe
4. The processes of growth and multiplication 4. ...
   A. have been replaced by others discovered by Darwin
   B. were the basis for the theory of gravitation
   C. are "the struggle for existence" and "natural selection"
   D. are scientific theories not yet proved
   E. are accepted as fundamental processes of nature
5. Darwin's treatise on evolution 5. ...
   A. traces life on the planets from the beginning of time to the present day
   B. was translated from the Greek
   C. contains an ancient philosophy in modern, scientific guise
   D. has had a profound effect on evolution
   E. has had little notice outside scientific circles
6. The theory of evolution 6. ...
   A. was first advanced in the "Origin of Species"
   B. was suppressed by the ancient Greeks
   C. did not get beyond the monasteries during the millennium
   D. is philosophical, not scientific
   E. was elaborated and revived by Darwin
7. Darwin has contributed GREATLY toward 7. ...
   A. a universal acceptance of the processes of nature
   B. reviving the Greek intellect
   C. ending the millennium of theological scholasticism
   D. a satisfactory explanation of scientific theory
   E. easing the struggle for existence

TEST 6

PASSAGE

The higher forms of plants and animals, such as seed plants and vertebrates, are similar or alike in many respects but decidedly different in others. For example, both of these groups of organisms carry on digestion, respiration, reproduction, conduction, growth, and exhibit sensitivity to various stimuli. On the other hand, a number of basic differences are evident. Plants have no excretory systems comparable to those of animals. Plants have no heart or similar pumping organ. Plants are very limited in their movements. Plants have nothing similar to the animal nervous system. In addition, animals can not synthesize carbohydrates from inorganic substances. Animals do not have special regions of growth, comparable to terminal and lateral meristems in plants, which persist throughout the life span of the organism. And,finally,the animal cell "wall" is only a membrane, while plant cell walls are more rigid, usually thicker, and may be composed of such substances as cellulose, lignin, pectin, cutin, and suberin. These characteristics are important to an understanding of living organisms and their functions and should, consequently, be carefully considered in plant and animal studies.

Questions 1-7.

1. Which of the following do animals lack? 1. ...
   A. Ability to react to stimuli
   B. Ability to conduct substances from one place to another
   C. Reproduction by gametes
   D. A cell membrane
   E. A terminal growth region
2. Which of the following statements is false? 2. ...
   A. Animal cell "walls" are composed of cellulose.
   B. Plants grow as long as they live.
   C. Plants produce sperms and eggs.
   D. All vertebrates have hearts.
   E. Wood is dead at maturity.
3. Respiration in plants takes place 3. ...
   A. only during the day
   B. only in the presence of carbon dioxide
   C. both day and night
   D. only at night
   E. only in the presence of certain stimuli
4. An example of a vertebrate is the 4. ...
   A. earthworm B. starfish C. amoeba
   D. cow E. insect
5. Which of the following statements is true? 5. ...
   A. All animals eat plants as a source of food.
   B. Respiration, in many ways, is the reverse of photosynthesis.
   C. Man is an invertebrate animal.
   D. Since plants have no hearts, they can not develop high pressures in their cells.
   E. Plants can not move.
6. Which of the following do plants lack? 6. ...
   A. A means of movement B. Pumping structures
   C. Special regions of growth
   D. Reproduction by gametes
   E. A digestive process
7. A substance that can be synthesized by green plants but NOT by animals is 7. ...
   A. protein B. cellulose C. carbon dioxide
   D. uric acid E. water

TEST 7

PASSAGE

Sodium chloride, being by far the largest constituent of the mineral matter of the blood, assumes special significance in the regulation of water exchanges in the organism. And, as Cannon has emphasized repeatedly, these latter are more extensive and more important than may at first thought appear. He points out "there are a number of circulations of the fluid out of the body and back again, without loss." Thus, by example, it is estimated that from a quart and one-half of water daily "leaves the body" when it enters the mouth as saliva; another one or two quarts are passed out as gastric juice; and perhaps the same amount is contained in the bile and the secretions of the pancreas and the intestinal wall. This large volume of water enters the digestive processes; and practically all of it is reabsorbed through the intestinal wall, where it performs the equally important function of carrying in the digested foodstuffs. These and other instances of what Cannon calls "the conservative use of water in our bodies" involve essentially osmotic pressure relationships in which the concentration of sodium chloride plays an important part.

Questions 1-11.

1. This passage implies that 1. ...
   - A. the contents of the alimentary canal are not to be considered within the body
   - B. sodium chloride does not actually enter the body
   - C. every particle of water ingested is used over and over again
   - D. water can not be absorbed by the body unless it contains sodium chloride
   - E. substances can pass through the intestinal wall in only one direction
2. According to this passage, which of the following processes requires MOST water? The 2. ...
   - A. absorption of digested foods
   - B. secretion of gastric juice
   - C. secretion of saliva
   - D. production of bile
   - E. concentration of sodium chloride solution
3. A body fluid that is NOT saline is 3. ...
   - A. blood B. urine C. bile
   - D. gastric juice E. saliva
4. An organ that functions as a storage reservoir from which large quantities of water are reabsorbed into the body is the 4. ...
   - A. kidney B. liver C. large intestine
   - D. mouth E. pancreas
5. Water is reabsorbed into the body by the process of 5. ...
   - A. secretion B. excretion C. digestion
   - D. osmosis E. oxidation
6. Digested food enters the body PRINCIPALLY through the 6. ...
   - A. mouth B. liver C. villi
   - D. pancreas E. stomach

7. The metallic element found in the blood in compound form and present there in larger quantities than any other metallic element is 7. ...
   A. iron B. calcium C. magnesium
   D. chlorine E. sodium
8. An organ that removes water from the body and prevents its reabsorption for use in the body processes is the 8. ...
   A. pancreas B. liver C. small intestine
   D. lungs E. large intestine
9. In which of the following processes is sodium chloride removed MOST rapidly from the body? 9. ...
   A. Digestion B. Breathing C. Oxidation
   D. Respiration E. Perspiration
10. Which of the following liquids would pass from the alimentary canal into the blood MOST rapidly? 10. ...
   A. A dilute solution of sodium chloride in water
   B. Gastric juice
   C. A concentrated solution of sodium chloride in water
   D. Digested food
   E. Distilled water
11. The reason why it is unsafe to drink ocean water even under conditions of extreme thirst is that it 11. ...
   A. would reduce the salinity of the blood to a dangerous level
   B. contains dangerous disease germs
   C. contains poisonous salts
   D. would greatly increase the salinity of the blood
   E. would cause salt crystals to form in the blood stream

TEST 8

PASSAGE

The discovery of antitoxin and its specific antagonistic effect upon toxin furnished an opportunity for the accurate investigation of the relationship of a bacterial antigen and its antibody. Toxin-antitoxin reactions were the first immunological processes to which experimental precision could be applied, and the discovery of principles of great importance resulted from such studies. A great deal of the work was done with diphtheria toxin and antitoxin and the facts elucidated with these materials are in principle applicable to similar substances.

The simplest assumption to account for the manner in which an antitoxin renders a toxin innocuous would be that the antitoxin destroys the toxin. Roux and Buchner, however, advanced the opinion that the antitoxin did not act directly upon the toxin, but affected it indirectly through the mediation of tissue cells. Ehrlich, on the other hand, conceived the reaction of toxin and antitoxin as a direct union, analogous to the chemical neutralization of an acid by a base.

The conception of toxin destruction was conclusively refuted by the experiments of Calmette. This observer, working with snake poison, found that the poison itself (unlike most other toxins) possessed the property of resisting heat to 100 degrees C, while its specific antitoxin, like other antitoxins, was destroyed at or about

70 degrees C. Nontoxic mixtures of the two substanues, when subjected to heat, regained their toxic properties. The natural inference from these observations was that the toxin in the original mixture had not been destroyed, but had been merely inactiviated by the presence of the antitoxin and again set free after destruction of the antitoxin by heat.

Questions 1-10.

1. Both toxins and antitoxins ORDINARILY 1. ...
   A. are completely destroyed at body temperatures
   B. are extremely resistant to heat
   C. can exist only in combination
   D. are destroyed at 180°F
   E. are products of nonliving processes
2. MOST toxins can be destroyed by 2. ...
   A. bacterial action B. salt solutions
   C. boiling D. diphtheria antitoxin
   E. other toxins
3. Very few disease organisms release a true toxin into the blood stream. It would follow, then, that 3. ...
   A. studies of snake venom reactions have no value
   B. studies of toxin-antitoxin reactions are of little importance
   C. the treatment of most diseases must depend upon information obtained from study of a few
   D. antitoxin plays an important part in the body defense against the great majority of germs
   E. only toxin producers are dangerous
4. A person becomes susceptible to infection again immediately after recovering from 4. ...
   A. mumps B. tetanus C. diphtheria
   D. smallpox E. tuberculosis
5. City people are more frequently immune to communicable diseases than country people are because 5. ...
   A. country people eat better food
   B. city doctors are better than country doctors
   C. the air is more healthful in the country
   D. country people have fewer contacts with disease carriers
   E. there are more doctors in the city than in the country
6. The substances that provide us with immunity to disease are found in the body in the 6. ...
   A. blood serum B. gastric juice C. urine
   D. white blood cells E. red blood cells
7. A person ill with diphtheria would MOST likely be treated with 7. ...
   A. diphtheria toxin B. diphtheria toxoid
   C. dead diphtheria germs D. diphtheria antitoxin
   E. live diphtheria germs
8. To determine susceptibility to diphtheria, an individual may be given the 8. ...
   A. Wassermann test B. Schick test
   C. Widal test D. Dick test
   E. Kahn test
9. Since few babies under six months of age contract diphtheria, young babies PROBABLY 9. ...
   A. are never exposed to diphtheria germs

B. have high body temperatures that destroy the toxin if acquired
C. acquire immunity from their mothers
D. acquire immunity from their fathers
E. are too young to become infected

10. Calmette's findings 10. ...
A. contradicted both Roux and Buchner's opinion and Ehrlich's conception
B. contradicted Roux and Buchner, but supported Ehrlich
C. contradicted Ehrlich, but supported Roux and Buchner
D. were consistent with both theories
E. had no bearing on the point at issue

TEST 9

PASSAGE

In the days of sailing ships, when voyages were long and uncertain, provisions for many months were stored without refrigeration in the holds of the ships. Naturally no fresh or perishable foods could be included. Toward the end of particularly long voyages the crews of such ships became ill and often many died from scurvy. Many men, both scientific and otherwise, tried to devise a cure for scurvy. Among the latter was John Hall, a son-in-law of William Shakespeare, who cured some cases of scurvy by administering a sour brew made from scurvy grass and water cress.

The next step was the suggestion of William Harvey that scurvy could be prevented by giving the men lemon juice. He thought that the beneficial substance was the acid contained in the fruit.

The third step was taken by Dr. James Lind, an English naval surgeon, who performed the following experiment with 12 sailors, all of whom were sick with scurvy: Each was given the same diet, except that four of the men received small amounts of dilute sulfuric acid, four others were given vinegar and the remaining four were given lemons. Only those who received the fruit recovered.

Questions 1-7.

1. Credit for solving the problem described above belongs to 1. ...
A. Hall, because he first devised a cure for scurvy
B. Harvey, because he first proposed a solution of the problem
C. Lind, because he proved the solution by means of an experiment
D. both Harvey and Lind, because they found that lemons are more effective than scurvy grass or water cress
E. all three men, because each made some contribution

2. A good substitute for lemons in the treatment of scurvy is 2. ...
A. fresh eggs B. tomato juice C. cod-liver oil
D. liver E. whole-wheat bread

3. The number of control groups that Dr. Lind used in his experiment was 3. ...
A. one B. two C. three D. four E. none

4. A substance that will turn blue litmus red is 4. ...
A. aniline B. lye C. ice
D. vinegar E. table salt

5. The hypothesis tested by Lind was: 5. ...
   A. Lemons contain some substance not present in vinegar.
   B. Citric acid is the most effective treatment for scurvy.
   C. Lemons contain some unknown acid that will cure scurvy.
   D. Some specific substance, rather than acids in general, is needed to cure scurvy.
   E. The substance needed to cure scurvy is found only in lemons.

6. A problem that Lind's experiment did NOT solve was: 6. ...
   A. Will citric acid alone cure scurvy?
   B. Will lemons cure scurvy?
   C. Will either sulfuric acid or vinegar cure scurvy?
   D. Are all substances that contain acids equally effective as a treatment for scurvy?
   E. Are lemons more effective than either vinegar or sulfuric acid in the treatment of scurvy?

7. The PRIMARY purpose of a controlled scientific experiment is to 7. ...
   A. get rid of superstitions
   B. prove a hypothesis is correct
   C. disprove a theory that is false
   D. determine whether a hypothesis is true or false
   E. discover new facts

TEST 10

PASSAGE

The formed elements of the blood are the red corpuscles or erythrocytes, the white corpuscles or leucocytes, the blood platelets, and the so-called blood dust or hemoconiae. Together, these constitute 30-40 per cent by volume of the whole blood, the remainder being taken up by the plasma. In man, there are normally 5,000,000 red cells per cubic millimeter of blood; the count is somewhat lower in women. Variations occur frequently, especially after exercise or a heavy meal, or at high altitudes. Except in camels, which have elliptical corpuscles, the shape of the mammalian corpuscle is that of a circular, nonnucleated, bi-concave disk. The average diameter usually given is 7.7 microns, a value obtained by examining dried preparations of blood and considered by Ponder to be too low. Ponder's own observations, made on red cells in the fresh state, show the human corpuscle to have an average diameter of 8.8 microns. When circulating in the blood vessels, the red cell does not maintain a fixed shape but changes its form constantly, especially in the small capillaries. The red blood corpuscles are continually undergoing destruction, new corpuscles being formed to replace them. The average life of red corpuscles has been estimated by various investigators to be between three and six weeks. Preceding destruction, changes in the composition of the cells are believed to occur which render them less resistant. In the process of destruction, the lipids of the membrane are dissolved and the hemoglobin which is liberated is the most important, though probably not the only, source of bilirubin. The belief that the liver is the only site of red cell destruction is no longer generally held. The leucocytes, of which there are several forms, usually number between 7000 and 9000 per cubic millimeter of blood. These increase in number in disease, particularly when there is bacterial infection.

Questions 1-10.

1. Leukemia is a disease involving the 1. ...
   A. red cells B. white cells C. plasma
   D. blood platelets E. blood dust
2. Are the erythrocytes in the blood increased in number after a heavy meal? The paragraph implies that this 2. ...
   A. is true B. holds only for camels
   C. is not true D. may be true
   E. depends on the number of white cells
3. When blood is dried, the red cells 3. ...
   A. contract B. remain the same size
   C. disintegrate D. expand
   E. become elliptical
4. Ponder is probably classified as a professional 4. ...
   A. pharmacist B. physicist C. psychologist
   D. physiologist E. psychiatrist
5. The term "erythema" when applied to skin conditions signifies 5. ...
   A. redness B. swelling C. irritation
   D. pain E. roughness
6. Lipids are insoluble in water and soluble in such solvents as ether, chloroform and benzene. It may be inferred that the membranes of red cells MOST closely resemble 6. ...
   A. egg white B. sugar C. bone
   D. butter E. cotton fiber
7. Analysis of a sample of blood yields cell counts of 4,800,000 erythrocytes and 16,000 leucocytes per cubic millimeter. These data suggest that the patient from whom the blood was taken 7. ...
   A. is anemic
   B. has been injuriously invaded by germs
   C. has been exposed to high-pressure air
   D. has a normal cell count
   E. has lost a great deal of blood
8. Bilirubin, a bile pigment, is 8. ...
   A. an end product of several different reactions
   B. formed only in the liver
   C. formed from the remnants of the cell membranes of erythrocytes
   D. derived from hemoglobin exclusively
   E. a precursor of hemoglobin
9. Bancroft found that the blood count of the natives in the Peruvian Andes differed from that usually accepted as normal. The blood PROBABLY differed in respect to 9. ...
   A. leucocytes B. blood platelets C. cell shapes
   D. erythrocytes E. hemoconiae
10. Hemoglobin is probably NEVER found 10. ...
    A. free in the blood stream
    B. in the red cells
    C. in women's blood
    D. in the blood after exercise
    E. in the leucocytes

TEST 11

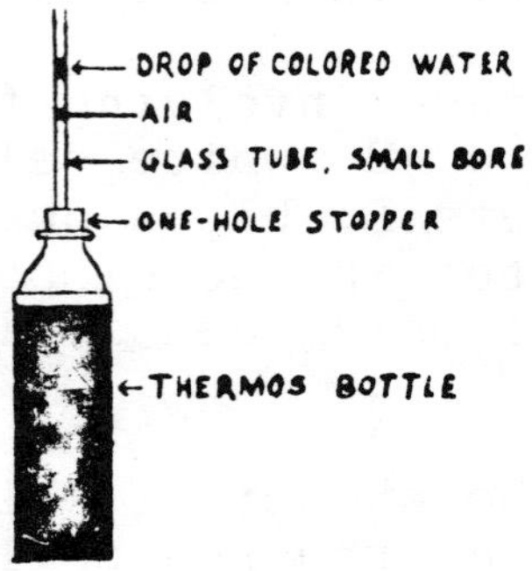

Questions 1-7.

1. The device shown in the diagram above indicates changes that are measured more accurately by a(n) 1. ...
   A. thermometer B. hygrometer C. anemometer
   D. hydrometer E. barometer
2. If the device is placed in a cold refrigerator for 72 hours, which of the following is MOST likely to happen? 2. ...
   A. The stopper will be forced out of the bottle.
   B. The drop of water will evaporate.
   C. The drop will move downward.
   D. The drop will move upward.
   E. No change will take place.
3. When the device was carried in an elevator from the first floor to the sixth floor of a building, the drop of colored water moved about 1/4 inch in the tube. Which of the following is MOST probably true? The drop moved 3. ...
   A. *downward* because there was a decrease in the air pressure
   B. *upward* because there was a decrease in the air pressure
   C. *downward* because there was an increase in the air temperature
   D. *upward* because there was an increase in the air temperature
   E. *downward* because there was an increase in the temperature and a decrease in the pressure
4. The part of a thermos bottle into which liquids are poured consists of 4. ...
   A. a single-walled, metal flask coated with silver
   B. two flasks, one of glass and one of silvered metal
   C. two silvered-glass flasks separated by a vacuum
   D. two silver flasks separated by a vacuum
   E. a single-walled, glass flask with a silver-colored coating
5. The thermos bottle is MOST similar in principle to 5. ...
   A. the freezing unit in an electric refrigerator
   B. radiant heaters
   C. solar heating systems
   D. storm windows
   E. a thermostatically controlled heating system
6. In a plane flying at an altitude where the air pressure is only half the normal pressure at sea level, the plane's altimeter should read, *approximately*, 6. ...
   A. 3000 feet B. 9000 feet C. 18000 feet
   D. 27000 feet E. 60000 feet

7. Which of the following is the POOREST conductor of heat? 7. ...
   A. Air under a pressure of 1.5 pounds per square inch
   B. Air under a pressure of 15 pounds per square inch
   C. Unsilvered glass
   D. Silvered glass
   E. Silver

TEST 12

PASSAGE

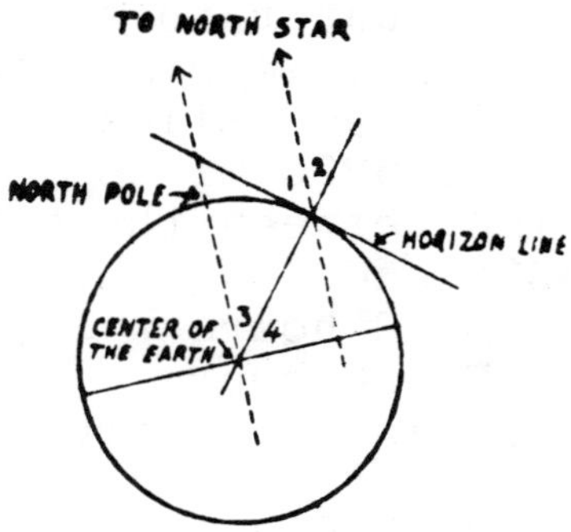

The latitude of any point on the earth's surface is the angle between a plumb line dropped to the center of the earth from that point and the plane of the earth's equator. Since it is impossible to go to the center of the earth to measure latitude, the latitude of any point may be determined indirectly as shown in the accompanying diagram.

It will be recalled that the axis of the earth, if extended outward, passes very near the North Star. Since the North Star is, for all practical purposes, infinitely distant, the line of sight to the North Star of an observer on the surface of the earth is virtually parallel with the earth's axis. Angle 1, then, in the diagram represents the angular distance of the North Star above the horizon. Angle 2 is equal to angle 3, because when two parallel lines are intersected by a straight line, the corresponding angles are equal. Angle 1 plus angle 2 is a right angle and so is angle 3 plus angle 4. Therefore, angle 1 equals angle 4 because when equals are subtracted from equals the results are equal.

Questions 1-10.

1. If an observer finds that the angular distance of the North Star above the horizon is 30°, his latitude is 1. ...
   A. 15°N B. 30°N C. 60°N D. 90°N E. 120°N
2. To an observer on the equator, the North Star would be 2. ...
   A. 30° above the horizon B. 60° above the horizon
   C. 90° above the horizon D. on the horizon
   E. below the horizon
3. To an observer on the Arctic Circle, the North Star would be 3. ...
   A. directly overhead B. 23 1/2° above the horizon
   C. 66 1/2° above the horizon
   D. on the horizon
   E. below the horizon

4. The distance around the earth along a certain parallel of latitude is 3600 miles. At that latitude, how many miles are there in one degree of longitude? 4. ...
   A. 1 mile B. 10 miles C. 30 miles
   D. 69 miles E. 100 miles
5. At which of the following latitudes would the sun be DIRECTLY overhead at noon on June 21? 5. ...
   A. 0° B. 23 1/2°S C. 23 1/2°N
   D. 66 1/2°N E. 66 1/2°S
6. On March 21 the number of hours of daylight at places on the Arctic Circle is 6. ...
   A. none B. 8 C. 12 D. 16 E. 24
7. The distance from the equator to the 45th parallel, measured along a meridian, is, *approximately*, 7. ...
   A. 450 miles B. 900 miles C. 1250 miles
   D. 3125 miles E. 6250 miles
8. The difference in time between the meridians that pass through longitude 45°E and longitude 105°W is 8. ...
   A. 6 hours B. 2 hours C. 8 hours
   D. 4 hours E. 10 hours
9. Which of the following is NOT a great circle or part of a great circle? 9. ...
   A. Arctic Circle B. 100th meridian C. Equator
   D. Shortest distance between New York and London
   E. Greenwich meridian
10. At which of the following places does the sun set EARLIEST on June 21? 10. ...
   A. Montreal, Canada B. Santiago, Chile
   C. Mexico City, Mexico D. Lima, Peru
   E. Manila, P.I.

KEY (CORRECT ANSWERS)

TEST 1
1. C
2. E
3. C
4. A
5. A
6. B
7. B
8. C

TEST 2
1. C
2. B

TEST 3
1. B
2. A
3. C
4. C
5. D
6. D
7. D
8. E
9. C

TEST 4
1. A
2. B
3. C
4. C
5. D

TEST 5
1. D
2. B
3. A
4. E
5. D
6. E
7. A

TEST 6
1. E
2. A
3. C
4. D
5. B
6. B
7. B

TEST 7
1. A
2. A
3. D
4. C
5. D
6. C
7. E
8. D
9. E
10. E

TEST 8
1. D
2. C
3. C
4. E
5. D
6. A
7. D
8. B
9. C
10. D

TEST 9
1. E
2. B
3. B
4. D
5. D
6. A
7. D

TEST 10
1. B
2. D
3. A
4. D
5. A
6. D
7. B
8. A
9. D
10. E

TEST 11
1. A
2. C
3. B
4. C
5. D
6. C
7. A

TEST 12
1. B
2. D
3. C
4. B
5. C
6. C
7. D
8. E
9. A
10. B

SCIENCE READING COMPREHENSION

EXAMINATION SECTION

DIRECTIONS FOR THIS SECTION:

This section consists of several reading passages, each followed by questions based on the text. Each question consists of a statement followed by several suggested answers, *only one* of which is correct. After reading each passage, choose the letter of the *BEST* answer among the suggested answers, basing your answer upon what is *stated* or *implied* in the passage, *and on your own understanding of science*.

Print the letter of the correct answer in the space at the right.

TEST 1

Questions 1-2.

This is a geological time-scale or time-table.

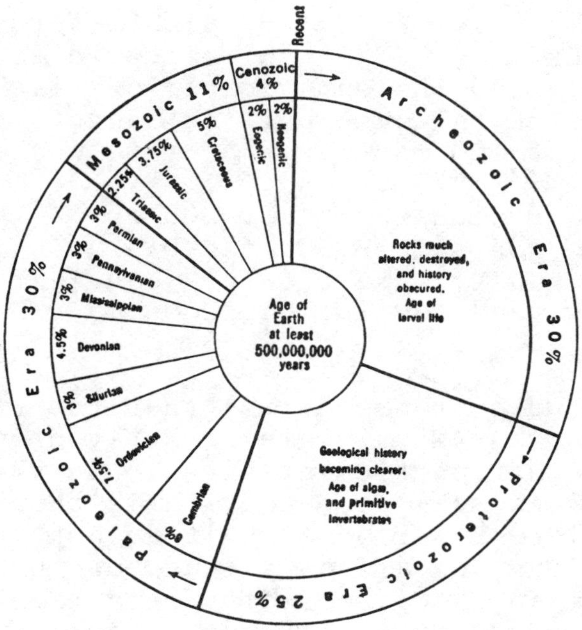

1. What is the missing word? The names of the periods in the Paleozoic era were generally adapted from the names of ______ in which the strata were first studied. 1. ...
   A. colleges B. laboratories
   C. regions D. states
2. From the information in the outer perimeter it seems reasonable to believe that 2. ...
   A. man did not exist until after the beginning of the Paleozoic era
   B. the Cenozoic era will ultimately be like the Archeozoic era
   C. the earth is at least 500,000,000 years old
   D. the percentage for the Archeozoic era ultimately will be less than 30%

Questions 3-7.

The diagram shows a gear system. Gear A has 48 teeth, B has 30 teeth, and C and D each have 6 teeth.

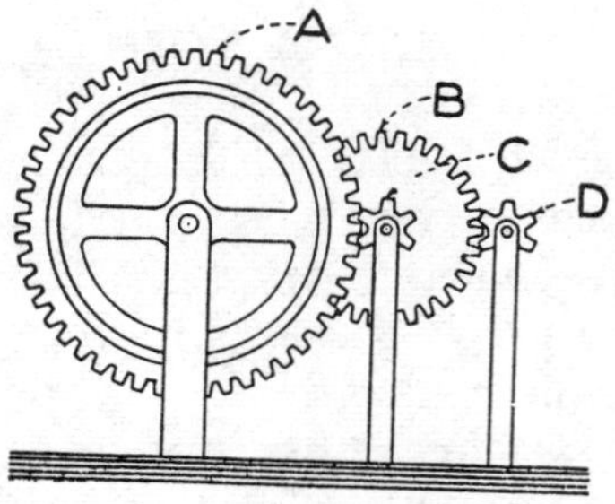

3. If gear A is the driver rotating clockwise at 50 rpm, at what rate does gear B rotate? 3. ...
   A. 50 rpm B. 250 rpm C. 400 rpm D. 1,200 rpm
4. The ratio of the speed of rotation of gear D relative to gear C is 4. ...
   A. 1:5 B. 5:1 C. 5:8 D. 8:1
5. This type of gear train is *most likely* to be found in a(n) 5. ...
   A. bicycle B. planimeter
   C. alarm clock D. electric motor
6. If gears A and B had the same number of teeth, and gears C and D each had just half as many as A, when gear D rotated at 100 rpm, at what rate would gear B rotate? 6. ...
   A. 50 rpm B. 100 rpm C. 200 rpm D. 400 rpm
7. If the teeth in gears A, B, C, and D are in the proportions 5, 4, 3, and 2,respectively, when gear A makes one revolution, how many revolutions does gear D make? 7. ...
   A. $1\frac{7}{8}$ B. $2\frac{1}{2}$ C. $3\frac{1}{3}$ D. $4\frac{2}{3}$

Questions 8-10.

Two hypotheses were proposed: (1) that the rate of depletion of the body reserves of a vitamin are directly proportional to the total reserves of that particular vitamin in the body, and,further, (2) when an animal is subjected to vitamin therapy, it should be possible to calculate a period of half adjustment.

It was thought that data from a study of the depletion of vitamin A reserves in the livers of steers might offer some light on the tenability of these hypotheses. Table 1 shows the slaughtering data and the average vitamin A content of the livers. The sample consisted of observations of 120 Hereford steers, about 18 months of age, taken from native grass pasture and placed on a fattening ration consistent with good feeding practice.

TABLE 1

Days in the feed lot	No. of animals slaughtered	Vitamin A reserves (µg. vitamin A/gram liver)
0	22	51.4
41	19	23.7
76	20	11.9
119	19	5.3
166	40	1.9

To determine the validity of these hypotheses, the data in Table 1 were subjected to analysis. Vitamin A reserves were plotted against days in the feed lot, and vitamin A values determined at intervals of 40 days. Table 2 gives the values obtained.

TABLE 2

Days in the feed lot	Vitamin A reserves (µg. vitamin A/gram liver)	Drop in 40 days (%)
0	51.4	..
40	24.2	47
80	11.1	46
120	5.2	47
160	2.2	42

8. The data of Tables 1 and 2 show that 8. ...
   A. both hypotheses are supported
   B. neither hypothesis is supported
   C. the first hypothesis is supported and the second is not
   D. the second hypothesis is supported and the first is not

9. The curve obtained by plotting the data in Table 1 would show for vitamin A reserves during the experimental period 9. ...
   A. a constant loss B. a decreasing loss
   C. an increasing loss D. no loss

10. Plotting days in the feed lot on the abscissa (with 0 at the left) and vitamin A reserves (Table 2) as ordinate (with 0 at the bottom), which curve would result? 10. ...

A. 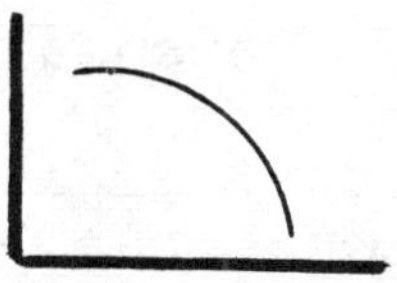

B. 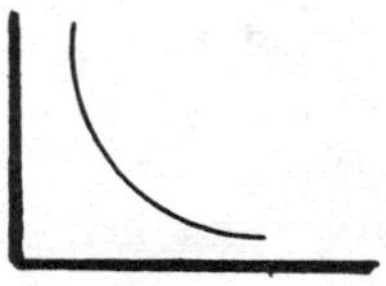

C. 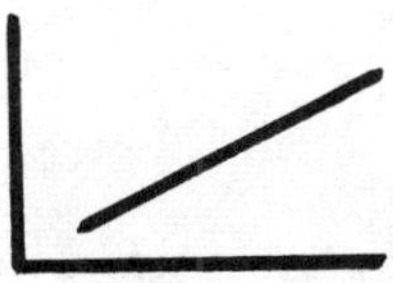

D. 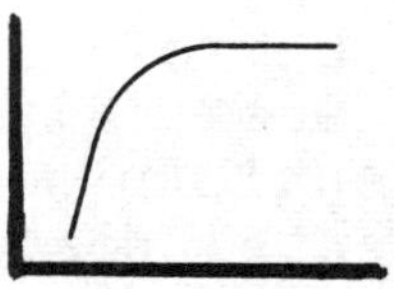

Questions 11-14.

The blood levels resulting from the injection of a new penicillin were of a shorter duration than those obtained under the same conditions from a commercial penicillin. This new penicillin (No. 128) had an activity of 3,500 units/mg. as compared with 2,300, 1,667, and 900 units/mg. for penicillins K, G, and X, respectively. An experiment was set up to determine whether the rate of excretion of a pure penicillin is a function of its potency in terms of units/mg., or, in other words, of the number of molecules injected. The penicillins used were analytically pure and were dissolved in normal saline at a concentration of 5,000 units/ml.

Each penicillin, on different days, was injected into each of the same four subjects. Twenty-five thousand units were injected intravenously into one arm, and blood samples withdrawn from the other arm at suitable intervals. Urinary excretion of the penicillins was measured at half-hourly intervals during the first two hours and hourly thereafter. The urine was assayed by the usual cylinder-plate method against *Staphylococcus aureus* 209P, and the blood levels were determined. A penicillin G standard was used in each case.

The duration of penicillin blood levels of at least 0.03 unit/ml. for each of the penicillins was as follows: penicillin G, 2-2.5 hours; penicillin 128, 1-1.25 hours; penicillin K, .5-.75 hour; and penicillin X, 4-4.5 hours. During the first two hours, the various penicillins were excreted in the following percentages: penicillin G, 83; penicillin 128, 58; penicillin K, 28; and penicillin X, 78. Penicillins G and X were excreted in the amount of approximately 80 percent, the difference between them being within experimental error. Penicillin K, however, was excreted to the extent of only about 30 percent.

11. At the concentrations in which penicillin G occurs in the blood, voiding by the kidneys in the first two hours — 11. ...
    A. almost completely removes it
    B. decreases its potency slightly
    C. has practically no effect on it
    D. increases its concentration

12. It would seem that penicillin K is — 12. ...
    A. destroyed rapidly in the body, and is therapeutically effective
    B. destroyed rapidly in the body, and is not therapeutically effective
    C. fairly stable in the body, and is therapeutically effective
    D. fairly stable in the body, and is not therapeutically effective

13. Apparently penicillins G and X are sufficiently stable that their excretion by the kidneys represents the limiting factor in the maintenance of — 13. ...
    A. a high rate of inactivation
    B. the number of molecules injected
    C. their sensitivity
    D. therapeutic blood levels

14. The experimental dosage of each of the penicillins was — 14. ...
    A. inversely proportional to the molecular weights of the penicillins used
    B. proportional to the body weights of the subjects
    C. proportional to the molecular weights of the penicillins used
    D. the same for all subjects

Questions 15-19.

A $2\frac{1}{2}$ inch cube, as shown in the diagram, is made of half-inch cubes. Any one cube may be located in terms of a coordinate system. For example, cube *a* is in the fifth layer from the left, the fourth layer from the bottom, and the second from the front. It is, therefore, located in the position 5,4,2.

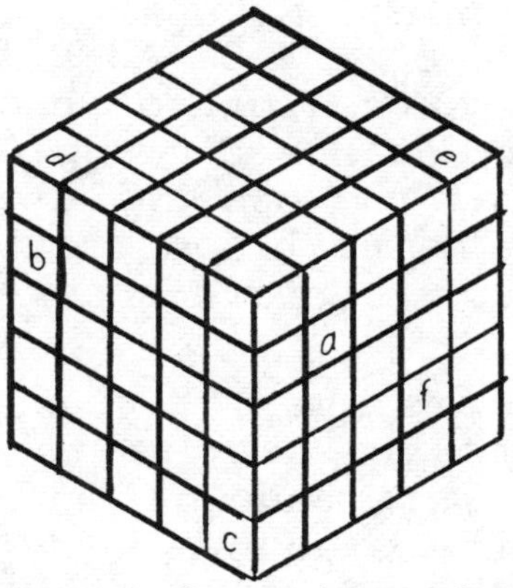

15. If the entire exterior surface is painted blue, what is the largest cube which can be built from the unpainted cubes? 15. ...
    A. 1-inch cube B. 1½-inch cube
    C. 2-inch cube D. 2½-inch cube
16. The coordinates of the cube nearest the center of the cube shown in the diagram are 16. ...
    A. 1,1,1 B. 2,2,2 C. 3,3,3 D. 5,5,5
17. What are the coordinates of the cube which would have two holes in it if a hole $\frac{1}{32}$ of an inch in diameter were drilled from cube 2,4,1 through cube 2,4,5 and a similar hole from cube 5,4,3 through 1,4,3? 17. ...
    A. 1,3,4 B. 2,4,3 C. 3,3,3 D. 5,4,1
18. If the layer containing cubes *b* and *c* is turned so that *b* is next to cube *a*, and the layer containing cubes *d* and *e* is turned so that cube *d* is located where cube *e* is shown in the diagram, what then are the coordinates of cube *a*? 18. ...
    A. 1,4,2 B. 5,1,1 C. 5,4,2 D. 5,5,1
19. If the layer containing cubes *d* and *e* is moved to the bottom of the cube, and then the layer containing cubes *b* and *c* is moved to the back of the cube, what then are the coordinates of cube *f*? 19. ...
    A. 4,3,4 B. 5,2,4 C. 5,3,3 D. 5,3,4

Questions 20-25.

The Table shows the observations regarding blood groups of 267 families of Danish subjects.

Parents	No. of Families	Offspring O	A	B	AB
O X O	41	126	1	0	0
A X A	22	10	70	0	0
O X A	68	69	102	0	0
B X B	1	1	0	1	0
O X B	13	18	0	29	0
A X B	22	13	16	13	26
O X AB	43	0	50	60	0
A X AB	42	0	59	21	33
B X AB	13	0	8	20	15
AB X AB	2	0	3	4	1
Totals	267	237	309	148	75

20. About what percent of parents had blood group O? 20. ...
    A. 30 B. 40 C. 50 D. 60
21. What combination of blood groupings of parents produced offspring of all four blood groups? 21. ...
    A. A X AB B. A X B C. AB X AB D. O X AB
22. If it is true that parents, both of blood group O, can produce offspring only of blood group O, which is probably the best explanation of the one child of such parents shown in the table as being blood group A? 22. ...
    A. Faulty test sera or uncertain paternity could cause such exceptions
    B. Most such tables are subject to clerical errors
    C. The number of families sampled was too small
    D. The observations were made on Danish families only
23. Children of group O were produced by how many combinations of parents neither of which had group O blood? 23. ...
    A. 0 B. 3 C. 5 D. 6
24. A study of 2,046 offspring of Japanese families showed 691 group O, 756 A, 476 B, and 123 AB. The proportion of Japanese offspring of group AB bears what relationship to the proportion of AB offspring in the Danish sample? 24. ...
    A. Equal B. Greater C. Less D. Non-comparable
25. The fact that there are so few families of AB X AB parentage is probably due to the fact that 25. ...
    A. personality adjustment of group AB is such that chances of marriage are decreased
    B. such combinations of men and women do not usually occur in the same communities
    C. such matings tend to be sterile
    D. there is a relatively low occurrence of blood group AB

KEY (CORRECT ANSWERS)

1. C
2. D
3. C
4. B
5. C
6. A
7. C
8. C
9. B
10. B
11. A
12. B
13. D
14. D
15. B
16. C
17. B
18. C
19. C
20. B
21. B
22. A
23. B
24. C
25. D

TEST 2

Questions 1-4.

The accompanying diagram represents a confined body of liquid connecting two cylinders of areas *a* and A respectively, each fitted with a piston. Upon applying a force *f* to the smaller piston, a greater force F will be exerted by the larger one, such that the pressures at the two pistons are equal.

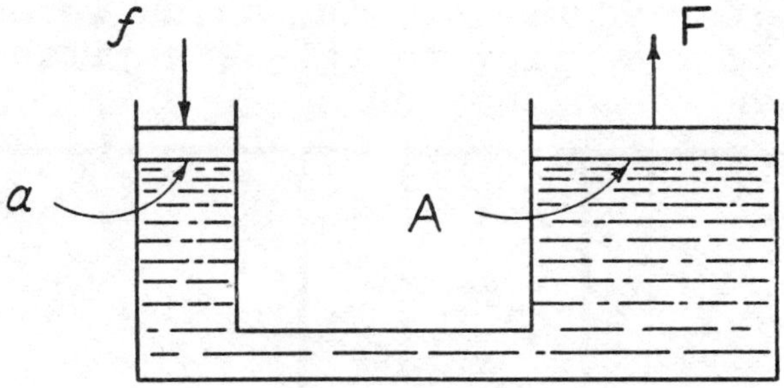

1. If the area *a* is one fifth as great as the area A, the ratio of *f* to F will be 1. ...
   A. 0.2 B. 0.5 C. 1.0 D. 5.0
2. Which of the following devices uses the principle described in the paragraph? 2. ...
   A. Hydraulic brakes B. Hydrometer
   C. Sonic depth finder D. Standpipe
3. The mechanical advantage of such a machine as the hydraulic press is the ratio of the force exerted by the machine to the force applied. Disregarding friction, the mechanical advantage is: 3. ...
   A. $\frac{A}{a}$ B. $\frac{f}{a}$ C. $\frac{F}{a}$ D. $\frac{f}{F}$
4. If the hydraulic pressure were transferred from the pressure cylinder to two cylinders, the relationship of force and area would be: 4. ...
   A. $\frac{f}{a} = \frac{F}{A} + \frac{F'}{A'}$ B. $\frac{f}{a} = \frac{F}{A} + \frac{F'}{A'}$
   C. $\frac{f}{a} = \frac{FXF'}{A+A'}$ D. $\frac{f}{a} = \frac{FF'}{AA'}$

Questions 5-9.

In a previous publication it was reported that intravenous injections of crystalline *L. casei* factor led to complete regressions of spontaneous breast cancers in mice, in about one-third of the animals. Drs. Hutchings and Stokstad indicate that the correct tentative designation of this substance is fermentation *L. casei* factor. The isolation of this compound was announced, and its microbiological activity and other properties were described by Hutchings. More recently, Angier reported the synthesis of a compound identical with the *L. casei* factor from liver. This substance differs in microbiological activity from that of the fermentation *L. casei* factor used in our previously reported experiments in that the liver *L. casei* factor is about 17 times as active for the test organism, *Streptococcus lactis R*, at half maximum growth.

Ninety-eight mice bearing single spontaneous breast cancers were selected for present studies. In each case a definite diagnosis of malignancy was established by biopsy. The animals were kept on a normal diet (Rockland mouse pellets). Three groups were formed. The first group, 39 tumor mice, received 5 μg. of liver *L. casei* factor; the second group, 31 mice, received 100 μg. of liver *L. casei* factor; and the third group, 28 mice, received 5 μg. of the crystalline fermentation *L. casei* factor. All substances were injected intravenously daily for a period of 4-6 weeks. As control, the data of 71 mice of the same strain, which were observed in the laboratory during a period prior to this experiment, were used. The results are presented in the table.

Group	No. of mice	Substance and dose (μg.)	No. of mice with complete regression of tumors	No. of mice with new tumors	No. of mice with lung metastases	Mean life span in days*
1	39	Liver *L. casei* factor(5 μg.)	1	12	19 among 32	75 ± 6
2	31	Liver *L. casei* factor (100μg.)	0	11	3 among 30	55 ± 6
3	28	Fermentation *L. casei* factor (5μg.)	11	2	†	After 100 days 23 mice alive
4	71	0	0	19	13 among 61	74 ± 6.2

*Life span calculated after start of experiment.

†An evaluation cannot be given since the majority of mice in this group are alive.

5. Which of the following statements is correct? 5. ...
   A. No null hypotheses were used in the experiment.
   B. The control data are inadequate because observations were made prior to the observations for the experimental data.
   C. The mice in the third group, treated with fermentation *L. casei* factor, were younger than those in the other groups.
   D. The numbers of mice for the four groups were not equal.
6. In producing regressions of tumors, the liver *L. casei* factor was 6. ...
   A. effective with many animals, ineffective with many others
   B. in general, effective
   C. in general, ineffective
   D. not used enough to give significant results

7. The fermentation *L. casei* factor led to regressions of tumors in practically 7. ...
   A. no cases B. one-fifth of the cases
   C. one-fourteenth of the cases
   D. one-third of the cases
8. The greatest percentage of mice showed lung metastases in group 8. ...
   A. 1 B. 2 C. 3 D. 4
9. Diagnosis of malignancy of the cancers was established by 9. ...
   A. examination of tissues removed from the living animal
   B. examination of tissues removed in autopsy
   C. palpation of the affected areas
   D. reaction of the cancers to diagnostic pharmaceutical

Questions 10-15.

Suppose a number system were instituted which had eight digits, □, Λ, Z, ≲, ⊁, S, ә, and ᒥ, corresponding respectively to the digits 0, 1, 2, 3, 4, 5, 6, and 7. The digit □ is used in the same fashion as the 0 in the decimal system, e.g., Λ□ = 8.

10. Which is equal to 8 X 8? 10. ...
    A. Λ□□ B. ә⊁ C. Λ□Λ D. S≲
11. What is the sum of ⊁ + ә + ≲ ? 11. ...
    A. ZΛ B. SV C. ≲⊁ D. Λә
12. Which of the following indicates three-quarters of an inch? 12. ...
    A. $\frac{S}{Λ□}$ inches B. $\frac{ә}{Λ□}$ inches
    C. $\frac{ᒥ}{Λ□}$ inches D. $\frac{ᒥS}{Λ□□}$ inches
13. What is the value of ΛZә − ⊁ᒥ + $\frac{Λ□}{Z}$? 13. ...
    A. ⊁ә B. Sᒥ C. ә≲ D. ᒥ□
14. What is the value of Λ□≲ә ? 14.
    A. 542 B. 829 C. 900 D. 1,036
15. How many feet are there in a mile? 15. ...
    A. ⊁Z⊁⊁ B. S≲□□ C. ƏV3Ə D. ΛZZ⊁□

Questions 16-21.

Silver pigment is deposited in the experimental rat in a way essentially similar to that in which it is deposited in man. In view of the efficacy of 2,3-dimercaptopropanol (BAL) in the treatment of poisoning with arsenic and mercury, it appeared desirable to study the effect of this agent on the experimental argyrosis of the rat.

The experiment was carried out on four rats, grouped in pairs and placed on a diet of dog pellets. The first pair received a solution of 1:1,000 silver nitrate in place of drinking water for a period of 456 days. During this time a total amount of 23.2 grams of silver nitrate was consumed by the two animals, or an average of 11.6 grams each. On the 457th day the silver nitrate solution was discontinued and replaced by water. At this time the eyes of both rats were distinctly pigmented, one slightly more so than the other. Eighteen days later the more deeply stained rat was started on treatment with intramuscular BAL. The BAL was given in a 1:50 dilution in cottonseed oil. A total of nine injections was given on alternate days, covering a period of 18 days. Each single dose was 10 times the minimal effective dose for the treatment of acute arsenic poisoning in the rat. The other rat was maintained as a control. The treated animal showed a weight loss of 30 grams over the period of therapy, but otherwise appeared healthy. The control animal lost 6 grams. Both animals were sacrificed on the 21st day, at which time the eyes of the treated rat were still darker than those of the control.

On histological examination, the eyes, thyroid, liver, pancreas, spleen, and kidneys contained an apparently identical amount of silver deposit. No lesions were found in either rat.

The second pair of rats received for a period of 514 days a 1:1,000 solution of silver chloride with added sodium thiosulfate (approximately 1:300) in place of drinking water. The total average silver chloride intake for each of the two animals was 12.9 grams. On the 515th day the silver chloride solution was replaced by drinking water. The eyes of the pair were also distinctly pigmented. Eighteen days later the more deeply stained rat was started on BAL therapy. The dose and manner of administration was as described above, with the exception that a total of 18 injections of BAL was given, covering a period of 38 days. The cage mate was kept as a control. During the period of treatment the treated animal lost 25 grams in weight, but otherwise appeared healthy; the control showed a 3-gram gain. On the 42nd day both were sacrificed, at which time the eyes of the treated rat still appeared darker than those of the control.

On histological examination, there were apparently identical amounts of silver deposits in the thyroid, kidneys, eyes, and choroid plexus of each rat. There were no lesions indicating any toxic effect in either rat.

16. These observations indicate that BAL is 16. ...
    A. capable of mobilizing mercury
    B. capable of mobilizing silver
    C. incapable of mobilizing mercury
    D. incapable of mobilizng silver

17. In the treatment of argyrosis in man, BAL probably would be 17. ...
    A. absolutely useless B. of considerable value
    C. of little or no value D. the basis for a cure

18. Treatment of the rats with BAL 18. ...
    A. eventually resulted in the deaths of the rats
    B. produced unusual chronic effects in the treated rats
    C. showed little effect except loss in body weight
    D. showed their great susceptibility to poisoning by BAL

19. The *null* hypothesis upon which the experiment is based may be stated as follows: 19. ...
    A. BAL will act in cases of silver poisoning in the same fashion as in cases of arsenic poisoning
    B. Silver pigment deposited in an experimental animal is as dangerous to that animal as equal amounts of mercuric deposits
    C. The proper dosage of BAL for rats is 10 times that for a cat, since the ratio of weight of cats to rats is 10
    D. Treatment of argyrosis by means of BAL will not alter the silver deposit in various organs of the animal

20. The method of examination of the various organs for silver was 20. ...
   A. electro-chemical B. micro-chemical
   C. not specifically described
   D. photometric

21. Which of the following statements is *most nearly TRUE?* 21. ...
   A. Rats require a dosage of BAL 10 times as great as for cats
   B. The cottonseed oil maintained the weight of the treated animal during therapy
   C. The experiment tended to show that BAL therapy was not effective in the treatment of experimental argyrosis
   D. The number of animals used in this study is too small to warrant drawing of any conclusions

Questions 22-25.

Subtilin, an antibiotic obtained from *Bacillus subtilis,* was found to be active *in vitro* against *Staphylococcus aureus, Lactobacillus casei, Micrococcus conglomeratus,* and *Streptococcus viridans.* Salle and Jann have indicated that it is also active *in vitro* against gram-positive bacteria including *Mycobacterium tuberculosis.* It was reported by them to have a cytotoxic index of about 20. Because of its favorable antibiotic activity it was desired to investigate possible modes of action against a variety of organisms. Effects on *Trypanosoma equiperdum, Leishmania donovani, Endamoeba histolytica, Lactobacillus plantarum,* and *Ascaris suis* were studied. In addition, physical behavior was considered in an effort to explain the biologic activity of subtilin and other antibiotics *in vitro* and *in vivo.*

Using the technic of Heilman and Herrell, subtilin, 0.05 percent in water or in 85 percent ethyl alcohol, showed immediate surface-tension-lowering effect. Gramicidin and gramicidin derivative (formaldehyde treated) exhibited similar properties. Lysozyme and streptomycin produced only slight effects, while penicillin did not alter surface tension. Figure 1 summarizes the findings. The Cenco-Du Noüy tensiometer was used.

EFFECT OF ANTIBIOTICS
ON SURFACE TENSION

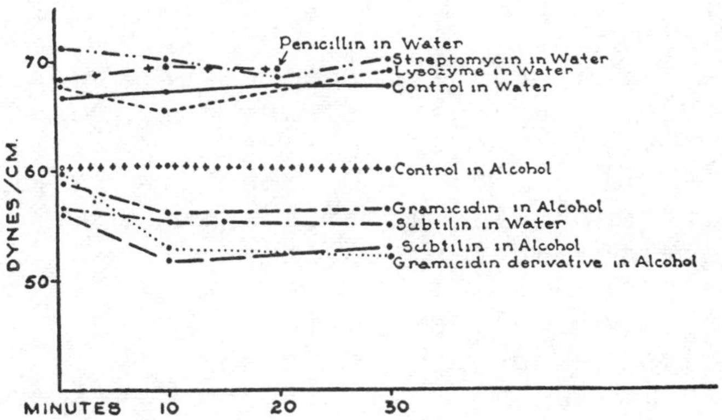

FIGURE 1

The hemolytic effect of gramicidin was compared with that of the other antibiotics. Confirming the studies of Lewis, *et al.*, gramicidin derivative proved less hemolytic. Subtilin had no immediate effect on red cells, but after 24 hours at 4° C. hemolysis occurred. Penicillin and streptomycin caused no hemolysis.

Brief exposure of *T. equiperdum* to subtilin dissolved in 0.45 percent sodium chloride solution resulted in immediate cytolysis when 1:2,000 dilution was used. Streptomycin and penicillin were not lytic. Survival of trypanosome-infected mice was not prolonged when 80 to 160 mg./kg. amounts of subtilin were given intraperitoneally.

Subtilin was not active *in vitro* or *in vivo* against *L. donovani*. Penicillin G in 1:1,000 dilution caused cytolysis of leishmania in 6 hours, and in 1:10,000, in 24 hours. *In vivo* it was not active. Neither streptomycin nor lysozyme was effective *in vitro*.

E. histolytica was killed *in vitro* in liquid liver medium at 1:400,000 dilution of subtilin, as well as the associated bacterium 't.' In egg slope medium it was active within the range of emetine hydrochloride, and on autoclaving solutions for 10 minutes, subtilin's activity was markedly enhanced. The gramicidins had similar activity in egg slope medium but were only one-fifth as active as subtilin in liquid liver medium. Streptomycin in 1:2,500 dilution killed the amoeba *in vitro*.

Against *L. plantarum* (342y) in liquid medium containing 1 percent dextrose and 1 percent Difco yeast extract (pH 6.8), a 1:80,000 dilution of subtilin inhibited growth after 48 hours at 37° C. Cholesterol did not enhance its activity, but para-aminobenzoic acid did. The gramicidins were active at 1:40,000 dilution and streptomycin at 1:10,000.

In vitro tests against *A. suis* revealed that none of the antibiotics studied was active.

The acute toxicity of subtilin in mice, on intravenous injection of 1 percent solution, was $^{LD}50$ (60 ± 3 mg./kg.); on subcutaneous injection, the $^{LD}50$ was 670 ± 30 mg./kg.; when given intragastrically, 5.0 grams/kg. killed. One percent solution instilled into the rabbit's eye was non-irritating.

Gramicidin, 1 percent in propylene glycol, given intravenously in mice had an $^{LD}50$ of 1.5 mg./kg. Gramicidin derivative was less toxic, $^{LD}60$ being 4.7 mg./kg. Lethal doses of the gramicidins killed within one minute, which precluded the possibility of delayed hemolysis, were responsible.

22. Against *L. plantarum, E. histolytica* and its associated bacterium 't' and *T. equiperdum* subtilin proved 22. ...
    A. active *in vitro* B. active *in vivo*
    C. inactive *in vitro* D. inactive *in vivo*
23. As compared with subtilin, gramicidin is 23. ...
    A. less hemolytic and less toxic
    B. less hemolytic and more toxic
    C. more hemolytic and less toxic
    D. more hemolytic and more toxic
24. Which of the following was shown to be *MOST* destructive of red blood cells? 24. ...
    A. Gramicidin B. Penicillin
    C. Streptomycin D. Subtilin

25. Which of the following statements is *BEST* borne out by the paragraph? 25. ...
   A. Subtilin is a member of a class of substances which tend to destroy life
   B. Subtilin is highly irritating to mucous membranes
   C. Subtilin is more active *in vitro* than *in vivo*
   D. Subtilin showed a greater surface tension in an alcohol solution than in aqueous solution

KEY (CORRECT ANSWERS)

1. A
2. A
3. A
4. B
5. D

6. C
7. D
8. A
9. A
10. A

11. B
12. B
13. C
14. A
15. D

16. D
17. C
18. C
19. D
20. C

21. C
22. A
23. B
24. D
25. A

SCIENCE READING COMPREHENSION

EXAMINATION SECTION

DIRECTIONS: This section consists of a long reading passage, followed by questions based on the text. Each question consists of a statement followed by several suggested answers, only one of which is correct. After reading the passage, choose the letter of the BEST answer among the suggested answers, basing your answer upon what is stated or implied in the passage, and on your own understanding of science. *PRINT THE LETTER OF THE CORRECT ANSWER IN THE SPACE AT THE RIGHT.*

PASSAGE

PHARMACOLOGICAL STUDIES OF STIMULANTS AND DEPRESSANTS

ABSTRACT

A group of experiments is described in which chimpanzees and orangutans are utilized as subjects in research projects designed to evaluate the effects of stimulant and depressant drugs on learning and performance. Efficiency of performance on a task which measures spaced responding was impaired when subjects smoked cigarettes containing Δ^5-tetrahydrocannabinol prior to testing. In a sequential learning task, these subjects also demonstrated reduced performance when stimulant drugs were orally administered before testing. Depressant drugs did not produce comparable decrements in sequential learning performance. Physical and behavioral tolerance and dependence on ethanol were investigated in rhesus monkey subjects using a variety of experimental procedures, including forced oral acceptance, intragastic intubation, intravenous infusion, and conditioned voluntary oral acceptance.

Chimpanzees, orangutans, and gorillas are the largest of all nonhuman primate species and constitute the great ape family. In our studies, we have generally utilized chimpanzees (Pan troglodytes) from the great ape colony of the Yerkes Regional Primate Research Center of Emory University. Chimpanzees tend to be inquisitive subjects that perform well on a wide variety of behavioral tasks. Although none of the research projects undertaken are terminal experiments, there are obviously greater risks in some procedures than others. For that reason, in studies involving surgical preparation, indwelling catheters, and the like, the rhesus monkey (Macaca mulatta) has been our primary subject.

LEARNING AND PERFORMANCE

With the chimpanzee, we have focused our attention on evaluating the effects of potentially psychoactive compounds on learning and performance. One of the earliest experiments of this type was designed to examine the effects of smoking cigarettes containing Δ^9-tetrahydrocannabinol (Δ^9-THC) on spaced responding. The behavioral task used involved lever pulling performance for M & M candy rewards on a DRL schedule (differential reinforcement low), in which the subject was required to pause for a minimum of either 10 sec. or 20 sec. before pulling a lever that would deliver an M & M candy reward. For example, on a DRL 10-sec. schedule, the subject was required to wait at least 10 sec. before responding to obtain the reward. If a response was made prior to the end of the 10 sec. interval, the timer was reset and the subject was again required to pause 10 sec. or more to obtain a reinforcement.

Prior to initiation of drug testing, pretraining on both the smoking and DRL task was completed. To facilitate absorption of the Δ^9-THC, two chimpanzees and one orangutan (Pongo pygmaeus) were trained to make long draws on a pipe that was inserted through the wall of the testing cage. One end of the pipe contained a lighted cigarette, and the subject was required to maintain constant negative pressure on the pipe for approximately 5 sec. or longer before an M & M candy reinforcer was delivered. On drug days, the cigarettes smoked by the subjects were injected with Δ^9-THC such that the total putative dose of the drug was varied from 1.8 mg/kg to 6.2 mg/kg. Following the smoking session, behavioral testing on the DRL task was initiated. As can be seen in Fig. 1, the results of this experiment indicated that the efficiency of responding (rewards obtained/total response) decreased below control levels when the cigarette contained Δ^9-THC. This reduction in performance was observed in all three subjects.

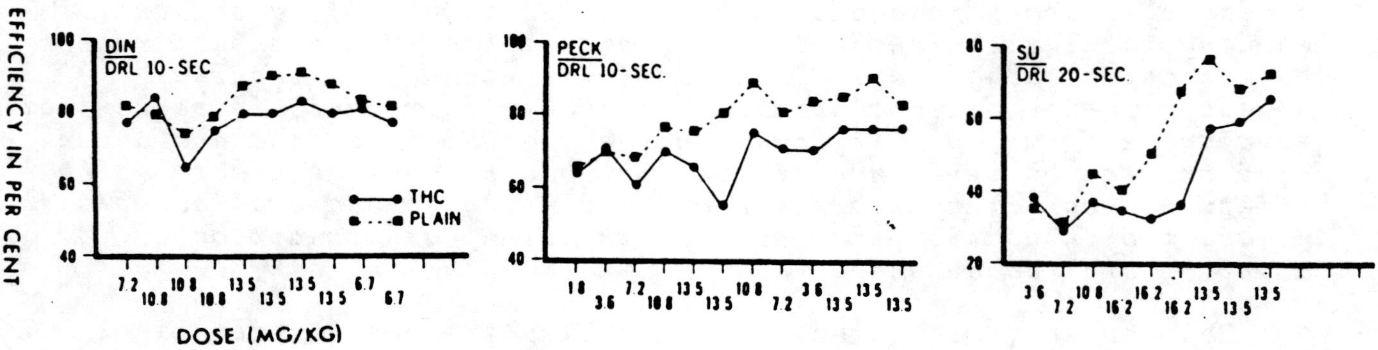

Figure 1. Efficiency of responding (reinforcements/ responses) per 30-min. DRL test session for three great apes. Doses of Δ^9-THC as indicated on the abscissa were administered every 3-4 days and performance on those days compared to intervening control days.

Although this approach demonstrated the feasibility of using large adult ape subjects (40-70 kg) for psychopharmacological research, two major problems remained. (a) Rigorous control over the dose of drug via inhalation proved very difficult, since variable amounts of inhalation by the animal were still possible. Further, routine monitoring of the blood concentrations of inhaled compounds was not practical because of the size of the subjects and the lack of practical analytical procedures for measuring substances such as Δ^9-THC in biological fluids. (b) Performance on the DRL task could not be directly related to the effects of drugs on the process of learning, since the subjects were all given extensive training on the task prior to drug testing. For these reasons, we shifted to oral administration of all drugs and adopted a sequential response task to assess the effects of drugs on learning.

This sequential response task was first described by Boren and Devine and is uniquely suited to the problem in at least three respects. First, the subject is required to learn a relatively complex sequential response chain rather than a simple visual discrimination or light tracking task. Second, a stimulus fading procedure is used so that learning is guided in a standardized manner. Initially, brightness cues are used to shape the animal's response. These cues are then gradually diminished so that the animal has to rely more and more on memory rather than brightness discrimination. This procedure has proved to be more efficient in sequential learning than nonfading techniques. Third, and most important, while the basic nature of the task is the same over sessions, the subject is required to learn a new sequence on each day. Thus, the learning deficit or enhancement associated with various orally administered drugs can be assessed using a nonhuman primate species closely related to man.

We have used a modified version of this task consisting of a manipulandum panel with six horizontally mounted Lindsley response levers. A transilluminated circular disk was mounted 10 cm above each of the six levers. These lights served as visual cues signaling the correct lever to pull at a given time. The saliency of these brightness cues was varied across eight levels of illumination, ranging from high contrast (the correct lever fully lighted with the other five off) to no contrast (all levers, including the correct one, at full brightness). Below the manipulandum panel was a food receptacle into which M & M candy reinforcers were delivered from a dispenser. These reinforcers were delivered each time the animal pulled the final lever in a correct sequence of levers. When an error was made, a 7-sec. timeout went into effect during which a buzzer was sounded and the house lights and all lever lights were extinguished. Each day testing began with maximum light cues followed by a gradual fading out of the discriminable brightness feature, thereby forcing the subject to learn the position of the correct levers. The length of the lever pulling sequence was also systematically increased from one lever to six levers. The fading procedure was first used with the shortest sequence length of one. Each correct lever response was followed by a reduction in the brightness cue by one level while each error resulted in the light cue "backing up" to the level used on the previous trial. At the eighth level, all stimulus lights were identically illuminated and consequently, no longer functioned as a cue. Therefore, a correct response at the eighth level indicated that the animal had learned the correct position of the lever(s). Thus, the brightness cue was systematically faded out through eight equal intensity changes, so that the stimulus lights provided no cue to the correct sequence of levers when acquisition of the behavioral chain was completed. When the subject correctly completed sequence one, the sequence was increased to a two-lever chain. The subject was now required to pull two levers in the correct sequence to obtain reinforcement. Again, maximal brightness cues were used on the initial trials but were progressively faded out with each correct response. When the subject successfully completed the sequence to two levers at the eighth level of illumination, demonstrating that he had learned to discriminate the correct two-lever sequence by position, the sequence was lengthened to three levers and the process repeated.

Daily test sessions were terminated either when 50 minutes had elapsed or when the subject has successfully completed a sequence of six levers, whichever occurred first. Since a new lever sequence was presented each day, a new sequence was learned each day. Thus, this task provided learning data for each day of testing. Therefore, learning (acquisition) on those days when a particular drug was administered could be compared with intervening control days when only placebo was given.

The primary dependent measure obtained from this task is the maximum sequence length completed during the 50-min. test sessions. In general, drugs that have a depressant or tranquilizing action (butabarbital, secobarbital, glutethimide, and diazepam) have little effect on learning as measured by the sequential task when the doses are kept below the level where obvious general physical impairment occurs. However, stimulants (benzphetamine, d-amphetamine, diethylpropion, phendimetrazine, and phentermine) do produce decreases in learning, depending on the potency of the drug and the size of dose, even though no overt symptoms of general impairment are present (see Fig. 2).

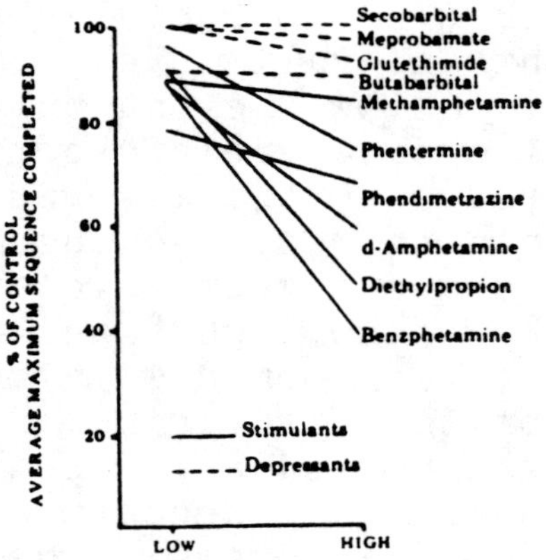

Figure 2. The effect of a series of drugs on learning as measured by the maximum sequence length achieved during a test session. Performance on drug testing days is indicated as a percent of that on the control days that immediately preceded the drug administration days.

ETHANOL TOLERANCE AND DEPENDENCE

In our laboratory, physical dependence on ethanol has been produced in young chimpanzees by including alcohol in their liquid diet in gradually increasing doses. With rhesus monkeys, ethanol physical dependence has been produced using this same procedure and also by using nasogastric intubation of ethanol in liquid diet two to three times per day, and by constant infusion of ethanol solutions through surgically implanted intrajugular catheters. All procedures have resulted in the production of physical dependence as evidenced by the emergence of withdrawal symptoms when blood ethanol concentrations decreased from previously elevated values achieved during the chronic administration period. In general, these studies demonstrated that chronic administration of ethanol in sufficient amounts and at appropriate intervals to maintain blood ethanol concentrations above zero for a period of 4 or more days was necessary to produce observable signs of physical dependence. Further, blood methanol was observed to accumulate during these periods of chronic ethanol administration, probably due to competitive inhibition of the enzyme system that catalyzes the metabolism of both alcohols. This buildup of methanol, which is toxic in primates, may have some significance in the development of physical dependence.

In addition to physical dependence, the addictive process is characterized by the development of tolerance to ethanol. Both metabolic and behavioral tolerance have been investigated in these animals. The rate of disappearance of ethanol from the blood was determined at frequent intervals during periods of chronic ethanol administration. In both chimpanzees and rhesus monkeys, disappearance rates increased with chronic administration and the magnitude of the increase was significantly and positively correlated with the quantity of ethanol administered. This effect was reversible as demonstrated by a return of disappearance rates to baseline values following termination of chronic ethanol administration.

Behavioral or functional tolerance associated with ethanol intake has also been investigated in our laboratory using rhesus monkeys that had been extensively trained on a two-choice discrimination reversal task. Performance of this task under baseline conditions or following administration of a placebo that was isocaloric to the ethanol dose was compared to performance 90-min. following the nasogastric administration of 3 q/kg of ethanol. Upon initiation of ethanol administration, performance decrements were significant. However, over a 36-day period during which this same dose of ethanol was given each day prior to testing, performance gradually returned to control levels, indicating the development of functional tolerance (see Fig. 3). Blood ethanol concentration measured at the end of each test session averaged 235 mg/dl and did not vary significantly, suggesting that the changes in performance were not due simply to increased disappearance rates and, consequently, lower blood ethanol concentration at time of testing. Subsequent testing demonstrated that this tolerance was retained at both a 24-day and a 1-year interval following the original alcohol test period.

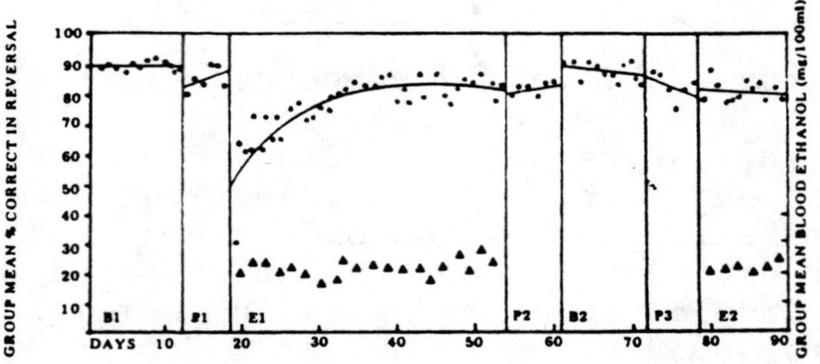

Figure 3. Group mean percentage of correct responses during trials 2-10 following cue reversal or a two choice discrimination-reversal task. Scores for individual animals were obtained by calculating the mean percentage of correct responses during reversal for each daily test session; equations for the lines were calculated using the method of least squares. Ethanol (3 g/kg) was administered nasogastrically 90 min. prior to the test session on days 19 through 54 and days 70 through 90 (E1 and E2). Group mean blood ethanol concentrations (▲) are shown for these days. Placebo solutions of isocaloric lactose were similarly administered during the 6-day placebo periods (P1, P2, and P3). During baseline testing (B1 and B2), no solutions were administered prior to testing.

In this series of studies, we have demonstrated the development of both physical dependence and tolerance to alcohol in nonhuman primates. These are two primary aspects of the addictive process and their development in nonhuman primates is a demonstration that these animals are suitable models for the systematic experimental investigation of alcoholism.

More recently, our efforts have been directed toward the investigation of behavioral dependence on alcohol in rhesus monkeys and on the development of procedures for quantitatively evaluating the severity of the withdrawal syndrome in dependent monkeys.

To study the development of behavioral dependence, we have designed an experiment that examines the effects of a conditioning procedure in which oral consumption of ethanol is accompanied by simultaneous intravenous (i.v.) ethanol infusion on voluntary oral intake. The taste of the drug is temporally paired with the apparently reinforcing pharmacological effects. Animals with intrajugular catheters were trained to make contact with a drinking tube to initiate the delivery of fluid both orally and i.v. During conditioning, 0.1 g/kg of ethanol was administered per response. Initially, the delivery was entirely by i.v. infusion, but gradually the dose was partitioned between the oral and i.v. components with the i.v. concentration decreasing as the oral concentration was increased, until the entire dose was delivered orally. A free choice between water and an 18% ethanol solution was then made available to the animal.

Of five monkeys for which data are available for the post-conditioning choice period, increased voluntary oral intake of ethanol was demonstrated in three animals. In one animal, intake exceeded 10.5 g/kg per day for 10 of the first 11 days following conditioning and withdrawal symptoms were observed on the day when intake decreased to 6.6 g/kg per day. Unfortunately, this animal died on the 14th day following conditioning. In a second animal, intake averaged 5-8 g/kg per day for 9 weeks following conditioning and in the third, the range was 3-5 g/kg per day for 2 weeks. In both these latter animals, ethanol intake declined following these periods of elevation, but was again increased following a 2-week period of forced ethanol intake. In the remaining two animals, intake was slightly elevated following conditioning, but returned to preconditioning levels within 2 weeks. Preconditioning mean ethanol intake in the entire group of monkeys did not exceed 1.5 g/kg per day at ethanol concentrations ranging from 1 to 12%. At concentrations of 12-18%, mean intake ranges from 1.5 to 2.5 g/kg per day. Thus, the quantity of ethanol consumed after conditioning by the three animals described above represents a considerable increase above control levels.

The development of methods for reproducibly and quantitatively assessing physical dependence during ethanol withdrawal has also been investigated using rhesus monkeys. Physiological tremor was chosen as the parameter to measure, since increased tremor is one of the earliest and most universal symptoms of ethanol withdrawal and since it could be recorded frequently during withdrawal with minimal disturbance to the animal. A transducer was strapped to the leg of a chair-restrained monkey and tremor was recorded on a paper chart for visual examination and on magnetic tape for further analysis by computer. Recordings were made each hour for a 33-hour withdrawal period that followed a 4-day period of ethanol administration. These tremor measurements were compared to control measurements from a 33-hour period following 4 days of chair restraint during which no ethanol was administered. After a 1-week recovery period, each animal began another cycle. Physical dependence was induced by constant infusion of ethanol solutions through intrajugular catheters to maintain blood ethanol concentration at one of four levels: 50, 100, 200, or 300 mg/dl. Each of these blood ethanol concentrations was examined in each animal in a counterbalanced order. During withdrawal, an observational score was also obtained each hour based on a rating scale of withdrawal symptoms.

These procedures have been followed with four rhesus monkeys, and the data from these studies are currently being evaluated. Analyses of variance have shown that baseline tremor measurements repeated in a single animal are statistically distinguishable, indicating that these measurements must be repeated before each ethanol administration period and used as a basis of comparison for the accompanying withdrawal period. During withdrawal, we generally observe an increase in tremor frequency and data analysis is in progress to statistically evaluate the observed differences and to determine the reproducibility of the procedure.

In the studies described above, we have attempted to develop procedures for using nonhuman primate subjects for systematically investigating the effect of stimulant and depressant drug on learning and the behavioral and physical aspects of ethanol usage. Although major research projects with chimpanzees and rhesus monkeys are necessarily restricted to relatively specialized institutional settings, these animals can prove extremely useful animal models of psychopharmacological processes that have major implications for serious public health problems in this country and throughout the world.

DIRECTIONS: Each question or incomplete statement is followed by several suggested answers or completions. Select the one that BEST answers the question or completes the statement. *PRINT THE LETTER OF THE CORRECT ANSWER IN THE SPACE AT THE RIGHT.*

1. The experiments in which ethanol was given both *orally* and *intravenously* were designed to study the development of 1.___
   A. metabolic tolerance B. behavioral tolerance
   C. behavioral dependence D. functional tolerance

2. In the experiments in which Δ^9-THC was smoked, the amounts of drug inhaled 2.___
   A. were controlled by forcing the subjects to maintain a constant pressure on the pipe for 5 seconds before getting a reward
   B. were controlled by using a 10 second differential reinforcement schedule
   C. were maintained constant by injecting measured amounts of the drug into the cigarettes
   D. proved to be impossible to control rigorously

3. In experiments in which physical dependence was studied, hourly comparisons of tremor were made between a subject 3.___
   A. after 4 days of chair restraint and the same subject after another 4 days of chair restraint and alcohol administration
   B. after four days of chair restraint and another subject similarly treated
   C. after four days of chair restraint and another subject after four days of chair restraint and alcohol administration
   D. with a blood ethanol level of 50 mg/dl and another subject with blood ethanol level of 300 mg/dl

4. According to this article, the BEST kind of task to be used in assessing the effects of drugs on learning would be one that is 4.___
   A. learned prior to drug administration
   B. basically a new procedure each time
   C. learned for the first time under the influence of the drug
   D. independent of any rewards

5. Given the design of these experiments, behavioral dependence could be said to have been established if, after a period of conditioning, the animals 5.___
   A. chose to drink a great deal of alcohol
   B. appeared to have an aversion to alcohol
   C. manifested withdrawal symptoms if alcohol were not available
   D. showed a rapid rate of ethanol metabolism

6. Metabolic studies of the blood of chimpanzees during chronic ethanol administration indicate 6.___
   A. ethanol accumulates in the blood
   B. the rate of methanol disappearance is increased
   C. the rate of ethanol disappearance is increased
   D. the magnitude of the increase in the rate of ethanol disappearance is inversely related to the quantity of ethanol given

7. In the two weeks following conditioning, ethanol ingestion 7.___
   A. was substantially greater in three animals than in the preconditioning period
   B. was approximately the same as in the preconditioning period
   C. could not be followed in more than one animal because the others died
   D. was very low, in the range of 1.5 g/kg/day

8. In these experiments, when the subjects that had been treated with a drug for several weeks demonstrated an accelerated rate of disappearance of that drug from the blood, it was considered evidence for 8.___
   A. functional tolerance
   B. behavioral tolerance
   C. metabolic tolerance
   D. addiction

9. The test that was used in the investigation of behavioral tolerance associated with chronic ethanol administration was 9.___
   A. not described in detail in the article
   B. the same as the task used in the tests involving Δ^9-THC
   C. a sequential response task
   D. a task on a differential reinforcement schedule

10. A _____ test was used in the investigation of behavioral tolerance associated with chronic ethanol administration. 10.___
   A. behavioral task on a differential reinforcement schedule
   B. sequential response task
   C. visual discrimination task
   D. two-choice discrimination-reversal task

11. The functional tolerance to ethanol that was developed 11.___
   A. persisted for as long as a year after the original testing (36-day) period
   B. could not be demonstrated 24 days after the 36-day test
   C. could not be clearly demonstrated during the 36-day period
   D. could only be demonstrated if alcohol continued to be given on a daily basis

12. Signs of physical dependence on ethanol were produced 12.___
   A. by nasogastric administration of 3 g/kg of ethanol
   B. by nasogastric administration of three doses of ethanol in one day
   C. by nasogastric administration of one dose of ethanol/day for three days
   D. when blood ethanol concentrations were maintained above zero for four or more days

13. When an error was made during an SRT training session, 13.___
   A. a buzzer delivered a shock to the animal
   B. an M & M candy reinforcer was retracted
   C. a 2-second timeout went into effect
   D. all the house lights and lever lights were extinguished

14. In testing for the development of behavioral tolerance in response to chronic ethanol administration, evidence was sought that 14.___
   A. performance continues to deteriorate throughout the course of the experiment
   B. after initial impairment, performance tends to improve even though blood levels of ethanol are held constant
   C. removal of alcohol leads to withdrawal symptoms
   D. blood levels of ethanol decrease even though equal doses of ethanol are given

15. One of the MAJOR objectives of the studies using ethanol was to 15.___
   A. demonstrate some of the characteristics of the addiction process
   B. determine what are lethal amounts of ethanol for non-human primates
   C. study behavior in intoxicated monkeys
   D. determine the rate of blood ethanol disappearance in addicted subjects

16. A MAJOR drawback to the use of chimpanzees and other large apes in psychopharmacologic investigation is 16.___
   A. their size
   B. their inquisitive nature
   C. that they are poor models for experiments on the effects of drugs on behavior
   D. that their use is restricted to specialized institutional settings

17. The sequential response task (SRT) proved to be a better measure of learning than the DRL spaced response test because SRT 17.___
   A. proved to be more appropriate to monkeys
   B. made it possible to compare learning acquisition on drug days with learning on placebo days
   C. was less distracting than the DRL spaced response test
   D. does not depend on visual cues, whereas the DRL spaced response test does

18. Following the period of ethanol administration, recordings of leg tremor were made during the succeeding 18.___
A. four days B. thirty-three hours
C. one week D. eleven days

19. Which of the following would be evidence of the development of behavioral dependence on alcohol? 19.___
A. A rapid rate of ethanol metabolism
B. Appearance of withdrawal symptoms when alcohol is not available
C. An aversion to alcohol on the part of the animals
D. A tendency to drink a great deal of alcohol

20. An integral procedure in training for sequential response task testing is the 20.___
A. use of a stimulus fading device
B. surgical preparation of the brain for placement of indwelling catheters
C. use of a candy reinforcer before and after each lever pull
D. use of a board having many levers, each a different color

21. Which of the following drugs was labeled a stimulant? 21.___
A. Ethanol B. Diethylpropion
C. Δ^9-THC D. Meprobamate

22. Which of the following statements CORRECTLY describes some aspect of sequential response task testing? 22.___
A. The subject is required to repeat the same task every day.
B. The test session is 50 minutes, or less if the subject has successfully learned the sequence of levers.
C. M & M candy reinforcers are delivered at 10 and 20 second intervals.
D. The six levers are uniformly illuminated.

23. In the ethanol ingestion experiments in which animals were conditioned, how many animals were available for post-conditioning testing? 23.___
A. One B. Five C. Six D. Eleven

24. In the experiments in which withdrawal was quantitatively assessed, physical dependence was produced in monkeys by 24.___
A. allowing them free access to ethanol in their drinking water
B. restraining them in a chair and forcing them to drink 18% ethanol
C. inducing a fine tremor of the leg
D. maintaining blood ethanol concentration at four levels, ranging between 50 and 300 mg/dl

25. According to this study, the BEST way to evaluate the effect of a drug on learning is to test the ability of the animal, while under the effect of the drug, to 25.___
A. learn a new task each test day
B. repeat the same task each test day

C. repeat the same task over a long period, with no intervening training
D. do the same task each test day, but at a different rate of speed

26. The reason for giving ethanol both orally and by intravenous infusion is to 26.___
A. make the animals more intoxicated than they would have been with oral ingestion alone
B. demonstrate that orally administered ethanol disappears more rapidly from the blood than intravenously administered ethanol
C. provide a reward for animals undergoing task training
D. temporally pair the taste of ethanol with the pharmacological effects produced by intravenous administration

27. The MAJOR point made in this report is that 27.___
A. learning ability is adversely affected by drugs
B. inhalation of a drug via smoking is not as reliable a way of delivering a drug as oral administration
C. nonhuman primates made good models for the study of effects of drugs on learning and behavior
D. monkeys become addicted to Δ^9-THC

28. Which of the following observations, made during or after chronic administration of ethanol, makes it possible to say that ethanol causes physical dependence? 28.___
A. Withdrawal symptoms occurred when blood levels of ethanol fell.
B. Methanol was observed to accumulate in the blood.
C. Rate of disappearance of ethanol from the blood increased.
D. Performance of discrimination-reversal tasks was adversely affected.

29. Which of the following terms is a synonym for *behavioral tolerance*? 29.___
A. Metabolic tolerance B. Physical dependence
C. Functional tolerance D. Discrimination tolerance

30. Nonhuman primates are good models for experiments on human alcohol use because 30.___
A. they develop a great fondness for alcohol
B. they can be given large quantities of alcohol over long periods of time without deleterious effects
C. it is possible and convenient to monitor blood ethanol levels from minute to minute
D. it was possible to demonstrate two primary aspects of the human addictive process in the nonhuman primates

31. The MAJOR disadvantage of the spaced task for studying the effects of drugs on learning is that it is 31.___
A. too simple
B. learned entirely before the administration of drugs and cannot be varied thereafter

C. too dependent on extraneous clues, like lights
D. too distracting for use in nonhuman primates

32. For experiments in which procedures were involved, the animal of choice was the — 32.___
A. chimpanzee
B. orangutan
C. gorilla
D. rhesus monkey

33. The use of large apes for research on the effects of drugs on behavior — 33.___
A. was first demonstrated in chimpanzees trained to do a sequential response task
B. was shown to be feasible in a limited number of experiments on Δ^9-THC treated chimpanzees
C. is severely limited by the natural inquisitiveness of large apes
D. is limited by the inability of large apes to learn sequential tasks

34. Nasogastric administration of 3 g/kg of ethanol every day for over a month led to — 34.___
A. a progressive and continuing decrease in performance levels
B. relatively constant blood ethanol levels at the end of each session
C. a decreased rate of disappearance of ethanol from the blood
D. a significant increase in body weight

35. To which of the following nonhuman primates does the name Pan Troglodyte apply? — 35.___
A. Chimpanzees
B. Orangutans
C. Gorillas
D. Rhesus monkeys

36. Metabolic tolerance to alcohol was established by the fact that during chronic administration of ethanol — 36.___
A. its rate of disappearance from the blood increased
B. methanol accumulated in the blood
C. ethanol was converted into methanol
D. the rate of ethanol disappearance from the blood increased and remained elevated long after termination of ethanol administration

37. A MAJOR advantage of the sequential response task in studies of the effects of drugs on learning is that — 37.___
A. while the basic nature of the task remains the same, the animal must learn a new procedure each day
B. the nature of the task forces the animal to rely more on brightness cues than on memory
C. it provides a good test of color discrimination
D. the six-lever sequence appears ideally suited to nonhuman primates

38. Figure 1 indicates that 38.___
   A. the great ape named *Din* has the lowest tolerance to THC
   B. in general, the efficiency in the response of all three apes was reduced when THC was taken
   C. the 20 second DRL was experimentally most effective
   D. the great ape named *Peck* initially had the most efficient responses

39. The experiments using ethanol demonstrate that 39.___
   A. ethanol severely impairs the learning of a sequential response task
   B. many aspects of human drug addiction can be reproduced and studied in nonhuman primates
   C. it is impossible to demonstrate true withdrawal in monkeys
   D. depressant drugs are antagonists of stimulant drugs

40. What was the MAJOR point made in this article? 40.___
   A. Learning ability is adversely affected by drugs.
   B. Smoking and drug usage is hazardous to the health of nonhuman primates and, therefore, of humans.
   C. Nonhuman primates make good models for the study of the effects of drugs on learning and behavior.
   D. Rhesus monkeys are more effective subjects for drug-effect studies than other primates.

41. Which of the following drugs produced a *decrease* in learning at dosage levels NOT associated with general physical impairment? 41.___
   A. Secobarbital B. Glutethimide
   C. Phentermine D. Butabarbital

42. Which of the following statements CORRECTLY describes a procedure in sequential response task testing? 42.___
   A. The subject is required to learn a new task sequence every day.
   B. The testing period is the length of time required to complete a sequence of six levers, no matter how long this takes.
   C. M & M candy reinforcers are delivered at 10 and 20 second intervals.
   D. The six levers are illuminated at an unvarying intensity of light.

43. At the end of the conditioning period in the ethanol ingestion experiments, 43.___
   A. all the ethanol was delivered orally
   B. all the ethanol was delivered intravenously
   C. 18% of the ethanol was delivered intravenously
   D. no ethanol was delivered

44. One of the MAJOR problems encountered in the experiments on the effect of smoking on spaced responding was the fact that 44.___
   A. large apes tend to be too inquisitive for this kind of study

B. the subjects were all given extensive training on the task prior to drug testing so that performance could not be directly related to the effects of drugs
C. the subjects refused to smoke cigarettes containing Δ^9-THC
D. the 10-second DRL schedule proved to be too short

45. An IMPORTANT part of the procedure for training for sequential task testing involves the 45.___
A. use of light cues of varying intensity
B. routine monitoring of blood concentrations of inhaled compounds
C. use of a candy reinforcer before and after each lever pull
D. use of transilluminated discs of various colors

46. Learning, as measured by sequential response task testing, is considered to have taken place when the animal 46.___
A. correctly pulls a number of levers in sequence with all stimulus lights identically illuminated
B. pulls the same number of levers in the same sequence one day after learning the sequence
C. no longer required the M & M candy reward to pull the levers in the correct sequence
D. correctly pulls a number of levers, each with a different brightness cue, in sequence

47. Alterations in blood methanol levels during chronic ethanol administration 47.___
A. led to a decrease in physical tolerance to ethanol
B. causes a change in the disappearance rate of ethanol in the blood
C. may be caused by competitive inhibition of the enzyme system that metabolizes both alcohols
D. were interpreted as evidence for physical dependence on methanol

48. Physical dependence on ethanol has been produced in chimpanzees by 48.___
A. administering ethanol by means of a nasogastric tube
B. infusing ethanol through surgically implanted catheters
C. substituting ethanol for the drinking water
D. including alcohol in their liquid diet in increasing doses

49. In the study of the development of behavioral tolerance, performance of a task by an ethanol-treated subject was compared with performance of that task by 49.___
A. other subjects given a placebo isocaloric with ethanol
B. the same subject given a placebo isocaloric with ethanol
C. other untreated subjects
D. untreated subjects 36 days later

50. The effects of administration of diazepam at doses that did not cause general physical impairment were similar to those produced by 50.___
   A. metamphetamine
   B. drugs having a tranquilizing effect
   C. doses that did cause general physical impairment
   D. drugs classified as stimulants

1. C	11. A	21. B	31. B	41. C
2. D	12. D	22. B	32. D	42. A
3. A	13. D	23. B	33. B	43. A
4. B	14. B	24. D	34. B	44. B
5. A	15. A	25. A	35. A	45. A
6. C	16. D	26. D	36. A	46. A
7. A	17. B	27. C	37. A	47. C
8. C	18. B	28. A	38. B	48. D
9. A	19. D	29. C	39. B	49. B
10. D	20. A	30. D	40. C	50. B

BASIC FUNDAMENTALS OF INORGANIC CHEMISTRY

CONCISE TEXT

CONTENTS

BASIC FUNDAMENTALS OF

INORGANIC CHEMISTRY

CONCISE TEXT

1. Chemistry explained. Chemistry is the science dealing with the composition of materials and the changes in composition which these materials undergo. Because it is such a tremendously large subject, chemistry is divided into many specialized fields–inorganic chemistry, dealing with the elements and mineral material; organic chemistry, dealing with material originating from living matter or from synthetic sources and composed largely of carbon; physical chemistry; biochemistry; etc. This chapter will be concerned with inorganic chemistry and will cover the basic elements and compounds of pharmaceutical significance.

2. Importance of chemistry. There is no denying that chemistry plays an important role in the lives of all human beings.

a. General importance. Chemistry answers many questions that arise in everyday life. It explains, for example, why substances burn, why ice melts, why water freezes, why antiseptics kill germs, why some soaps are ineffective in hard water, and why butter turns rancid. Many of the daily phenomena you witness can be explained by chemistry.

b. Importance to the pharmacist. Besides the general importance in everyday life, chemistry is particularly important to the pharmacist. Here are just a few of the many reasons that the pharmacist studies chemistry.

(1) Body chemistry. In order to understand the actions of medicinals on the body, we must know the normal and abnormal chemistry of the body.

(2) Actions of chemical compounds. Different chemical compounds bring about different responses in the body. From a knowledge of the body chemistry and the chemistry of the medicinal compounds, we are able to understand the curative effects of drugs which we will be compounding and dispensing.

(3) Predicting reactions. In the compounding of medicinals, chemical reactions are frequent. In order to be able to mix ingredients in the proper order, to add the proper augmentative ingredients, to prevent or modify undesirable reactions, the pharmacist must be aware of the possible chemical reactions which can occur. The study of chemistry gives us this knowledge.

3. Matter. In chemistry we are concerned with matter. It is one of the basic considerations of both chemistry and physics.

a. Definition of matter. Matter is anything which occupies space and has weight. If you look about, you will see matter. The desk, the books, the walls, the clothing you wear, you yourself; all are composed of matter. You may say that if something occupies space it must have weight; and conversely if something has weight, it must occupy space. This is essentially true.

b. Matter versus energy. Besides matter, there are many things around us that we sense or feel. Electricity, rays of light or sound–these things are not material and yet they exist. Since they do not occupy space or have weight, they are not matter. They are forms of energy. Before the atomic theory was formulated, it was thought that matter and energy were completely different things. Matter was thought to be indestructible and, certainly, energy could never be transposed into matter. The thinking has been greatly altered in the past few years. With the advent of the atomic bomb and nuclear fission, it is now possible to convert matter to energy and energy to matter.

c. Physical states of matter. Matter exists in one of three physical states—as a solid, a liquid, or a gas. Liquids and gases taken together are called fluids.

(1) Solids. Solids have a definite shape and volume. They are rigid. Examples of solids are blocks of wood, pieces of steel, rocks, and sand.

(2) Liquids. Liquids have a definite volume but take the shape of any container into which they are placed. Water, mercury, alcohol, and oils are liquids.

(3) Gases. Gases do not have a definite shape nor a definite volume. They assume not only the shape of their container, but also the volume. Gases may be expanded or compressed, depending upon the temperature and pressure in their container. Thus, the amount of air forced into an automobile tire would, if released, expand to fill a large weather balloon. For this reason, gases must be measured at specified temperatures and pressures.

d. Properties of matter. Matter possesses two types of properties—physical and chemical. Characteristics such as smell, color, shape, freezing point, boiling point, and solubility are said to be physical properties of matter. Energy content; reactions with other substances; reactions due to light, heat, and electricity are chemical properties. From the physical and chemical properties exhibited by a substance, it is possible to isolate, identify, and classify the particular substance.

e. Classification of matter. Matter is either homogeneous, that is, uniform throughout, or it is heterogeneous or not uniform.

(1) Homogeneous matter. Pure elements and compounds are homogeneous. They are uniform throughout.

(a) Elements. An element is matter which cannot be broken down into simpler matter by present ordinary chemical means. Examples of elements are oxygen, iron, gold, mercury, hydrogen, carbon, and the others listed in table 3-1.

(b) Compounds. A compound is matter composed of two or more elements combined chemically in definite proportions to form a molecule. Compounds may be decomposed into their component elements by chemical means. The compound formed from two or more elements does not have the properties of its parent elements. Hydrogen, one of the parent elements making up water, is a gas which burns in the presence of oxygen. Oxygen, also a gas, which supports combustion, is the other parent element. Water, the compound formed from the two gaseous elements, is a liquid. It does not burn nor support combustion; on the contrary, it is the first thing one thinks of when there is a fire to be extinguished. Sodium chloride, another compound, is harmless, commonly used table salt. Its parent elements are not harmless, however. Table salt, a crystalline white solid, is formed from the parent elements of sodium and chlorine, both very poisonous elements.

(2) Heterogeneous matter. Impure substances are mixtures of elements or compounds. They are heterogeneous, that is, not uniform. These mixtures can be separated into the pure matter of which they are composed by physical means. The properties of mixtures are the sum total of the individual properties of their components. A combination of sand and water is a mixture. This mixture can be separated by purely physical means. If the mixture is filtered, the water passes through, leaving the sand as a residue on the filter paper.

f. Elements. More than 100 different elements have been identified to date. Table 1 lists these elements, their symbols, atomic numbers, and atomic weights. The elements most frequently used in pharmacy and medicine are marked with an asterisk. About 33 elements can be said to have wide use in our field.

(1) Elemental symbols. Symbols are widely used to represent one atom of an element. Much unnecessary writing is eliminated by use of the proper symbol. As you will see when we discuss formulas and reactions later in this chapter, these symbols are invaluable in describing chemical reactions. The symbol for one atom of an element is generally formed from the first or first two letters of the name; the first letter in capitals and the second, if it occurs, in the lower case. Thus, the symbol for Carbon is C; for Iodine, I; for Aluminum, Al; for Lithium, Li; and for Silicon, Si. Frequently, the symbol or abbreviation will be derived from the Latin name for the element such as Au for gold, from aurum; Ag for silver, from argentum; Na for sodium, from natrium; and K for potassium, from kalium. It is extremely important that you know the symbols for the more common elements. You should be able to list the symbols from memory if you are given the names of the elements.

Table 1. Elements, Symbols, Atomic Numbers, Atomic Weights in Alphabetical Order

ELEMENT	SYMB.	AT. NO.	AT. WT.	ELEMENT	SYMB.	AT. NO.	AT. WT.	ELEMENT	SYMB.	AT. NO.	AT. WT.
Actinium	Ac	89	227.00	Hafnium	Hf	72	178.49	Praseodymium	Pr	59	140.907
* Aluminum	Al	13	26.98	Helium	He	2	4.0026	Promethium	Pm	61	147.00
Americium	Am	95	243.00	Holmium	Ho	67	164.94	Protoactinium	Pa	91	231.00
Antimony	Sb	51	121.75	* Hydrogen	H	1	1.00797	* Radium	Ra	88	226.00
Argon	Ar	18	39.948	Indium	In	49	114.82	Radon	Rn	86	222.00
* Arsenic	As	33	74.92	* Iodine	I	53	126.9044	Rhenium	Re	75	186.2
Astatine	At	85	210.00	Iridium	Ir	77	192.2	Rhodium	Rh	45	102.905
* Barium	Ba	56	137.34	* Iron	Fe	26	55.847	Rubidium	Rb	37	85.47
Berkelium	Bk	97	247.00	Krypton	Kr	36	83.80	Ruthenium	Ru	44	101.07
Beryllium	Be	4	9.0122	Lanthanum	La	57	138.91	Samarium	Sm	62	150.35
* Bismuth	Bi	83	208.980	Lawrencium	Lw	103	257.00	Scandium	Sc	21	44.956
* Boron	B	5	10.811	* Lead	Pb	82	207.19	* Selenium	Se	34	78.96
* Bromine	Br	35	79.909	* Lithium	Li	3	6.939	* Silicon	Si	14	28.086
Cadmium	Cd	48	112.40	Lutetium	Lu	71	174.97	* Silver	Ag	47	107.870
* Calcium	Ca	20	40.08	* Magnesium	Mg	12	24.312	* Sodium	Na	11	22.9898
Californium	Cf	98	249.00	* Manganese	Mn	25	54.9380	* Strontium	Sr	38	87.62
* Carbon	C	6	12.011	Mendelevium	Md	101	256.00	* Sulfur	S	16	32.064
Cerium	Ce	58	140.12	* Mercury	Hg	80	200.59	Tantalum	Ta	73	180.948
Cesium	Cs	55	132.905	Molybdenum	Mo	42	95.94	Technetium	Tc	43	99.00
* Chlorine	Cl	17	35.453	Neodymium	Nd	60	144.24	Tellurium	Te	52	127.60
Chromium	Cr	24	51.996	Neon	Ne	10	20.183	Terbium	Tb	65	158.924
* Cobalt	Co	27	58.9332	Neptunium	Np	93	237.00	Thallium	Tl	81	204.37
* Copper	Cu	29	63.54	Nickel	Ni	28	58.71	Thorium	Th	90	232.038
Curium	Cm	96	247.00	Niobium	Nb	41	92.906	Thulium	Tm	69	168.934
Dysphrosium	Dy	66	162.50	* Nitrogen	N	7	14.0067	Tin	Sn	50	118.69
Einsteinium	Es	99	254.00	Nobelium	No	102	254.00	Titanium	Ti	22	47.90
Erbium	Er	68	167.26	Osmium	Os	76	190.2	Tungsten	W	74	183.85
Europium	Eu	63	151.96	* Oxygen	O	8	15.9994	Uranium	U	92	238.03
Fermium	Fm	100	253.00	Palladium	Pd	46	106.4	Vanadium	V	23	50.942
* Fluorine	F	9	18.998	* Phosphorus	P	15	30.9738	Xenon	Xe	54	131.30
Francium	Fr	87	223.00	Platinum	Pt	78	195.09	Ytterbium	Yb	70	173.04
Gadolinium	Gd	64	157.25	Plutonium	Pu	94	242.00	Yttrium	Y	39	88.905
Gallium	Ga	31	69.72	Polonium	Po	84	210.00	* Zinc	Zn	30	65.37
Germanium	Ge	32	72.59	* Potassium	K	19	39.102	Zirconium	Zr	40	91.22
* Gold	Au	79	196.967								

* Denotes elements most common to pharmacy and medicine.

(2) Classification of elements. Elements can be classified as metals, nonmetals, or metalloids.

(a) Metals. Metals are lustrous elements which can conduct heat and electricity and can also reflect heat and light. Some metals can be drawn out into fine wires (ductile) while others can be hammered into thin sheets (malleable). Metals have a positive valence. More will be said about valence and metals later in this chapter. Some examples of metals are aluminum, copper, calcium, gold, iron, lead, silver, tin, and zinc.

(b) Nonmetals. Nonmetals are almost direct opposites of metals. They do not conduct heat or electricity well. They cannot be drawn into wire or hammered into sheets because of their brittleness. Sulfur, iodine, and carbon are solid nonmetals; bromine is a liquid nonmetal; oxygen, nitrogen, and chlorine are gaseous nonmetals.

(c) Metalloids. Metalloids exhibit some of the properties of metals and some of the properties of nonmetals. Arsenic and antimony are examples of this category. Arsenic resembles the metals in being lustrous, but it does not resemble the metals in being brittle. Antimony, an almost silver-white, hard, lustrous substance, appears to be a metal. However, it is a metalloid because it also has the nonmetal's brittleness.

(3) Compounds.

(a) Definition. Compounds are composed of two or more elements combined in a definite proportion by weight. By combining one atom of carbon with two atoms of oxygen we get the compound, carbon dioxide. This chemical action is represented by the formula

$$C + O_2 \longrightarrow CO_2$$

Similarly, by combining one atom of sodium (Na) and one atom of chlorine (Cl), we form the compound sodium chloride (NaCl).

(b) Acid-base system. There are several systems by which compounds can be classified, but generally a system is based on the principle of grouping together the like properties or like origins. The system based on properties is the "acid-base" system. In this system, we categorize compounds into three groups–acids, bases, and salts.

1. Acids. Acids are compounds containing hydrogen. During certain reactions this hydrogen can be easily replaced by a metal. Hydrochloric acid (HCl) is an acid.

2. Bases. Bases are compounds which will react with acids to form salts and water. Sodium hydroxide (NaOH) is a base.

3. Salts. Salts are compounds formed from the reaction of acids with bases. Sodium chloride (NaCl) is a salt.

(c) Inorganic and organic compounds. Based upon origin, compounds may be classified as organic or inorganic. The organic compounds are those derived from carbon, i.e., fuel oil, gasoline, kerosene, and petroleum. The inorganic compounds are not derived from carbon, i.e., water, aluminum hydroxide, and potassium permanganate.

g. Energy. Energy is the ability to do work. It is a universal property of matter. Basically, there are two types of energy, potential and kinetic.

(1) Potential energy. Potential energy is energy at rest. It is also called energy of position. It is inherent, stored, or available. The energy stored in fuels, the water behind a dam, the wound spring of an alarm clock are examples of matter with potential energy. In order to accomplish work, this potential energy must be converted to kinetic energy.

(2) Kinetic energy. Kinetic energy is energy in motion. Running water, burning coal or fuel, a running clock—all display kinetic energy.

(3) Forms of energy. Energy, either potential or kinetic, can take various forms. Mechanical energy, chemical energy, atomic energy, heat energy, and light energy are all forms of energy. One form can readily be converted to another. Think of a steam engine providing mechanical energy to turn a dynamo. The steam is produced by the burning of some fuel (heat energy) to vaporize water into steam. The steam produced drives a shaft which turns a wheel (mechanical energy). The wheel in turn causes a dynamo to produce electrical energy which can be utilized to operate a lamp (light energy) or an electric heater (heat energy) or a motor (mechanical energy). The cycle can go on and on.

h. Some basic laws of chemistry. Now that you have learned what matter and energy are, let us look at some laws governing them. The balancing of chemical equations, which we will discuss later, is based upon these laws.

(1) Law of constant composition. Substances reacting to form compounds do so in a

definite ratio by weight. Thus, for any specimen of a given compound, the elements and their quantities will be exactly the same. Thus, any 58.5 Gm. specimen of sodium chloride will contain 23 grams of sodium and 35.5 grams of chlorine.

(2) Law of conservation of mass. Mass can neither be gained nor lost in a chemical reaction. You have learned that sodium (Na) and chlorine (Cl) react to form sodium chloride; and they react in a definite proportion by weight. Thus, 46 grams of sodium reacted with 71 grams of chlorine will produce 117 grams of sodium chloride. There has been neither gain nor loss in the total weight: 46 + 71 = 117.

(3) Law of conservation of energy. Energy, like mass, cannot be created or destroyed by chemical means. It is possible, however, to convert one form of energy to another. When coal is burned in the presence of oxygen, the carbon and oxygen unite in definite proportions by weight and no mass is gained or lost. However, there is a change in the form of energy. Chemical energy possessed by the carbon and oxygen is converted through this reaction into heat energy, but no energy has been created or destroyed.

(4) Matter and energy related. We have stated that neither matter nor energy can be created or destroyed. Matter can be converted to energy and energy to matter, as Albert Einstein theorized and experiments later proved. This is because matter and energy are two forms of the same thing.

i. Changes in matter. You previously learned that matter has physical and chemical energy. Changes in matter, be they physical or chemical changes, are caused by energy changes.

(1) Physical changes in matter.

(a) Solid to liquid to gas. The physical state of matter can be changed by varying the temperature and pressure in the environment. At temperatures above 0° C. (32° F.), ice will turn into a liquid; at temperatures above 100° C. (212° F.), this liquid will become a gas. Most substances follow this pattern from solid to liquid to gas, and return in reverse order.

(b) Solid to gas. Certain substances, because of their nature, do not pass through the liquid state. They go directly from solids to gases and on cooling back to solids. Dry ice, when warmed, evaporates into a gas (carbon dioxide). It never becomes a liquid. When a substance goes directly from the solid state to the gaseous state without passing through the liquid the process is known as *sublimation.*

(2) Chemical changes in matter. A chemical change is a change in composition. When matter changes chemically, it loses its original identity and a new substance, or substances, is formed. The burning of coal produces water and carbon dioxide. Such chemical changes are termed *reactions.*

(3) Importance of such changes. These changes in matter are extremely important to us as pharmacists in the formation of new and useful products and dosage forms. Changes in matter may also bring about or eliminate certain compounding problems which will be discussed later.

j. Atomic structure. The atom is the smallest particle of an element that can enter into combination with other elements. It is the smallest particle of an element which can display the chemical properties of that element. Thus, an atom of sodium and an atom of chlorine, each having its own identity, can combine chemically to form the compound sodium chloride which has properties different from either the sodium or the chlorine that make it up. The simplest atom, that of hydrogen, is made up of a nucleus (center) which contains one *proton.* Around this proton nucleus orbits an *electron,* much the same as the earth circles the sun (fig. 1).

(1) The proton. The proton is that portion of the atom's nucleus which has a charge

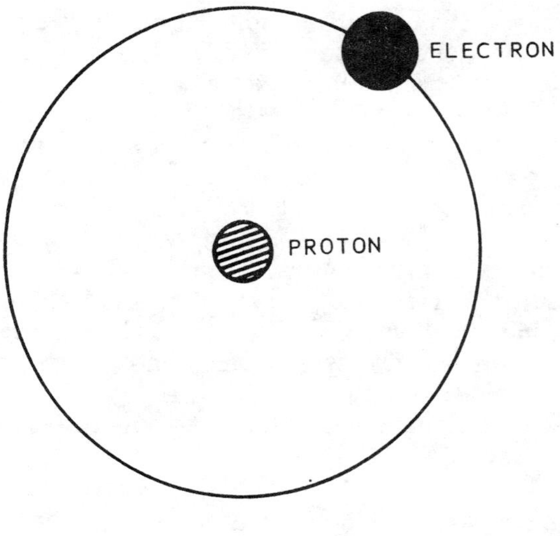

Figure 1. Structure of the hydrogen atom.

of plus one and a mass of approximately one on the atomic weight scale. It is the unit of positive electricity.

(2) The electron. The electron, the unit of negative electricity, carries a charge of minus one. It has a mass of 1/1837, that of a proton, and therefore contributes very little toward the weight of the atom. The electrons orbit in definite paths about the nucleus, and are held in this orbit by the electrostatic attraction between the positive protons and the negative electrons. Since matter is normally electrically neutral, the number of protons within the nucleus is equal to the number of orbiting electrons.

(3) The neutron. Another particle found in the atomic nucleus of all atoms except simple hydrogen is the neutron. As its name suggests, it is neutral, having no charge of electricity. The neutron has a mass approximately the same as that of a proton, and together with the proton makes up the entire nucleus of the atom. Since the electron is of negligible weight, the mass of an atom is concentrated mainly in the nucleus.

k. Atomic weights. Long ago, chemists determined that oxygen was 16 times heavier than hydrogen. To establish a table of relative weights for the elements so they could determine reactions, they arbitrarily assigned the relative weight of 16 to oxygen, so that hydrogen which was 1/16th as heavy as oxygen would have a value not less than one. Hydrogen, the lightest of the elements, has a value of 1. A helium atom was determined to weigh one-fourth as much as oxygen, and therefore its relative weight is ¼ of 16 or 4. With meticulous calculation, the remaining elements were compared and assigned atomic weights. In 1930, physicists adopted oxygen with a weight of 16 as the standard, but subsequent research disclosed that carbon, with a weight of 12, was much more advantageous. As a result, the International Union of Pure and Applied Physics adopted it in 1960. The International Union of Pure and Applied Chemistry followed suit in 1961 and published a revised table of atomic weights on the basis of an assigned value of 12 for carbon. It was recommended that the new table have universal use beginning January 1, 1962. Today, the standard element is carbon and the atomic weight assigned to it is 12. An atom of one element is different from an atom of another element, and there are as many different atoms as there are elements. The atoms of each element have a definite average weight. These atomic weights are set down in table 3-1.

l. Atomic number. The atomic number of an element is equal to the number of protons in the nucleus. You can see from the table of elements that each element has an atomic number different from the next by 1. The atomic numbers range from 1 for hydrogen to 103 for lawrencium. It is the number of protons, and thus the atomic number which identifies the element.

m. Determining the number of neutrons in an atom. The only substantial weight in an atom, aside from the protons, is due to the neutrons; thus, by subtracting the atomic number which represents the number of protons from the atomic weight which represents both protons and neutrons, you can determine the number of neutrons in any atom. Using helium as an example, you find from the table that it has an atomic number of 2, but an atomic weight of 4. By subtracting 2 from 4, you find that helium has 2 neutrons in its nucleus. Lithium has an atomic number of 3 and an atomic weight of 7. It, then, must have 4 neutrons.

n. Isotopes. Elements may exist in several forms, differing only in weight, not in atomic number. Each form contains the same number of protons and electrons, but varies in the number of neutrons. Some of these different forms are naturally occurring; others are artificially prepared. These different forms of the same element are called *isotopes.* They do not differ in chemical properties. *For example,* hydrogen exists in three isotopic forms. The most common is the isotopic form to which we generally allude, having one proton, one electron, and no neutrons. The second form consists of one proton, one electron, and one neutron. This second form of hydrogen is often referred to as heavy hydrogen, and chemists have named it *deuterium.* The third form has one proton, two neutrons, and one electron. This form is called *tritium.*

o. Electron shells. The electrons orbiting around the nucleus of an atom have a definite pattern.

(1) Energy levels. There are various energy levels at which these electrons can revolve. The first or innermost shell is called the K shell. The second and more distant from the nucleus is

the L shell; then the M, N, etc. These shells are sometimes numbered, the K shell being shell 1 and L being 2.

(2) Saturation of orbits. There is a limit or saturation point at each level and generally one level must be saturated before another is started. The limits to the number of electrons possible in the respective shells are as follows:

K–limit of 2 orbiting electrons
L–limit of 8 orbiting electrons
M–limit of 18 orbiting electrons
N–limit of 32 orbiting electrons
O–limit of 32 orbiting electrons
P–limit of 18 orbiting electrons
Q–limit of 8 orbiting electrons

(3) Electron configuration. Knowing this, we can determine the exact configuration of the electrons revolving about any given elemental nucleus. *For example,* helium has two electrons and therefore only one shell. Both of helium's electrons orbit at the K level of energy. Lithium has 3 protons (atomic number = 3), and therefore 3 orbiting electrons. Two of these electrons are in the K shells, giving it saturation; the remaining electron is in the L shell. Sodium has an atomic number of 11 and thus has 11 protons and 11 electrons. To meet the saturation requirements, 2 must be at the K level, 8 at the L level, and the remaining 1 at the M level.

p. Periodic table and law. To study chemistry element by element and compound by compound would be a nearly impossible feat. For this reason, chemists have grouped the elements according to their properties and by studying one member of the group thoroughly, the remaining members may be compared to it. This grouping of elements is called the periodic table.

(1) Periodic table. Table 2 shows a modified version of the periodic table. This table is invaluable to us because of the wide variety of information it offers. Contained in this table are the elements grouped by properties and atomic number; and the atomic numbers, atomic weights, and even the electron configuration of the atoms.

(2) Periodic law. The periodic law, based upon the periodic table, can be correctly stated as follows: The chemical properties of elements are periodic functions of their atomic numbers. That is, chemical properties recur at intervals.

q. How to use the periodic table. Figure 2 illustrates the significance of the numbers and

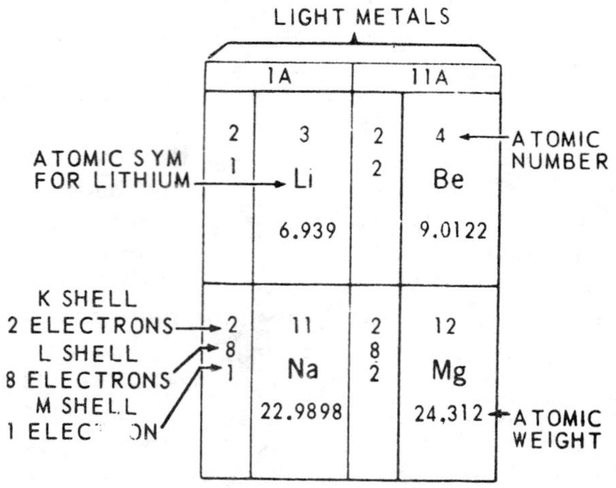

Figure [illegible]. Identifying the components of the periodic table.

letters in the periodic chart. The groups are specified at the tops of the columns (IA, IIA). The narrow column at the left of each element contains a number or series of numbers which outline the electron distribution. The uppermost number is the K shell; below it, the L shell; and so on. The larger blocks contain, in the center, the chemical symbol for the particular element. This is why you must memorize the elemental symbols. Above the symbol is the number representing the atomic number of the element. At present the numbers progress from 1 to 103. Below the symbol appears another number which is the atomic weight of the element. At the tops of the columns are descriptions, categorizing the elements into light metals, transition heavy metals, nonmetals, and inert gases.

4. Formation of compounds. Now that you are familiar with the structure of atoms, we may progress to molecules and compounds. Atoms of elements can combine to form molecules. A molecule is the smallest particle of a compound that can exist and retain the properties of that compound.

a. Valence.

(1) Definition. The capacity of an element to combine with another element to form a molecule is called *valence.* It is the electrons in the outermost shell which determine this combining capacity and for this reason the electrons of the outermost shell are called *valence electrons.*

Table 2. Periodic Table of the Elements

1 H 1.00797 (1)	2 He 4.0026 (2)

LIGHT METALS — TRANSITION HEAVY METALS — NON METALS — INERT GASES

I A	II A	III B	IV B	V B	VI B	VII B	VIII B			I B	II B	III A	IV A	V A	VI A	VII A	VIII A
																	2 He 4.0026 (2)
3 Li 6.939 (2-1)	4 Be 9.0122 (2-2)											5 B 10.811 (2-3)	6 C 12.01115 (2-4)	7 N 14.0067 (2-5)	8 O 15.9994 (2-6)	9 F 18.9984 (2-7)	10 Ne 20.183 (2-8)
11 Na 22.9898 (2-8-1)	12 Mg 24.312 (2-8-2)											13 Al 26.9815 (2-8-3)	14 Si 28.086 (2-8-4)	15 P 30.9738 (2-8-5)	16 S 32.064 (2-8-6)	17 Cl 35.453 (2-8-7)	18 Ar 39.948 (2-8-8)
19 K 39.102 (2-8-8-1)	20 Ca 40.08 (2-8-8-2)	21 Sc 44.956 (2-8-9-2)	22 Ti 47.90 (2-8-10-2)	23 V 50.942 (2-8-11-2)	24 Cr 51.996 (2-8-13-1)	25 Mn 54.9380 (2-8-13-2)	26 Fe 55.847 (2-8-14-2)	27 Co 58.9332 (2-8-15-2)	28 Ni 58.71 (2-8-16-2)	29 Cu 63.54 (2-8-18-1)	30 Zn 65.37 (2-8-18-2)	31 Ga 69.72 (2-8-18-3)	32 Ge 72.59 (2-8-18-4)	33 As 74.9216 (2-8-18-5)	34 Se 78.96 (2-8-18-6)	35 Br 79.909 (2-8-18-7)	36 Kr 83.80 (2-8-18-8)
37 Rb 85.47 (2-8-18-8-1)	38 Sr 87.62 (2-8-18-8-2)	39 Y 88.905 (2-8-18-9-2)	40 Zr 91.22 (2-8-18-10-2)	41 Cb(Nb) 92.906 (2-8-18-12-1)	42 Mo 95.94 (2-8-18-13-1)	43 Tc 99 (2-8-18-13-2)	44 Ru 101.07 (2-8-18-15-1)	45 Rh 102.905 (2-8-18-16-1)	46 Pd 106.4 (2-8-18-18)	47 Ag 107.870 (2-8-18-18-1)	48 Cd 112.40 (2-8-18-18-2)	49 In 114.82 (2-8-18-18-3)	50 Sn 118.69 (2-8-18-18-4)	51 Sb 121.75 (2-8-18-18-5)	52 Te 127.60 (2-8-18-18-6)	53 I 126.044 (2-8-18-18-7)	54 Xe 131.30 (2-8-18-18-8)
55 Cs 132.905 (2-8-18-18-8-1)	56 Ba 137.34 (2-8-18-18-8-2)	57–71 LANTHANIDE SERIES	72 Hf 178.49 (2-8-18-32-10-2)	73 Ta 180.948 (2-8-18-32-11-2)	74 W 183.85 (2-8-18-32-12-2)	75 Re 186.2 (2-8-18-32-13-2)	76 Os 190.2 (2-8-18-32-14-2)	77 Ir 192.2 (2-8-18-32-17)	78 Pt 195.09 (2-8-18-32-17-1)	79 Au 196.967 (2-8-18-32-18-1)	80 Hg 200.59 (2-8-18-32-18-2)	81 Tl 204.37 (2-8-18-32-18-3)	82 Pb 207.19 (2-8-18-32-18-4)	83 Bi 208.980 (2-8-18-32-18-5)	84 Po 210 (2-8-18-32-18-6)	85 At 210 (2-8-18-32-18-7)	86 Rn 222 (2-8-18-32-18-8)
87 Fr 223 (2-8-18-32-18-8-1)	88 Ra 226 (2-8-18-32-18-8-2)	89– ACTINIDE SERIES															

LANTHANIDE SERIES	57 La 138.91 (2-8-18-18-9-2)	58 Ce 140.12 (2-8-18-19-9-2)	59 Pr 140.07 (2-8-18-20-9-2)	60 Nd 144.24 (2-8-18-22-8-2)	61 Pm 147 (2-8-18-23-8-2)	62 Sm 150.35 (2-8-18-24-8-2)	63 Eu 151.96 (2-8-18-25-8-2)	64 Gd 157.25 (2-8-18-25-9-2)	65 Tb 158.924 (2-8-18-26-9-2)	66 Dy 162.50 (2-8-18-28-8-2)	67 Ho 164.930 (2-8-18-29-8-2)	68 Er 167.26 (2-8-18-30-8-2)	69 Tm 169.934 (2-8-18-31-8-2)	70 Yb 173.04 (2-8-18-32-8-2)	71 Lu 174.97 (2-8-18-32-9-2)
ACTINIDE SERIES	89 Ac 227 (2-8-18-32-18-9-2)	90 Th 232.038 (2-8-18-32-19-9-2)	91 Pa 231 (2-8-18-32-20-9-2)	92 U 238.03 (2-8-18-32-21-9-2)	93 Np 237 (2-8-18-32-22-9-2)	94 Pu 242 (2-8-18-32-23-9-2)	95 Am 243 (2-8-18-32-24-9-2)	96 Cm 247 (2-8-18-32-25-9-2)	97 Bk 247 (2-8-18-32-26-9-2)	98 Cf 249 (2-8-18-32-27-9-2)	99 Es 254 (2-8-18-32-28-9-2)	100 Fm 253 (2-8-18-32-29-9-2)	101 Mv 256 (2-8-18-32-30-9-2)	102 No 254 (2-8-18-32-31-9-2)	103 Lw 257 (2-8-18-32-32-9-2)

(2) Chemical bonding. When elements combine to form chemical compounds, the valence electrons may be transferred from one atom to another or there may be a mutual sharing of the valence electrons. In either case, a *chemical bond* is produced. Both atoms involved in the reaction attain a completed outer shell, and stability results. Those elements whose outer shell is not complete may react with others; those elements with completed outer shells, such as the inert gases, do not usually react. There are three types of chemical bond—electrovalent, covalent, and coordinate covalent. The differences are explained as follows:

(a) Electrovalent (ionic) bond. In electrovalent bonding, electrons from the valence orbit are transferred from one atom to another. A compound is formed from the two elements bound together by the electrovalent bond. This occurs in the reaction between sodium and chlorine. Sodium reacts with chlorine to yield sodium chloride (NaCl). Sodium has only 1 electron in its outermost shell; chlorine has 7. In seeking stability, each needs 8 electrons in the outer shell. The single valence electron of the sodium atom is given up and accepted into the valence shell of chlorine. The compound formed now has 8 electrons in the outer shell and is now stable (fig. 3).

(b) Covalent bond. In covalent bonding, each atom donates one or more valence electrons to be shared equally by the two. An example of covalent bonding is the reaction between hydrogen and chlorine. An atom of hydrogen reacts with an atom of chlorine to yield a molecule of HCl. The hydrogen donates 1 valence electron and the chlorine 7 to make a covalently bonded stable compound with 8 electrons in the outermost orbit (fig 4).

(c) Coordinate covalent bond. This bond is essentially the same as the covalent bond except *one* atom donates all the electrons to be shared. An example of coordinate covalent bonding is represented by the compound formed from sulfur and oxygen in figure 5. In this reaction, the sulfur atom provides 2 electrons each to 3 atoms of oxygen. The oxygen atom provides none to the bond. A stable compound with 8 valence electrons in the outer rings, sulfur trioxide, is formed by coordinate covalent bonding.

(3) Variable valence. Most elements have only one possible valence, but a few may have two or more valences because under certain circumstances their electrons move back and forth between their valence shell and the next innermost shell. Compounds resulting from the combination

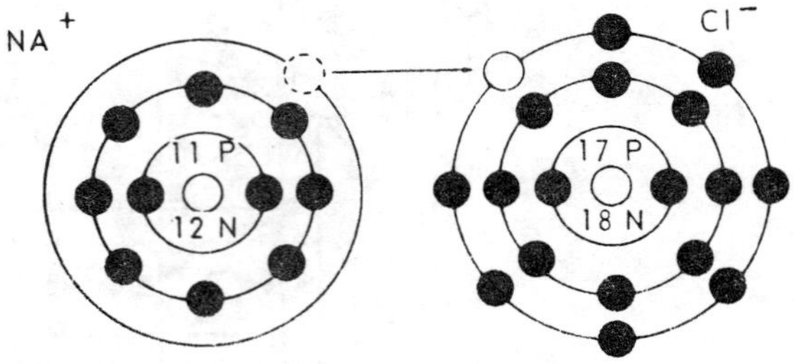

Figure 3. Formation of a sodium chloride (NaCl) molecule.

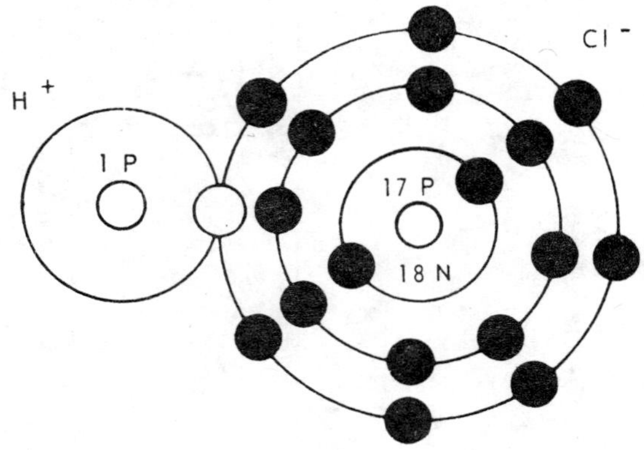

Figure 4. Formation of a hydrogen chloride (HCl) molecule.

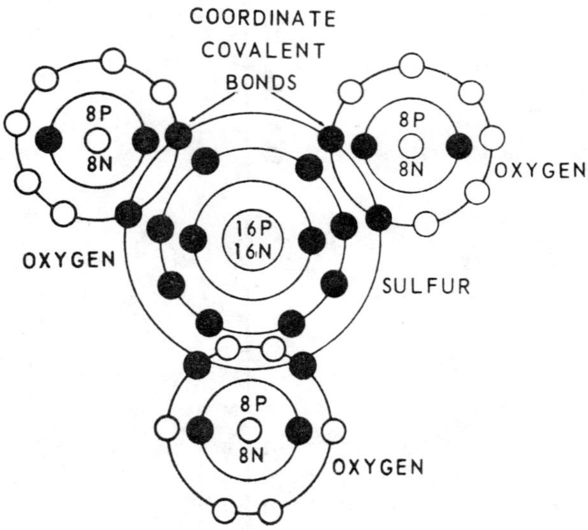

Figure 5. Formation of a sulfur trioxide (SO_3) molecule.

of such elements are named to indicate which valence state is involved. Compounds containing the lower valence state are named by adding "ous" to the end of the name, whereas those of the higher valence state have "ic" added to the end. Thus, mercur*ous* chloride (HgCl) has mercury exhibiting a valence state of 1, while mercur*ic* chloride ($HgCl_2$) exhibits the valence state of 2.

(4) Valences of common elements and radicals. Table . 3 shows the valence or valences of the most common elements and radicals. *Radicals* are groups of atoms which act and react as a single atom. Examples of radicals are NH_4 (ammonium), PO_4 (phosphate), and NO_3 (nitrate). In order to be able to write formulas and predict reactions, you must commit to memory the valences of the most important elements and radicals; these are listed in table 3-3.

b. Formulas and the naming of compounds. Formulas are combinations of symbols representing compounds. Compounds are named from the formulas, and the formulas are derived on the basis of the valences of the two (or more) elements entering into the reactions.

(1) Formulas. The valences of two or more elements combining chemically to form a compound determine the formula for the compound formed. The compound must be electrically neutral and therefore must have as many negative charges as positive. In the reaction between sodium (Na) and chlorine (Cl), the sodium has a valence of +1 and the chlorine a valence of −1. They are equal and opposite, yielding an electrically neutral compound in the ratio of 1:1. Therefore, the formula is correct as NaCl.

(a) Subscripts. What, then, would be the correct formula for aluminum hydroxide? Aluminum has a valence of +3 and the hydroxide radical a valence of −1. It is easy to visualize that it will take 3 hydroxides to be equally opposite to one aluminum. The formula must be $Al(OH)_3$. The subscript 3 following the OH in parentheses indicates that there are 3 OH groups. If the OH were not placed in parentheses, the 3 would appear to belong only to the H. It is very important when radicals are taken more than once that they be inclosed in parentheses. In formulas such as for aluminum bromide, where no radicals appear, no parentheses are needed, for example, $AlBr_3$.

(b) Rule of crossing valences. A convenient rule for determining what subscriptions are necessary in writing formulas is the rule of

Table 3. Valences

Name	Symbol	Valence
Acetate	$C_2H_3O_2$	−1
Aluminum	Al	+3
Ammonium	NH_4	+1
Antimony	Sb	+3, +5
Arsenic	As	+3, +5
Barium	Ba	+2
Bicarbonate	HCO_3	−1
Bismuth	Bi	+3
Bromine	Br	−1*
Calcium	Ca	+2
Carbon	C	+4, −4
Carbonate	CO_3	−2
Chlorine	Cl	−1*
Copper	Cu	+1, +2
Fluorine	F	−1*
Gold	Au	+1, +3
Hydrogen	H	+1
Hydroxide	OH	−1
Iodine	I	−1*
Iron	Fe	+2, +3
Lead	Pb	+2
Lithium	Li	+1
Magnesium	Mg	+2
Manganese	Mn	+2
Mercury	Hg	+1, +2
Nickel	Ni	+2
Nitrate	NO_3	−1
Nitrogen	N	+3, +5
Oxygen	O	−2
Permanganate	MnO_4	−2
Phosphate	PO_4	−3
Phosphorus	P	−3
Potassium	K	+1
Silver	Ag	+1
Sodium	Na	+1
Strontium	Sr	+1
Sulfate	SO_4	−2
Sulfur	S	−2
Zinc	Zn	+2

*Usually 1, but may react with other valences (such as +1, +3, +5, +7).

crossing valences. Zinc chloride is used as an example.

- *Step 1.* List the valences for the elements involved.

Zinc has a valence of +2
Chlorine has a valence of −1

- *Step 2.* Write the formula, inserting the valences.

$$Zn^{+2}Cl^{-1}$$

- *Step 3.* Take the valence of the element at the left (Zn) and make it the subscript of the element at the right (Cl). In like manner, take the valence of the element at the right and make it the subscript of the element at the left. Thus–

$$Zn_1Cl_2$$

- *Step 4.* Since it is understood by simply writing the elemental symbol that 1 atom is present, the subscript 1 is omitted. Thus the correctly written compound becomes–

$$ZnCl_2$$

This rule works for binary and tertiary compounds alike. A *binary* compound is formed from two elements; a *tertiary* from three elements and involves a radical, as with $Al(OH)_3$.

(c) Empirical formula. The usual formula for inorganic compounds expresses the simplest ratio of elements in the compound. This is called the empirical formula. Sometimes the simplest formula does not give a true picture of the molecule. Then it is necessary to modify the formula to fit the situation. This is usually done by the use of a molecular formula.

(d) Molecular formula. The molecular formula expresses the actual numbers of atoms that occur in the molecule. For example, calomel or mercurous chloride has the empirical formula HgCl. However, each molecule contains two atoms of mercury and two atoms of chlorine. Therefore, the molecular formula becomes Hg_2Cl_2. (Other examples: hydrogen, H_2; oxygen, O_2; chlorine, Cl_2; iodine, I_2; nitrogen, N_2; and phosphorus, P_4.)

(2) Acids, bases, and salts. We have briefly defined acids, bases, and salts in previous pages. Before continuing, it is necessary to define them more concretely.

(a) Acids. Acids are compounds containing hydrogen which can be easily replaced by a metal. An acid is a hydrogen compound giving on ionization no other positive ion except the hydrogen ion. For example, hydrochloric acid (HCl) on ionization yields an H^+ and a Cl^- ion. The only positive (+) ion is the hydrogen ion. It is an acid. Similarly, nitric acid (NHO_3) ionizes, yielding H^+ and NO_3^- ions. The only positive ion is the hydrogen ion again, and the compound is an acid. When sodium chloride ionizes, it yields Na^+ and Cl^- ions. There is a positive ion which is NOT a hydrogen ion and the compound is therefore NOT an acid.

(b) Bases. Bases are compounds which will react with acids to form salts and water. A base gives hydroxyl (OH^-) ions upon ionization and no other negative ion. Sodium hydroxide (NaOH) on ionization yields Na^+ and OH^- ions. The only negative ion is the hydroxyl ion. Similarly, potassium hydroxide (KOH) ionizes to K^+ and OH^- and since there are no negative ions other than the OH, the compound is a base.

(c) Salts. Salts are compounds formed from the reaction of acids with bases. Salts furnish positive ions *other* than hydrogen, and negative ions *other* than hydroxyl. Magnesium sulfate ($MgSO_4$) ionizes to Mg^+ and SO_4^-. The Mg^+ is a positive ion other than hydrogen and the SO_4^- is a negative ion other than hydroxyl. Magnesium sulfate is a salt. The same can be shown for sodium chloride, aluminum bromide, sodium sulfate, or any other salt.

(3) Nomenclature for compounds. The names given to compounds are derived from the elements forming them.

(a) General nomenclature. In the reaction between sodium and chlorine, the product is named sodium chloride. To obtain the product name, state the name of the metal in its entirety and add the name of the nonmetal after changing its ending to *ide.* Thus we obtain potassium brom*ide* (from the combination of potassium and bromine) and aluminum hydroxide (from the combination of aluminum and the hydroxyl radical).

(b) Naming compounds formed from elements of varying valence. There are slight variations from the rule for elements with variable valences. The product for iron and chlorine could be either ferrous chloride or ferric chloride, depending upon the valence of the iron. The lower valence state is always identified with the ending *ous,* the higher state with *ic.* We have previously cited the example of mercurous chloride and mercuric chloride.

(c) Naming radicals. Another slight variation from the basic rule involves radicals. Observe the names of the following radicals:

Sulfite SO_3	Chlorite ClO_2	Nitrite NO_2
Sulfate SO_4	Chlorate ClO_3	Nitrate NO_3

(d) Prefixes. Another system for naming binary compounds is by use of a prefix attached to the second element to indicate the number of atoms present. Thus we have carbon monoxide and carbon dioxide. These prefixes are as follows:

1 = mono
2 = di
3 = tri
4 = tetra
5 = penta

Two other prefixes which will come up occasionally are *hypo,* meaning lower or less than, and *hyper* meaning more or higher.

(e) Naming acids. Because acids always have hydrogen for the positive portion of the molecule, they are named differently from salts or bases. Acids may also be binary or tertiary, and the method of naming differs.

1. In the binary acids, *hydro* is used as a prefix and *ic* as a suffix. Thus HCl is named *hydro*chlor*ic* acid, H_2S is hydrosulfuric acid and HBr is hydrobromic acid. This rule holds true for all the binary acids.

2. Tertiary acids are named according to the amount of oxygen they contain. (An exception to this rule exists with HCN. Although a tertiary acid, it is named like a binary acid. It is called hydrocyanic acid.) The rules are as follows:

- Acids which contain as much oxygen as they normally can are given the ending *ic* (sulfuric acid–H_2SO_4).
- Acids containing one less oxygen than normal are given the ending *ous* (sulfurous acid–H_2SO_3).
- Acids containing two less oxygens than normal are prefixed *hypo* in addition to the *ous* ending (hypochlorous acid–HClO).
- Acids containing one more oxygen atom than normal are prefixed *per* in addition to the *ic* ending (perchloric acid–$HClO_4$).

(4) Law of definite proportions. As you learned earlier in this chapter, every compound has a definite composition by weight. Because of the valence of elements and the sharing or transfer of electrons, the proportion in which elements can combine is rigidly controlled. Evidence of this is the reaction between hydrogen and chlorine. The hydrogen atom has only one electron to share and the chlorine atom needs to share only one to complete its outermost electron ring. The combination must be one to one. It cannot be otherwise. And because the ratio is one to one, the formula must always be HCl.

(5) Law of multiple proportions. When two or more elements unite to form two or more compounds, if the amount of one element is constant, the weights of the other element in the series of compounds will be in the ratio of small whole numbers. This sounds like quite a mouthful, but an example should clarify it. Because of variable valences, carbon and oxygen can combine to yield carbon monoxide (CO), carbon dioxide (CO_2) and carbonic acid (H_2CO_3).

28 Gm. of CO contains ---------------- 12 Gm. C and 16 Gm. O
44 Gm. of CO_2 contains -------------- 12 Gm. C and 32 Gm. O
62 Gm. of H_2CO_3 contains ---------- 12 Gm. C and 48 Gm. O

In each of these members of the series, the weight of carbon remained constant at 12 Gm., but the amounts of oxygen were in the ratio of small whole numbers, 1 to 2 to 3.

c. Chemical equations and reactions. Chemical equations are abbreviated ways of writing chemical reactions. They save much writing and effort and give as much, if not more, information than a verbally stated reaction. Chemical equations show (1) the kinds of atoms or molecules reacting; (2) the products formed; (3) the number of atoms entering into the reaction; (4) the number of molecules formed in the product; and (5) the proportion in which the substances react to give definite products. Four types of chemical reaction are possible. They are combination reactions, decomposition reactions, single replacement reactions, and double replacement reactions. ($\triangle$ stands for heat; $\uparrow$ = given off as a gas.)

(1) Combination reactions. The general equation representing combination reactions is A + B = AB. A specific example of the combination reaction is the formula for a metal reacting with oxygen to yield a metallic oxide:

$$2Mg + O_2 \longrightarrow 2\,MgO$$

(2) Decomposition reactions. The general equation representing decomposition reactions is AB $\longrightarrow$ A + B. The following examples show some possibilities [heat ($\triangle$) hastens speed of reaction].

$$CaCO_3 \xrightarrow{\Delta} CaO + CO_2\uparrow$$

$$Ca(OH)_2 \xrightarrow{\Delta} CaO + H_2O$$

$$2KClO_3 \xrightarrow{\Delta} 2KCl + 3O_2\uparrow$$

$$H_2CO_3 \xrightarrow{\Delta} H_2O + CO_2\uparrow$$

$$2HgO \xrightarrow{\Delta} 2Hg + O_2\uparrow$$

(3) Single replacement reactions. The general equation for a single replacement reaction is $A + BC \longrightarrow AC + B$. A more specific example is the reaction between zinc and copper sulfate:

$$Zn + CuSO_4 \longrightarrow ZnSO_4 + Cu$$

In this type of reaction, a more active metal replaces a less active one. This depends upon electromotive force which for the purposes of pharmacy need not be discussed.

(4) Double replacement reactions. The general equation for the double replacement reaction is $AB + CD \longrightarrow AD + CB$. A more specific example is the reaction which occurs between barium chloride and copper sulfate:

$$BaCl_2 + CuSO_4 \longrightarrow BaSO_4 + CuCl_2$$

The double replacement reaction is the most commonly occurring reaction. The double replacement reaction can be further subdivided into classes, of which the following three are the most common:

(a) Acid-base. An acid reacts with a base to give a salt and water. Example:

$$HCl + NaOH \longrightarrow NaCl + H_2O$$

(b) Precipitation reaction. Precipitation is the falling out of solution of a substance, usually a solid, as the result of some physical or chemical change which has taken place. In the precipitation reaction, two soluble substances in solution react to form one or more insoluble substances which precipitate from solution and settle. This is indicated in an equation by an arrow pointing downward ($\downarrow$) after the formula for the precipitated material:

$$BaCl_2 + Na_2SO_4 \longrightarrow BaSO_4\downarrow + 2NaCl$$

(c) Oxidation-reduction reactions. You have probably always thought of oxidation as the phenomenon which takes place in the rusting of iron or the burning of combustibles, where a substance chemically combines with oxygen. Actually, *oxidation includes any reaction in which an atom or ion loses electrons and therefore gains in valence. Reduction is the opposite, and results in a gain in electrons and a loss of valence.* Oxidation and reduction occur simultaneously, NEVER separately. Let's look at some of the possible valence states of sulfur.

SO_3	SO_2	S	H_2S	(Compound or element)
+6	+4	0	−2	(Valence state)

← oxidation reduction →

In this illustration, the arrows point toward the direction of the reaction. Going from right to left (from H_2S to SO_3), oxidation is occurring. Going from left to right (SO_3 toward H_2S), reduction is occurring. You can see that sulfur dioxide (SO_2) going to sulfur trioxide (SO_3) presents a gain in valence or a loss of electrons and is, according to our definition, oxidized. Going from elemental sulfur (S) to hydrogen sulfide (H_2S), there is a loss of valence or a gain in electrons and the sulfur is reduced. The processes of oxidation and reduction are reactions and can be better illustrated by using equations. We are considering oxidation-reduction under double replacement reactions, even though single replacement reactions are *all* redox reactions. (Redox is a commonly used abbreviation for oxidation-reduction.) Follow the equations below and see what happens during a single replacement reaction.

1. $Zn + CuSO_4 \longrightarrow ZnSO_4 + Cu$

Elemental zinc (being natural) has no charge. In the copper sulfate molecule, copper has a valence of +2 and sulfate a valence of −2, thus giving the molecule electrical neutrality. Zinc sulfate in the product combines zinc with a valence of +2 and a sulfate with a valence of −2. The elemental copper formed has a valence state of 0, since it is elemental and neutral. This can be represented in the following manner so that the whole picture is clearly visible at one time.

$$\overset{0}{Zn} + \overset{+2}{Cu}\overset{-2}{SO_4} \longrightarrow \overset{+2}{Zn}\overset{-2}{SO_4} + \overset{0}{Cu}$$

Zinc has gone from a valence state of 0 to a valence state of +2–a gain in valence, a loss of electrons. This is oxidation. Copper has gone from a +2 valence to a 0 valence state–a loss in valence, a gain in electrons. This is reduction. The zinc was oxidized. The copper was reduced. The substance oxidized is the reducing agent (zinc in this case), and the substance reduced is the oxidizing agent (copper in this case). Not nearly so hard as it sounded in the beginning, is it? Let's try another.

2. $\overset{0}{Mg} + 2\overset{+1}{H}\overset{-1}{Cl} \longrightarrow \overset{+2}{Mg}\overset{-2}{Cl_2} + \overset{0}{H_2}$

The magnesium is oxidized; the hydrogen is reduced. How do you know?

$$\overset{0}{H_2} + \overset{+2\,-2}{CuO} \longrightarrow \overset{0}{Cu} + \overset{+2\,-2}{H_2O}$$

3. $H_2 + CuO \longrightarrow Cu + H_2O$

The hydrogen is oxidized and the copper reduced. Do you agree?

d. *Writing chemical equations.* The writing of chemical equations, as we have previously stated, is accomplished by using symbols, coefficients (prefixed numbers which multiply the symbol or formula to which attached), subscripts, and various other signs and figures. Up to this point in showing reactions we have made no attempt to show how to balance the equations. That is, we have not taken into consideration how many parts of each element react and how many parts are formed. But in order to write correct equations to represent chemical reactions, you must know the symbols for the elements involved, their respective valences, and diatomic molecules. You must be able to change the elements to their symbols and predict the results of the reaction.

(1) Diatomic molecules. The atoms of the common gases form two-atomed molecules by covalence. They occur in the free state, not alone, but in the molecular or diatomic state. Following are the common diatomic molecules as they exist free in nature.

H_2 N_2 Cl_2 I_2 O_2 F_2 Br_2

When equations containing these gases are written, they must be written in their diatomic state.

(2) Coefficients and subscripts. What is the difference between a coefficient and a subscript? Look at the following equation:

$$2H_2 + O_2 \longrightarrow 2H_2O$$

The coefficients before H_2 and H_2O multiply each by 2. In this equation, it means that 2 diatomic molecules of hydrogen react with 1 of oxygen to yield 2 molecules of water. Coefficients are placed in front of the symbol or formula they multiply and pertain to the whole formula rather than a single part. The subscripts for hydrogen and oxygen in the preceding equation multiply only the symbol (or, in other cases, radical) which they follow. They do not pertain to the entire formula. It is very important that coefficients and subscripts not be confused.

(3) Steps in equation writing. The most effective and safest way to write chemical equations is to follow this sequence:

(a) Write the word equation—this is a statement of the reaction. *Example:* Hydrogen reacts with chlorine to form ______.

(b) Predict the outcome of the reaction. What do the reactants react to form? Thus, hydrogen reacts with chlorine to form hydrochloric acid.

(c) Transpose the proper symbols and formulas for the words in the equation. Be careful to observe the valence laws. Do not forget subscripts.

(d) Check for diatomic molecules. They must be written in their diatomic form, not as atoms.

(e) Balance the equation by placing coefficients in front of the symbols and formulas so that the numbers of each element and radical are the same on each side of the equation. *Subscript numbers given to formulas to agree with valence must not be changed in balancing.* This is a common error among students.

(4) Examples. In order to get a clearer view of equations and how they are written, some specific examples will be beneficial. Follow through the steps in equation writing for the examples given below.

(a) Hydrogen plus chlorine.

• *Step 1.* Write the word equation: Hydrogen reacts with chlorine.

• *Step 2.* Predict the results: Hydrogen reacts with chlorine to yield hydrochloric acid.

• *Step 3.* Transpose into proper symbols and formulas. The proper symbols are H for hydrogen and Cl for chlorine. The valence of H is +1; Cl is −1. To this point, the equation becomes:

$$H + Cl \longrightarrow HCl$$

• *Step 4.* Check for diatomic molecules. Hydrogen and chlorine are both diatomic—H_2 and Cl_2. The formula to this point now becomes—

$$H_2 + Cl_2 \longrightarrow HCl$$

From what you have already learned, this would appear to be a correct expression for the reaction between hydrogen and chlorine. IT IS NOT! You still must balance the equation.

• *Step 5.* Balance the equation. Notice in the equation as written in step 4 that there are two hydrogens on the left (H_2) and two chlorines (Cl_2); but on the right there is only one of each. The equation is not balanced. The law of conservation of matter states that the amount of the products must be equal to the amount of the reactants. By placing a coefficient of 2 before HCl, the sides become equal. Remember that we never change subscripts to balance. The correct, balanced equation is: $H_2 + Cl_2 \longrightarrow 2HCl$. Expressed in words, the equation means that one molecule of hydrogen reacts with one molecule of chlorine to yield two molecules of hydrochloric acid.

(b) Write the equation for the reaction occurring between zinc and silver nitrate.

- *Step 1.* Write the word equation: Zinc reacts with silver nitrate.

- *Step 2.* Predict the results: Zinc reacts with silver nitrate to produce zinc nitrate and silver.

- *Step 3.* Transpose into proper symbols—

$$\overset{0}{Zn} + \overset{+1\,-1}{AgNO_3} \longrightarrow \overset{+2\,-1}{ZnNO_3} + \overset{0}{Ag}$$

The valences have been added for your convenience at this time. Notice that in the product, Zn has a valence state of +2 and the nitrate radical has a valence of only −1. This is in violation of our rule of valences since the molecule would, under these circumstances, have a collective charge of +1. In order to give the molecule a neutral charge, the valences must be equal and opposite. Thus, the equation at this point should be:

$$\overset{0}{Zn} + \overset{+1\,-1}{AgNO_3} \longrightarrow \overset{+2\,-2}{Zn(NO_3)_2} + \overset{0}{Ag}$$

- *Step 4.* Check for diatomic molecules. There are none in this equation.

- *Step 5.* Balance the equation, using coefficients. On the left, you have one zinc and on the right, one zinc. This checks. One silver on the left, one on the right; this checks. One nitrate on the left, but two on the right—this must be corrected. Placing a coefficient of 2 before the $AgNO_3$, you arrive at—

$$Zn + 2AgNO_3 \longrightarrow Zn\,(NO_3)_2 + Ag$$

Now check again to see if this has done the trick. One zinc left and one right. Two silvers left, but only one right. The equation still needs further correction. Adding a coefficient of 2 to the Ag, you have—

$$Zn + 2AgNO_3 \longrightarrow Zn\,(NO_3)_2 + 2Ag$$

Once again, check to see if the equation is balanced. One zinc left and one right. Two silvers left and two right. Two nitrates left and two right. The equation is now balanced and correct. In some reactions, a precipitate forms or a gas is evolved. These can be shown in the equation by arrows pointing up ($\uparrow$) for the gases bubbling off, or down ($\downarrow$) for a precipitate settling. The arrows follow the substance involved. Thus, in our previous example, the silver is precipitated from the solution, and the equation would be—

$$Zn + 2AgNO_3 \longrightarrow Zn\,(NO_3)_2 + 2Ag\downarrow$$

(c) Potassium iodide plus chlorine.

- *Step 1.* Potassium iodide reacts with chlorine.

- *Step 2.* Potassium iodide reacts with chlorine to yield potassium chloride and iodine.

- *Step 3.* $KI + Cl \longrightarrow KCl + I$

- *Step 4.* $KI + Cl_2 \longrightarrow KCl + I_2$

- *Step 5.* $\overset{+1-1}{2KI} + \overset{0}{Cl_2} \longrightarrow \overset{+1\,-1}{KCl} + \overset{0}{I_2}$

$$2KI + Cl_2 \longrightarrow 2KCl + I_2\downarrow$$

(d) Practice chemical equations. Before going on to new material, work and balance as many of the following chemical equations as you can, using the correct chemical symbols and formulas.

1. Combination reactions.

A + B . . . . .) AB

- Hydrogen + oxygen . . . .)
- Carbon + oxygen . . . .)
- Sodium + chlorine . . . .)
- Magnesium + oxygen . . . .)
- Iron + sulfur . . . .)
- Sodium + oxygen . . . .)
- Hydrogen + chlorine . . . .)

2. *Single replacement reactions.*

A + BC . . . . .) AC + B

- Zinc + sulfuric acid . . . .)
- Sodium + water . . . .)
- Potassium iodide + chloride . . . .)
- Magnesium + hydrochloric acid . . . .)
- Sodium + hydrochloric acid . . . .)
- Aluminum + sulfuric acid . . . .)

3. *Decomposition reactions.*

AB . . . . .) A + B

- Sulfuric acid + heat . . . .)
- Barium carbonate + heat . . . .)
- Mercuric hydroxide + heat . . . .)
- Ammonium hydroxide + heat . . . .)
- Carbonic acid + heat . . . .)
- Nickel chlorate + heat . . . .)
- Mercuric oxide + heat . . . .)

4. *Double replacement reactions.*

AB + CD . . . . .) AD + CB

- Cupric hydroxide + acetic acid . . . .)
- Nickel chloride + ammonium carbonate . . . . .)
- Sodium carbonate + hydrochloric acid . . . . . .)
- Ammonium acetate + magnesium hydroxide . .)
- Barium chloride + magnesium sulfate . . . .)
- Ferric chloride + ammonium sulfate . . . .)
- Silver nitrate + zinc chloride . . . .)
- Silver nitrate + hydrochloric acid . . . .)
- Ammonium chloride + nitric acid . . . .)
- Sodium hydroxide + hydrochloric acid . . . . . .)

e. Molecular weights. Turn back and review quickly what has been said about atomic weights. *Molecular weight* is the sum of the atomic weights in the formula. For this reason, it is also commonly called formula weight. What is the molecular weight of CO_2? Turning to your periodic chart of the elements, or table of symbols and atomic weights, you will see that carbon has an atomic weight of 12.0000 and oxygen an atomic weight of 15.9994. Therefore, the molecular weight of carbon dioxide is found by adding the atomic weights.

$$\begin{aligned} C &= 12.0000 \\ O_2 &= \underline{31.9988}\ (15.9994 \times 2) \\ &\ 43.9988 \text{ molecular weight (m.w.) of carbon dioxide } (CO_2) \end{aligned}$$

The same follows with more complex substances. What would be the formula weight for Na_2SO_4?

Na = 22.9898	therefore,	Na_2 =	45.9796 (22.9898 x 2)
S = 32.064		S =	32.064
O = 15.9994		O_4 =	63.9976 (15.9994 x 4)
			142.0412 m.w. of Na_2SO_4

Some molecules have water of crystallization and their formulas are expressed with a number of water molecules following the formula—

$$AlK(SO_4)_2 \cdot 12H_2O$$

The water is an integral part of the molecule in these cases and must be calculated in determining the molecular weight. Thus, to determine the molecular weight of the above chemical—

Al = 26.98	x	1 =	26.98
K = 39.102	x	1 =	39.102
S = 32.064	x	2 =	64.128
O = 15.9994	x	20 =	319.988
H = 1.00797	x	24 =	24.1913
			474.3893 = m.w.

Atomic weights and molecular weights are abstract numbers. They are relative and have no exact units. They are not grams, ounces, pounds, or tons. In order to give them units, we may express them in grams and thereby have a *gram atomic weight* or *gram molecular weight.*

f. Avogadro's law. Avogadro's law states that *at the same temperature and pressure, equal volumes of all gases contain the same number of molecules.* It is not important to the chemist to know exactly how many molecules are present in a given quantity of gas, but it is extremely important that equal volumes contain equal numbers of molecules, because it follows that the number of molecules will have the same ratio as the quantities.

g. Percent composition. The percentage of each element making up a compound can be readily determined, if we know the correct formula. This can be accomplished by first calculating the molecular weight of the compound, then dividing the atomic weight of the substance concerned (or its multiple) by the molecular weight. The result is the percentage in decimal form; multiplying by 100 gives the percent. Find the percent composition of Na_2HPO_4. Using the method previously taught, we calculate the molecular or formula weight to be 141.958, or rounded off, 142. For the sake of brevity, we are rounding off the atomic and molecular weights to the nearest whole number.

Na (at. wt. 23) – Percent Na =

$$\frac{2 \times 23}{142} \times 100 = 32.4\ \%$$

H (at. wt. 1) – Percent H =

$$\frac{1}{142} \times 100 = 0.71\%$$

P (at. wt. 31) – Percent P =

$$\frac{31}{142} \times 100 = 21.82\%$$

O (at. wt. 16) – Percent O =

$$\frac{4 \times 16}{142} \times 100 = \underline{45.07\%}$$

TOTAL 100.00%

The significance of percent composition is important to chemists because it enables them to predict how much of a product can be made from a quantity of ingredients. This is called yield determination. Naturally, if the amount of yield is known, the amounts of the respective ingredients necessary can be determined from that. To the pharmacist, percent composition has importance in determining how much of a salt to use to obtain a specified amount of an element. A prescription calling for a solution to contain so much fluorine is made from a quantity of sodium fluoride (NaF) by determining the percent composition of the fluorine and, based upon this determination, calculating the amount of NaF which would be equal to fluorine needed.

5. Solutions. A solution is a homogeneous body, the composition of which can be varied within wide limits. Solutions are like compounds in that they are homogeneous. They are like mixtures in that their compositions are variable. All solutions consist of two phases, namely, solute (that which is dissolved) and solvent (that in which the solute is dissolved). Usually (there are exceptions) the constituent present in the larger quantity is the solvent. In true solutions, the dissolved particles are molecular in size.

a. Types of solutions. Solutions may be thought of as being of three types: gaseous, liquid, or solid.

(1) Gaseous solutions. Gases mix with one another in all proportions to form homogeneous mixtures, which may be called solutions. *Example:* Dry air is a solution containing about 78-percent nitrogen and 21-percent oxygen, the other 1 percent consisting of carbon dioxide, and the rare gases, helium, neon, argon, etc.

(2) Liquid solutions. Gases, liquids, and solids dissolved in liquid solvents are called liquid solutions. *Example:* Pure HC1 is a gas which dissolves readily in water to form an aqueous solution of hydrochloric acid. Oils form liquid solutions in chloroform. Salts, sugars, and bases dissolved in water are also liquid solutions.

(3) Solid solutions. In these solutions, gases, liquids, and solids are dissolved with solids. *Example:* Hydrogen dissolves in solid palladium. Certain alloys are solid solutions of one metal in another.

b. Molar (M) solutions. A molar solution, or a 1-molar solution, consists of one gram molecular weight of solute dissolved in *enough water to make 1 liter of finished solution.* Molarity, then, is the number of molecular weights dissolved in enough water to make a finished solution of 1000 ml. Molar solutions may have as a solute a solid, a liquid, or a gas.

(1) Finding the gram molecular weight. Going back to gram molecular weights (GMW), we said that one gram molecular weight of a substance is its molecular weight expressed in grams. Thus a GMW of NaOH would be (Na = 22.9898, O = 15.9994, and H = 1.00797) 39.997 *grams.* For the sake of simplicity, let's round that number off to 40 grams; this is the gram molecular weight of NaOH. Then, .5 GMW of NaOH would be 20 grams, 2 GMW would be 80 grams, and so forth. A *mole* is one gram molecular weight of a substance. Thus, a mole of NaOH is 40 grams of NaOH; half mole (.5 mole) is 20 grams, 2 moles is 80 grams, and so on.

(2) Finding the molarity of a solution. To find the molarity of a solution, divide the number of gram molecular weights in that solution by the number of liters of total solution. The formula may be written:

$$M = \frac{\text{Moles}}{\text{Liters}}$$

Since most problems are stated in terms of the weight of solute and require you to determine the number of gram molecular weights (moles), the following formula will be of benefit:

$$\text{Number of GMW} = \frac{\text{Weight of solute}}{\text{Molecular weight}}$$

(3) Example: What is the molarity of a solution containing 29.25 grams of sodium chloride in 500 ml. of total solution?

- *Step 1.* Find the number of moles (GMW).

  The molecular weight of NaCl = 58.4

  $$\text{Moles} = \frac{\text{Weight of solute}}{\text{Molecular weight}}$$

  $$\text{Moles} = \frac{29.95}{58.4} = .5 \text{ moles (GMW)}$$

- *Step 2.* Find the molarity.

  $$\text{M (molarity)} = \frac{\text{Moles}}{\text{Liters}}$$

  500 ml. = .5 liter

  $$M = \frac{.5}{.5} = 1 \text{ Molar or } 1M$$

(4) Example: How many grams of sodium chloride are necessary to make 2000 ml. of a .25 M solution?

- *Step 1.* Find the moles.

$$M = \frac{\text{Moles}}{\text{Liters}}$$

$$.25 = \frac{x}{2} \ (2000 \text{ ml.} = 2 \text{ liters})$$

$$x = .5 \text{ moles}$$

- *Step 2.* Find the number of grams. If 1 mole is 58.4 grams, then .5 mole is 58.4 x .5 = 29.20 grams, answer

(5) Example: How much 1-molar solution can be made from 175.5 grams of sodium chloride?

- *Step 1.* Find the number of moles.

$$\text{Moles} = \frac{\text{Weight of solute}}{\text{Molecular weight}}$$

$$\text{Moles} = \frac{175.5}{58.4}$$

$$\text{Moles} = 3$$

- *Step 2.* Find the number of liters.

$$M = \frac{\text{Moles}}{\text{Liters}}$$

$$1M = \frac{3}{x}$$

$$x = 3 \text{ liters or } 3000 \text{ ml., answer}$$

The problems illustrated have been approximated or calculated to work out to easy numbers with few decimal points. In practice, you will find that most of your answers will have to be carried to several decimal places.

c. *Molal solutions.* Of particular use to chemists, but little use to pharmacists, is the molal solution. Do not confuse it with molar solutions. A *molal* solution is made by dissolving one mole of solute in exactly 1000 grams of solvent. The resulting solution measures more than 1000 ml.

d. *Normal solutions.* A normal solution is made by dissolving one *gram equivalent weight* (GEW) of solvent in enough water to make 1000 ml. of total finished solution. What, then, is a gram equivalent weight? An equivalent weight of an element is the weight of that element which combines with 1 gram of hydrogen, or the weight of the element which replaces 1 gram of hydrogen.

$$2Al + 6HCl \longrightarrow 2AlCl_3 + 3H_2$$

In the equation above, 2 atoms of aluminum displaced 6 atoms of hydrogen. The ratio here is 2:6, or 1:3. Looking up the atomic weight of aluminum in our table, we find it to be 27 (26.9815). Since it takes 1 aluminum to replace 3 hydrogens, by dividing 27 by 3, we have 9 atomic weight units to replace 1 hydrogen. Therefore, 9 grams of aluminum will replace 1 gram of hydrogen. This is the *equivalent weight.* This seems like quite a procedure to have to go through to find the equivalent weight, but fortunately from this knowledge we can derive a formula. Looking a bit further, we see that this 3 by which we divided the atomic weight of the aluminum is also aluminum's positive valence. Thus–

$$\text{Equivalent weight} = \frac{\text{atomic weight}}{\text{positive valence}}$$

(1) Example: What is the equivalent weight of magnesium oxide?

- *Step 1.* Magnesium Oxide = MgO.

atomic weight of Mg = 24
atomic weight of O = 16
40 = m.w.

- *Step 2.* Find the positive valence.

$$\overset{+2}{Mg}\overset{-2}{O}$$

Therefore the total positive valence is 2.

- *Step 3.* Divide the molecular weight by the positive valence.

$$\frac{40}{2} = 20 \text{ the equivalent weight (e.w.)}$$

The gram equivalent weight of magnesium oxide, then, would be 20 grams.

(2) Example: What is the gram equivalent weight of ammonium nitrate?

- *Step 1.* Ammonium nitrate = NH_4NO_3.

atomic weight of N = 14
H_4 = 4 (1 x 4)
N = 14
O = 48
80 = m. w.

• *Step 2.* Find the total positive valence.

$$\overset{+1}{NH_4}\,\overset{-1}{NO_3}$$

Therefore the positive valence is 1.

• *Step 3.* Divide the molecular weight by the positive valence.

$$\frac{80}{1} = 80 \text{ e.w.}$$

• *Step 4.* Express the equivalent weight in grams.
80 grams = the gram equivalent weight, answer.

(3) Example: What is the gram equivalent weight of $Al_2(SO_4)_3$?

• *Step 1.* $Al_2(SO_4)_3$.

atomic weight of Al = 27 x 2 = 54
S = 32 x 3 = 96
O = 16 x 12 = 192
342 m.w.

• *Step 2.* Find the positive valence.

$$\overset{+6}{Al_2}\,\overset{-6}{(SO_4)_3}$$

Therefore the positive valence is 6.

• *Step 3.* Divide the molecular weight by the positive valence.

$$\frac{342}{6} = 57 \text{ e.w.}$$

• *Step 4.* Express the e.w. in grams.
57 grams = gram equivalent weight, answer.

Now that you can determine the gram equivalent weight of a compound, you should be able to prepare normal solutions. We said that a 1 normal (1N) solution contains 1 gram equivalent weight in 1 liter of solution. Two gram equivalent weights in 1 liter of finished solution would be 2N, etc. Then the formula is:

$$\text{Normality (N)} = \frac{\text{gram equivalent weights}}{\text{liters}}$$

(4) Example: What is the normality of a solution containing 98 grams of H_2SO_4 in 600 ml. of total solution?

• *Step 1.* Find the gram equivalent weight of H_2SO_4.

atomic weight of H = 1 x 2 = 2
S = 32 x 1 = 32
O_4 = 16 x 4 = 64
98 m.w.

$$\overset{+2}{H_2}\,\overset{-2}{SO_4}$$

H_2SO_4, therefore positive valence is 2

$$\frac{98}{2} = 49, \text{ therefore 1 GEW} = 49 \text{ grams}$$

• *Step 2.* Since you have 98 grams of H_2SO_4, divide by 49 to find how many gram equivalent weights you have.

$$49\overline{)98}\quad = 2$$

98

You then have 2 gram equivalent weights of H_2SO_4.

• *Step 3.* Substitute in formula.

$$N = \frac{GEW}{L}$$

$$N = \frac{2}{.6}$$

$$.6\overline{)2.000} = 6\overline{)20.000} = 3.333$$

18
20
18
20
18
20
18
2

The normality is 3.333; you have a 3.333 normal solution.

(5) Example: How many grams of calcium chloride will it take to prepare 200 ml. of a 1.5N solution?

• *Step 1.* Calcium chloride = $CaCl_2$.

atomic weight Ca = 40
Cl = 71
111 = m.w.

$$\overset{+2}{Ca}\,\overset{-2}{Cl_2}$$

$CaCl_2$, therefore total positive valence is 2

$$\frac{111}{2} = 55.5 = \text{e.w., } 55.5 \text{ grams} = \text{GEW}$$

• *Step 2.*

$$N = \frac{GEW}{L}$$

Substitute in formula:

$$1.5 = \frac{x}{.2}$$

x = .3; you need .3 gram equivalent weights

• *Step 3.* Compute. Since you need .3 gram equivalent weights, and a gram equivalent weight of $CaCl_2$ is 55.5 grams, .3 x 55.5 = 16.65 grams of $CaCl_2$ needed to make 200 ml. of 1.5 normal solution.

6. Titration. Normal solutions are used in a method of analysis known as *titration.* Since normal solutions are made with equivalent weights, normal acid solutions neutralize normal base solutions milliliter for milliliter. Or, equal volumes of equally normal solutions are equal. This leads to the formula $N \times V = N_1 \times V_1$ where

N = normality of the acid solution
V = volume of acid solution
N_1 = normality of the basic solution
V_1 = volume of the basic solution

Hence, if we have a known volume of solution, we may determine its normality by reacting it with an opposite solution of known normality. An indicator solution (one which changes color at definite degrees of acidity or alkalinity) is used which exhibits a color change at neutrality, and this is the point at which the reaction is complete. This point is called the end point.

a. Steps in titration. To walk through a sample titration without being able to demonstrate it is like trying to teach you to drive without an automobile. If you possibly can, procure the necessary apparatus and chemicals and follow the procedure yourself. Figure 6 shows titration equipment. The following procedure takes you through the steps for determining the normality of an unknown sodium hydroxide solution. The same technique and steps would apply to a titration for determining the normality of an acid solution.

• *Step 1.* Carefully prepare a .1N solution of hydrochloric acid. Using a pipette, measure accurately 10.0 ml. of the solution into a clean dry flask. Any error you make in preparing the acid solution or measuring out the 10 ml., or any foreign substance in the flask will cause error of equal degree in the calculation of the base. This is the first half of your formula, N x V, or 0.1 x 10.

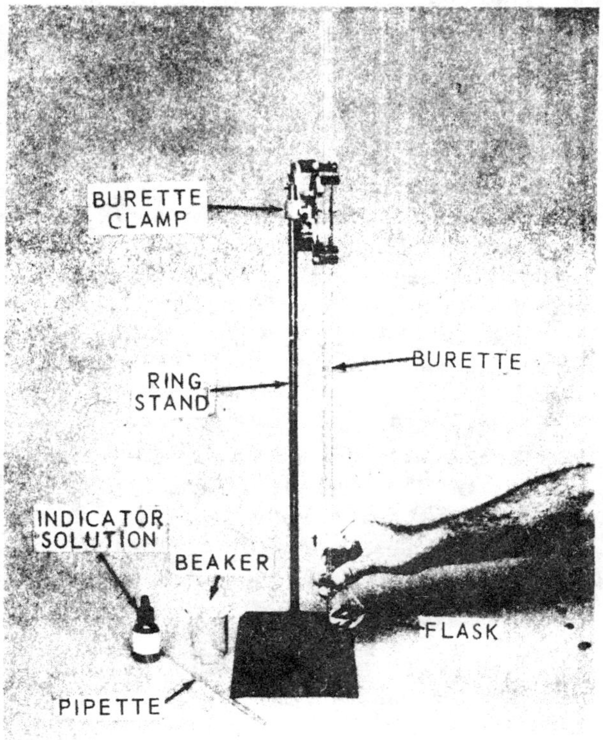

Figure 6. Titration equipment.

• *Step 2.* Add 2 drops of phenolphthalein test solution and about 50 ml. of distilled water to the flask to give volume. This will NOT affect the amount of acid in the flask.

• *Step 3.* Prepare a solution of NaOH in water. This is to be your unknown, so just dump in a quantity of the sodium hydroxide pellets. Make sure they are completely dissolved. Using a clean, dry, 50-ml. burette, rinse it first with distilled water and then with a quantity of the unknown solution. Make sure to allow some of the unknown to run through the stopcock so that the entire burette is moistened by the solution. Now, with the burette securely fastened to a ringstand, pour in approximately 50 ml. of unknown NaOH solution, opening the stopcock briefly to make sure the solution gets all the way to the bottom. Burettes are calibrated from the point at the end. Now record the level of the unknown in the burette. Assume here that you see a reading of 46.5 ml. This is the starting point.

• *Step 4.* Open the stopcock and allow the unknown solution to flow into the known acid solution slowly, constantly swirling the flask. Near the end point of the reaction, the solution surrounding the droplet of base solution will turn pink and swirl until it disappears. At this point you must proceed VERY slowly, drop by drop, thoroughly mixing after each drop until the pink color generated remains for 30 seconds or more before disappearing. This is the end point, for another drop or two will color the solution permanently pink and it will have an excess of base.

• *Step 5.* Read the level of the base left in the burette and subtract this amount from the starting figure. Say that the final reading was 20.5 ml. Subtracting 20.5 from your original 46.5 ml., you see that you have used 26.0 ml. to neutralize the acid. You now have enough information to substitute in your formula.

b. *Calculating the unknown normality.* To calculate the unknown normality, substitute the titration finding in the following formula:

$$N \times V = N_1 \times V_1$$

$$0.1 \times 10 = N_1 \times 26.0$$

Solve the equation and you will have the normality of the unknown solution.

$$1 = N_1 \times 26$$

$$\frac{1}{26} = N_1$$

$$N_1 = 26\overline{)1.00000} = .03846$$

$$\begin{array}{r} 78 \\ \hline 220 \\ 208 \\ \hline 120 \\ 104 \\ \hline 160 \\ 156 \\ \hline \end{array}$$

N of unknown = 0.0385N

7. Oxygen, hydrogen, water, and the peroxides. Oxygen and hydrogen were discovered at approximately the same time in history. They are extremely important elements to us. Two common chemical compounds containing oxygen and hydrogen are water and the peroxides.

a. *Oxygen (O, diatomic O_2) valence – 2.* Oxygen, the most abundant of all the elements, has been given the symbol O and is a nonmetal.

(1) *Physical properties.* Oxygen is a colorless, odorless, tasteless gas which, when liquefied, has a pale blue color. It is slightly soluble in water, and less soluble in sea water. It is interesting to note that more oxygen is soluble in cold than in warm water, and thus when tap water is heated, bubbles of oxygen can be seen collecting on the sides of the container. It is heavier than air.

(2) *Occurrence and preparation.*

(a) *Uncombined.* In a free or uncombined form, oxygen makes up one-fifth of the earth's atmosphere, and there is a small amount dissolved in water. This is important because, with few exceptions, all life requires oxygen. Fish extract the dissolved oxygen from water to sustain their existence. This can be proved by placing a fish in boiled and cooled water. Oxygen has been driven off by the boiling and the fish will die.

(b) *Combined.* Oxygen also occurs in combined forms which make up approximately 50 percent of the earth's crust. Water is 89 percent oxygen by weight. Oxides of metals and nonmetals are widely distributed in nature, for example, the oxides of iron, tin, aluminum, manganese, and zinc; sea sand and quartz are both silicon dioxides; and then there is carbon dioxide. Carbonates, nitrates, sulfates, and complex silicates also contain goodly quantities of combined oxygen.

(c) *Historical preparation.* Although people have been aware of the existence of oxygen since about the eighth century, it was not actually discovered until 1774, when Joseph Priestly heated mercuric oxide in an inverted tube by concentrating the rays of sunlight with a magnifying glass. The mercuric oxide was decomposed to metallic mercury and free oxygen.

$$2HgO \xrightarrow[\Delta]{} 2Hg + O_2\uparrow$$

Δ represents the application of heat. In addition to preparing oxygen, Priestly demonstrated that a candle burned more brightly in concentrations of this gas and that mice became brisk and frisky in an atmosphere of it.

(d) *Modern methods of preparation.* Commercially, or in the laboratory, oxygen can be prepared by–

• Heating a mixture of potassium chlorate and manganese dioxide.

$$2KClO_3 + MnO_2 \xrightarrow[\Delta]{} 2KCl + 3O_2\uparrow$$

- Electrolysis of water.
- Distillation of liquid air.

(3) Chemical properties and reactions. Oxygen is a very active nonmetal, and its activity increases with increasing temperature. Oxygen combines by the process of oxidation with all the nonmetals except the halides and inert gases to form oxides. Oxides are compounds of oxygen and other elements. Oxides thus formed when dissolved in water form acids and are therefore called acid anhydrides (acids without water). Oxygen also combines with most of the metals, slowly at low temperatures and rapidly, even explosively, at high temperatures. Oxides of alkali metals and alkaline earth metals (calcium, barium, strontium) when dissolved in water form metallic hydroxides and are therefore called basic anhydrides. Oxygen supports combustion, but is itself nonflammable. Oxidation is generally a slow process, as evidenced by the rusting of iron. Combustion is a similar but more rapid reaction. Combustion or burning is a chemical reaction which occurs so rapidly that appreciable light and heat are given off.

(4) Uses of oxygen. No life process in the animal kingdom can be carried on without oxygen. Medically, oxygen is used in pure form or mixed with other gases for treatment of respiratory failure. Also of medical significance is the purifying property of oxygen. Sunlight and oxygen are excellent antibacterial agents. Sanitation departments and waterworks make use of this knowledge by a process known as aeration, or spraying the waste or water to be purified into the air in fountains or cascades. Besides purifying the water, this process makes the water taste better. Boiled water, which contains little oxygen, tastes flat. Another extremely important use of oxygen is in syntheses of many compounds and medicinals.

(5) Ozone. Ozone (O_3), a bluish-colored pungent smelling gas, is an allotropic form of oxygen. When a chemical element exists in more than one form, we have the phenomenon of allotropism (from the Greek, "other form"). Sulfur, carbon, and phosphorous are other elements which exhibit allotropism. The different allotropic forms are given different names to distinguish them, as with carbon graphite and diamond.

(6) Nascent oxygen (O). When ozone decomposes, it breaks down to O_2 and O. This monoatomic oxygen is called nascent oxygen. It is another allotropic form of oxygen. Bleaching and disinfectant properties are features of nascent oxygen, and it is these characteristics which make hydrogen peroxide and sodium perborate effective medicinal agents. These agents will be discussed later in their appropriate places.

b. Hydrogen (H, diatomic H_2; valence + 1). Hydrogen, symbol H, is a nonmetallic, gaseous chemical element, the lightest known.

(1) Physical characteristics. Hydrogen is a colorless, odorless, tasteless gas with the lowest molecular weight (hydrogen occurs in diatomic form, H_2) and the least density of any substance. It has the second lowest boiling point and melting point and is less soluble in water than oxygen. A rather interesting property is hydrogen's adsorption by certain metals. At a temperature of 25° C., one volume of palladium will adsorb (accumulate on its surface) 600 or more volumes of hydrogen, at the same time generating copious amounts of heat.

(2) Occurrence and preparation. Hydrogen occurs in nature in the diatomic state (H_2). There is a small percentage in the atmosphere in the free state, but the majority occurs combined. Water is made up of one-ninth hydrogen; all acids, all body tissue, and all fuels such as gas, wood, coal, and oil contain hydrogen. Hydrogen may be prepared by the following reactions:

(a) $Fe + H_2SO_4 \longrightarrow FeSO_4 + H_2\uparrow$

(b) Active metal + water yields metallic hydroxide + H_2

$$2Na + 2HOH \longrightarrow 2NaOH + H_2\uparrow$$

(c) Steam over hot carbon

$$C + HOH \longrightarrow CO\uparrow + H_2\uparrow$$

(d) Electrolysis of water

$$2HOH \xrightarrow{e} 2H_2\uparrow + O_2\uparrow$$

(e is symbol for electrical current or energy)

(3) Chemical properties and reactions. Hydrogen burns in oxygen with a very hot, pale blue flame, yielding only water. Hydrogen does not support combustion. It is a good reducing agent. At room temperature, hydrogen is not very active, but at extremely elevated temperatures, it reacts with many elements directly. It reacts directly with the halides and, using chlorine as an example, forms HCl, a gas which when dissolved in water produces hydrochloric acid. Hydrogen reacts with sulfur to produce hydrogen sulfide (H_2S) and with nitrogen to produce a very important compound, ammonia (NH_3).

(4) Uses of hydrogen. Because it is a reducing agent, hydrogen is sometimes used to replace the atmosphere when working on oxidation-prone chemicals and drugs. As previously stated, hydrogen is used in the manufacture of ammonia which has many uses in the field of pharmacy and medicine.

c. Water. Composed exclusively of hydrogen and oxygen, water (H_2O) is our most abundant compound and most useful liquid.

(1) Physical properties. Pure water is colorless, odorless, and tasteless. It has a freezing point of 0° C., a boiling point of 100° C., and is most dense at a temperature of 4° C., at which temperature 1 ml. weighs 1 gram. Large bodies of water may appear bluish or greenish in color, due mostly to impurities and reflected light. These impurities may be suspended solids, dissolved salts, dissolved greases, and dissolved organic matter.

(2) Occurrence and preparation. Three-fourths of the earth's surface is covered by water. Moreover, most organic material has high quantities of water in its composition. The human body is roughly 70-percent water. Water is prepared from the direct chemical combination of hydrogen and oxygen. This reaction is slow, except at temperatures of about 500° C., when explosion occurs.

(3) Structure. The molecular structure of water is a triangle, the hydrogen atoms bonded at an angle of 104.31°.

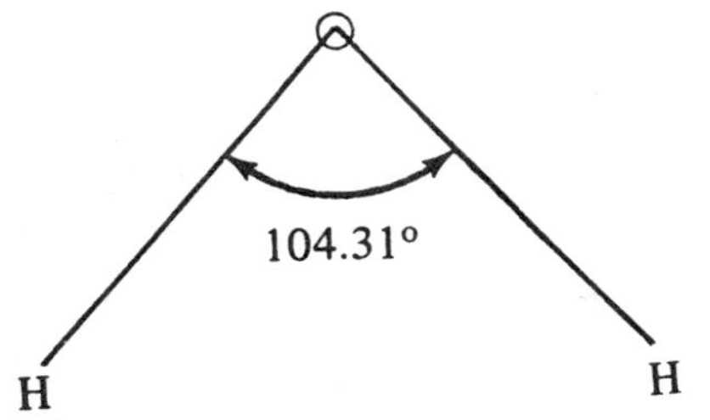

Because of this molecular structure, water is a *dipolar molecule* or *dipole.* That is, the hydrogens with their plus charges are toward one end, and the oxygen with its negative charge is toward the other. It can then be compared to a bar magnet, one end of which has a positive pole and the other a negative pole. This polarity causes the positive hydrogens of one molecule to become loosely associated with the oxygen of another molecule and clusters are formed.

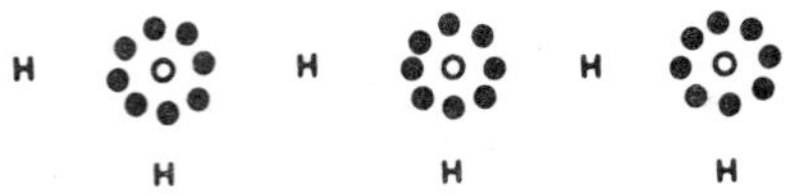

When water freezes, the hydrogen bonds form slightly farther apart than at 4° C., and since the molecule is expanded, density is reduced and ice floats. It is the polarity of water that makes it such an efficient solvent and has led to water being spoken of as the "universal solvent."

(4) Water purification. To make water suitable for its many uses, it must be purified.

(a) Impurities in water. The impurities in water may be either dissolved or suspended. Before looking at the actual ways of purifying water, let's see what impurities are found in water that would make it unsuitable for drinking and other purposes.

1. Organic impurities. Some impurities of water are organic in nature. Examples of organic matter would be bacteria, sewage, and other forms of animal or vegetable matter. If the amount of organic matter in water is high, it becomes a media for the breeding of bacteria. Such water is not fit for drinking. Although some bacteria are not harmful to the human body, others are pathogenic, producing diseases such as typhoid, cholera, and dysentery. Drinkable or *potable* water must be clear and colorless, with a pleasing taste, and must be free of harmful bacteria and other harmful organisms.

2. Inorganic impurities. Depending upon the composition of the earth and the rock through which the water runs, various minerals will be dissolved in it. Large quantities of calcium, magnesium, iron, chlorine, sulfate, or bicarbonate ions in the water produce what is commonly referred to as "hard water." Bicarbonate ions produce temporary hardening because when bicarbonate is heated ($HCO_3 \xrightarrow[\triangle]{} \triangle CO_2 + H_2O$), the bicarbonate breaks down into carbon dioxide and water. The expression "hard water" probably originated because it is hard to get a lather or suds from most soaps in hard water. Conversely, water which lathers well with soaps has been named "soft" water. The terminology is misleading.

3. Soaps and hard water. Most soaps contain sodium stearate, which is soluble in water. When such soaps come into contact with the ions in hard water, a double replacement reaction takes place and an insoluble stearate is formed which is sticky and feels greasy.

Thus, until all the "hard" ions have been reacted, it is impossible to get a lasting suds or lather.

(b) Methods of purification. The purification of drinking water generally consists of sedimentation, filtration, aeration, and chlorination.

1. Sedimentation. Running water from the source is allowed to collect and stand in reservoirs or tanks. The particles of material in suspension settle to the bottom. The upper portions of the water are drawn off and passed through a filtration apparatus.

2. Filtration. Most waterworks use a sand filter consisting of tanks or concrete basins at the bottoms of which are a layer of filtering sand, a layer of charcoal, a layer of fine gravel, one of coarse gravel, and finally at the very bottom, a layer of stones and an outlet for the water that has filtered through. Sediment which has not settled out in the sedimentation tank is removed by this filtering.

3. Aeration. The water, previously settled out and filtered, is blown into the air where it is exposed to oxygen and sunlight. Bacteria are destroyed by oxidation and sunlight.

4. Chlorination. Chlorine, which we will study with the halogens, has bactericidal effects and is widely used in purifying public drinking water. Water for medicinal use is purified still further. The USP contains monographs for water, water for injection, sterile water for injection, and purified water.

- *Water, USP.* This water, although not further purified after the normal drinking water purification, must meet the standard of the USP and the United States Public Health Service.
- *Water for injection, USP.* Water for injection is water purified by distillation. It contains no added substance. The USP cautions that "Water for Injection is intended for use as a solvent only in parenteral solutions that are to be sterilized after preparation."
- *Sterile water for injection, USP.* "Sterile Water for Injection" is water for injection sterilized and suitably packaged. It may contain a bacteriostatic agent when in containers of 30 ml size or smaller, in which case it is exempt from the requirements of the tests for Ammonia and Oxidizable substances."
- *Purified water, USP.* "Purified Water is water obtained by distillation or ion-exchange treatment.... Caution: Do *not* use purified water in preparations intended for parenteral administration. For such purposes use Water for Injection, Bacteriostatic Water for Injection, or Sterile Water for Injection." In the manufacture of pharmaceutical preparations, tap water is never used. The lowest grade of water which may be used in pharmacy is Purified Water, USP.

(5) Chemical properties and reactions. Water is an extremely stable compound. The following properties are true of water:

(a) Water is not decomposed by heat in wide ranges, only 2 percent being broken down at temperatures of 2000° C.

(b) Metals above cobalt in the electromotive series will replace hydrogen from water and form bases.

$$2Na + 2HOH \longrightarrow 2NaOH + H_2\uparrow$$

(c) Oxides of the very active metals react with water to form hydroxides. Sodium, potassium, and calcium oxides will undergo this reaction with water.

$$CaO + HOH \longrightarrow Ca(OH)_2$$

Remember that oxides which react with water to form bases are called *basic anhydrides.*

(d) Oxides of the nonmetals react with water to form acids. These oxides are called *acid anhydrides.*

$$CO_2 + HOH \longrightarrow H_2CO_3 \text{ (carbonic acid)}$$

(e) When a substance contains water in a definite proportion by weight, that water is said to be water of hydration. When a crystal combines with water in definite proportions by weight, the water is said to be water of crystallization. This water is essential for the structure of the crystal and removal of it results in the destruction of the crystal and formation of an amorphic (without shape) powder. The blue crystals or chunks of copper sulfate have a formula $CuSO_4 \cdot 5H_2O$. The dot in the formula shows that the attachment between the five waters of crystallization and the molecule of $CuSO_4$ is rather a loose one. Water of hydration or crystallization can be driven off by elevating the temperature slightly above the boiling point of water. Such compounds which have lost their water of hydration or crystallization are said to be *anhydrous* (without water). This process of driving off the water of crystallization *completely* is known as *exsiccation.*

(f) Substances which lose part or all of their water of hydration when exposed to the atmosphere are called *efflorescent* substances.

(g) Substances which absorb water from the atmosphere when allowed to stand and become moist, but not liquid, are said to be *hygroscopic.*

(h) Substances which absorb water from the air and then dissolve in that water to form liquids are said to be *deliquescent.*

(i) When unusually large crystals are formed, or the crystallization takes place very rapidly, water may be mechanically retained within the structure of the crystal. This water is not chemically bound. It is called *interstitial* water.

(6) Uses. Water is the most widely used solvent in medicine and pharmacy. It is commonly used as a standard as in specific gravity, measuring heat (amount necessary to raise the temperature of 1 gram of water 1 degree Centigrade is 1 cálorie), and in the calibration of thermometers and other measuring devices. Water is also used in many reactions.

d. Peroxides. Peroxides are derivatives of H_2O_2 (hydrogen peroxide), and all contain a covalent bonding between the oxygens. The structure of hydrogen peroxide is

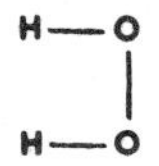

(1) Physical characteristics of hydrogen peroxide. Pure hydrogen peroxide is a thick, syrupy liquid which mixes with water in any proportion and has bitter taste.

(2) Occurrence and preparation. Being very unstable, hydrogen peroxide is not naturally occurring. For quite some time, it was prepared by reaction of barium peroxide and cold, dilute sulfuric acid.

$$BaO_2 + H_2SO_4 \longrightarrow BaSO_4 + H_2O_2$$

Commercial manufacturers use electrolysis to produce persulfuric acid which reacts with the water in the solution to yield sulfuric acid and hydrogen peroxide. These are separated by distillation under reduced pressure.

(3) Chemical properties and reactions. Hydrogen peroxide is a powerful oxidizing agent. It is decomposed by alkalies and is unstable in water solutions. Light catalyzes its decomposition. In contact with organic material, because it is an oxidizing agent, it is reduced to nascent oxygen and water.

(4) Uses. In 3-percent concentrations, hydrogen peroxide is used as an antiseptic solution. This solution must be stored in dark bottles to protect it from light. Besides destroying bacteria, in higher concentrations of 20 to 30 percent, it destroys the color in some organic matter and is therefore used to bleach hair, wool, silk, ivory, and feathers. Peroxide has been used for a source of oxygen in rocket propulsion.

8. Acids, bases, and salts. Acids, bases, and salts are three very important classes of chemical compounds. Lemon juice and vinegar are mild acids found in the home. Much stronger acids are found in the pharmacy. Strong acids, such as hydrochloric, sulfuric, and nitric, are corrosive; that is, they gnaw at or eat away metals and tissue. Household ammonia and milk of magnesia are bases found in the home. The stronger bases in pharmacy such as sodium hydroxide are caustic, that is, they destroy tissue. Acids react with bases to form a salt and water. Sodium chloride, common table salt, is the most widely used of the salts.

a. Acids. An acid is a substance containing hydrogen which in water solution forms no positive ions other than hydrogen ions. It is a proton donor. Hydrogen chloride ionizes in water as illustrated by the equation $HCl \longrightarrow H^+ + Cl^-$. Since the only positive ions in solution are hydrogen ions, it fits the definition of an acid. A hydrogen ion is nothing more than a proton, so acids are said to give up protons. They are proton donors. In the formula above we showed H^+ existing alone, and this is the way chemists simplify ionization for practical purposes. Actually, the hydrogen ion associates with a water molecule to form H_3O^+, the hydronium ion.

(1) General properties of acids. Acids have the following common properties:

- Taste sour.
- Affect some indicators.
- Neutralize bases to form salts.
- React with some metals to form salts.
- React with some metallic oxides to form salts.
- React with carbonates to form carbon dioxide and water.
- Are generally soluble in water.

(2) General methods of preparation of acids. Generally, acids may be prepared by the following methods:

(a) Reacting water with a nonmetallic oxide (acid anhydride):

$$CO_2 + H_2O \longrightarrow H_2CO_3$$

(b) Reacting sulfuric acid with the salt of the acid desired:

Sulfuric Acid		Sodium Chloride		Sodium Bisulfate		Hydrochloric Acid
H_2SO_4	+	NaCl	$\longrightarrow$	$NaHSO_4$	+	HCl

(3) Classification of the acids. Acids may be classified according to the number of hydrogen ions (protons) furnished by each molecule.

- Monobasic acids give 1 proton or hydrogen ion per molecule. *Example:* HCl, HNO_3
- Dibasic acids give 2 protons or hydrogen ions per molecule. *Example:* H_2SO_4, H_2CO_3
- Tribasic acids give 3 protons or hydrogen ions per molecule. *Example:* H_3PO_4, H_3BO_4

b. Bases. A base is a substance containing the hydroxyl group (OH) which, when dissolved in water, forms no negative ions other than OH^- ions. Bases are proton acceptors. Sodium hydroxide ionizes in water solution to Na^+ and OH^-. The only negative ion is the hydroxyl ion. When acids and bases react in a reaction called neutralization, the proton (H^+ ion) reacts with the proton acceptor (OH^- ion) to form water.

(1) General properties of bases. Bases have the following common properties:

- Taste bitter (those that are soluble).
- If solution, feel slick and slippery like soap.
- Affect some indicators.
- React with acids to produce salts.
- React with nonmetallic oxides to form salts.

(2) General methods of preparation of bases. Generally, bases may be prepared by the following methods:

(a) Some active metals react with water to form bases.

$$2Na + 2HOH \longrightarrow 2NaOH + H_2\uparrow$$

(b) Some metallic oxides react with water to form bases.

$$CaO + HOH \longrightarrow Ca(OH)_2$$

(c) Insoluble bases can be made from soluble ones. When salts of calcium, magnesium, iron, chlorine, sulfate, or bicarbonate come in contact with the soluble bases, double replacement reactions occur, forming insoluble bases which precipitate.

Example:

$$FeCl_3 + 3NaOH \longrightarrow Fe(OH)_3\downarrow + 3NaCl$$

(3) Nomenclature of the bases. Naming the bases is most simple. Name the metallic ion and follow it by the word hydroxide and you have the chemical name for the base.

$Zn(OH)_2$ = zinc hydroxide
NaOH = sodium hydroxide
KOH = potassium hydroxide

(4) Classification of the bases. Bases can be classified according to the number of protons they will accept.

- Monoacidic bases take up 1 proton or hydrogen ion. *Example:* KOH, NaOH
- Diacidic bases take up 2 protons or hydrogen ions. *Example:* $Ca(OH)_2$
- Triacidic bases take up 3 protons or hydrogen ions. *Example:* $Fe(OH)_3$

The classes of acids and bases are more readily understood when the student considers that one molecule of a diacid base will react with two molecules of a monobasic acid or that one molecule of a tribasic acid will combine with three molecules of a monoacid base.

c. Relations between acids and bases. In some acids the protons are more readily given up than in others. The strength of an acid depends on the ease with which this occurs. A strong acid gives up its protons easily. A weak acid does so with difficulty. Conversely, a strong base readily accepts a proton while a weak base does not accept protons readily. Table 4 shows the relationship between some strong and weak acids and bases.

Table 4. Relative Strength of Some Acids and Bases

Bases	Strength	Acids
NaOH KOH	Strong	HCl H_2SO_4 HNO_3
$Ca(OH)_2$ $Mg(OH)_2$	Moderate	H_3PO_4
NH_4OH $Zn(OH)_2$	Weak	HCN $H(C_2H_3O_2)$

d. Salts. A compound whose water solution contains a positive ion other than a hydrogen ion, and a negative ion other than a hydroxyl ion is a *salt.* Salts are produced in addition to water when acids neutralize bases. The most common salt is table salt or sodium chloride (NaCl).

(1) Properties of salts. Because there are hundreds of possible salts with greatly varying properties, it is impossible to list any general properties which more than a few salts would exhibit. One important property, which differs among the salts, but can be set up in table form is solubility. This is an important property of any compound.

- Na, K, NH_4 compounds are soluble.
- NO_3, OAC, ClO_3 (nitrates, acetates, chlorates) are soluble.
- Chlorides *except* Ag, Hg, Pb are soluble.
- Sulfates *except* Ba, Ca, Sr, Pb are soluble.
- Carbonates, phosphates, and silicates are *insoluble except* Na, K, and NH_4.
- Sulfides are *insoluble.*

(2) General methods of preparation of salts. Salts may be prepared by the following methods:

- Direct union.

$$2Na + Cl_2 \longrightarrow 2NaCl$$

- Replacement of hydrogen from acid.

$$Zn + H_2SO_4 \longrightarrow ZnSO_4 + H_2\uparrow$$

- Acid reacting with metallic oxide.

$$2HCl + HgO \longrightarrow HgCl_2 + HOH$$

- Base plus a nonmetal.

$$2NaOH + CO_2 \longrightarrow Na_2CO_3 + HOH$$

- Double replacement.

$$AgNO_3 + NaCl \longrightarrow AgCl\downarrow + NaNO_3$$

- Acid plus carbonate.

$$ZnCO_3 + H_2SO_4 \longrightarrow ZnSO_4 + HOH + CO_2\uparrow$$

- Neutralization. Acid plus base yields salt plus water.

$$HCl + NaOH \longrightarrow NaCl + HOH$$

(3) Nomenclature of salts. Generally, the names of salts are derived from the ions forming them, as in NaCl, sodium chloride; $ZnSO_4$, zinc sulfate; and AgCl, silver chloride. If the element has a varying valence, the lower valence state is the *ous* form; the higher, the *ic* form. Thus, in $FeCl_2$, the iron has a valence of +2 and is the ferr*ous* chloride. $FeCl_3$ gives a valence of +3 and thus makes the name ferr*ic* chloride.

e. *Hydrolysis.* Hydrolysis is a decomposition due to the incorporation and splitting of water. The two resulting products divide the water, the hydrogen ion attaching to one end and the hydroxyl ion to the other.

(1) Nonhydrolyzing salts. Salts may partially decompose in water solution by the process of hydrolysis. Sodium chloride, when dissolved in water, does not hydrolyze. This is because it is a salt formed from the neutralization of a *strong* acid and a *strong* base. Potassium chloride, potassium nitrate, potassium sulfate, and sodium nitrate are also formed from *strong* acids and *strong* bases and do not hydrolyze.

(2) Hydrolyzing salts. Salt formed from a strong acid and a weak base, from a strong base and weak acid, or from a weak acid and weak base hydrolyze.

(a) Strong base–weak acid. Sodium carbonate, formed from a *strong* base and a *weak* acid, hydrolyzes in water solution. On testing this solution with litmus indicator, red litmus turns blue, a reaction signifying the presence of a base. You would not normally expect that the solution of a neutral salt in neutral water would produce a basic solution. The following reactions explain why the salt solution exhibits a basic nature.

$$\begin{array}{lcccc} Na_2CO_3 & \longrightarrow & 2Na^+ & + & CO_3^{=} \\ & & + & & + \\ 2HOH & \longrightarrow & 2OH^- & + & 2H^+ \\ & & \downarrow & & \downarrow \\ & & 2NaOH & & H_2CO_3 \end{array}$$

Sodium carbonate dissociates in the first equation and water ionizes in the second. The vertical reactions between the sodium ions and the hydroxyl ions and between the carbonate ions and the hydrogen ions show the formation of sodium hydroxide, a strong base, and carbonic acid, a weak acid. The strong base dominates. A salt formed from a *strong base* and a *weak acid* partially hydrolyzes in water, yielding a solution which is *basic* to litmus.

(b) Strong acid–weak base. Zinc chloride, formed from a strong acid and a weak base, hydrolyzes in water solution. On testing this solution with litmus, blue litmus turns red, signifying an acid solution. Again, a neutral salt dissolved in neutral water produces other than a neutral solution. The following reactions explain why the salt solution exhibits an acidic nature.

$$\begin{array}{lcccc} ZnCl_2 & \longrightarrow & Zn^{++} & + & 2Cl^- \\ & & + & & \\ 2HOH & \longrightarrow & 2OH^- & + & 2H^+ \\ & & \downarrow\uparrow & & \downarrow \\ & & Zn(OH)_2 & & 2HCl \end{array}$$

The vertical reactions in this case show the formation of a strong acid and a weak base, with the acid predominating. A salt formed from a *strong acid* and a *weak base* partially hydrolyzes in water, yielding a solution which is acid in reaction.

(c) Weak acid–weak base. Aluminum sulfide, formed from a very weak acid and a very weak base, hydrolyzes in water solution. Notice the reactions that occur below.

$$\begin{array}{lcccc} Al_2S_3 & \longrightarrow & 2Al^{+++} & + & 3S^{=} \\ & & + & & + \\ 6HOH & \rightleftharpoons & 6OH^- & & 6H^+ \\ & & \downarrow\uparrow & & \downarrow\uparrow \\ & & 2Al(OH)_3\downarrow & & 3H_2S\downarrow\uparrow \end{array}$$

The salts of very *weak* acids and very *weak* bases hydrolyze almost completely when dissolved in water. In the case above, the aluminum hydroxide formed is precipitated and therefore the aluminum and hydroxide ions are removed from the water. Hydrogen sulfide is given off as a gas and thus both the hydrogen and the sulfide ions are removed. This hydrolysis, then, runs to completion.

9. Ionization and pH. Dissociation is the ionization of a substance in solution into its constituent ions. pH is the symbol expressing the hydrogen ion concentration of a solution and therefore its acidity or alkalinity.

a. Electrolytes. Water solutions of certain substances have the ability to conduct electricity. Such substances are called *electrolytes.* A nonelectrolyte, then, is a compound whose water solution does NOT conduct electricity. When substances are dissolved in water, the freezing point of the solution is lower than that of water alone; also, the boiling point is higher than for water alone. Electrolytes lower freezing points and raise boiling points of solutions two to three times as much as nonelectrolytes do.

b. Theory of ionization. The theory of ionization which explains the behavior of electrolytes was first proposed by Svante Arrhenius. Arrhenius' theory states that–

- Electrolytes in solution exist in the form of ions.
- An *ion* is an atom or group of atoms which carry an electrical charge.
- In aqueous solutions of electrolytes, there are an equal number of positive and negative charges.

(1) Structure of water review. Let's review the structure of water. We said that water consists of two atoms of hydrogen covalently bonded to one atom of oxygen at an angle of 104.31°. We further said that because of this angle, the end toward the hydrogens was positively charged and the end toward the oxygen was negatively charged. Molecules, which like water molecules have distinct poles, are called *dipoles* or *polar molecules.* Compounds that do not exhibit this unsymmetrical charge are *nonpolar compounds.*

(2) Ion formation. At the beginning of this chapter, we explained that in electrovalent bonding one atom gives up an electron and another accepts it. Each atom, at this time, gains a charge. Since atoms are electrically neutral, these charged atoms are no longer atoms, but *ions.* Perhaps this will be clearer if you look at sodium and chlorine. As elements, both of these substances are electrically neutral. When they interact, sodium donates an electron and chlorine accepts it, forming a compound which is stable. Both outer electron shells are now completed. In giving an electron, the sodium, now an ion, has a charge of plus one; and the chlorine, now a chloride ion, has a charge of minus one. Notice that the charge of the ion equals its valence. Better stated, the charge *is* the valence.

c. Dissociation of electrovalent compounds. Sodium chloride has a crystalline structure due to the attraction between the ions. When added to water, the polarity of the water reduces the attraction of the two ions for each other and causes them to break away from their crystalline structure. This process is known as *dissociation.* Electrovalent compounds dissociate completely when dissolved. Thus, 100 percent of the sodium chloride that dissolves in water is dissociated.

d. Ionization and dissociation differentiated.

(1) Ionization is the breakup of a substance into ions.

(2) Dissociation is the separation of the ions of electrovalent compounds by the action of the solvent.

e. Electrolyte strength. The strength of an electrolyte is determined by its ability to produce ions. Strong electrolytes are ionized almost completely. Hydrochloric acid and sodium hydroxide are strong electrolytes. Weak electrolytes are those which produce relatively few ions. Acetic acid and ammonium hydroxide are weak electrolytes. Do not confuse weak and strong with dilute and concentrated. These terms are confusing and warrant explanation. Weak and strong refer to the amount of ionization, NOT to the degree of concentration in solution. Dilute and concentrated refer to the amount of solute in a solvent.

f. Electrolysis. When studying oxygen and hydrogen we explained one method of preparation as the decomposition of water by electrolysis. You should now be able to thoroughly appreciate this reaction. Water ionizes only very slightly, something like two parts in one billion, so in order for an electric current to be passed between two electrodes placed in the water, we must add a substance to supply ions. Although many agents can be used, sulfuric acid is the most common one.

$$2H_2O \longrightarrow 2H_2 + O_2$$

(1) Formation of hydrogen. When a source of direct current is applied to the electrodes in the solution, the very few hydrogen ions from the water itself and the ions of hydrogen from the sulfuric acid, carrying a charge of +1, are attracted toward the negative electrode which is called the cathode. These ions are called cations. When they contact the electrode, they gain an electron, become neutral, and form hydrogen atoms. Two of these newly formed hydrogen atoms combine to form a molecule, and these molecules bubble up as hydrogen gas.

(2) Formation of oxygen. Also in this solution are the negative ions, a very few of OH^- from the slight ionization of the water and many more of $SO_4^=$ from the sulfuric acid. Despite the difference in number, the OH^- ions give up electrons more easily and so they are the ions discharged. These ions, called anions, are attracted to the positive electrode, which is called the anode; give up an electron; and become neutral atoms and are liberated as molecules of oxygen.

g. pH.

(1) Definition. pH is the negative common logarithm of a hydrogen ion concentration expressed in moles per liter. pH is dependent upon solubility and ionization of the substance. pH derives its name from the combination of "p," for the power of the negative exponent, and "H" for the hydrogen ion concentration expressed in moles per liter. A solution, then, which has 1×10^{-6} moles of hydrogen ion per liter, has a pH of 6. A solution with 1×10^{-14} moles of hydrogen ion per liter has a pH of 14. The pharmacist should know how pH is measured and what the reading obtained means.

(2) pH values. A pH reading of 7 is neutral, neither acidic nor basic. Anything above 7, ranging up to 14, is basic. The higher the number above 7, the stronger (more highly ionized) is the base. Below 7 and ranging down to 1 is acid, the stronger acids being lower numbers.

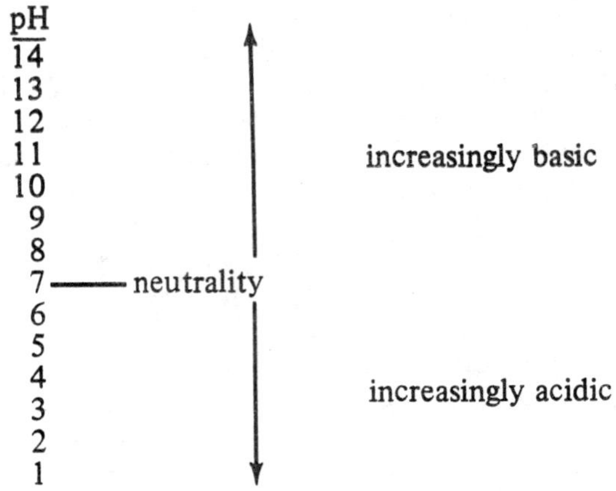

h. Measurement of pH. pH is measured by using one or more of the hundreds of organic indicators. These compounds are capable of changing color when exposed to different pH values. Some indicate only whether a solution is acidic or basic, but do not tell the degree. Others will give a fairly accurate estimate of the pH itself by the color or degree of color it attains in the solution. Below are some examples of indicators and what happens to their colors under different conditions.

(1) Litmus. Litmus paper is an indicator paper with the coloring property from a lichen. Blue litmus paper coming into contact with acids turns red. Red litmus paper turns blue on contact with bases. This is a very popular test to distinguish between acids and bases. No indication is given as to the strength of the acid or base, however.

(2) Impregnated paper. There are other papers impregnated with organic indicators which when touched by a drop of solution produce a range of colors. These colors are matched with a chart to give the corresponding pH value.

(3) Indicator solutions. There are various indicator solutions which when placed in an unknown solution produce a color which is compared to a colorimetric pH chart.

(4) Phenolphthalein. Phenolphthalein, previously mentioned in titrations, is an indicator which is colorless in acid solutions and pink or red in alkaline solution.

(5) pH meter. For very accurate measurement of pH, an expensive machine called a pH meter is available to chemists. Such devices are not necessary to the general pharmacist. They are, however, used frequently in industry and research.

i. Buffers. A substance which resists a change in pH is called a buffer.

(1) Use of buffers. The activity of many drugs is destroyed or severely lessened at certain pH ranges, with maximum efficiency being at a specific pH. Such medications must be buffered to assure that the patient derives all possible benefits from the drug.

(2) Other pH adjusting substances. Other substances, although not considered buffers, are used to promote the proper pH. *For example,* mandelic acid or sodium phosphate is given in conjunction with methenamine to assure an acid urine. Methenamine, a urinary antiseptic, breaks down into formaldehyde in acid urine, killing the unwanted organisms. Urine, normally acid, may be alkaline under certain conditions so, to assure acidity, the acid substances are given.

(3) Buffer pairs. Buffering agents may consist either of a weak acid and one of its salts, or a weak base and one of its salts. Such agents are called buffer pairs. These pairs resist change in pH by reacting with increased acid or base and neutralizing it.

j. Total acidity. Total acidity refers to the amount of ionizable hydrogen a substance contains. Thus 10 ml. of a 1N HCl solution contains the same total acidity as does 10 ml. of 1N acetic acid. And 10 ml. of a 1N acid contains the same total acidity as 20 ml. of a .5N acid.

10. Alkali metals. The alkali metals are those from group 1A on the periodic table. They have been so named because hydroxides of these metals form the strongest alkalies known. In this group are lithium, sodium, potassium, rubidium, cesium, and francium. Of these, the first three are of importance to pharmacists.

a. General properties of the alkali metals. All the alkali metals have a valence of +1, and have one valence electron in the outermost ring. They all react with water to yield hydrogen and a base. They form oxides, peroxides, bases, sulfates, hydroxides, and halides. Because these metals are so reactive, they occur in nature in the combined form only, and when pure must be stored under petrolatum or some other appropriate substance which will exclude air. The alkali metals are soft, being easily cut with a knife; have a low specific gravity, low melting points and boiling points; and may be prepared from the electrolysis of their fused chloride.

b. Pharmaceutically important alkali metals. Sodium and potassium are extremely important to pharmacists. Hardly a day will pass that you will not see some medication in the form of sodium or potassium salt. Lithium is also used in medicine, but much less frequently. We will discuss these three elements, not in the order of their importance, but in order of the periodic table.

(1) Lithium (Li, +1) and its compounds. Lithium, occurring in nature in the form of silicates and phosphates, looks like stone and was accordingly named from the Greek word lithos, meaning stone. Certain waters containing lithium are called lithia waters.

(a) Lithium metal. Lithium metal, like the other alkali metals, is prepared from the fused chloride by electrolysis. This metal, although less prone to oxidation than sodium and potassium, must be stored under hydrocarbon oils or sealed hermetically to preserve it. It is a silver-white substance with definite metallic luster. Salts of lithium when moistened with hydrochloric acid and flamed on platinum wire give distinct crimson red color to the flame.

(b) Soaps. Soaps made from lithium are among the insoluble soaps. The soaps prepared from sodium and potassium are soluble.

(c) Medical uses. Medically, the lithium ion (Li^+) is depressant to nerve centers and to circulation. It also has slight diuretic action. Lithium is eliminated from the body by the kidney and intestinal tract. The only official compound of lithium is lithium bromide. This product was once widely used as a sedative, but has proved to be quite toxic and has fallen into disuse. Another lithium salt that is in use is lithium carbonate (Li_2CO_3). It is being used for depressive states.

(2) Sodium (Na, +1) and its compounds. The symbol (Na) for sodium is derived from the Latin, natrium. Its English name comes from Italian, referring to soda, an ash used in the manufacture of glass. Sodium also has a valence of +1.

(a) Properties. A very soft metal, sodium can be easily cut with a knife and has a silver-white luster that tarnishes almost immediately on exposure to air. It floats in water, melting and spinning as it reacts. The nature of its reaction with water is thus–

$$2Na + 2H_2O \longrightarrow 2NaOH + H_2$$

Because of its extreme activity in air, sodium must be stored under kerosene or petroleum oils. It will combine, if exposed, with most of the nonmetallic elements and all of the common acids.

(b) Occurrence and preparation. Sodium occurs naturally only in the combined state. The most commonly occurring compound of sodium is sodium chloride or common salt. Sodium is prepared by electrolysis after the sodium chloride has first been fused. Chlorine is an important byproduct of this reaction.

(c) Important compounds of sodium.

1. Sodium chloride (NaCl). Great volumes of sodium chloride are dissolved in sea and inland (salt lake) waters. Solid massive deposits are also located throughout the world. This compound is mined from these deposits in huge quantities. Some deposits are over a half mile thick. Sodium chloride is probably one of the most important of the salts you will study. It is the predominant ion in the extracellular fluid of the tissues, and quite necessary to life. In fact, when you get to isotonic solutions and their manufacture, you will see that sodium chloride solutions of a certain percent are isotonic when they have the same electrolyte concentration as extracellular fluid. *Hypotonic,* then, is less concentrated than the extracellular fluids; *hypertonic,* more concentrated. Because this salt is predominant in extracellular fluid and can be made isotonic, it is used medicinally as an electrolyte replenisher and blood volume builder for burn patients or for those who have lost considerable quantities of body fluids. Many insoluble medicinals are reacted with sodium to produce the related soluble sodium salt.

- *Sodium Chloride Injection, USP.* Sterile, isotonic solution for injection as a fluid and electrolyte replenisher. It is given IV (intravenously) in quantities from 500 to 5000 ml.
- *Sodium Chloride Solution, USP.* A physiological salt solution NOT for injection. It is intended for topical use. As with the sterile solution for injection, the concentration of NaCl is 0.9 percent.

2. Sodium acetate ($C_2H_3NaO_2 \cdot 3H_2O$). Sodium acetate is used in pharmacy as a buffering agent in combination with acetic acid, and as a systemic antacid in cases of acidosis. Also, because of its alkalizing properties, it is used to produce an assuredly alkaline urine in conjunction with medications with urinary antiseptics which are most active in alkaline media. Sodium acetate undergoes hydrolysis to yield sodium hydroxide and acetic acid.

3. Sodium bicarbonate (baking soda, $NaHCO_3$). This compound neutralizes acidity but may cause stomach ulceration because, after frequent use, the stomach becomes sensitized and secretes even more hydrochloric acid. It is also used in cases of systemic acidosis to regulate the body toward normal balance. This compound is particularly useful in conjunction with the sulfonamide drugs which tend to crystallize in acid urine. Not only are these drugs more active in alkaline media, but they are less likely to form crystals in the urinary tract. The newer, more soluble sulfa drugs do not seem to produce crystalluria when water intakes are adequate.

4. Sodium biphosphate (sodium acid phosphate, sodium dihydrogen phosphate, $NaH_2PO_4H_2O$). When given internally, this compound assures a distinctly acid urine and is therefore commonly co-prescribed with methenamine. A mixture of sodium biphosphate and sodium phosphate is used as a saline cathartic taken both internally and as an enema. The most common trade name of this product is Fleet's Phospho-soda. The enema, a disposable package also manufactured by Fleet, is called a Fleet enema.

5. Sodium bisulfite (sodium acid sulfite, sodium hydrogen sulfite, $NaHSO_3$). This compound is used mainly as an antioxidant.

6. Sodium bromide (NaBr). Sodium bromide is the choice when bromides must be administered. It is the least toxic of the bromide salts. Mainly used as a sedative, the dose is 1 Gm.

7. Monohydrated sodium carbonate ($Na_2CO_3 \cdot H_2O$). Sodium carbonate, monohydrated, has been called washing soda. It is used in lotions for certain skin conditions. Its mode of action is to react with the skin oils and scaly skin, forming soaps that can be easily washed away.

8. Sodium citrate ($C_6H_5Na_3O_7 \cdot 2H_2O$). A white or colorless crystalline powder, sodium citrate is used in the preparation of anticoagulant sodium citrate solution and anticoagulant acid citrate dextrose solution. This substance is the one used in blood-drawing apparatus to prevent coagulation. However, it has a peculiarity when administered *intravenously,* it has the opposite effect and PROMOTES coagulation. Administered orally, sodium citrate is a useful expectorant. It is used pharmaceutically as a solubilizer (increase the solubility) of certain substances, especially aspirin and the salicylates. It also has the ability to prevent discoloration of certain products, such as glycerite or tannic acid.

9. *Sodium nitrite ($NaNO_2$).* This is a white or slightly yellow granular powder, deliquescent in air, used as a preservative, a rust inhibitor in cold sterilization solutions, and an antidote in cyanide poisoning.

10. *Sodium hydroxide (caustic soda, NaOH).* Sodium hydroxide is a strong base used in the manufacture of several pharmaceutical preparations. It occurs in white fused masses which may be compressed into pellets, flakes, or sticks.

(3) Potassium (K, +1) and its compounds. The name potassium is derived from the English word potash, referring to the ashes produced from burning vegetable matter in pots. The symbol K is from the Latin, kalium.

(a) Potassium in the body. Potassium is the predominant cation in the intracellular fluid. (Remember, Na was the predominant cation in the extracellular fluid.) These ions in solution easily pass through a semipermeable membrane. Lack of the potassium ion in the body causes general weakness, cardiac (heart) depression, feeble muscle action, and low blood pressure. The potassium ion is essential for the metabolism of carbohydrates. Potassium salts are the best of the osmotic diuretics (medications to increase the flow of urine by the passing of fluid from body tissues to the more concentrated areas developed by the potassium salts).

(b) Compounds of potassium.

1. *Potassium acetate ($C_2H_3KO_2$).* A deliquescent, colorless, crystalline powder, potassium acetate is used as a diuretic and a systemic and urinary alkalizer.

2. *Potassium bitartrate (cream of tartar, $C_4H_5KO_6$).* The main use of this substance is as a cathartic (laxative). It has also been used as a surgical dusting powder because of its bacteriostatic action.

3. *Potassium bromide (KBr).* Potassium bromide is one of the official bromides used as sedatives. Sodium bromide is preferred to this salt, however, because it is less toxic. The usual dose of potassium bromide is 1 Gm.

4. *Potassium chloride (KCl).* Like sodium chloride, potassium chloride is an electrolyte replenisher, particularly indicated where sodium salts are contraindicated. It may be given orally or as an injection by slow infusion.

5. *Potassium permanganate ($KMnO_4$).* The dark purple crystals of potassium permanganate are stable in air and, generally, when dissolved in water are an oxidizing anti-infective. The potassium permanganate liberates nascent oxygen in contact with organic substances, which is its mode of action in killing bacteria and fungal organisms. Because it is a powerful oxidizing agent, care must be used in avoiding its contact in concentrated amounts with organic substances. Serious explosions can result. DO NOT MIX WITH GLYCERIN!

6. *Sulfurated potash.* Sulfurated potash is a mixture consisting mainly of potassium polysulfides and potassium thiosulfate. It may be referred to as potassium sulfide, but you should be aware that this name is not completely true. This chemical is used in the preparation of White Lotion, USP, a preparation used for topical application as an astringent for certain skin conditions. The action of this preparation is based on the hydrogen sulfide produced.

11. **Alkaline earth metals.** The alkaline earth metals are sometimes called the calcium family. In the periodic table, group IIA, beryllium, magnesium, calcium, strontium, barium, and radium, are listed together. There are certain differences in these elements and because of these differences, calcium, barium, and strontium certainly qualify as alkaline earth metals, but the others, although similar in some respects, differ in many chemical respects, more nearly resembling other classes. Radium, because of its unusual property of being radioactive, will not be discussed in this text, although it does have some medical application. Magnesium will be discussed with the alkaline earth metals, although it is similar in many ways to zinc and cadmium.

a. *General.* The elements are referred to as alkaline earth metals because they react with water to form a base and hydrogen.

(1) Valence and activity. All the elements in this group are divalent (+2 valence) and for the most part, the bonding is ionic with a tendency toward covalence. The activity of these elements increases as the atomic weight increases:

beryllium → magnesium → calcium
strontium → barium → increasing activity

(2) Reactions. Although less active than the alkali metals, all the alkaline earth metals except beryllium are attacked by oxygen. Magnesium in the presence of oxygen forms a

protective coating of magnesium oxide (MgO) and the reaction halts as soon as this coating prevents the element within from coming in contact with the air.

(3) Solubility. The salts of the alkaline earth metals are not as soluble as those of the alkali metals and generally decrease in solubility with increase in atomic weight. The hydroxides, however, are exceptions to this solubility rule, increasing in solubility as the atomic weight increases. Thus–

- Generally, salt solubility, decreasing Ca ⟶ Sr ⟶ Ba.
- Hydroxide solubility, decreasing Ba ⟶ Sr ⟶ Ca.

The most soluble salts are formed when these elements react with elements having a valence of −1.

(4) Occurrence and preparation. Because of their activity, these metals are not found free in nature, but their carbonates, sulfates, and phosphates are quite abundant. The elemental form may be liberated by electrolysis of the fused chloride.

b. Calcium (Ca, +2) and its compounds. The name and symbol for calcium are both derived from the Latin, calx, meaning lime. This element occurs combined in nature in marble, limestone, and chalk.

(1) Calcium in the body. Calcium is an extremely important element to man, for it plays an important role in the function of the voluntary and autonomic nervous systems. It is a factor in heart function and in blood coagulation; blood will not coagulate in the absence of calcium. Calcium is the basis for the skeletal system and similar tissue. Bone is made up principally of calcium phosphate and calcium carbonate. Ionic calcium is present in all extracellular fluid. A reduction of ionic calcium in the blood causes hypocalcemic tetany (low-calcium spasms). Conversely, an increase in calcium ions in the blood acts as a nerve sedative and is therefore of benefit in those allergic manifestations such as eczema and pruritis caused by stimulation of the vagus nerve.

(2) Compounds of calcium.

(a) Calcium bromide ($CaBr_2 \cdot H_2O$). Calcium bromide has the same action of sedation as the other bromides. Sodium bromide is the preferred salt because it is least toxic. The usual dose is 1 gram.

(b) Calcium bromidio galacto gluconate. Calcium bromidio galacto gluconate, a complex calcium and bromide containing salt, is employed in the treatment of eczema. It is less toxic than the other bromides.

(c) Precipitated calcium carbonate (precipitated chalk, $CaCO_3$). Calcium carbonate is used mainly as an antacid and is of the nonsystemic type (does not cause systemic alkalosis). It has protective qualities also, and is sometimes used in diarrhea mixtures. It may be used as a dusting powder to adsorb moisture. Notice the word *ad*sorb. The moisture is not absorbed.

(d) Prepared chalk (chalk, drop chalk, $CaCO_3$). Prepared chalk is an official form of chalk freed from *most* of its impurities by elutriation. The elutriation removes gritty particles making it easier to suspend. Since the elutriation does not purify the chalk of insoluble fine particles, this product is not as chemically pure as precipitated calcium carbonate. Prepared chalk is used as an antacid and antidiarrheal in the dose of 1 Gm.

(e) Calcium chloride ($CaCl_2$). Calcium chloride is used to produce diuresis, to increase acidity, and to provide a source of calcium in cases of hypocalcemic tetany. Sometimes it is used as a muscle sedative in cases of lead poisoning. Calcium chloride is a constituent in Ringer's solution, an electrolyte replenisher.

(f) Calcium gluconate. Calcium gluconate may be administered either orally or by intravenous injection for low-calcium tetany. It is less irritating than calcium chloride and is therefore much more commonly used for this purpose. It also is frequently used as a dietary supplement where increased calcium is indicated, as in pregnancy. Calcium gluconate is employed in the treatment of black widow spider bite to help control the muscle spasm pain.

(g) Calcium hydroxide [slaked lime, $Ca(OH)_2$]. Calcium hydroxide is primarily important in the manufacture of calcium hydroxide solution (lime water). This solution is used in a great number of external preparations as an astringent, protective, and emulsifying agent (especially with a fixed oil and fatty acid, as in calamine liniment). Although too weak to serve as an effective antacid for adults, it is effectively used with infants. It also provides a small amount of necessary calcium for infants.

c. Magnesium (Mg, +2) and its compounds. Magnesium, like the other alkaline earth metals, is found naturally only in combination with mineral substances such as talc, soapstone, and meerschaum, and in some mineral waters. The magnesium ion, essential to human life, is an enzyme system activator, important to the neuromuscular system. It is not readily absorbed in the gastrointestinal tract and its absorption is enhanced by acidity and retarded by alkalinity. Alkalies, in fact, precipitate the magnesium ion. Magnesium products are generally employed in medicine as saline cathartics (magnesium sulfate) and antacids (magnesium hydroxide). Since the magnesium ion is excreted by the kidneys, impaired renal function is a definite contraindication for its use, as toxic quantities may be accumulated. The soluble salts may be used externally as anti-inflammatory agents, working by osmotic pressure. The more important compounds of magnesium are—

(1) Magnesium carbonate ($MgCO_3 \cdot Mg(OH)_2 \cdot 5H_2O$). Magnesium carbonate is generally used as an antacid and cathartic. It may be combined with other substances (such as calcium carbonate) to overcome their constipating effect. It should never be used to counteract the effects of acid poisoning because CO_2 is liberated on contact with acids. The added gas content may easily rupture the stomach or intestine. Magnesium carbonate is also used in pharmacy to clarify turbid liquids and to help prevent eutectic mixtures by absorbing liquids.

(2) Magnesium hydroxide ($Mg(OH)_2$). Magnesium hydroxide, although an antacid and cathartic itself, is mainly used in pharmacy in the manufacture of Milk of Magnesia, USP, which contains 7 to 8 percent of $Mg(OH)_2$ as the active ingredient. Milk of magnesia is widely used in hospitals and nursing homes as a nonsystemic antacid and cathartic. Its action depends upon the dose, 4 ml. being the antacid dose and 15 ml. the cathartic dose. Less frequently, this product may be used as an alkaline mouthwash.

(3) Milk of magnesia (magnesium hydroxide mixture). Milk of magnesia is a popularly used household antacid and cathartic. Five ml. function as an antacid, 15 to 30 as a cathartic. Since hydroxides react with glass, 0.1 percent of citric acid may be added as a preventative.

(4) Magnesium oxide (MgO). Two forms of magnesium oxide are common to pharmacy, the light and the heavy. The light magnesium oxide is 4 to 5 times as bulky as the heavy form. Magnesium oxide is generally used as an antacid or in the preparation of mixtures which prove to be eutectic.

(5) Tribasic magnesium phosphate ($Mg_3(PO_4)_2 \cdot 5H_2O$). This compound is used as a nonsystemic antacid which is mildly cathartic.

(6) Magnesium sulfate ($MgSO_4 \cdot 7H_2O$). Magnesium sulfate, also called Epsom salts, Seidlitz salt, Crab Orchard salt, is extremely soluble; one gram dissolves in 1 ml. of water. Externally, the salt solution is used as an anti-inflammatory agent; the hypertonic solution promotes osmosis of fluid from the tissues. Internally, as a saline cathartic, it works by the same principle since it is not absorbed from the intestine. It has been used orally for seasickness, but we have newer products which produce better results. When given intramuscularly, it acts as an anticonvulsant and has been used for eclampsia, tetanus, and muscular relaxation during obstetrical procedures.

(7) Magnesium trisilicate. Magnesium trisilicate is an extremely effective antacid. In the stomach it combines with hydrochloric acid to yield magnesium chloride, which precipitates out, and trisilicic acid, a gelatinous mass. Because of magnesium chloride's saline cathartic effect and the soothing gelatinous trisilicic acid mass, this is an ingredient often added to aluminum hydroxide for ulcers, to overcome the constipation.

d. Barium (Ba, +2) and its compounds. Barium occurs naturally in the form of barium sulfate and barium carbonate. Its name is derived from the Greek "barus," meaning heavy. The barium ion, a protein precipitant, is extremely toxic. Therefore, any barium salt which is soluble is *poisonous.* Barium sulfate, which is insoluble, may be and is used internally. It is a radiopaque substance used in X-ray or fluoroscope examinations of the gastrointestinal tract. Magnesium sulfate (Epsom salts) is the most readily available antidote for barium poisoning; it acts to form the insoluble sulfate which precipitates.

12. Halogens. The halogens and their halide derivatives are of great pharmaceutical importance. The word halogen means "to produce," and is quite descriptive for this class of elements for they all react to produce salt-like products. The halogens are the most active of the nonmetals. The important elements in this group which we will discuss are fluorine, chlorine, bromine, and iodine. All the halogens exhibit a negative valence of one

(−1), and exist in the diatomic state; for example, F_2, Cl_2, Br_2, and I_2. However, they can exhibit valences of +1, +3, +5, and +7. Halogens exhibit an important relationship in their atomic weights, solubility, activity, and physical state. This relationship may be stated: As the molecular weight of the halogen increases, the activity decreases, the solubility decreases, and the physical state becomes more dense.

	Atomic Weight	Activity	Solubility	Dense	
Fluorine (F_2)	Increases ↓	Decreases ↓	Decreases ↓	More ↓	Gas
Chlorine (Cl_2)					Gas
Bromine (Br_2)					Liquids
Iodine (I_2)					Solid

By knowing the key, you can determine which halogens will replace others; the more active ones are able to replace less active ones in compounds.

a. Fluorine (F, −1) and fluorides. Fluorine, the most active member of the halogen family, is a yellow-green gas. It is so active that it is difficult to contain; it even reacts with glass to frost it. The fluoride ion is extremely toxic to the body; it reacts with calcium to form CaF_2 which is excreted from the body. The resulting calcium deficiency is evidenced by violent spasms. It also destroys enzymes. The main use of fluorine is in the manufacture of fluorides, the most important of which to medicine is sodium fluoride.

(1) Sodium fluoride (NaF). Sodium fluoride, a white odorless powder, has been used for years as a roach powder and for mothproofing textiles. In the recent past, it was discovered that sodium fluoride is very effective as a dental prophylactic. A concentration of one part per million of sodium fluoride in drinking water results in more than 50-percent reduction in dental caries in permanent teeth. Repeated 2-percent solution applications to children's teeth have resulted in caries reductions of 40 percent. Sodium fluoride is extremely poisonous, however, and the small amount added to water must be carefully regulated. In acid medium, sodium fluoride reacts to form hydrofluoric acid which is also poisonous and very caustic.

(2) Dental prophylactic tablet. This tablet for dental prophylaxis of caries contains calcium fluoride, ascorbic acid, and vitamin D. Where drinking water has been fluoridated, this tablet is contraindicated.

b. Chlorine (Cl, −1, +1, +3, +5, +7) and chlorides. Because of its greenish-yellow color, it was called chlorine, a name derived from a Greek word meaning "greenish yellow." It is found in the combined state in sea water and in solid deposits of sodium chloride. Chlorine gas has a characteristically suffocating odor. Although less active than fluorine, chlorine is a very active element and combines vigorously with a variety of elements and compounds. It acts as a powerful oxidizing agent. The chloride ion is important and essential to life and is found in the extracellular fluid. It is important to osmotic pressure control. Chlorine derivatives are used as diuretics and electrolyte replenishers internally, and as bleaching agents and purifying substances elsewhere. Some of the important chlorine derivatives are–

(1) Sodium chloride and potassium chloride. These have been previously discussed as electrolyte replenishers under the metals from which they are prepared.

(2) Hydrochloric acid (muriatic acid, spirit of salt, HCl). This strong acid is used commercially in manufacturing and by plumbers and masons for cleaning. The only pharmaceutical significance other than manufacturing is in the preparation of diluted hydrochloric acid.

(3) Diluted hydrochloric acid. This acid is made by adding 234 ml. of hydrochloric acid to enough water to make 1000 ml. of finished product. Diluted hydrochloric acid is used in drop dosage mixed with larger amounts of water to treat gastric achlorhydria. It is sipped with a straw to keep the acid from contacting the teeth and decomposing the enamel. *Achlorhydria* refers to a condition where hydrochloric acid is absent from the secretions of gastric juices. It is prescribed in conjunction with iron preparations in the treatment of anemia.

(4) Chlorox. Chlorox (not official) is a solution of about 5-percent sodium hypochlorite and is used as an antiseptic and deodorant in douches, gargles, and wet dressings.

c. Bromine (Br, −1, +1, +3, +5, +7) and its derivatives. The name bromine is from a Greek word which means "stench." It could not be better named, for if you ever smell bromine, you will never forget its odor! It is a liquid at ordinary room temperature. Extreme care must be used when working with bromine. The main effect of the bromide ion on the body is as a central nervous system depressant, working directly on the cortex of the brain. The following bromides are official sedatives:

(1) Ammonium bromide.

(2) Calcium bromide.

(3) Lithium bromide.

(4) Potassium bromide.

(5) Sodium bromide (the agent of choice when using a single bromide).

(6) Three bromides elixir (contains ammonium, potassium, and sodium bromide).

d. *Iodine (I, −1, +1, +3, +5, +7) and its derivatives.* Iodine is the least active and the only solid among the halogens.

(1) *Occurrence.* Iodine occurs combined in nature as iodides in marine algae and weeds.

(2) *Properties.* Iodine is quite insoluble in water, but by making a water solution of an iodine such as potassium iodide, the iodine becomes soluble in this solution. Iodine is one of the substances previously mentioned that sublime (change directly from a solid to a gas without passing through the liquid state) and this is a method for purifying it. Iodine solutions coming in contact with starch give a profuse blue color which is an accepted test for both iodine and starch.

(3) *Uses.* Iodine is a powerful oxidizing agent and protoplasmic poison and is thus employed as an antiseptic. A 2-percent tincture (alcoholic solution) is used topically as an antiseptic of very effective degree. A 7-percent tincture is available for disinfecting inanimate objects and is sometimes used on horses and cattle. Because of its strong oxidizing properties, metal spatulas must never be used when working with iodine. Iodine is also necessary to the proper function of the thyroid gland.

(4) *Official compounds.* Some official iodine preparations are—

(a) Saturated solution of potassium iodide (SSKI). Saturated solution of potassium iodide is a 100-percent solution, that is, it contains 1000 grams of KI in 1000 ml. of total solution. This solution is an excellent source of iodine for the prevention and treatment of goiter. As an expectorant, it liquefies clots of sputum. It is effective in the treatment of asthma and bronchitis. The usual dose of SSKI is 0.3 ml. (approximately 5 minims).

(b) Iodine.

(c) Iodine ampuls.

(d) Iodine solution.

(e) Strong iodine solution.

(f) Iodine tincture.

(g) Strong iodine tincture.

(h) Dilute hydriodic acid.

(i) Hydriodic acid syrup.

13. Sulfur (S, +2, +4, +6, −2) and its compounds. Sulfur is a yellow brittle solid often found in the free state in the earth. It may also be found in the combined state as sulfides and sulfates.

a. *Elemental sulfur (S).* Sulfur is one of the elements spewed forth by volcanic eruptions.

(1) *Properties.* Sulfur, a yellow solid, is practically insoluble in water, but is soluble in carbon disulfide and carbon tetrachloride. It either dissolves in or unites with strong bases and is precipitated from such solutions by acids. When heated to liquidity, most substances become thinner as the temperature is increased. Sulfur, on the contrary, becomes thicker, up to about 250° C. Above this temperature, it becomes thinner. Heating changes its color from light yellow to reddish brown to black. When heated, sulfur burns to unite with oxygen and yields sulfur dioxide and sulfur trioxide. It can be forced to react with some nonmetals like hydrogen, carbon, and chlorine. As you can see from these combinations, sulfur can react with elements having a valence of +6, +4, or −2.

(2) *Uses.*

(a) *Industrial.* Sulfur is used in industry in the manufacture of sulfur dioxide, carbon disulfide, sulfuric acid, matches, black powder, certain insecticides and fungicides for plant spray, and in the vulcanization of rubber.

(b) *Medicinal.* In medicine, the sulfide ion acts as a cathartic by forming H_2S which is irritating to the intestine. It is incorporated into ointments and creams as a parasiticide and keratolytic. A keratolytic is an agent which breaks down the epidermis and causes it to slough off. The sulfate ion ($SO_4^{=}$) acts as an osmotic diuretic and saline cathartic.

(3) *Types of sulfur.* Three different varieties of sulfur are used in the pharmacy. They are precipitated sulfur, sublimed sulfur (flowers of sulfur), and washed sulfur. The first is prepared by precipitation, the second by sublimation, and the third by washing sublimed sulfur with a mixture of water and diluted ammonia solution.

b. Compounds of sulfur. The following are important pharmaceutical sulfur compounds:

(1) Sulfuric acid (oil of vitriol, H_2SO_4). Sulfuric acid is used in the manufacture of many sulfate salts and in the synthesis of the sulfonamides. If you are ever called upon to handle sulfuric acid, use extreme caution. When mixing the acid with other liquids, ALWAYS add the acid to the other liquid with extreme care. If water is added to the acid, it splatters and may cause burns.

(2) Sodium bisulfite. Sodium bisulfite is used as an antioxidant and stabilizing agent. It is added to epinephrine solutions in small amounts of the hydrochloride salt to stabilize it.

(3) Sulfur ointment. Sulfur ointment contain 10-percent precipitated sulfur incorporated into a base of white ointment. Its main use is as a scabacide.

(4) Sulfur resorcinol lotion. Sulfur resorcinol lotion, although not official, is widely used in the military. It has a variety of names including Sulforcin lotion, S-R lotion, and SulfoRes Lotion.

14. Nitrogen (N, +1, +3, +5, −3), phosphorus (P, +3, +5, −3), and their compounds. Nitrogen and phosphorus are the first and second members of group V in the periodic table of the elements.

a. Nitrogen. Nitrogen is the only gaseous member of the group V elements, all the others being solids. It exists in the diatomic state, the 2 atoms bonded by 6 electrons in the form of 2 triple bonds. Nitrogen is colorless, odorless, and tasteless. It is quite inactive except under forced conditions.

(1) Occurrence and preparation. Free nitrogen constitutes approximately 79 percent of the earth's atmosphere. It also occurs in combination with other elements in the form of nitrates and in plant and animal protein. Nitrogen is commercially prepared by distillation of liquid air. In laboratory situations, it may be prepared from air or from ammonium nitrate. In the first instance, a piece of phosphorus is burned in a crucible floating in water and covered by a bell jar. The oxygen is combined and an atmosphere of nitrogen remains. Gentle heating of ammonium nitrate produces nitrogen gas and water; the nitrogen is collected in a water-displacement, gas-collecting apparatus.

(2) Nitrogen fixation. Nitrogen fixation is a process, either natural or synthetic, in which nitrogen is combined chemically with other elements.

(a) Naturally occurring nitrogen fixing. You are probably aware that certain crops grown year after year in the same soil deplete the land so that it is not suitable for further use. This is because these crops have extracted all the fixed nitrogen, leaving behind little or none so that future growth may be inhibited. Such nitrogen-depleting crops are wheat, corn, and oats.

1. Nitrogen-fixing bacteria. You are, no doubt, also aware that farmers rotate their crops each year or every other year. The purpose of this rotation is to grow plants which have the power to replace nitrogen to the land. It is not the plant which accomplishes the nitrogen fixing, but bacteria that live in nodules (swellings) on the roots of vegetables of the bean and pea family. These are the nitrogen-fixing bacteria. If the soil is alkaline, these bacteria take nitrogen from the air and combine it into nitrogen compounds. Clover and alfalfa contain these nitrogen-fixing properties.

2. Electrical-discharge nitrogen fixing. Another naturally occurring phenomenon that restores nitrogen to the soil is a chemical reaction taking place during discharge of lightning in electrical storms. The electrical discharges furnish energy in sufficient quantities to cause some of the atmospheric nitrogen to be reacted with oxygen in minute particles. These are trapped by moisture and fall to earth in the rain. Millions of tons of nitrogen are donated to the earth's soils yearly by this process.

(b) Artificial or synthetic nitrogen fixing. The chief method of artificial nitrogen fixing is to react nitrogen with hydrogen, using a catalyst, to yield ammonia. The ammonia is oxidized to nitric acid, which is further reacted to nitrates. The nitrates are added in varying amounts to fertilizers, assuring maximum productivity of the treated soil.

(3) Uses of free nitrogen. Free nitrogen is the starting point for the synthesis of many nitrogen-containing compounds, an example of which is the previously mentioned nitrates. Further, being a relatively inert gas, it is used to package substances in an oxygen-free atmosphere to prevent oxidation. Many of the ampuls of injectable medicinals are packaged in an atmosphere of nitrogen. Nitrogen is also used to fill lightbulbs. Medically, liquid nitrogen is used to remove warts.

(4) Nitrogen compounds. The following nitrogen compounds are important:

(a) Ammonia (NH_3). Ammonia, a colorless gas with a characteristic odor, is very soluble in water. It is used in the manufacture of many nitrogen-containing compounds.

(b) Strong ammonia solution (stronger ammonia water, stronger ammonium hydroxide solution). This solution of ammonia in water contains between 27 percent and 30 percent of ammonia by weight. Upon exposure to the atmosphere, it gives off an extremely irritating odor and loses strength. This solution is used in chemistry and manufacturing; weaker dilutions are used in pharmaceutical preparations and for household cleaning.

(c) Diluted ammonia solution (ammonia water, diluted ammonium hydroxide solution). This solution is made by diluting 398 ml. of strong ammonia solution with enough water to make 1000 ml. of finished product. The dilute solution is used in the manufacture of aromatic ammonia spirit, more commonly referred to as smelling salts. Given orally, and highly diluted with water, it acts as a reflex stimulant.

(d) Ammonium bromide (NH_4Br). Here is another bromide compound used, like the others, for CNS depression.

(e) Ammonium chloride (NH_4Cl). Ammonium chloride is used commercially in the manufacture of dry cells, in soldering, and in certain iron cements. Pharmaceutically it acts as an expectorant; a diuretic alone, or potentiating when used in conjunction with mercurials; and a systemic acidifier.

(f) Nitrous oxide (N_2O). Nitrous oxide (you may have heard it called "laughing gas") is a general inhalation anesthetic. It is frequently used for dental surgery where deep surgical anesthesia is not required. It is relatively safe from explosion because it does not burn, but it does support combustion.

b. Phosphorus. Phosphorus occurs in two allotropic forms, white and red phosphorus. Their properties are widely different.

(1) Properties of phosphorus.

(a) White phosphorus. White phosphorus when fresh and pure is colorless, but may shortly attain a very pale yellow color and be referred to sometimes as yellow phosphorus. It is a waxy, translucent solid with a low kindling point, burning at a temperature of only 35° C. (95° F.). White phosphorus is extremely poisonous to the body, must be stored under water to prevent reaction, and should never be handled with the bare hands as it can produce severe burns that heal slowly.

(b) Red phosphorus. Red phosphorus is nonpoisonous, not combustible in air, except at high temperatures (250° C.). This is the form used in the manufacture of safety matches.

(2) Occurrence and preparation.

(a) Occurrence. Because of its activity, phosphorus is not found free in nature. It occurs mainly in phosphate formations, probably from the bones of prehistoric animals. Bones and teeth contain large amounts of calcium phosphate. Phosphorus is also found combined in protoplasm, nerve tissue, and egg yolks.

(b) Preparation. White phosphorus is manufactured in an arc furnace from calcium phosphate. The uncombined phosphorus thus produced comes off in the form of a gas and is condensed under water in molds in the form of sticks. Red phosphorus is prepared by allowing white phosphorus to stand for several days in an atmosphere of CO_2 at 215° C. to 250° C.

(3) Uses. Red phosphorus is mainly used in the match and fertilizer industry. White phosphorus is used in incendiary bombs, tracer bullets, and rat poisons. Trisodium phosphate is used as a water softener and detergent. Ammonium phosphate is used for fireproofing, and several other phosphates and hypophosphates are used in medicine. Dilute phosphoric acid is an antidote for lead poisoning.

15. Zinc, manganese, aluminum, and their compounds. Zinc, manganese, and aluminum are common metals. Zinc is used in the manufacture of galvanized iron. Aluminum is replacing copper in many instances in electrical conductors and in cookware. Manganese is used in the manufacture of extraordinarily hard steel.

a. Zinc (Zn, +2). Zinc is a divalent (+2), active metal, known to the world for centuries.

(1) Occurrence and preparation. Zinc occurs in the combined state in the form of oxides, silicates, and sulfides. Zinc has been extracted from the ores in which it occurs by two processes; the older process of reducing the ore with coal, and the newer, more satisfactory method of electrolysis. The electrolytic process of zinc extraction is preferred because the zinc obtained is of a higher purity than that obtained from the reduction

method. In this process, the ore is roasted and treated with sulfuric acid to remove the zinc as zinc sulfate in solution. An electric current causes the zinc to deposit on an aluminum cathode sheet from which it is easily stripped off.

(2) *Properties of zinc.*

(a) *Physical.* Zinc is a bluish-white metallic substance which, in pure form, is quite brittle at room temperature. When heated it becomes malleable and ductile, and can be pounded into sheets or drawn into wire. Upon cooling it does not regain its brittleness.

(b) *Chemical.* Zinc is not attacked by dry air, but moist air will react and coat the metal with a covering of zinc carbonate. This coating is adhering and somewhat impervious, protecting the zinc beneath. Zinc burns in the presence of oxygen to form zinc oxide. The zinc ion is precipitated by basic sulfides.

(3) *Importance.* Zinc is essential in the enzyme structure of red blood corpuscles and enzyme systems of the body. It is involved in acceleration of carbon dioxide exchange in the body. The zinc ion is not used medically or pharmaceutically INTERNALLY because it precipitates protein, but it is used externally as an astringent, mild antiseptic, and corrosive.

(4) *Compounds of zinc.* The following compounds and official preparations contain zinc:

(a) *Zinc chloride ($ZnCl_2$).* Zinc chloride is a white crystalline, very deliquescent powder. It hydrolyzes in solution, producing zinc hydroxide and hydrochloric acid, making the solution acid to litmus. Preparations containing this agent are available in 1- to 2-percent concentrations for application to skin, and in 0.2- to 0.5-percent concentrations for application to mucous membranes. Lavoris is a mouthwash containing small amounts of zinc chloride.

(b) *Zinc oxide (ZnO).* Zinc oxide is a white, very fine, nongritty powder. It is insoluble in both water and alcohol, but soluble in dilute acids. It is protective, mildly antiseptic, and astringent in action and is incorporated into a host of ointments, pastes, creams, and lotions, as well as talcs for external use in the treatment of skin conditions such as eczema, impetigo, psoriasis, ringworm, and ulcers. Dentally, it is used as a cement.

(c) *Calamine.* Calamine is a mixture of zinc oxide and ferric oxide, generally in quantities of 98 percent and 2 percent, respectively. Its chief use in preparations is in treatment of sunburn and ivy poisonings; it is also used to impart color to the product. Its action is astringent. Neocalamine is a mixture of zinc oxide and red and yellow ferric oxides. Its action is exactly the same as calamine.

(d) *Calamine lotion, phenolated calamine lotion, and calamine ointment.* These are preparations containing calamine.

(e) *Medicinal zinc peroxide.* This fine, white, odorless powder is practically insoluble in water and organic solvents, but is freely soluble in mineral acids. Medicinal zinc peroxide is classified as an anti-infective. Used as a paste and smeared on gauze and placed over a wound, the water reacts with the zinc peroxide, liberating zinc oxide and hydrogen peroxide. The hydrogen peroxide further decomposes to water and nascent oxygen. Its action, then, is due to oxidation.

(f) *Zinc stearate.* Zinc stearate, a white bulky powder, feels waxy to the touch and adheres well to skin. Its action is astringent and mildly antiseptic. At one time it was used as a substitute for talc as an astringent, antiseptic dusting powder. It is no longer used for this purpose because of the incidence of pulmonary disorders attributed to the use of this preparation.

(g) *Zinc sulfate ($ZnSO_4 \cdot 7H_2O$).* This compound occurs as colorless prisms or needles. It is classified as an ophthalmic astringent, which is its primary use, generally as a 0.2-percent aqueous sterile solution. Zincfrin is an example of such an eye preparation. It may be used either alone or in combination and has mildly antiseptic properties. Zinc sulfate has been used internally in certain poisonings as an emetic. Although it is very toxic (protein precipitant), it produces vomiting so rapidly that it has little time in the stomach to cause the body any harm. Its protein precipitant action can be effectively demonstrated by making a strong solution of zinc sulfate in water and breaking a raw egg into it. The white, or protein portion of the egg, turns solid as if it were being cooked.

(h) *White lotion.* White lotion is a preparation made from zinc sulfate and sulfurated potash. A chemical reaction takes place in the manufacture, yielding zinc sulfide. When applied to the skin, this lotion is astringent and protective. Hydrogen sulfide is liberated when this product comes into contact with the skin.

b. *Manganese (Mn, +2, +3, +4, +6, +7).* Manganese, a steel-gray, hard, brittle metal acts with varying valences of +2, +3, +4, +6, and +7. Almost every organ in the body contains manganese ions, but when administered orally, there is no effect. It has been used as a tonic and iron synergist, with questionable results.

c. *Aluminum (Al, +3).*

(1) Occurrence and preparation. Aluminum is the third most abundant element. In nature it occurs only in the combined state, with such substances as feldspar, mica, clay, emery, corundum, rubies, sapphires; and in ores from which it is commercially extracted, such as bauxite and cryolite.

(2) Uses. Topically applied, dilute solutions of aluminum ions cause a constricting of the blood vessels. This is the basis for its use as an antiperspirant. In greater concentrations, it is a protein precipitant and is used as an antiseptic and deodorant.

(3) Chemical property. Aluminum salts undergo hydrolysis to yield acid solutions.

(4) Compounds of aluminum.

(a) Aluminum chloride ($AlCl_3$). Twenty- to thirty-percent solutions of aluminum chloride (generally $Al(OH)Cl_2$) are used for their astringent and anhydrotic (reduction of perspiration) effects in most of the antiperspirant and deodorant preparations. The basic salt is preferred because it is not acid and consequently is less harmful to the clothing.

(b) Aluminum hydroxide ($Al(OH)_3$). In the form of a gel, this substance is official in the USP. The preparation may contain various flavoring agents and a preservative of benzoic acid or sodium benzoate. Aluminum hydroxide gel is used as a nonsystemic antacid in the treatment of peptic ulcers. Excess hydrochloric acid is neutralized by the $Al(OH)_3$, yielding $AlCl_3$ which is astringent and actually tends to shrink the ulcerated area.

(c) Aluminum hydroxide and magnesium trisilicate gel. This product, much like plain aluminum hydroxide gel, acts as an antacid, adsorbent, and demulcent. The addition of magnesium trisilicate counteracts the constipating effects of the aluminum hydroxide by acting as a mild saline cathartic. The trisilicic acid formed is gelatinous, acting as a bulk and demulcent. Since these aluminum gels are generally used over prolonged periods and are known to interfere with absorption of phosphorus in the gastrointestinal tract, aluminum phosphate gel may be used.

(d) Aluminum silicates.

1. Bentonite is a brown powder of hydrated aluminum silicate used in the preparation of bentonite magma (a suspending agent for insoluble medicaments), as an emulsifier for oils, as a base for plasters and ointments, and as a protective colloid for suspension stabilization.

2. Kaolin is a clay-like hydrated aluminum silicate often employed in the making of pottery. Its medicinal use is as an adsorbent for the control of certain types of diarrhea, as a protective in ulcerative colitis, and as a clarifying and filtering agent. Kaopectate and a number of other products combining kaolin with pectin in a thick suspension are common diarrhea mixtures.

3. Pumice is a gritty substance of volcanic origin consisting of the silicates of aluminum, potassium, and sodium. It is used as a filtering and distributing agent in medicinals, as a cleansing agent (through its grittiness) in hand soaps, and as an abrasive in dentistry and metal polishing.

(e) Alum. Alum may be either potassium alum ($AlK(SO_4)_2 \cdot 12H_2O$) or ammonium alum ($AlNH_4(SO_4)_2 \cdot 12H_2O$), but the package must specify which is contained. Alum is an astringent in acid solutions and is slightly bacteriostatic. It is used in astringent lotions and douches and is the active ingredient in styptic pencils and powders.

16. Compounds of carbon, boron, and silicon. Carbon, boron, and silicon are nonmetals. The black soot from chimneys, charred wood, and diamonds are forms of carbon. Glass is a mixture of silicates. Borax, a compound of boron, is used in making glass.

a. *Carbon (C, +4, −4).* Carbon, a very widely distributed element, is a component of all organic material. It also occurs in the free state as diamond, coal, graphite, lignite, and peat. There are more compounds of carbon than of any other element. This is due to the fact that carbon has the power to form indefinitely long chains. Carbon is the basis for organic chemistry which is discussed in the following chapter. Although carbon generally has a valence of +4 and may act as a metal or nonmetal, there are relatively few inorganic compounds of carbon.

(1) Activated charcoal. Activated charcoal is a fine, black, odorless, tasteless powder containing some impurities. It is the residue from the destructive distillation of organic materials. It is mainly used as an adsorbent for clarifying solutions, in universal antidote, and in some

mixtures to relieve stomach gas. Its adsorptive properties are greatly reduced or absent when it is wet. Sometimes it is used on dressings to adsorb the odor from foul-smelling wounds. Activated charcoal is specially treated to increase adsorptive properties and should not be replaced by other, less active forms such as animal charcoal, wood charcoal, or burned toast.

(2) Carbon dioxide (CO_2) (carbonic acid gas). This colorless, odorless gas is an acidic anhydride, forming carbonic acid in solution. Carbon dioxide is a product of the burning of coke or coal, the breakdown of carbonates, and the fermentation of sugar. It is used in the carbonation of soda water for beverages; in the liquid state and solid state (dry ice) it is employed as a refrigerant. It is manufactured in certain fire extinguishers as a propellant and in others as the actual smothering agent. It is used to replace oxygen in atmospheres for preparation and storage of materials to which oxygen is detrimental. Medically, carbon dioxide is used as a respiratory stimulant in operative procedures by inhalation. It has been used in high concentrations as a respiratory depressant in hiccoughs, and as an expectorant. Presently, some experimentation is being conducted using 30-percent concentrations of CO_2 for treatment of delirium tremens and other emotional and psycho-disturbances.

(3) Carbonic acid-bicarbonate buffer pair. Letting HA be any strong acid and BOH any strong base, the carbonic acid-bicarbonate buffering system works in the following manner:

(a) Buffering of the base.

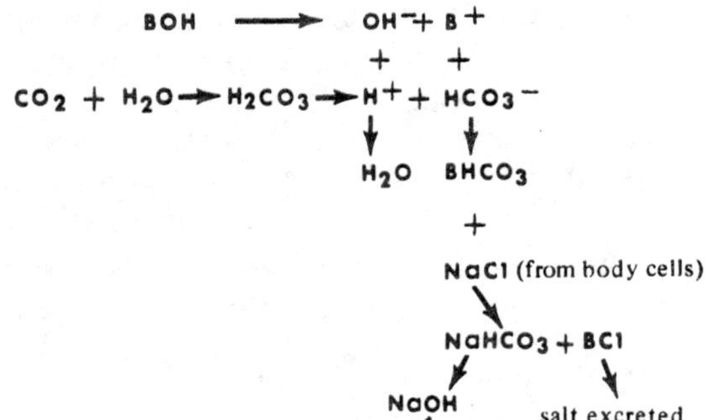

(b) Buffering of the acid.

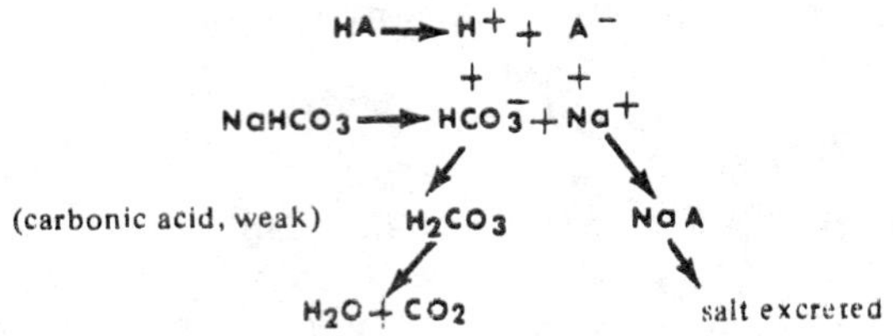

(4) Carbon monoxide (CO). When carbon or carbon-containing substances are incompletely oxidized, carbon monoxide is formed. This gas is odorless and very poisonous. It accounts for many intentional and accidental poisoning deaths each year, mainly from the exhaust fumes of internal combustion engines and coal gas. The bloodstream has a particular affinity for carbon monoxide; this affinity results in oxygen being replaced by carbon monoxide. Death, then, is a result of anoxia.

b. Silicon (Si, +4, –4). Silicon is the second most abundant element on earth, occurring in combined form in nearly every mineral substance. Like carbon, silicons can form chains, but only to the extent of 6 links. Large oral doses are irritant to the organs. Products of silicon have been discussed with the compounds of aluminum for the most part, but below are two silicons which are not in combination with aluminum.

(1) Purified siliceous earth. Purified siliceous earth also has the common names of purified infusorial earth, purified kieselguhr, and terra silicea purificata. Because it has the ability to absorb and retain about 4 times its own weight of moisture, it is very effective as an absorbing agent. It is also an effective filtering agent.

(2) Talc (purified talc, talcum). Talc is mainly magnesium silicate, sometimes containing small amounts of aluminum silicate. It is used as a dusting powder, filtering agent, protective agent, and inert ingredient.

c. Boron (B, +3, –3). Because boron is a heavy metal and a protoplasmic poison, no soluble boron derivative can be safely employed internally or topically where there is possibility of absorption. Pharmaceutically, boron is significant in the following preparations:

(1) Boric acid (H_2BO_3, boracic acid).

(a) Properties. Boric acid is a scaly, crystalline crystal or powder. The crystal form is more easily soluble than the finer powder

form. As you will learn in "Manufacturing Pharmacy," this is directly opposite to the rule that the finer the subdivision of a substance, the more rapidly soluble it becomes. In solution, boric acid is weakly acidic, but the addition of glycerin makes it more strongly acid.

(b) Uses. Boric acid is mildly antiseptic, maintaining sterility, but not being able to sterilize a septic field. It is nonirritating and can thus be used in ophthalmic preparations. It is used in the form of ointments and solutions for external or topical application only. It was once widely used in baby preparations for diaper rash and heat rash, but has become less popular after several instances of poisoning from absorbed boric acid.

(c) Boric acid solution. Boric acid solution, more commonly referred to as saturated solution of boric acid or SSBA, is a 5-percent solution in purified water. Since the solubility of boric acid is 1:18 in water (5.5 percent), this is not a truly saturated solution. On chilling or evaporation of the liquid, boric acid tends to crystallize out of solution. Solution of boric acid should only be dispensed when clear and free of crystal deposits. This solution is intended for treatment of inflammation.

(d) Isotonic boric acid solution. A 2.2-percent solution in sterile water is isotonic and may be used as an eyewash or drop.

(2) Sodium borate (borax, sodium tetraborate, $Na_2B_4O_7 \cdot 10H_2O$).

(a) Properties. Sodium borate is a colorless crystal or white powder, odorless, and efflorescent in warm, dry air. In solution, it is hydrolyzed to sodium metaborate, then to sodium hydroxide and boric acid, producing an alkaline solution. Since zinc salts are precipitated in an alkaline medium, boric acid should replace borax when combining zinc preparations with boron ones, or enough glycerin should be added to acidify. Addition of glycerin, making the solution acidic, makes it incompatible with carbonates and bicarbonates.

(b) Uses. Sodium borate is used in making wet dressings, in eyewash preparations, and in the manufacture of rose water ointment.

(3) Sodium perborate ($NaBO_3 \cdot 4H_2O$). Sodium perborate undergoes hydrolysis to form hydrogen perioxide, which further breaks down to water and nascent oxygen, making it an oxidant and local anti-infective. It was widely used by dentists in the treatment of Vincent's angina (trench mouth) for some time, but has fallen into disuse. Sodium perborate must not be used, except on the advice and under the supervision of medical or dental personnel because, after prolonged use, it may destroy healthy tissue.

17. **Compounds of iron, arsenic, and antimony.** Iron is the second most plentiful metal. The earth's core is believed to be molten iron. Arsenic and antimony are found in ores of other metals to a much smaller extent.

a. Iron (Fe, +2, +3). Iron is an extremely common element, found in the form of its oxides and sulfides.

(1) Ferrous iron. The ferrous iron (Fe^{++}) is essential to the hemoglobin of blood and has to do with the transportation of oxygen to the tissues. Deficiencies of iron therefore cause inadequate formation of blood cells and the body suffers from general weakness. Such deficiencies can be treated by administering iron salts. Sometimes the iron salts are given in conjunction with ascorbic acid or copper to enhance their combination into the hemoglobin.

(2) Ferric iron. The ferric iron (Fe^{+++}) is mainly used externally because it is a protoplasmic poison. Its action externally is as an astringent and antiseptic.

(3) Reduced iron. Reduced iron (pure iron treated with hydrogen) has been used in years past as a source of iron in deficiency anemias, but the ferrous salts have proved to be much more efficient.

(4) Iron compounds.

(a) Ferrous sulfate (iron sulfate, $FeSO_4 \cdot 7H_2O$). This is the salt of iron most commonly administered for iron-deficiency anemias. It is irritating to the stomach and is often given in coated tablets to help alleviate this irritation. Its main use is as a hematinic, given 300 mg. 3 times a day. In solution, this salt is used as a disinfectant, in the tanning of leather, in the making of iron inks, in photography, and in manufacture of other iron salts.

(b) Ferrous carbonate pills (Blaud's pills, chalybeate pills, ferruginous pills). These pills, used for many years in the past, are falling into disuse now. Their main use was as a hematinic.

(c) Ferrous gluconate ($C_{12}H_{22}FeO_{14} \cdot 2H_2O$). Used in the same manner as the strictly inorganic salts of iron as a hematinic, this salt is much less irritating to the gastric mucosa. It is available in the form of tablets, elixir, and injection.

(d) *Ferrous fumarate* ($FeC_4H_2O_4$). Of all the salts of iron used to date, this one causes the least amount of irritation. Also important about this iron product is the fact that its stability to oxidation or hydration is far superior to that of ferrous sulfate or ferrous gluconate, even in hot, humid climates. It is therapeutically equivalent to the sulfate or the gluconate salts in that it is equivalent to 33 percent iron ($FeSO_4$ = 31%).

(e) *Ferric chloride* ($FeCl_3$). Ferric chloride is used medicinally as an astringent and styptic.

(f) *Iron, quinine, and strychnine elixir (elixir IQ and S).* This preparation was widely used in bygone years as a hematinic and bitter tonic. It is an irrational mixture, because the amount of iron is not high enough to be of therapeutic value in anemia, and the strychnine is useless.

(5) *Iron incompatibility.* Iron is incompatible with tannins, yielding a black precipitate of iron tannate. This reaction was used for centuries in the manufacture of a crude ink.

b. *Arsenic (As, +3, +5, −3).* Arsenic is a protoplasmic poison and is lethal if taken in sufficient quantities. It was at one time used extensively as a tonic and in the treatment of anemias; it was even tried as a possible anti-cancer drug. Today, because of its toxicity and its questionable value, arsenic compounds are rarely used. About its only value today is in the treatment of psoriasis and in chronic myelogenous leukemia. Arsenic trioxide and potassium arsenite solution (Fowler's solution) are official.

c. *Antimony (Sb, +3, +5, −3).* Antimony, a metalloid, derives its symbol, Sb, from the Latin stibium. Its English name is thought to come from "anti," meaning "against" and "moine" meaning "monk" because legend has it that the alleged discoverer of antimony used it to poison certain monks. The antimony ion has the normal heavy metal effect of being a protoplasmic poison. Topically, it is irritant and internally it acts as an expectorant and as an emetic.

(1) *Antimony potassium tartrate (tartar emetic).* Tartar emetic is used as an anti-schistosomal. It is administered by injection. Orally, small doses can be used as expectorants and large doses as emetics.

(2) *Stibophen.* Stibophen, like tartar emetic, is used in the treatment of tropical diseases caused by protozoa, such as leishmaniasis (kala-azar) and schistosomiasis.

18. Miscellaneous inorganic compounds of medicinal significance. Grouped under this broad catchall title are many chemical elements and compounds which are noteworthy in the pharmaceutical profession.

a. *Bismuth (Bi, +3, +5).* Bismuth occurs free in nature or in the combined state. Elemental bismuth is of little value, but its salts have some importance in pharmacy and medicine. The bismuth ions are protoplasmic poisons to the body. The official inorganic bismuth preparations include–

(1) *Bismuth subcarbonate.* Bismuth subcarbonate is frequently used internally as an astringent, adsorbent, protective, and antacid. It is insoluble and not toxic for this reason. Because of these actions, bismuth subcarbonate is employed in the treatment of diarrheas, dysentery, enteritis, and ulcerative colitis.

(2) *Bismuth subnitrate.* Bismuth subnitrate was used frequently at one time, but the nitrate ions caused considerable irritation and it was superseded by bismuth subcarbonate, whose action is almost identical to that of bismuth subnitrate.

b. *Lead (Pb, +2, +4).* Lead and lead compounds are poisonous and are no longer used in pharmacy. You should recognize the element as a dangerous poison. Since lead is stored in bone tissue, a chronic poisoning is likely to develop in people coming in contact with lead products over long periods of time, or inhaling fumes of lead-bearing substances. Lead is an ingredient in many types of paint and there have been a number of poisonings resulting from infants chewing on painted surfaces. Painter's colic is a chronic lead poisoning due to continuous inhalation of the paint fumes. People handling gasoline containing tetraethyl lead day after day are subject to chronic lead poisoning by absorption through the skin. The signs and symptoms and treatment of lead poisoning are discussed in the chapter on pharmacology and toxicology.

c. *Mercury (Hg, +1, +2).* Mercury, a silvery-white liquid metal, is used as an indicator in thermometers, barometers, and similar instruments. In dentistry it is used in combination with silver for filling dental caries. Mercury gives off an unnoticeable vapor at room temperature which can be toxic after long exposure in concentrations as low as 1 part in 50 million of air. Metallic mercury vaporizes when heated and emits an ultraviolet light. It is used in mercury lamps. It is also used in the manufacture of medicinal mercury compounds.

(1) Mercury ions. The mercurous ion (Hg) builds up toxicity after long use and can be employed for its diuretic and cathartic effects. The mercuric ion (Hg^{++}) is a protoplasmic poison, extremely and immediately toxic in the body. It is employed as an antiseptic, fungicide, and germicide.

(2) Official inorganic preparations. Official inorganic preparations of mercury include—

(a) Ammoniated mercury, used in the manufacture of ointments.

(b) Ammoniated mercury ointment, a 5-percent ointment of ammoniated mercury used in the treatment of crab louse, impetigo, pruritis ani, psoriasis, and ringworm.

(c) Ammoniated mercury ophthalmic ointment, a 3-percent ointment intended for application to eyelids.

(d) Mild mercurial ointment (blue ointment), used topically for crab louse infestation.

(e) Red mercuric iodide, an antibacterial.

(f) Yellow mercuric oxide, used in the manufacture of yellow mercuric oxide ointments.

(g) Yellow mercuric oxide ointment, a preparation intended for local antibacterial action in opthalmic ointments.

OFFICIAL CAUTION

During its manufacture and storage, yellow mercuric oxide ointment must not come into contact with metallic utensils or containers except those made of stainless steel, tin, or tin-coated materials.

(h) Mild mercurous chloride (calomel, mercurous chloride), intended to be used internally as a cathartic and diuretic.

(i) Mild mercurous chloride ointment, a local antibacterial ointment.

(j) Mercury bichloride (corrosive sublimate, mercuric chloride), a powder to be used in a 1:1000 solution for disinfection of inanimate objects. This substance is extremely poisonous and never is intended for internal use.

(k) Mercury bichloride ophthalmic ointment, an ophthalmic antibacterial ointment.

(l) Mercury bichloride large poison tablets, which are of distinctive color, not white; of angular or irregular shape, not discoid. They must be bottled in distinctively shaped bottles and clearly marked poison in red on the label. There are explicit directions for these tablets for they are poisonous and not intended to be taken internally. They are used in the manufacture of disinfectant solutions.

(m) Mercury oleate, classified as a pharmaceutical necessity, that is, it is needed in the preparation of other products. Mercury oleate must not be dispensed if the globules of mercury have separated.

d. Silver (Ag, +1). Silver is a heavy metal protoplasmic poison. It is toxic in the body and intended medicinally for use in external preparations for its antiseptic or caustic effects. Official inorganic silver compounds include—

(1) Silver nitrate ($AgNO_3$), a local anti-infective agent and caustic, intended for external use in solutions of 0.1 to 10 percent.

(2) Silver nitrate ophthalmic solution, a 1-percent solution of silver nitrate, applied to the conjunctiva to combat local infections.

(3) Toughened silver nitrate (fused silver nitrate, lunar caustic, silver nitrate pencils), a caustic, used topically as required.

e. Copper (Cu, +1, +2). Copper has a multitude of commercial uses, but only limited medicinal uses. Copper ions are protoplasmic poisons and copper compounds, and thus are used for their astringent and antiseptic action. Copper is added to hematinic and vitamin preparations because it is essential for normal hemoglobin formation. The only official copper compound is cupric sulfate (copper sulfate, $CuSO_4$). Sometimes called blue vitriol, this crystal is used in lakes to prevent the growth of algae commonly referred to as "working." It is also classified as an astringent and emetic.

f. Gold (Au, +1, +3). Gold has been known and treasured since the earliest recorded history. The alchemists have worked endlessly searching for methods of converting other metals to gold. The symbol, Au, comes from Latin, aurum, meaning "shining dawn," and in several languages the word gold or like words mean "yellow." Because of its beauty and value, it was thought that such an element would have to be of great therapeutic value in the treatment of disease, and it has been tried for many disorders. The official inorganic gold compounds include–

(1) Gold sodium thiosulfate ($Na_3Au(S_2O_3)_2 \cdot 2H_2O$). This compound is also official in the form of a sterile solution for injection. In this form it is primarily used in the treatment of rheumatic-type diseases. Used topically the compound has had satisfactory results in the treatment of some dermatological disorders, including lupus erythematosus.

(2) Radiogold solution (sterile radioactive gold colloid, sterile radiogold (Au^{198}) colloid). This radioactive, sterile solution for injection of gold is sometimes used as a neoplastic suppressant, that is, to prevent the formation of new tissue as in cancerous growths. It is administered by intracavity injection in doses of 30 to 150 millicuries.

OFFICIAL CAUTION

In making dosage calculations, correct for radioactive decay. The half-life of Au^{198} is 2.70 days. Any change from the natural deep-cherry-red color of the solution indicates that the gold is no longer in stable colloid form.

g. *Selenium.* Selenium is somewhat similar in nature to sulfur and is important in pharmacy as selenium sulfide, used topically for certain conditions of dermatitis. Human toxicity resembles that of dermatitis associated with arsenic toxicity. Selenium compounds must never be allowed to come in contact with the eyes.

ANSWER SHEET

O. ____________ PART ______ TITLE OF POSITION ______________________________
(AS GIVEN IN EXAMINATION ANNOUNCEMENT - INCLUDE OPTION, IF ANY)

OF EXAMINATION ______________________________ ______________ DATE ______________
(CITY OR TOWN) (STATE)

RATING

USE THE SPECIAL PENCIL. MAKE GLOSSY BLACK MARKS.

1 A B C D E	26 A B C D E	51 A B C D E	76 A B C D E	101 A B C D E
2 A B C D E	27 A B C D E	52 A B C D E	77 A B C D E	102 A B C D E
3 A B C D E	28 A B C D E	53 A B C D E	78 A B C D E	103 A B C D E
4 A B C D E	29 A B C D E	54 A B C D E	79 A B C D E	104 A B C D E
5 A B C D E	30 A B C D E	55 A B C D E	80 A B C D E	105 A B C D E
6 A B C D E	31 A B C D E	56 A B C D E	81 A B C D E	106 A B C D E
7 A B C D E	32 A B C D E	57 A B C D E	82 A B C D E	107 A B C D E
8 A B C D E	33 A B C D E	58 A B C D E	83 A B C D E	108 A B C D E
9 A B C D E	34 A B C D E	59 A B C D E	84 A B C D E	109 A B C D E
10 A B C D E	35 A B C D E	60 A B C D E	85 A B C D E	110 A B C D E

Make only ONE mark for each answer. Additional and stray marks may be counted as mistakes. In making corrections, erase errors COMPLETELY.

11 A B C D E	36 A B C D E	61 A B C D E	86 A B C D E	111 A B C D E
12 A B C D E	37 A B C D E	62 A B C D E	87 A B C D E	112 A B C D E
13 A B C D E	38 A B C D E	63 A B C D E	88 A B C D E	113 A B C D E
14 A B C D E	39 A B C D E	64 A B C D E	89 A B C D E	114 A B C D E
15 A B C D E	40 A B C D E	65 A B C D E	90 A B C D E	115 A B C D E
16 A B C D E	41 A B C D E	66 A B C D E	91 A B C D E	116 A B C D E
17 A B C D E	42 A B C D E	67 A B C D E	92 A B C D E	117 A B C D E
18 A B C D E	43 A B C D E	68 A B C D E	93 A B C D E	118 A B C D E
19 A B C D E	44 A B C D E	69 A B C D E	94 A B C D E	119 A B C D E
20 A B C D E	45 A B C D E	70 A B C D E	95 A B C D E	120 A B C D E
21 A B C D E	46 A B C D E	71 A B C D E	96 A B C D E	121 A B C D E
22 A B C D E	47 A B C D E	72 A B C D E	97 A B C D E	122 A B C D E
23 A B C D E	48 A B C D E	73 A B C D E	98 A B C D E	123 A B C D E
24 A B C D E	49 A B C D E	74 A B C D E	99 A B C D E	124 A B C D E
25 A B C D E	50 A B C D E	75 A B C D E	100 A B C D E	125 A B C D E

ANSWER SHEET

TEST NO. ________________ PART ______ TITLE OF POSITION ______________________________
(AS GIVEN IN EXAMINATION ANNOUNCEMENT - INCLUDE OPTION, IF ANY)

PLACE OF EXAMINATION ______________________________ ______________ DATE ________
(CITY OR TOWN) (STATE)

RATING

USE THE SPECIAL PENCIL. MAKE GLOSSY BLACK MARKS.

Each question: A B C D E

1	26	51	76	101
2	27	52	77	102
3	28	53	78	103
4	29	54	79	104
5	30	55	80	105
6	31	56	81	106
7	32	57	82	107
8	33	58	83	108
9	34	59	84	109
10	35	60	85	110

Make only ONE mark for each answer. Additional and stray marks may be counted as mistakes. In making corrections, erase errors COMPLETELY.

Each question: A B C D E

11	36	61	86	111
12	37	62	87	112
13	38	63	88	113
14	39	64	89	114
15	40	65	90	115
16	41	66	91	116
17	42	67	92	117
18	43	68	93	118
19	44	69	94	119
20	45	70	95	120
21	46	71	96	121
22	47	72	97	122
23	48	73	98	123
24	49	74	99	124
25	50	75	100	125

BASIC FUNDAMENTALS OF ORGANIC CHEMISTRY

CONCISE TEXT

CONTENTS

BASIC FUNDAMENTALS of ORGANIC CHEMISTRY

CONCISE TEXT

For years, chemistry was divided into two main categories—inorganic chemistry, dealing with substances of mineral origin, and organic chemistry, dealing with those derived from living organisms. It was widely accepted that some "vital force" was necessary in the making of organic compounds and although man could manufacture inorganic compounds, he would have to be satisfied with a role of merely analyzing substances of organic nature, leaving their manufacture up to the plants and animals with the "vital force." Since the synthesis of urea, a recognized organic substance, chemists have had to modify their thinking and organic chemistry has become the study of the compounds of carbon, regardless of whether or not they are derived from plants or animals. Since then, scientists have been able to produce hundreds of thousands of organic compounds.

1. The importance of organic chemistry

a. Organic substances important to life. From the simplest, one-celled organisms to the grossly complex human being, all living organisms are made up of organic materials. Protoplasm, the basis for life itself, is a highly complex mixture of organic compounds. Organic chemistry is of primary importance, then, in the composition and function of living things. Most of the things essential in our everyday life are also of organic nature.

(1) Food. Fundamental to our existence is the food which we ingest to produce energy and growth. Our food is organic in nature. Further, the foods required by the plants and animals which supply us our food are organic. Proteins ... carbohydrates ... fats ... vitamins ... these are all organic compounds.

(2) Housing. Many of the materials used in the construction of our houses and the furnishings within are organic. Wood ... plastic ... rubber ... all are organic.

(3) Clothing. It is hard to find a single garment or article of clothing that is not of organic material. Cotton ... wool ... silk ... rubber ... nylon ... leather ... plastic ... dacron, and many, many other synthetic materials make up almost 100 percent of our garments.

b. Organic substances important to health. A great majority of the items used by man to promote and sustain health are organic in nature.

(1) Medicinals. List every medicinal you and your family have ever taken, touched, heard of, or seen. When you have finished, you will have a lengthy list; more than 90 percent of the items will be organic or have organic ingredients. Less than 10 percent of our medicinal agents are of inorganic origin.

(2) Agents related to medicine and pharmacy. In addition to the medications given to treat and prevent disease, there are many adjunct items. Sterile dressings, sutures, and prostheses may also be of organic origin. More than a million organic compounds have been made and studied. Infinitely more are possible, whereas inorganic compounds synthesized and studied number only about 50,000. In years to come, there will be a far greater spread between the number of organic and inorganic compounds. This is so because carbon has the ability to form infinitely long and high molecular weight chains.

c. Advances in medicine and pharmacy. In the past 35 years, more advances have been made in medicine than since the beginning of civilization, and the vast majority of these have been through the efforts conducted in organic synthesis. Certainly, then, the field of organic chemistry is important to man, and even more important to the pharmacist and physician.

2. Sources of organic compounds. Before the synthesis of urea by Wohler in 1828, all the organic compounds in use were naturally occurring and produced by the plant or animal kingdom. Today, we have three possible sources for organic substances: natural, synthetic, and semisynthetic.

a. Natural. Mother nature has been kind to us in supplying many useful organic substances "readymade." Proteins, carbohydrates, and fats, our important food substances, along with vitamins, essential food supplements, are all naturally occurring in plant and animal life. Fibrous material for clothing manufacture is available, as are alkaloidal drugs, fuels, and building materials. We need only harvest and process these naturally occurring products.

b. Synthetic. The synthetic organic products used widely today may be compounded by chemical action of naturally occurring organic substances to produce new substances, or they may be entirely synthesized from raw elements. Organic chemists have been able to make in the laboratory not only exact duplicates of organic compounds occurring in nature, but also myriads of new compounds which do not occur naturally.

c. Semisynthetic. Some of the medicinal agents used today are neither natural nor synthetic, but combinations of the two. These may be thought of as semisynthetic compounds. The most impressive of these semisynthetics are the antibiotics. In 1928, Sir Alexander Fleming noticed that a foreign mold in a culture plate caused the inhibition of a staphylococcus culture. Through subculturing, he isolated penicillin, a widely used antibiotic. A number of the antibiotics used today are synthetic; others must still be derived semisynthetically with the help of the microorganisms.

3. Important basic principles of organic chemistry. Before we can learn about the organic compounds important to pharmacy, it is necessary that we know some basic principles and properties pertaining to all organic substances.

a. General properties of organic compounds. With a field so large, it is difficult to classify the hundreds of thousands of compounds that have been isolated and studied to date. They differ widely in structure, action, and use. The following general statements, however, apply to all organic compounds:

(1) The number of organic compounds possible is almost limitless, whereas inorganic compounds are held within a restricted field.

(2) Molecular structure of organic substances is far more complex than the structure of inorganic materials.

(3) Organic compounds favor covalent bonding, while most inorganic bonding is of the electrovalent type.

(4) Organic compounds are generally insoluble in water, but soluble in the organic solvents such as alcohol, carbon tetrachloride, carbon disulfide, chloroform, or ether.

(5) Most organic compounds are thermolabile; that is, they are sensitive to destruction by heat.

(6) Organic reactions are difficult to predict. You remember that in inorganic chemistry, reactions took place rapidly, yielding definite products. Organic reactions may take hours or even days and the yield of intended products is rarely more than 50 percent. There may be many compounds formed in a single reaction.

b. Unique properties of carbon. The unique properties of carbon compared to the other elements is the basis and reason for organic chemistry. Carbon, the first member of the fourth group in the periodic table, has six protons, six neutrons, and six orbital electrons. The electron configuration, as you should imagine, is two electrons in the K shell and four in the L shell. If you look carefully at the periodic table, you will see that carbon is the lowest atomic weight element exactly midway between two inert elements. In reacting, carbon can attain stability either by accepting four electrons *or* losing four electrons, and because of this it is equally liable to be oxidized or reduced. Actually, since carbon forms compounds by covalent bonding, the electrons are neither gained nor lost, but shared.

c. Purification of organic compounds. The purity of organic compounds may be determined by a number of tests, including specific gravity determination, refraction index, crystal form, and other physical constants. The customary way of determining the purity of organic compounds, however, is by determination of their boiling and melting points. Impurities lower melting points and make the range in temperature between starting and completion of melting rather wide. Moreover, the boiling point of pure organic compounds is constant. Variations from this constant indicate impurities.

(1) Purification by crystallization. Crystallization is the method generally employed for the purification of solid organic substances. A solvent is chosen in which the solid is much more soluble when the solvent is hot than cold. The substance to be purified is dissolved in the hot

solvent and any insoluble material is filtered off. The solution is then cooled, depositing crystals of the pure substance. The liquid is filtered off; the crystals are washed with more pure solvent and dried.

(2) Purification of extraction with an immiscible solvent. Liquids containing small amounts of impurities can be effectively purified by extracting the impurities with another solvent. The solvent chosen for the extraction should be immiscible with the liquid to be purified. It must also be one in which the impurity is much more soluble than in the liquid to be purified. The two liquids are shaken together and the impurity transfers to the liquid in which it is more soluble. Upon standing, the two liquids separate into layers which can then be separated by physical means.

(3) Fractional distillation. Mixtures of liquids or solutions of solids in liquids may be purified by fractional distillation. The impure substance is placed in a flask and by slowly increasing the temperature, the different substances are distilled off. The collecting vessels are changed with each rise in the temperature fraction to receive the various substances.

(4) Other methods. Other methods for eliminating impurities from organic substances are steam distillation and sublimation.

d. Tests for organic compounds. To determine if a compound is organic, it generally suffices to heat the compound. If it decomposes at a relatively low temperature, leaving a black, charred residue, it is very probably an organic compound. Compounds which sublime cannot be tested in this manner. Specific procedures for the qualitative and quantitative analysis of organic compounds are of no practical value to you as a pharmacy technician and will not be covered here. Most texts on organic chemistry and all laboratory manuals in the field will answer any questions you may have on the analysis of organic materials.

e. Skeleton structure. As previously stated, carbon possesses the ability to link together to form complex molecules. These molecules may form continuous chains, branching chains, closed chains (rings), or rings with separating elements other than carbon. The following are examples of these structures:

(1) Continuous or straight chain.

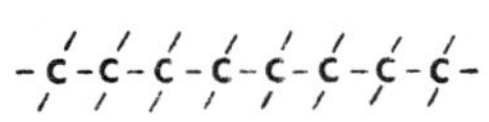

(2) Branching chain.

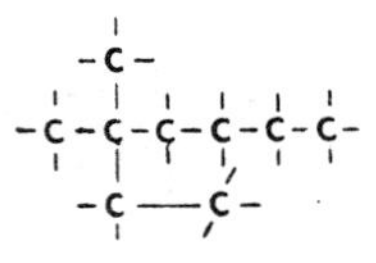

(3) Closed chains or rings.

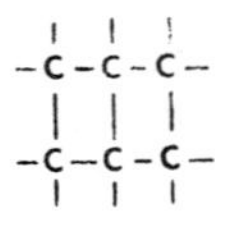

(4) Rings including other elements.

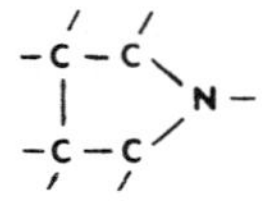

f. Bonds.

(1) Valence bonds. The study of organic compounds is immeasurably simplified by the graphic representation of their formulas. In writing these formulas, lines or dots (called bonds) are commonly used to show how the atoms are joined together in the molecule. These bonds represent the valence, and the number of bonds attached to each element symbol represents the valence of that atom in the molecule. Thus, in the formula—

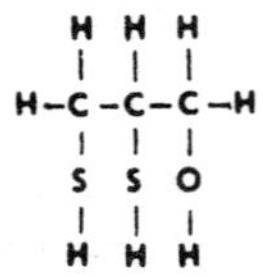

the valence of each C atom is 4, that of the S atom is 2, each 0 atom has a valence of 2, and each H atom has a valence of 1. It is also written—

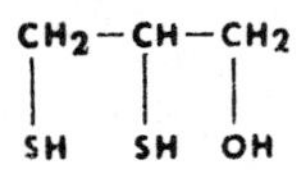

to represent the same formula. These written formulas show not only that the elements are bonded together, but how they are bonded. Therefore, it is advisable to include here a brief description of the more important kinds of valence bonds in terms of their electron meanings.

(2) Electrovalent bond. This type of bond is most frequently seen in electrolytes such as sodium chloride, NaCl. An actual electron transfer from one atom to another occurs in the electrovalent bond. In sodium chloride, the Na atom loses, transfers, or gives its single valence electron to the Cl atom.

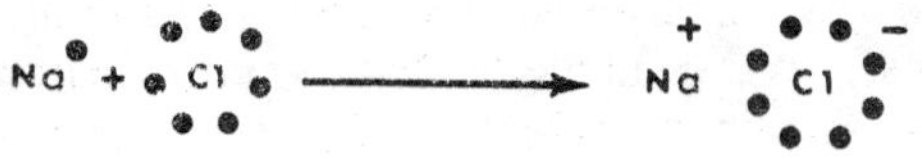

Since the Na atom loses a negative charge, it takes on a positive charge of one. The chlorine atom, gaining the electron, takes on a negative charge of one. The two elements, Na and Cl, are held together by the attraction of the opposite charges. These charged particles in solution will transmit an electric current and therefore are termed electrolytes. The electrovalent bond is not very common in organic molecules. An example of a bond which is at least partly electrovalent is the bond between the O and the H in carboxylic acids and phenols.

(3) Covalent bond. This is the type of bond found in organic compounds between carbon atoms and in such inorganic molecules as H_2O, H_2, or Cl_2.

(a) Sharing electron pairs. In the covalent bond, the atoms involved "share," rather than transfer, one or more pairs of electrons. In the case of the chlorine molecule, each element has seven outer electrons. Two atoms are combined to form a stable molecule, with each atom sharing two electrons (one from each atom).

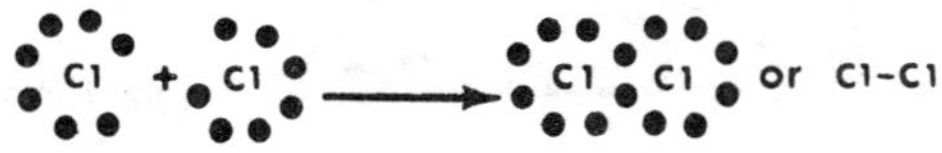

(b) Single, double, and triple bonds. A single bond between two C atoms signifies a covalence of one or a sharing of two electrons, one from each atom. In the same way, a double bond between two C atoms (C=C) signifies a covalence of two or a sharing of four electrons, two from each C atom. A triple bond (C≡C) would then show a covalence of three or a sharing of six electrons, three from each atom.

(c) Illustration of covalent bonding. To illustrate this bonding, the following electron formulas are shown. The electrons belonging originally to C are designated by circles, those originally part of H by dots, and those belonging originally to O by ■■.

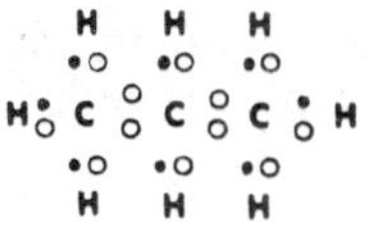

Propane

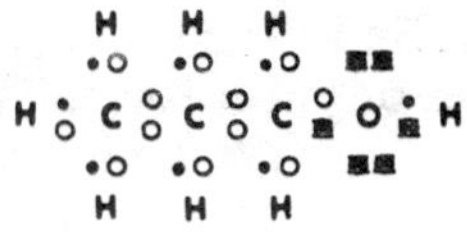

Propanol

Note that in both molecules, each element has attained a stable configuration. Hydrogen has attained two electrons in the outer orbit and both carbon and oxygen have eight electrons in their outer orbits.

g. Isomerism. Compounds that have the same composition; that is, the same number and kind of atoms but in different arrangement, are called isomers. Below are diagrams for three isomers of the same formula (octane). Eighteen are possible. For the sake of simplicity, the hydrogen atoms normally saturating the carbon atoms have not been shown.

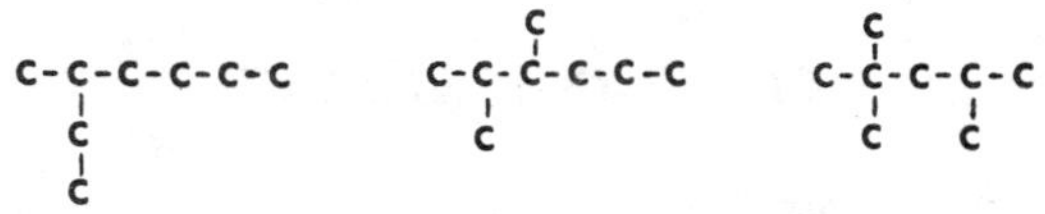

The atoms of octane can be arranged in 18 different ways, although there are always the same number and kind of atoms. Each different arrangement is an isomer. Each has the formula C_8H_{18}. As the complexity of the organic material involved increases, so does the number of possible isomers. These isomers are not identical in their properties or actions and consequently there are billions of possible arrangements for the hundreds of thousands of organic structures known.

h. Graphic formula. The best way to show the complete atomic relationships of the molecule is by graphic formulas. The formulas shown in the explanation of isomerism are examples of graphic formulas, except that the hydrogen atoms have been omitted. The following is an example of a full graphic formula:

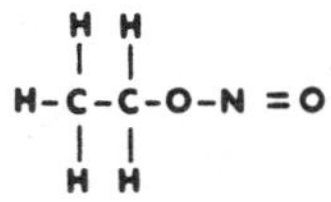

i. Linear formula. A linear formula is a simplification of a graphic formula. Although the linear formula is easier to write, unlike the graphic formula it does not show the complete molecular structure. In most cases, the graphic formula is preferred. The following examples compare three types of linear formulas with a graphic formula:

(1) Graphic formula.

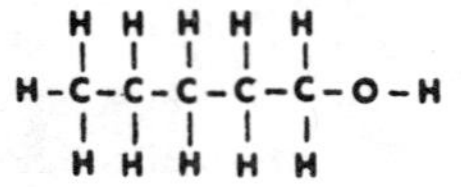

(2) Linear formula (dashes represent bonds).

$$CH_3-CH_2-CH_2-CH_2-CH_2-OH$$

(3) Linear formula (dots represent bonds).

$$CH_3 \cdot CH_2 \cdot CH_2 \cdot CH_2 \cdot CH_2 \cdot OH$$

(4) Linear formula (bonds not shown).

$$CH_3\,CH_2\,CH_2\,CH_2\,CH_2\,OH$$

j Classification of organic compounds. Practically all organic compounds are grouped into the following classes:

(1) Hydrocarbons
(2) Alcohols and phenols
(3) Aldehydes
(4) Ketones
(5) Acids
(6) Esters
(7) Ethers
(8) Carbohydrates
(9) Alkaloids
(10) Nitrogenous products

These ten classes may be broadly considered as derivatives of either methane or benzene. The methane derivatives, which are straight or branched chain compounds, are termed aliphatic compounds. The benzene derivatives are cyclic compounds and are classified as aromatic compounds.

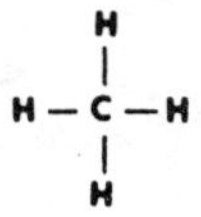

Methane

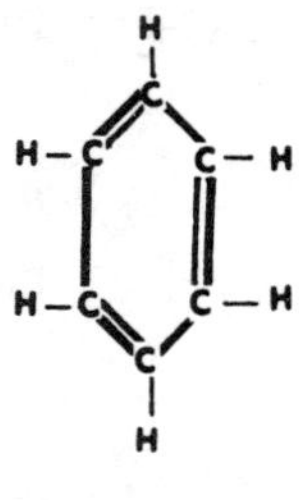

Benzene

4. Hydrocarbons. Compounds composed solely of carbon and hydrogen are called hydrocarbons. They may be either aliphatic, that is, straight or branched formations, or cyclic, i.e., arranged into a ring or closed cycle.

a. Terminal carbon atoms. The straight chain hydrocarbons have two terminal carbon atoms; the branched chain hydrocarbons have three terminal carbon atoms or more; and the closed ring or cyclic hydrocarbons have no terminal carbon atoms, since each carbon is joined to another in the ring. The following structures illustrate the terminal carbon atoms in the various formations.

(1) Straight chain hydrocarbon showing two terminal carbons.

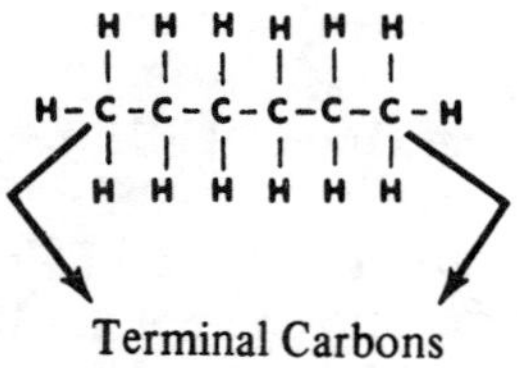

(2) Branched chain with three terminal carbons.

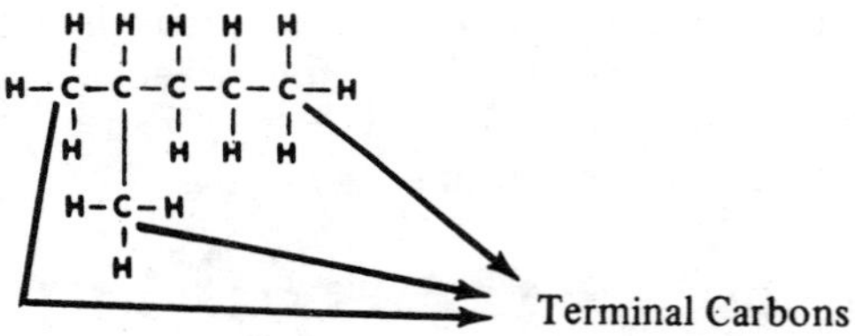

(3) Branched chain with four terminal carbons.

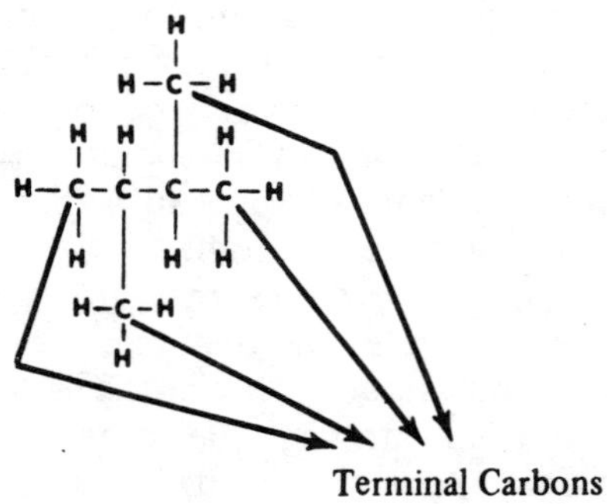

(4) Cyclic hydrocarbon showing no terminal carbons.

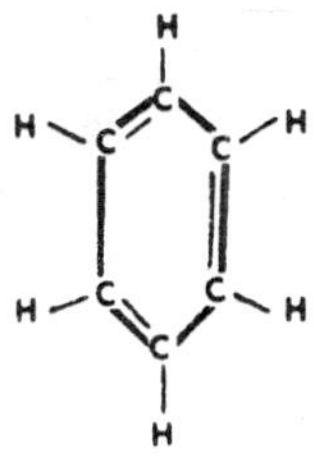

b. Aliphatic hydrocarbons. We will discuss in this portion of the chapter only the aliphatic hydrocarbons. The cyclic hydrocarbons will be discussed later with other cyclic compounds.

(1) Alkanes (paraffins, methane series, saturated hydrocarbons). This is the basic group of the hydrocarbons. They are composed solely of carbon-hydrogen bonds and carbon-carbon single bonds. Because they contain only single bonds, they are referred to as "saturated hydrocarbons." This is a very stable bond and not reactive. The term paraffin comes from this property. The Latin word "parum" means "little" and "affinis" means affinity. Paraffins do not easily react with other chemicals.

(a) Homologous series. The alkanes form a homologous series. Each member differs from the preceding one by the addition of CH_2. Members next to each other are called homologs. Ethane and methane differ by CH_2 and are homologs of each other. The smallest alkane is methane, thus the term "methane series." The following list of the first ten alkanes form the basis for all other organic compounds and should be learned.

- methane, CH_4
- ethane, C_2H_6
- propane, C_3H_8
- butane, C_4H_{10}
- pentane, C_5H_{12}
- hexane, C_6H_{14}
- heptane, C_7H_{16}
- octane, C_8H_{18}
- nonane, C_9H_{20}
- decane, $C_{10}H_{22}$

(b) Naming simple alkanes. Looking at the first ten members, you can see a pattern developing. All alkanes end in -ane. This indicates a saturated hydrocarbon. The first four members have common names but starting with the fifth member, pentane, the name indicates how many carbon atoms are present. For example, the Greek word for the number of carbon atoms is followed by "ane": hexane has six carbons (hexa) each connected to another by a single bond (ane).

(c) General formula of alkanes. All alkanes conform to the general formula C_nH_{2n+2} (where n = the number of carbon atoms). If we know the number of carbon atoms, we can determine the number of hydrogen atoms in the alkane. Example: What would be the formula for eicosane (eico stands for 20) according to the general formula?

$$n = 20$$

$$C_nH_{2n+2}$$

$$C_{20}H_{2\times 20+2} = C_{20}H_{42}$$

(d) Empirical formula. The formula above tells us only how many carbon and hydrogen atoms are present; it does not tell us how they are arranged. It is called an empirical formula. In order to identify the exact compound, we must use either a graphic formula or a linear formula. This is necessary as several isomers may exist.

(e) Isomers. Isomerism is possible from the fourth member of this series on. These are structural isomers; that is, they differ in arrangement of the atoms. Thus, butane may exist in the two following isomeric forms:

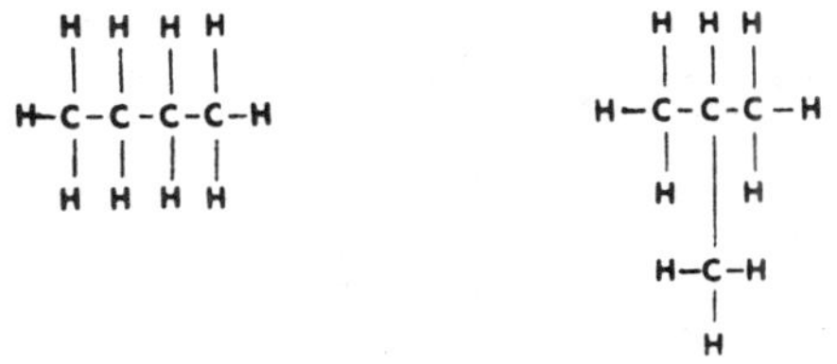

Both compounds have the empirical formula C_4H_{10}, but differ in arrangement. As the length of the carbon chain increases, the number of isomeric possibilities increases.

(f) Nomenclature of the alkanes. Because of the vast number of possible isomeric structures, it is necessary to have a system for naming these compounds. It would be hopeless to try to remember common names for all the members. The International Union of Chemists has devised the following system for naming any alkane.

1. All the straight chain alkanes have the ending *ane,* and except for the first four members, are named for the number of carbon atoms they possess.

2. Groups branching off a

straight chain are named by using the stem of the alkane with the same number of carbon atoms, and changing its *ane* ending to *yl.* Thus we have the following groups or radicals: CH_3 = Meth*yl*, same number of C atoms as meth*ane*; C_2H_5 = eth*yl*, same number of C atoms as eth*ane*, and so on.

3. Branching alkanes are named on the basis of the longest straight chain they contain. The groups or radicals attached are listed alphabetically, preceding the base name. If the same radical appears more than once, it is given a prefix to show the number of times; for example, "di" for twice, "tri" for thrice, and "penta" for five times.

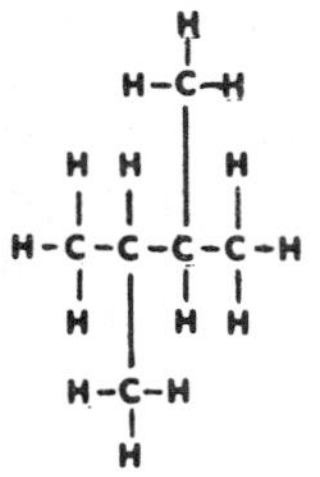

In the preceding graphic formula we have a branching chain isomer of hexane. The longest straight chain consists of four carbon atoms and therefore will be named on the basis of butane. There are two methyl groups attached and consequently this structure will be dimethyl butane.

4. It is important to know just where these methyl groups are attached, so the chain must be numbered. Only the longest chain is numbered, and always from the most branched end. In the case above, both ends are equally branched, so it makes no difference from which end you number.

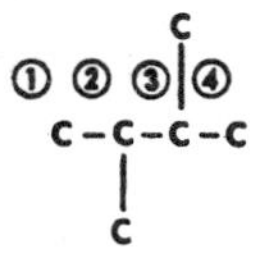

We can now further identify the compound as 2,3-dimethyl butane. How would you name the following compound?

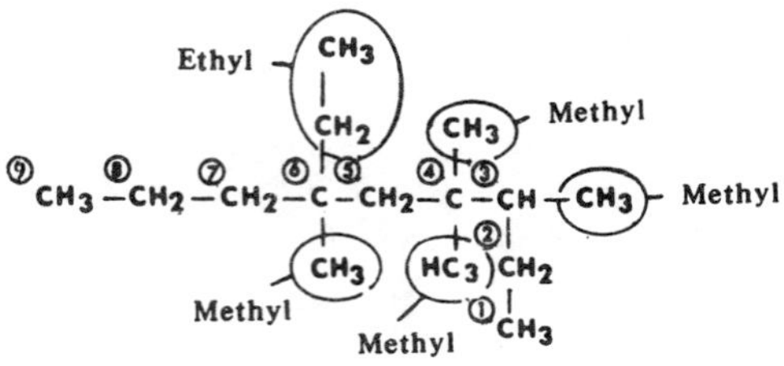

This compound is numbered for you, and the longest chain is 9 carbon atoms long. It will, then, be named as a nonane. Its name–6-ethyl-3, 4, 4, 6-tetramethylnonane.

5. In the event it is not obvious which end of the chain is most branching, number from both ends, name the compound both ways, and the compound whose numbers total the smaller figure when added will be the correct name. To illustrate this, let's number the above compound from the other end and see which is correct.

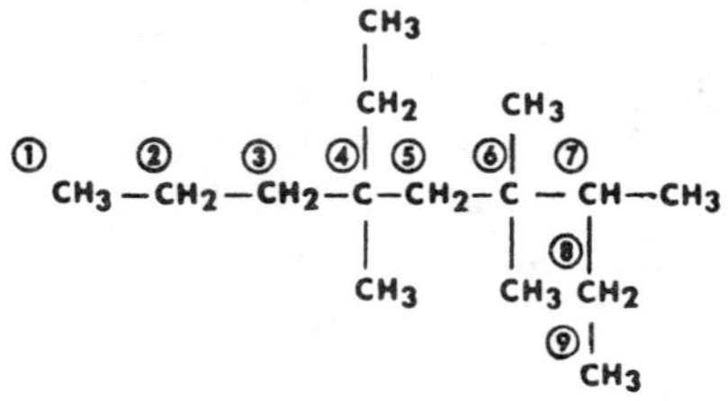

Numbered in this fashion, the name would be 4-ethyl-4, 6, 6, 7-tetramethylnonane. Adding the numbers 4, 4, 6, 6, and 7, we get a total of 27. The previous name's numbers (6, 3, 4, 4, and 6) when totaled give a sum of 23. Since 23 is the lower number, that name is correct.

6. Just as we can name a structure from its formula, we can construct the graphic formula, given its name. To illustrate, let's draw the formula for 2, 4-dimethyl hexane. This name tells us that the longest chain is six carbons long, and that there are two methyl groups attached, one at the number two carbon and one at the number four carbon. Thus we draw the structure–

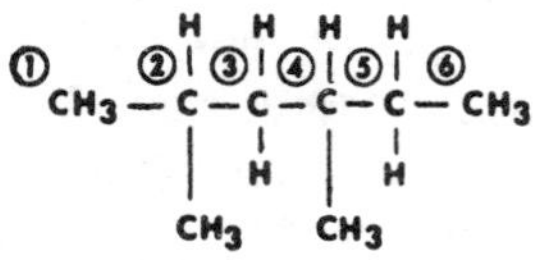

(2) Alkenes (ethylene series, olefins, unsaturated hydrocarbons). The first member of

the alkene series is ethylene (C_2H_4), which is also called ethene. You should guess from the number of carbons and hydrogens in this compound that the general formula for the alkenes is C_nH_{2n}. The number of hydrogen atoms is exactly twice the number of carbons.

(a) Reason for the general formula. The general formula for the alkenes (C_nH_{2n}) has two less hydrogens than that for the alkanes (C_nH_{2n+2}). This is because the alkenes are unsaturated; somewhere in the molecule a double bond exists. For each double bond, two pairs of electrons are required. Thus, bonds which were attached to a hydrogen in the alkanes are paired between two carbons in the alkenes, causing two less hydrogen atoms in the alkene molecule.

(b) Reactivity. Because the alkenes are unsaturated, having at least one double bond which is strained and unstable when compared to a single bond, they are quite reactive. Unsaturated compounds seek to gain saturation and thus enter into chemical reaction easily.

(c) Alkene nomenclature. Alkenes are named from the corresponding alkane; that is, from the alkane having the same carbon content. In adapting the proper alkane name to fit its corresponding alkene, the *ane* ending is dropped and *ene* or *ylene* is added. There is no alkene corresponding to methane, so the alkene series progresses in the following manner:

- Ethylene or ethene (C_2H_4)
- Propylene or propene (C_3H_6)
- Butylene or butene (C_4H_8)
- Pentylene or pentene (C_5H_{10})
- Hexylene or hexene (C_6H_{12})

(d) Naming complex alkenes. Naming alkenes is basically the same as naming the alkanes. The longest chain containing the double bond is selected as the base. The chain is numbered from the end that gives the double bonded carbon atoms the lowest numbers. The number of the carbon closest to the end of the chain is prefixed to the base name to indicate where the double bond is located. Radicals attached to the chain are named in the same manner as the alkanes. The formula below would be named 3-methyl-2-pentene:

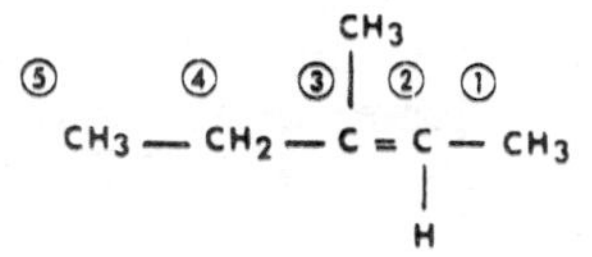

(3) Alkynes (alkines). This homologous series contains a triple bond and has the general formula C_nH_{2n-2}. The alkynes are even more unstable than the alkenes because of the triple bond. They react explosively. The first and simplest member of this group is ethyne, generally called by its common name, acetylene.

$$HC{\equiv}CH$$

Nomenclature for the alkynes is basically the same as for the alkenes.

(4) Occurrence of the hydrocarbons in nature. Petroleum, or crude oil as it is sometimes called, is a mixture of hydrocarbons varying greatly in composition. It is obtained from beneath the surface of the ground, and is the result of decomposition of various forms of marine life over thousands of years.

(a) Gaseous hydrocarbons. The first four alkanes (methane, ethane, propane, and butane) are gases. Natural gas is a mixture of about 80 percent methane with small amounts of ethane and propane. As the number of carbons increase, the compounds become denser, and pentane is the first liquid member of the series.

(b) Pentane and hexane. The first fraction to be distilled from crude oil is a mixture of pentane and hexane, two very volatile liquids. This combination of hydrocarbons is commercially known as petroleum benzin or petroleum ether, and is generally the substance used in cleaning fluids and lighter fluids.

(c) Heptane, octane, and nonane. The next fraction to distill off from the petroleum is a combination of heptane, octane, and nonane. This is the mixture known as gasoline. Normal heptane, the worst possible gasoline, has an octane rating of 0. The best gasoline is isooctane (2, 2, 4-trimethylpentane) and has an octane rating of 100.

(d) Kerosene. The next fraction to come off is not so volatile as the previous ones. This mixture has 10 or 11 carbon atoms and is commercially sold as kerosene. It is used as a fuel for heaters, kerosene stoves, and lanterns.

(e) Fuel oil and dieselene (diesel oil). These are the next mixtures to be distilled from the petroleum and they range from 12 to 16 carbon atoms in composition.

(f) Other fractions. Progressing in molecular composition and at the same time becoming thicker and more nearly solid are—

1. Light lubrication oils (*Example:* 3-in-1 oil).

2. Light motor oil.

3. Heavy motor oil.

4. Transmission grease.

5. Axle grease.

6. Petroleum tar.

7. Waxes or paraffins. Those fractions containing 30 or more carbon atoms are solids.

(5) Pharmaceutical products of the hydrocarbons.

(a) Ethylene (ethene) $CH_2 = CH_2$, C_2H_4. Ethylene, a very volatile gas, is highly flammable when mixed with oxygen. In concentrations of 85-90 percent, it is used as a surgical anesthetic that is powerful enough to permit any level of surgery. Because it is highly combustible, it must not be used near an open flame and extreme precautions must be taken against ignition by static electricity. Ethylene is used in the synthesis of ethyl alcohol and ethylene glycol and, because it destroys chlorophyll, it is used in the artificial ripening of oranges, lemons, and other fruits.

(b) Cyclopropane (trimethylene), C_3H_6.

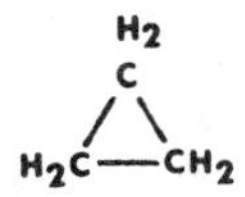

Although this is not an aliphatic hydrocarbon, it is usually considered with the aliphatics because it resembles them in properties and uses. This gas is also used as a general inhalation anesthetic, and since it is effective in concentrations of only 15-20 percent, it is safer for the patient than ethylene. It, too, is explosive and every precaution must be taken to prevent open flames or sparks from occurring in the operating room where it is being used.

(c) Ichthammol (ammonium ichthosulfonate). Ichthammol is a black, tarlike substance of natural occurrence. It can be manufactured by destructive distillation of bituminous substance, sulfonation, and neutralization of the product with ammonia. It is water miscible and is often incorporated into ointments for its anti-infective and irritant properties.

(d) Paraffin. Paraffin is a purified mixture of solid hydrocarbons obtained from petroleum. It is a waxy substance, insoluble in water and mainly used in pharmacy to stiffen ointments and suppositories. It is classified as a pharmaceutical necessity.

(e) Petrolatum (petroleum jelly; yellow petrolatum). Petrolatum is a purified mixture of semisolid hydrocarbons obtained from petroleum. It may contain a stabilizer. Petrolatum differs from automobile grease only in purity. The solid and liquid hydrocarbons making up this intermediate may contain impurities which are unsaturated. These will oxidize and become rancid. To prevent rancidity, some vitamin E is generally added in the processing. Petrolatum is used as an ointment base, emollient, and protective.

(f) White petrolatum (white petroleum jelly; petrolatum album). This substance is nothing more than yellow petrolatum which has been decolorized. It, too, is used as an ointment base and protective. It is also employed in the cosmetic industry.

(g) Mineral oil (heavy liquid petrolatum; liquid paraffin; white mineral oil). This is a viscous, clear liquid, containing hydrocarbon chains in the range of 18 to 24 carbon atoms. It is frequently used as a laxative because it acts as an intestinal lubricant. Since it is generally taken every day to promote regularity and soften the stool, and because it dissolves oil-soluble vitamins and allows them to be excreted, this preparation should only be administered at bedtime when it will not interfere with the assimilation of foods.

(h) Light liquid petrolatum (light liquid paraffin; light mineral oil). Light liquid petrolatum is not intended for internal use. It is the main ingredient in baby oils which may also contain rose oil for its pleasant scent and lanolin for its softening action. It is also used in the cosmetic industry. In the past, many nose drops and sprays used light mineral oil as a base, mainly because the ingredients were soluble in it. These are no longer widely used because the oil slicks down the hair-like structure (cilia) in the nostrils and allows bacteria to pass freely into the lungs. There is also the danger of children aspirating the oil into the lungs and developing lipoid (fatty) pneumonia.

5. Derivatives of the aliphatic hydrocarbons. By substituting chemically an element such as chlorine, or a radical such as hydroxyl, OH, for one or more of the hydrogen atoms of a hydrocarbon, hydrocarbon derivatives are achieved. Many of these substitution products are important in medicine. Notice in the following graphic formulas how elements have been substituted for hydrogen in methane to arrive at some important medicinal products.

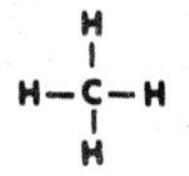

Methane

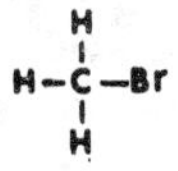

Methyl Bromide

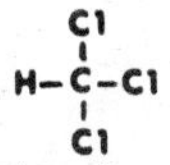

Chloroform

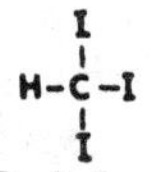

Iodoform

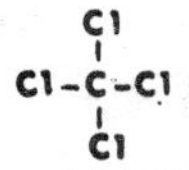

Carbon Tetrachloride

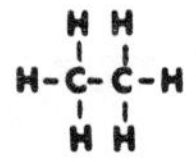

Ethane

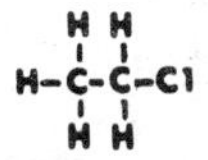

Ethyl Chloride

a. Ethyl chloride, CH_3CH_2Cl. Local anesthetic spray.

b. Butyl chloride (n-butyl chloride) $CH_3CH_2CH_2CH_2Cl$. An anthelmintic agent.

c. Carbon tetrachloride CCl_4 *(tetrachloromethane).* Solvent, anthelmintic, fire extinguishing agent.

d. Chloroform, $CHCl_3$. General anesthetic, carminative, solvent for extraction of alkaloids, irritant in liniments, and sedative expectorant in cough mixtures.

e. Trichloroethylene (Trilene).

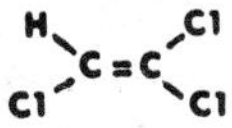

Trilene is an inhalation-type anesthetic.

f. Halothane (Fluothane) $CF_3CBrClH$. An inhalation anesthetic.

g. Iodoform (triiodomethane) CHI_3. An antibacterial used to impregnate gauze packing and dressings.

6. Aliphatic alcohols. Among the many important oxygen-containing compounds in the field of organic chemistry are the alcohols.

a. Structure. The general structure of the aliphatic alcohols can be represented by the formula R–OH; R being the hydrocarbon chain, and OH the alcohol group. Up to this point, you have been taught that an OH group signifies an alkali or base. In organic chemistry, the OH takes on a different meaning and lends far different characteristics and properties to the compound containing it. It is important that you thoroughly understand at this point that the OH group is now characteristic of the alcohol. It is this group which gives the compound its chemical properties as well as its therapeutic effects. Alcohols may contain one or more OH groups.

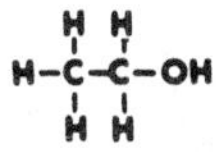

Ethyl Alcohol

b. Placement of alcohol group. Alcohols containing one hydroxyl group are called monohydric or monohydroxy alcohols, and those containing two or more OH groups are polyhydric or polyhydroxy alcohols. The placement of the alcohol group on the hydrocarbon chain greatly affects the nature of the compound. The alcohol groups may attach to a primary carbon atom (a carbon atom attached to only one other carbon), a secondary carbon atom (a carbon atom attached to two other carbons), or a tertiary carbon atom (a carbon atom attached to three other carbons). The alcohol formed when the hydroxyl group attaches to a primary carbon atom is a primary (1°) alcohol; to a secondary carbon atom, a secondary (2°) alcohol, and so on. In the graphic formulas below are shown the primary, secondary, and tertiary carbon atoms and the alcohol which results from attachment to each.

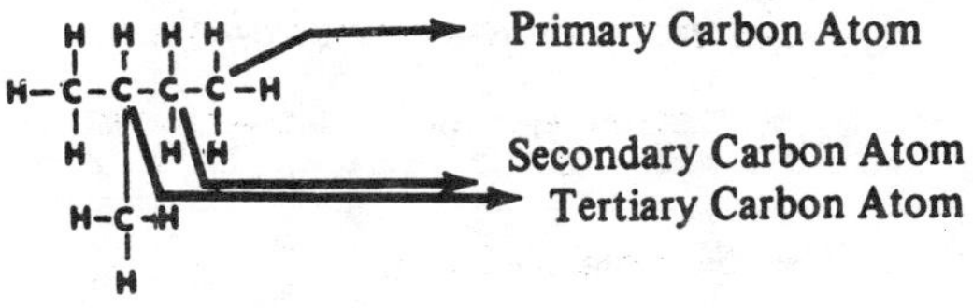

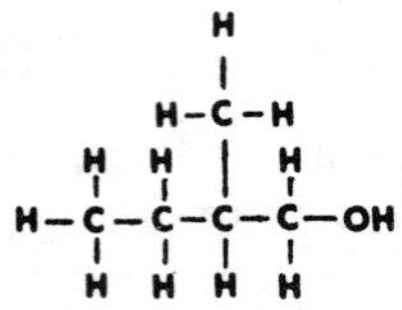

Primary (1°)
Alcohol

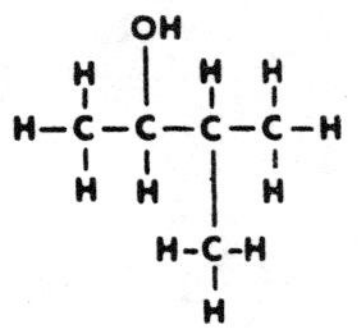

Secondary (2°)
Alcohol

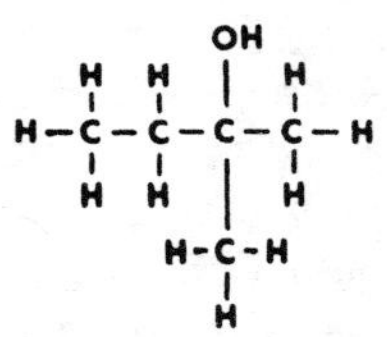

Tertiary (3°)
Alcohol

c. ***General formulas for alcohols.***

- Primary Alcohol $R-CH_2OH$
- Secondary Alcohol 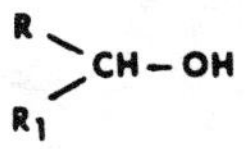
- Tertiary Alcohol 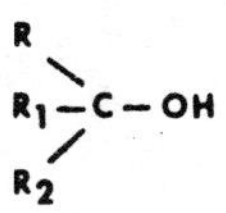

d. Properties. The following general properties can be stated for alcohols:

(1) Most monohydric alcohols are lighter than water; that is, they have specific gravities less than 1.000.

(2) Normal aliphatic alcohols are liquids up to 11 carbons in the chain and solids after 13.

(3) Addition of more OH groups increases the specific gravity and they become heavier than water. Alcohols also become sweeter as more OH groups are added to them. Sugar is a polyhydric alcohol.

(4) The alcohols are chemically neutral, that is, neither basic nor acidic. They do resemble bases in that they react with acids to form salts.

(5) Alcohols are miscible with water, but as the length of the chain increases, the solubility decreases. Solubility increases, however, as the number of hydroxy groups increases.

e. Nomenclature.

(1) Common name system. The common names of the alcohols are formed by taking the name of the radical and adding the word "alcohol." Thus, CH_3OH, containing a methyl radical, is called methyl alcohol. C_2H_5OH, containing an ethyl radical, is called ethyl alcohol. The common name system is satisfactory up to five carbon atoms in the radical. Beyond that it becomes too complicated for general use.

(2) International Union of Chemists (IUC) system. The IUC has established a system for naming the alcohols which is far superior to the common name method. This system is based upon ending the name with "ol." Taking the stem from the longest continuous carbon chain which contains the OH radical, the "e" is dropped and "ol" is added. Refer back to the nomenclature for the alkanes. By the IUC method, methyl alcohol becomes methanol and ethyl alcohol becomes ethanol.

f. Occurrence. Alcohols occur in nature as such (glycerin and mannitol) and with other radicals attached (glucose). Esterified alcohols are widely distributed in nature as volatile oils, fixed oils, fats, and waxes.

g. Preparation.

(1) Primary alcohols. Primary alcohols are prepared by the hydrolysis of the corresponding alkyl halide (halogen derivative) as in

$$C_2H_5Br + HOH \xrightarrow{NaOH} NaBr + HOH + C_2H_5OH$$

(2) Secondary alcohols. Secondary alcohols are prepared by the hydration of alkenes, by the reduction of ketones, or by the fermentation of sugars.

(3) Tertiary alcohols. Tertiary alcohols are made by the hydration of alkenes.

h. Reactions. The following are typical reactions which alcohols undergo:

(1) Hydrogen replaced by a metal to form salts.

$$2ROH + 2Na \longrightarrow H_2 + 2RONa$$

(2) Reaction with acids to form esters.

$$ROH + H_2SO_4 \longrightarrow ROSO_3H + HOH$$

(3) Replacement of the hydroxyl group by a halogen.

$$ROH + HCl \xrightarrow{ZnCl_2} HOH + RCl$$

(4) Oxidation to form an aldehyde and a molecule of water.

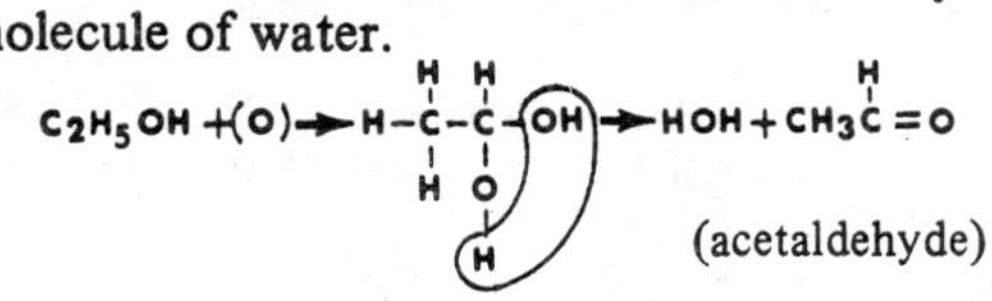

(acetaldehyde)

i. Alcohols used in pharmacy.

(1) Methyl alcohol (methanol; wood alcohol) CH_3OH. Because it was manufactured by the destructive distillation of wood, methanol was given the common name of wood alcohol. Today, it is primarily synthesized directly from carbon monoxide and hydrogen. Extremely poisonous both internally and externally, this alcohol is used in pharmacy only as a solvent, a denaturing agent, a fuel for alcohol lamps, and as a starting point for the synthesis of other organic compounds.

(2) Alcohol [ethanol, ethyl alcohol, spiritus vini rectificatus (SVR)] C_2H_5OH. Alcohol is manufactured by the process of fermentation, an enzymatic decomposition of carbohydrates. When alcohol is called for in a prescription or formula, this is the alcohol to be used unless otherwise specified.

(a) Uses. Ethyl alcohol is found in beverages, and although large quantities are toxic, it is intended for internal administration as well as external. It is used as a vehicle for liquid medications, as a preservative, and as a rub. It is a starting point in the manufacture of ether.

(b) Composition. In its official form, alcohol is a mixture of 95 percent C_2H_5OH and 5 percent water by volume. It is 95 percent pure or 190 proof.

(3) Diluted alcohol (diluted ethanol). Diluted alcohol is a mixture of equal volumes of ethyl alcohol and distilled water. This mixture is accompanied by a rise in temperature and a contraction in the total volume. When 500 ml. of alcohol and 500 ml. of water are mixed, the resulting volume is NOT 1000 ml., but closer to 970 ml., a loss of approximately 3 percent. Diluted alcohol is useful as a solvent because it combines the solvent properties of both alcohol and water.

(4) Alcohol rubbing compound (rubbing alcohol). Rubbing alcohol is 70 percent absolute ethyl alcohol, and 30 percent water and denaturants. The denaturants make it unsuitable for drinking and consequently it need not be controlled on stock record cards. Rubbing alcohol is used externally only.

(5) Isopropyl alcohol (isopropanol; 2-propanol) $CH_3CH(OH)CH_3$. This alcohol, produced synthetically as a byproduct in the hydrocracking of petroleum, is described by the National Formulary as a pharmaceutical necessity. It is supplied in a 99-percent strength to be used either full strength or diluted as desired. It is most commonly used in a 70-percent concentration, for external use only.

(6) Denatured alcohol. Ethyl alcohol rendered unfit for human consumption is termed denatured alcohol. There are 50 or more formulas for accomplishing this denaturation. The additives may be poisonous or may be substances which promote vomiting on internal ingestion. It is used as a solvent and as a fuel in alcohol burners and lamps.

(7) Glycerin (glycerol).

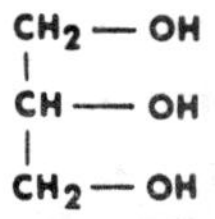

Glycerin is a clear, colorless, viscous liquid, sweet to the taste. As can be seen from the formula, it is a trihydric alcohol and is miscible with water in all proportions, as well as with other alcohols.

(a) Sources. Glycerin is a byproduct of the soap industry. A fat or oil reacted with an alkali such as sodium hydroxide yields a soap plus glycerin. It is also produced by

the fermentation of sugar and chemically from propylene, a byproduct of the petroleum industry.

(b) Reactions. When glycerin is heated to a very high temperature, it is dehydrated to acrolein, a substance with a very irritating odor. The fumes resulting from the burning of animal or vegetable fats smell of acrolein. Glycerin is very easily oxidized and when combined with oxidizing agents such as permanganates may explode. This is an incompatibility for glycerin about which more will be said in chapter 8.

(c) Uses. Glycerin has many uses in medicinal preparations.

- Glycerin is a good solvent.
- Glycerin is slightly antiseptic and in high concentrations may be used to prevent microbial growth in some preparations.
- Glycerin is humectant and emollient; that is, in preparations for external use, it moistens and lubricates the skin.
- Glycerin is used in some internal preparations as a sweetening agent.
- Glycerin is the active ingredient in glycerin suppositories.
- Glycerin in combination with water can be used as a permanent or reusable refrigerant. Packed in hermetically sealed containers, teething rings, ice collars, or caps, it can be chilled or frozen repeatedly.

(8) Ethylene glycol:

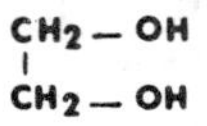

Ethylene glycol is a dihydric alcohol, toxic to the body. It is mainly used as a solvent in manufacturing procedures but must be carefully removed if the product is intended for internal use. Commercially, it is used as a permanent antifreeze.

(9) Propylene glycol (1, 2-propanediol).

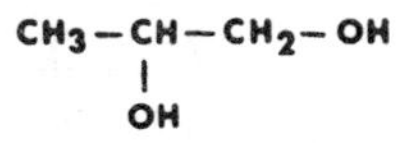

Propylene glycol is a relatively nontoxic substance and is often used as a substitute for glycerin. It is not quite as sweet as glycerin.

7. **Ethers.** Another class of oxygen derivatives of the hydrocarbons is the ethers. These are the dehydration products of two molecules of alcohol.

a. Structure. The general formula for an ether is ROR (the R represents an alkyl radical). The R's may be the same or they may be different. If the R's are the same, the ether is a simple ether and if they are different, it is a mixed ether. Study the following examples:

$CH_3-O-CH_3 \longleftrightarrow$ Dimethyl ether, a simple ether

$C_2H_5-O-CH_2CH_2CH_3 \longleftrightarrow$ Ethyl n-propyl ether a mixed ether

b. Graphic versus empirical formula. We have previously stated that the graphic formula was preferable over the empirical formula, as it completely identified the substance. This can now be illustrated by the comparison of dimethyl ether and ethyl alcohol. The following are graphic formulas for these two different compounds:

Ethyl Alcohol　　　　Dimethyl Ether

These formulas show at once that the compounds are different. One is an alcohol, the other an ether. The empirical formula, however, for both these compounds is C_2H_6O. Given only the empirical formula and no other information, it would be impossible to determine which compound was being considered. Ethyl alcohol and dimethyl ether are structural isomers.

c. Properties. Except for the saturated hydrocarbons, ethers are one of the most chemically inert classes of organic compounds. They do react, however, with bromine and chlorine to form halogenated ethers. Because of this stability, ethers are fine solvents. Ethers are more volatile than their isomeric alcohol counterpart and they decrease in volatility, inflammability, and water solubility as the molecular weight increases. Ethers are miscible with all organic solvents and with the volatile and fixed oils.

d. Preparation. Alcohols dehydrated in the presence of sulfuric acid at a temperature of approximately 135° C. (etherifying temperature) react to form the corresponding ether. A mixture of alcohols will logically form a mixture of ethers. The following equations illustrate the reactions taking place in the preparation of ether.

$$C_2H_5OH + H_2SO_4 \xrightarrow{\Delta} C_2H_5HSO_4 + HOH$$

Ethyl Alcohol + Sulfuric Acid → Ethyl Sulfuric Acid + Water

$$C_2H_5HSO_4 + C_2H_5-OH \longrightarrow C_2H_5-O-C_2H_5 + H_2SO_4$$

Ethyl Sulfuric Acid	+ Ethyl Alcohol	Ethyl Ether	+ Sulfuric Acid

A modification of the preceding process uses as a starting point, ethylene which is reacted with sulfuric acid to produce ethylsulfuric acid, and then proceeds as above.

e. Important ethers.

(1) Ether (diethyl ether; ethyl ether) C_2H_5-O-C_2H_5. Ether contains 96-98 percent ethyl ether; the remainder is alcohol and water. It is widely used as a general inhalation anesthetic. Since ether is highly volatile and flammable, the monograph bears this official caution–"Ether is highly volatile and flammable. Its vapor, when mixed with air and ignited, may explode." When ether is exposed to air, toxic oxidation products may form. The USP contains an official caution note relative to this danger: "Ether to be used for anesthesia must be preserved in tight containers of not more than 3-kg. capacity, and is not to be used for anesthesia if it has been removed from the original container longer than 24 hours. Ether to be used for anesthesia may, however, be shipped in larger containers for repackaging in containers as directed above, provided the ether at the time of repackaging meets the requirements of the tests of this pharmacopeia."

(2) Ethyl oxide (solvent ether) C_2H_5-O-C_2H_5. This product is chemically the same as ether for anesthesia EXCEPT that it is not as pure and free of oxidation products. It bears the official caution–"Ethyl oxide must not be used for anesthesia. Ethyl oxide is highly flammable. Do not use where it may be ignited." This commercial grade of ether is used as a solvent and as a motor ether for priming the carburetors of gasoline and diesel engines.

(3) Vinyl ether (divinyl oxide) CH_2=CH-O-CH=CH_2. Vinyl ether has two points of unsaturation, one at each side of the oxygen atom. The CH_2=CH group is known as the vinyl radical. This is a quite popular inhalation anesthetic. Because of its volatility, it cannot be used in the tropics. Vinyl ether bears this caution–"Do not use Vinyl Ether for anesthesia if the original container has been opened longer than 48 hours."

8. **Aldehydes.** Aldehydes are the oxidation products of *primary* alcohols.

a. Structure. Aldehydes have the general structure of R-CHO or R-C(=O)-H and are recognizable by the carbonyl group (C=O) plus a hydrogen and either another hydrogen or an alkyl radical in the general formula.

b. Nomenclature. Although the IUC has set up a system for naming the aldehydes, as for other compounds, because of the widely accepted usage of common names in pharmacy and even by organic chemists, we will pass over the IUC method fleetingly and use the common names.

(1) IUC nomenclature. The IUC method for naming the aldehydes is to use the hydrocarbon base, as with compounds previously discussed and drop the *e* and add *al* in its place. Thus the name for the simplest aldehyde is methanal (IUC) or, by common name, formaldehyde.

$$H-\overset{\overset{\displaystyle O}{\|}}{C}-H$$

Formaldehyde (Methanal)

(2) Common names. The common names of the aldehydes are taken from the acid formed from the oxidation of that aldehyde. *For example,* oxidation of H-C(=O)-H yields formic acid and therefore it is named formaldehyde. Oxidation of CH_3-C(=O)-H yields acetic acid, and thus it is named acetaldehyde. The same follows for propionaldehyde and butyraldehyde.

c. Properties. Formaldehyde, a gas with an extremely disagreeable odor, produces a painful choking sensation in the respiratory tract. Acetaldehyde's odor is not quite so disagreeable. The lower liquid members of the aldehyde family have pungent odors and as they progress toward higher molecular weights, the odors become more agreeable and finally very pleasant. These high molecular weight aldehydes are the substances which lend the fragrance to plants. Often they are employed in the manufacture of perfumes. Octalaldehyde, for example, has the odor of rose or jasmine; nonylaldehyde, the odor of rose; and decylaldehyde, the odor of orange. The first two aldehydes in the series are water soluble. As the number of carbons in the chain increases, the water solubility falls off rapidly. They are soluble, however, in the organic solvents.

d. Reactions. Some of the more important reactions that aldehydes undergo are the following:

(1) Oxidation. Aldehydes may be readily oxidized to their corresponding acid (one with the same number of carbons). This, in fact, is a test for aldehydes.

(2) Addition. Because of the unsaturation at the carbonyl group, aldehydes readily undergo addition reactions. A great number of different additions can take place and the following illustrates one such reaction.

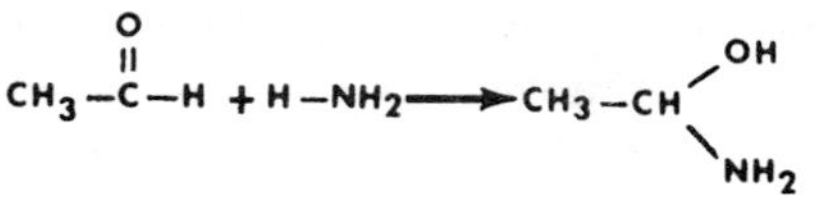

Acetaldehyde - ammonia

(3) Polymerization. A team of individual molecules of the same substance joining together without the formation of additional products is known as polymerization. Aldehydes tend to undergo this joining.

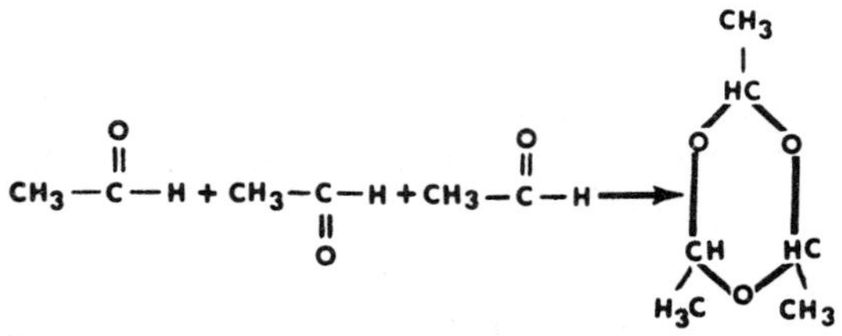

Paraldehyde

(4) Reduction. Since aldehydes are the oxidation products of primary alcohols, they can be reduced back to the corresponding primary alcohol.

$$RCHO \xrightarrow{2H} RCH_2OH$$

(5) Halogen replacement. Halogens may replace certain hydrogen atoms in the aldehyde molecule. This is illustrated in the following reaction.

$$3Cl_2 + CH_3CHO \longrightarrow 3HCl + Cl_3CCHO$$

(Trichloroacetaldehyde)

This reaction is important because addition of water to the molecule of trichloroacetaldehyde gives an important pharmaceutical product–chloral hydrate.

$$Cl_3CCHO + HOH \longrightarrow Cl_3CCH(OH)_2$$

(Chloral hydrate)

(6) Condensation. The "aldol condensation reaction" results in the addition of an aldehyde to itself or to another aldehyde in the presence of a weak base. This reaction is extremely important in synthetic work and is a means of forming extremely complex molecules from those already existing in nature. An example of an aldol condensation reaction is–

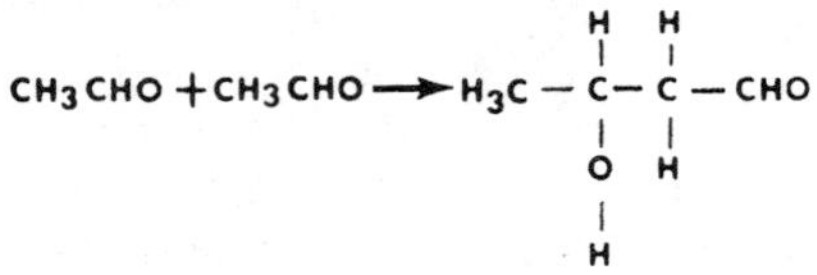

(an aldol)

(7) Silver mirror reaction. When a mixture of formaldehyde and ammoniacal silver nitrate is warmed, silver is deposited on the surface of the vessel in which the reaction is taking place. It is this reaction which is used in the mirror-making industry.

$$HCHO + 2AgNO_3 + NH_4OH \longrightarrow HCOONH_4 + 2Ag + 2H_2O$$

e. Occurrence. The simpler aldehydes are not found to a significant extent in nature but some longer chain aldehydes are constituents in plant and flower oils.

f. Preparation. Aldehydes may be prepared from their corresponding primary alcohol by the processes of dehydrogenation or oxidation. Acetaldehyde has a special method of preparation from acetylene.

(1) Dehydrogenation.

$$CH_3OH \xrightarrow[200-350^o]{Cu} H_2 + H_2C = 0$$

(2) Oxidation.

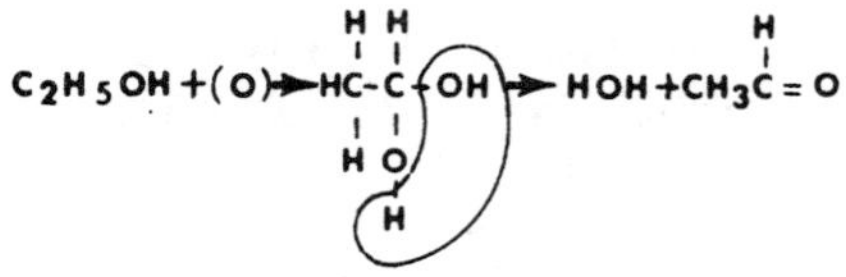

(acetaldehyde)

(3) Preparation of acetaldehyde from acetylene.

$$C_2H_2 + HOH \xrightarrow{Cat} CH_3CHO$$

The catalysts in this reaction are mercuric sulfate and sulfuric acid.

g. Important aldehydes.

(1) Formaldehyde solution. Formaldehyde solution, also known as Formalin, is a 37-percent solution of formaldehyde gas (HCHO) in water (w/w). Methyl alcohol is added to prevent polymerization. This solution is used full strength or diluted up to 1:10 for disinfection of inanimate objects. It is an ingredient in embalming fluids where it functions as a tissue preservative. Specimens are frequently preserved in formaldehyde solution.

(2) Paraldehyde.

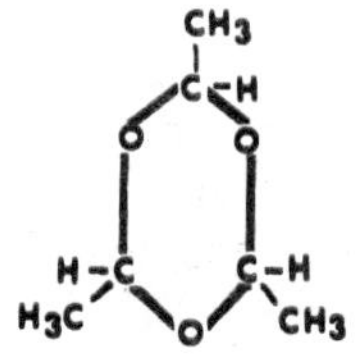

Paraldehyde is a clear, colorless liquid having a strong, characteristic, pungent odor. Some people seem to like the odor; others find it obnoxious. It is used as a sedative or hypnotic; its widest use is in the treatment of delirium tremens. It may be administered orally, rectally, or by injection. The USP states: "Paraldehyde is subject to oxidation to form acetic acid. Preserve in well filled, tight, light resistant containers holding not more than 30 ml., at a temperature not exceeding 25 C." Paraldehyde must not be used if it has a brownish color or the odor of acetic acid. Because of the oxidation to acetic acid any unused paraldehyde should be discarded 24 hours after the container has been opened.

(3) Chloral hydrate (chloral) $Cl_3CCH(OH)_2$. Chloral hydrate is a white or colorless crystal with a sweet and slightly acrid odor. This odor can also be classified as characteristic. It is used as a sedative and hypnotic.

9. Ketones. Ketones are to secondary alcohols what aldehydes are to primary alcohols. In other words, ketones are oxidation products of secondary alcohols.

a. Structure. Ketones are similar in structure to the aldehydes as represented below in their general formulas.

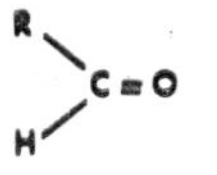

Aldehyde

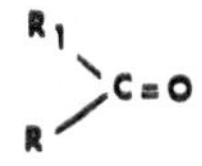

Ketone

The difference, as you can see, between an aldehyde and a ketone is an additional radical in place of the hydrogen on the aldehyde.

b. Properties. Acetone, the first member of the ketone series, is a clear, colorless liquid with an odor similar to nail polish. The higher members of the series are colorless liquids or solids.

c. Reactions. Due to the absence of the hydrogen, ketones are less reactive than the aldehydes. They undergo oxidation less readily and, unlike the aldehydes, ketones are not reducing agents. They may be oxidized by powerful oxidizing agents into acids with less carbons than the ketones themselves. This is due to the splitting between carbon atoms as illustrated in the following reaction:

$$CH_3\overset{O}{\overset{\|}{C}}CH_3 + 4(O) \longrightarrow CO_2 + HOH + CH_3COOH \quad \text{(acetic acid)}$$

In other respects, the reactions of the ketones follow the same pattern as the aldehydes.

d. Nomenclature. Like the aldehydes, ketones are given both common and IUC names.

(1) Common name. The names of both groups attached to the carbonyl group are followed by the word "ketone." Thus, $CH_3\text{-}\overset{O}{\overset{\|}{C}}\text{-}CH_2\text{-}CH_3$ is called methyl ethyl ketone.

(2) IUC name. As with other compounds, the IUC system bases its name for ketones on the hydrocarbon name of the longest chain containing the carbonyl group. The *e* is dropped from the hydrocarbon name and *one* is added in its place. The position of the carbonyl group is indicated by number. Thus–

$$CH_3-\overset{O}{\overset{\|}{C}}-CH_3 \quad \text{is Propanone}$$

$$CH_3-\overset{O}{\overset{\|}{C}}-CH_2-CH_3 \quad \text{is 2-Butanone}$$

e. Preparation. Just as oxidation of the corresponding primary alcohol yielded an aldehyde, oxidation of the corresponding secondary alcohol yields the ketone. Although there are other methods of preparation, for our purposes and needs this one will suffice.

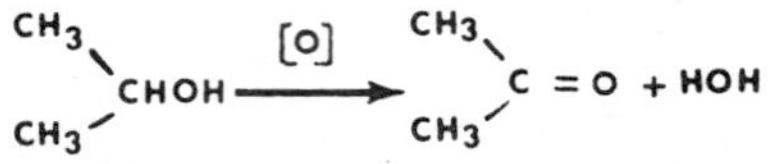

Isopropyl Alcohol Dimethylketone

f. Important ketones.

(1) Acetone (dimethyl ketone) CH_3COCH_3. Acetone is an excellent organic solvent, easily dissolving fats, resins, pyroxylin, and similar substances. It is widely used in organic syntheses, i.e., in the manufacture of chloroform, chlorobutanol, and ascorbic acid. Acetone is a colorless, extremely volatile and flammable liquid, having a characteristic odor. Acetone is readily miscible with water, alcohol, chloroform, ether, and most volatile oils. Because of its extremely inflammable nature, the NF bears this official caution: "Acetone is very flammable. Do not use where it may be ignited."

(2) Camphor (2-camphanone) $C_{10}H_{16}O$. Camphor is a colorless crystal, granule, or mass with a very penetrating odor which probably accounts for its use in nasal preparations. It is not soluble in water, but is very soluble in alcohol, chloroform, and ether. It occurs naturally in turpentine oil and is synthetically produced from pinene. It is commonly referred to as gum camphor because of its gummy nature and lauryl camphor from the plant from which it is extracted.

(a) Uses. Camphor is a mild anesthetic, mild antiseptic, rubefacient (reddens the skin), circulatory and respiratory stimulant, and expectorant. It is mainly used in preparations for external application for its rubefacient action and in some nasal solutions for its penetrating odor. A good deal of the therapeutic qualities of camphor may be psychological, due to its odor. Camphor is an ingredient in paregoric (Camphorated Tincture of Opium).

(b) Eutexia. When camphor is rubbed with chloral hydrate, thymol, menthol, phenol, and many other solids, the resulting mixture liquefies spontaneously. This mixture of two or more ingredients resulting in spontaneous liquefaction at room temperature is called a eutectic mixture.

(3) Rotenone, $C_{23}H_{22}O_6$. Rotenone is a ketone which is very toxic to insects and fish. It is used as an insecticide and as an agent to purge ponds and lakes of unwanted marine life. It is interesting to note that only one part in twenty million will kill goldfish in 3 hours. Oddly enough, rotenone is practically nontoxic to man.

10. Aliphatic monocarboxylic acids. Of the many types of organic acids, the two most important ones are carboxylic acids and their derivatives. Carboxylic acids may contain one or more carboxyl groups (COOH) and the number contained is signified by the prefixes mono, di, tri, or poly. The word carboxyl is derived from carbonyl and hydroxyl, showing that a carboxyl group is a combination of the two.

a. Structure. Monocarboxylic acids have the general formula of RCOOH, or graphically, $R\text{-}\overset{\overset{\displaystyle O}{\|}}{C}\text{-}OH$. An example of a true monocarboxylic acid, illustrating the general formula, is that of acetic acid, graphically shown below.

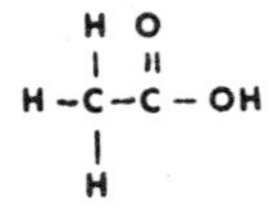

b. Properties. The monocarboxylic acids are colorless. The first nine normal members of the series are liquids; higher members are solids. The first three members have painful, stinging odors; the succeeding members to C_{10} have foul, rancid odors; those above C_{10} are odorless, or nearly so. The solubility of these acids ranges from completely water soluble (C_1 to C_3), decreasing rapidly from C_4 upward, until those over C_{12} are, for all intents and purposes, insoluble in water. The solid acids are greasy and wax-like to the touch and because many of them are actually prepared from fats, they are frequently called the "fatty acids." Acetic acid, when frozen, appears ice-like and so acquires the name "glacial" acetic acid. The organic acids ionize only slightly in solution and consequently are weak acids.

c. Reactions. The monocarboxylic acids undergo a variety of reactions. They are altered either in the hydrocarbon chain to yield substituted acids, or at the carboxyl group to yield acid derivatives. Halogen acids, hydroxy acids, and amino acids are substituted acids, while salts, esters, and amides are acid derivatives.

d. Occurrence. Organic acids are widely distributed in nature both in the free and the combined form. They are found in resins, carbohydrate derivatives, proteins, salts, human tissues, and fats. The substance injected by many insects, including the ant, bee, and wasp, is formic acid.

e. Preparation. There are a variety of methods for preparation of the carboxylic acids, most of which have oxidation or hydrolysis as one of the steps involved.

(1) Oxidation. You have learned that the hydrocarbons can be oxidized to alcohols, further to aldehydes, and now the aldehydes can be even further oxidized to organic acids. Still further oxidation results in breaking up of the molecule into carbon dioxide and water. Notice the progressive oxidation stages in the reaction below.

$$\underset{\text{Ethane}}{CH_3CH_3} \xrightarrow{[O]} \underset{\text{Ethyl Alcohol}}{CH_3CH_2OH} \xrightarrow{[O]} \underset{\text{Acetaldehyde}}{CH_3\overset{O}{\overset{\|}{C}}H} \xrightarrow{[O]} \underset{\text{Acetic Acid}}{CH_3\overset{O}{\overset{\|}{C}}{-}OH} \xrightarrow{[O]} \underset{\text{Carbon Dioxide}}{CO_2} + \underset{\text{Water}}{HOH}$$

(2) Hydrolysis. Esters of the carboxylic acids on hydrolysis yield carboxylic acids.

$$\underset{\text{Methylacetate}}{CH_3{-}\overset{O}{\overset{\|}{C}}{-}O{-}CH_3} + \underset{\text{Water}}{HOH} \rightarrow \underset{\text{Acetic Acid}}{CH_3{-}\overset{O}{\overset{\|}{C}}{-}OH} + \underset{\text{Methanol}}{CH_3{-}OH}$$

f. The important aliphatic monocarboxylic acids.

(1) Acetic acid (ethanoic acid) CH_3COOH.

$$CH_3{-}\overset{O}{\overset{\|}{C}}{-}OH$$

Acetic acid is a 36- to 37-percent solution of CH_3COOH by weight in water. It is a clear, colorless liquid with a strong, characteristic odor. It is miscible with water, alcohol, and glycerin. Acetic acid is used as a solvent and as the substance diluted to yield diluted acetic acid. It is mainly official because it is pharmaceutically essential for the compounding of aluminum subacetate solution. It is extremely important as a starting point in the synthesis of acetates, sulfa drugs, and acetanilid.

(2) Diluted acetic acid. This product is made by adding enough water to 158 ml. of acetic acid to make 1000 ml., yielding a 6-percent solution. Diluted acetic acid is bactericidal and spermatocidal in 1-percent concentrations and has been used as a wetting solution for surgical dressings, as well as a contraceptive and antibacterial douche.

(3) Glacial acetic acid. Glacial acetic acid is similar to, but more concentrated than, acetic acid. It is 99 percent by weight.

(4) Oleic acid, $CH_3(CH_2)_7CH = CH(CH_2)_7COOH$. Oleic acid, obtained from tallow (abdominal fat of the sheep or ox), may contain some of the other fatty acids such as linolenic and stearic acids also present in tallow. It is mainly used as a pharmaceutical necessity in the manufacture of oleates, medicinal soft soap, and benzyl benzoate lotion.

(5) Undecylenic acid (10-undecenoic acid), $CH_2 = CH(CH_2)_8COOH$. Undecylenic acid is an excellent fungistatic agent. It is used externally in a 1-percent to 10-percent concentration in ointments, liquids, and powders, to treat athlete's foot, ringworm, and similar infestations.

(6) Stearic acid. Stearic acid is a mixture of solid organic acids consisting mainly of stearic acid ($HC_{18}H_{35}O_2$) and palmitic acid ($HC_{16}H_{31}O_2$). It is obtained from tallow. The chief use of stearic acid in pharmacy is in the preparation of sodium stearate, a solidifying agent in glycerin suppositories.

11. Salts of the monocarboxylic acids. Salts of organic acids occur from the reaction between an organic acid and a metal, or the salt of a weaker acid such as a carbonate, oxide, or hydroxide.

$$\underset{\text{Acetic Acid}}{CH_3{-}\overset{O}{\overset{\|}{C}}{-}OH} + \underset{\text{Sodium Hydroxide}}{NaOH} \rightarrow \underset{\text{Water}}{HOH} + \underset{\text{Sodium Acetate}}{CH_3{-}\overset{O}{\overset{\|}{C}}{-}ONa}$$

Although organic substances in general are not widely water soluble, the salts of organic acids are. Some of the more important salts of monocarboxylic acids are–

a. Potassium acetate, CH_3COOK. Potassium acetate is used as a systemic and urinary alkalizer.

b. Sodium acetate, CH_3COONa. Sodium acetate is used as a systemic and urinary alkalizer.

c. Zinc undecylenate $[CH_2 = CH(CH_2)_8COO]_2Zn$. Used alone and in combination with undecylenic acid and other substances, this salt is effective in the treatment of athlete's foot and other fungal infections. It may be found in the form of a 20-percent ointment, liquid, or powder for topical application. A commercially marketed preparation for the treatment of such infections combines zinc undecylenate and undecylenic acid.

d. Mercury oleate. This compound, containing the equivalent of 25-percent mercuric oxide, is intended for the manufacture of Mercurial Ointment which is used as a parasiticide. Many commercial patent remedies for the treatment of psoriasis contain oleate of mercury as their active ingredient. Siroil and Riasol are examples.

12. Esters. Esters are products formed from the reaction between an alcohol and either an acid, an acid chloride, or an acid anhydride. The hydrogen of the carboxyl group is replaced by a radical.

a. Structure. The general graphic formula for esters of the organic monocarboxylic acid is—

$$\overset{O}{\overset{\|}{RC}}-OR_1$$

b. Properties. Esters may be either liquids or solids, all of which are colorless and essentially insoluble in water. The liquid members have strong and unusual odors, mostly quite pleasant.

c. Reactions. Esters are capable of many reactions, including hydrolysis, reduction, and reaction with ammonia to form amides. Examples of these reactions are enumerated below.

(1) Hydrolysis.

$$\underset{\text{ester}}{RCOOR_1} + \underset{\text{water}}{HOH} \longrightarrow \underset{\text{acid}}{RCOOH} + \underset{\text{alcohol}}{R_1OH}$$

(2) Reduction.

$$\underset{\text{ester}}{RCOOR_1} \xrightarrow{4H} \underset{\text{alcohol}}{RCH_2OH} + \underset{\text{alcohol}}{R_1OH}$$

(3) Reaction with ammonia.

$$\underset{\text{ester}}{RCOOR_1} + \underset{\text{ammonia}}{HNH_2} \longrightarrow \underset{\text{alcohol}}{R_1OH} + \underset{\text{amide}}{RCONH_2}$$

These reactions are important to pharmacy in producing compounds that otherwise are hard or impossible to obtain.

d. Occurrence. Esters occur in nature, widely distributed in fruits, flowers, and other parts of plants and animals. Esters are the forms in which the naturally occurring fatty acids exist. Esters impart the odor to many fruits and flowers. *For example,* amyl acetate has the odor of banana; amyl butyrate, the odor of apricot; octyl acetate, the odor of orange; and ethyl butyrate, the odor of pineapple.

e. Preparation.

(1) Reaction between alcohol and acid.

$$RCOOH + R_1OH \longrightarrow HOH + RCOOR_1$$

This reaction progresses very slowly, but more rapid and better yields can be obtained by (2) below.

(2) Reaction between alcohol and acid anhydride.

$$(RCO)_2O + ROH \longrightarrow RCOOH + RCOOR$$

(3) Reaction between alcohol and acid chloride.

$$RCOCl + ROH \longrightarrow HCl + RCOOR$$

f. Uses. The uses of esters vary widely. Some are used in manufacture of insecticides, others in the making of perfumes and flavors, some as solvents, some in plastics, and still others in explosives and medicine.

g. Important esters. Most of the important esters will be discussed later in the chapter with other classes to which they are related. Three products are listed below which are esters of inorganic acids.

(1) Ethyl nitrite spirit (sweet spirit of nitre; spirit of nitrous ether). Ethyl nitrite spirit is a solution in alcohol containing 4 percent of C_2H_5ONO. It was once mainly used as a diuretic and diaphoretic but today is considered less reliable than other more recent agents.

(2) Amyl nitrite, $CH_3CH(CH_3)CH_2CH_2ONO$. This very volatile liquid is inhaled in the treatment of attacks of angina pectoris. It is very flammable and should not be used where it is likely to be ignited.

(3) *Glyceryl trinitrate tablets (nitroglycerin; Trinitrin).* These tablets produce coronary artery dilation and are therefore useful in the treatment of attacks of angina pectoris.

13. Fats and fixed oils. Fats and fixed oils are much alike. Chemically, their structure is essentially the same in that both are glyceryl esters of fatty acids. The differentiation between a fat and an oil rests in the physical state of the substance at normal temperatures. A solid glyceryl ester of a fatty acid is a fat and a liquid glyceryl ester of a fatty acid is a fixed oil.

a. *Structure.* The following formulas depict a molecule of glycerol, three molecules of fatty acid (stearic in this case), and finally the fat molecule, stearin, an ester of the two.

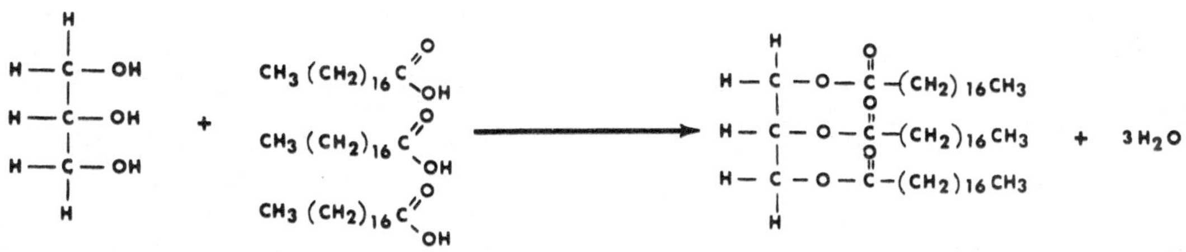

Glycerol | Stearic Acid (3 Molecules) | Stearin | Water

(1) *Mixed esters.* Stearin contains glycerol plus three molecules of stearic acid. It is quite possible that more than one fatty acid may join with a single molecule of glycerol to give a *mixed ester.* In fact, most of the naturally occurring fats and oils are mixtures of mixed esters of glycerol and fatty acids.

(2) *Carbon chains.* Most of the fats and fixed oils contain carbon chains of even numbers ranging from C_{10} to C_{16}. The four most common fatty acids combined with glycerol to form the fats and fixed oils in nature are all chains with 18 carbon atoms. Stearic, oleic, linoleic, and linolenic acids all have 18 carbon atoms, but differ in saturation. Stearic acid has no double bonds; oleic has one; linoleic has two double bonds; and linolenic has three.

b. *Properties.* Previously we said that at normal temperatures fats are solids and oils are liquids. This is a rather vague description because what is an oil in torrid climates might well be a fat in the Arctic. Since the glycerol portion of the molecule is common to all, it is the fatty acid composition which determines the properties of the particular fat or oil. The chain may be either short or long, completely saturated, partially unsaturated, or completely unsaturated. Long chain (high molecular weight) fatty acids in the molecule tend to make it insoluble in water and solid. Short chains tend toward liquidity and water solubility. Partially or completely unsaturated chains are more likely to be oils; those which are nearly saturated will be fats.

c. *Classes of fixed oils.* The fixed oils are sometimes grouped into classes by the amount of saturation they possess. The characteristics of these groups are reflected in their names.

(1) *Drying oils.* These oils contain fatty acids with many double bonds (highly unsaturated). They easily combine with oxygen and quickly dry into a hard, resinous coat. These oils give paint its drying properties. This drying process is an exothermic reaction, that is, reaction giving off heat, and can lead to spontaneous combustion. Rags or other combustible material, soaked with these drying oils and confined, become warmer and warmer as the oils dry and heat is liberated. Finally, the cloth reaches its ignition temperature and a fire results. A good example of a drying oil is linseed oil.

(2) *Semidrying oils.* Corn oil is a good example of a semidrying oil. There is less unsaturation in these oils and they oxidize to a gummy, resinous mass but do not harden completely.

(3) *Nondrying oils.* The nondrying oils, on exposure to the atmosphere, remain sticky and do not dry; they have the least number of double

bonds. Olive oil is nondrying.

d. Occurrence. As a general rule, it can be stated that fats occur in the animal kingdom and oils in the plant kingdom. There is some overlapping, but for the most part this is the case. The fats and fixed oils are gathered by expression, a procedure of compressing by hydrolic pressure the ground-up plant or animal tissue. Animal fats are often collected from the process of rendering in which the fatty tissue is heated until the fat melts and is collected.

e. Reactions. Fats and oils undergo definite chemical reactions and yield some very important products.

(1) Hydrolysis. Listed first, because it is of the most significance in nature, is the reaction of hydrolysis in which fats and oils react with water to form fatty acids and glycerol. When butter becomes rancid, the molecule has been broken down by hydrolysis to fatty acids, one of which is butyric acid. Butyric acid is the foul-smelling substance liberated in rancidity of butter and other fats and oils. Hydrolysis takes place slowly, unless in the presence of catalysts. Acids, bases, and certain digestive enzymes catalyze this reaction. When fats or oils are hydrolyzed in the presence of an alkali, the resulting products are glycerol and the metallic salt of the acid. The metallic salt of a fatty acid is a soap; this process then is termed saponification. More will be said about soaps and saponification later in the chapter.

(2) Oxidation. Short-chained acids, aldehydes, and ketones are produced when a fat or oil undergoes oxidation. In rancidity, this process is closely related to hydrolysis. Oxidation is hastened by light, heat, moisture, and metals.

(3) Hydrogenation. The unsaturated fats and oils may add hydrogen atoms at the point of unsaturation to become more nearly saturated. It is by this process that liquid cooking oils are solidified to yield a solid cooking fat that is more stable than lard or butter.

f. Uses. The fats and fixed oils are important to life and health from many standpoints. First, and probably foremost, they are essential foods (foods necessary to the proper function of the human body). Absence of fats and oils from the diet results in skin conditions, emaciation, and death. From the medical and pharmaceutical standpoint, fats and oils are used as laxatives, as bases for ointments and oleaginous preparations, as sources of vitamins, and in the manufacture of other pharmaceutically important preparations. The salts of several of the fatty acids are fungicidal. Other derivatives are soaps, detergents, and bactericides.

g. Pharmaceutically important fats and oils.

(1) Expressed almond oil (almond oil; sweet almond oil). Almond oil is not the flavorful part of constituent of almonds; therefore, the common name of sweet almond oil is misleading. Almond oil is an emollient, used in hand creams and lotions such as rose water ointment, and in the cosmetic industry.

(2) Castor oil (oleum ricini). This thick oil from the castor bean is an effective cathartic because of the liberation of ricinoleic acid in the intestine. This acid is irritating and produces catharsis. Castor oil is also used as a lubricating oil and a constitutent of collodion to make it flexible.

(3) Corn oil (oleum maydis). Corn oil is official mainly for its use as a vehicle for injections where the active ingredient is oil soluble. Many hormone injections which we will discuss later in the chapter are dissolved in corn oil for administration by injection. Corn oil is a good food substance. There are several patented products on the market which are emulsions of corn oil. These are used to supply extra calories to the debilitated and to those who wish to gain weight. Corn oil is also used as a liquid cooking substance and in the manufacture of soaps.

(4) Cottonseed oil (oleum gosypii seminis). This is another oil suitable for the vehicle in injections. It is taken internally as a cathartic, to increase caloric intake, and to decrease gastric secretion and motility. Cottonseed oil is used in the manufacture of soaps, glycerin, oleomargarine (and other lard substitutes), lubricating agents, and cosmetics. In the liquid form, it is widely used as a cooking and salad oil. Hydrogenated into a solid state, it becomes similar to shortening.

(5) Linseed oil. Linseed oil, no longer official, is expressed from flaxseed. It is mainly used in the preparation of liniments. Flaxseed is a greasy seed which can be used to clean handmade gelatin capsules before dispensing. It is used in the form of meal, combined with water, as a poultice to draw pus from wounds. The commercial linseed oil purchased in hardware and paint stores has been boiled with lead oxide and is poisonous; it is not suitable for medicinal use.

(6) Olive oil (sweet oil). Olive oil is an emollient substance used in the manufacture of lotions, emulsions, ointments, liniments, and plasters. It has good food properties and can be used as a caloric booster. It is frequently used as a salad oil. Sweet oil, used as a mild eardrop in children for many years, is nothing more than olive oil. Its soothing effects to earaches are due to its emollient action and its ability to dissolve encrusted wax.

(7) Peanut oil (arachis oil; oleum arachis). Peanut oil is used mainly in the preparation of oil soluble substances for injection. It is also used in the manufacture of liniments and ointments. Peanut oil is a frequently used base in the preparation of oleaginous nose drops.

(8) Sesame oil (oleum sesami). Sesame oil is used in the manufacture of injections; in liniments, emulsions, oleomargarine, cosmetics; and as a food. Because it is more quickly saponifiable and does not rapidly turn rancid, sesame oil has replaced cottonseed oil in many products.

(9) Cod liver oil. As the name suggests, this fixed oil is extracted from the livers of codfish. It has a high nutrient value and supplies rich quantities of vitamins A and D. (Vitamins A and D are treated more thoroughly in chapter 9.) It is more widely used today in the veterinary field because animals seem to relish the fishy taste. Applied topically in the form of ointments, this oil has excellent emollient properties and is quite healing, especially to diaper rash. White's A and D ointment contains vitamins A and D and has the same uses.

(10) Theobroma oil (cacao butter; cocoa butter). Despite the official name, theobroma oil is a fat. At room temperature, it is a brittle, waxy solid with a strong chocolate odor. At body temperature, it melts rapidly, becoming a loose liquid, and is therefore widely used as a base for suppositories. Cocoa butter is also used as an emollient when applied to the skin for inflammation. It is incorporated into many skin creams.

14. Waxes. The waxes, although closely related to the fats and oils, differ from them in that instead of glycerol, they are composed of high-molecular-weight monohydric alcohols in combination with fatty acids. The two more commonly occurring alcohols are lauryl and cetyl.

a. Occurrence. Waxes occur in the leaves of plants, are excreted by some insects, and are found in the head of the sperm whale.

b. Properties. Generally, waxes are harder substances than fats, having higher melting points and are brittle and less greasy.

c. Important official waxes.

(1) Anhydrous lanolin (wool fat; refined wool fat; adeps lanae). Wool fat is a fat-like wax extracted from the wool and/or skin of sheep. It resembles closely the natural human body oils. It contains cholesterol (a sterol) which gives it the property of being able to absorb large quantities of water (up to about one-third its own weight). For this reason it may be incorporated into ointment bases to allow absorption of aqueous solutions of ingredients. Because it has been found that many people are allergic to lanolin, this substance has been deleted from many preparations and has been replaced by a suitable amount of cholesterol.

(2) Lanolin (hydrous wool fat; adeps lanae hydrosus). Hydrous wool fat is wool fat containing between 25- and 30-percent water. When water is added to anhydrous lanolin, the sticky, yellowish-brown, translucent mass becomes a yellow, creamy, opaque ointment. This substance, because it contains water, is used more for its emollient properties than for its water absorbent qualities. It does, however, possess the ability to absorb still more water. Be careful at this point to fix firmly in your mind the official and common names of these two closely related compounds and know the difference between them.

(3) Spermaceti (cetaceum). Spermaceti is a waxy substance obtained from the head of the sperm whale. This wax is used to thicken the consistency of ointments. It is used in both ointments and suppositories to elevate their melting points. There is little or no absorption of spermaceti through the skin. It is found in the formula for cold cream.

(4) Yellow wax (beeswax). As the common name implies, this substance is the purified wax obtained from the honeycomb of the bee. Like other waxes, this wax is used to raise melting points of ointments and stiffen their consistency. It is officially used in the preparation of yellow ointment.

(5) White wax (bleached beeswax; cera alba). This wax differs from yellow wax only in being bleached. It is officially used in the preparation of white ointment and is more widely employed in pharmacy than the yellow variety.

15. Sterols. Another group of lipid compounds is the sterols. These are high molecular weight cyclic alcohols—specifically, tetracyclic, unsaturated, secondary alcohols. They are derived from the unsaponifiable portion of fats.

a. Classification. Depending upon their source, sterols are grouped into the following categories:

(1) Zoosterols (from animals).
(2) Phytosterols (from plants).
(3) Mycosterols (from fungi).

b. Official products.

(1) Cholesterol (cholesterin), $C_{27}H_{46}O$. Cholesterol is found in all animal tissue, mainly in nerve and brain tissues. This substance can be acquired by the body indirectly from the foods consumed, or directly by manufacture within the body. A great deal of research is being conducted at present to determine the relationship between cholesterol levels in the blood and heart disease. This would be an interesting area for outside reading. Pharmaceutically, cholesterol is of importance because of the water-absorbing qualities it imparts to ointments. The USP categorizes this substance as a pharmaceutical necessity for hydrophilic petrolatum.

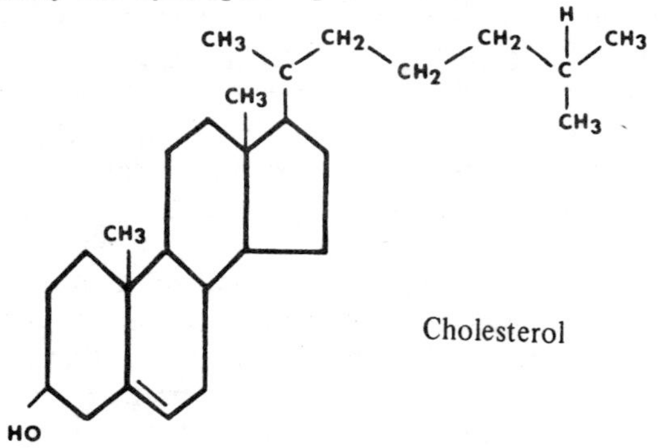

Cholesterol

(2) Hydrophilic petrolatum. This is a combination of stearyl alcohol, white wax, white petrolatum, and cholesterol. It is intended for use as a protective and water-absorbable ointment base.

16. Surface tension and surface active agents. Before discussing the surface active agents, or surfactants, as they are frequently called, it is necessary that you know what surface tension is and how it acts.

a. Surface tension. Surface tension is a property of liquids in which the exposed surface tends to contract to the smallest possible area. This property is attributable to the molecular forces of attraction within the liquid. You have seen surface tension at work if you have noticed the collection of droplets of water on a newly waxed automobile. The drops tend to pull themselves together into a spherical shape as if they were contained in a plastic film. It is surface tension which makes water spread out on a clean glass surface. In the first instance, the water and wax are immiscible substances, and there is no attraction of one for the other. Consequently, the cohesive properties of the water pull it together into a globule. There is, however, an affinity of water for clean, glass surfaces. The water spreads out, but the surface tension prevents the water film from being broken.

b. Surfactants (surface active agents). Surfactants are those substances intended to modify the surface tensions of liquids in contact with other liquids or solids. Try a couple of experiments first to show the effects of surface tension, and then the effect of a surfactant on this surface tension.

(1) Experiment one. In a bottle half full of water, add some mineral oil, replace the cap and shake the liquids briskly. Set the bottle down and watch. Shaking the liquids has caused them to mix temporarily, but because of their surface tensions they quickly separate into two distinct layers. Now repeat the procedure, adding a quantity of liquid detergent. This time, upon standing, the liquids do not separate as quickly. The surface tension has been modified by the detergent. The oil particles were able to be reduced to a much smaller size and the two liquids mixed. The resulting mixture is an emulsion. An emulsion can be defined on this basis as being a heterogeneous mixture of two or more immiscible liquids. Never confuse an emulsion with a solution.

(2) Experiment two. Soak a cloth in oil, allowing the oil to be well soaked into the rag. Wring it out and immerse it into a container of pure water. When you remove it from the water and allow the water to run off, it will be apparent that no water has soaked into the pores of the fiber. The oil has prevented the wetting of the material because of the surface tensions of the two liquids. The same oily cloth immersed in a solution of soapy water or water to which a detergent has been added will become wet, and if agitated in the solution for a time, the oil will be washed away. It

is this principle of surface activation which allows greasy dishware to be washed clean in the kitchen.

c. *Mixing immiscible liquids.* There are many instances in pharmacy when it is necessary to mix two otherwise immiscible liquids. Emulsions, lotions, creams, and some of the ointments you will prepare in the pharmacy will employ a surfactant and a special mixing procedure to allow you to accomplish proper incorporation.

d. *Classes of surfactants.* Surface active agents can be divided into three classes: cationic (positively charged ion is responsible for the action), anionic (negatively charged ion is responsible for the action), and non-ionic (the whole molecule is active).

(1) Cationic surfactants. The activity of the cationic surfactants is due to the positive ion in colloidal solution. Most frequently used members of this group are the quaternary ammonium compounds and pyridinium salts. Examples of these types of compounds are shown with the individual agents in *(a)* below. For more detail about each, refer to chapter 9. These cationic agents are unusual in that they display, besides their surface active properties, strong germicidal ability and make extremely useful antiseptics. Sometimes they are keratolytic and have the ability to penetrate dead skin.

(a) Important cationic surfactants.

1. *Benzalkonium chloride solution* (Zephiran Chloride solution).

2. *Benzalkonium chloride tincture* (Zephiran Chloride tincture).

3. *Benzethonium Chloride solution* (Phemerol chloride solution).

4. *Cetylpyridinium chloride* (Ceepryn Chloride).

(b) Incompatibilities. These products, as well as the other cationic surfactants, are incompatible with soap and other anionic surfactants. Soap inactivates the cationic surfactants and destroys their antibacterial properties.

(c) Properties. Most of these preparations are odorless, colorless, nonirritating, and, in germicidal concentrations, nontoxic. They are very stable, nonvolatile compounds and may be safely boiled or autoclaved.

(2) Anionic surfactants. Anionic surfactants owe their action to the negatively charged portion of the molecule. These agents are incompatible with the cationic surfactants. This class of surface active agents includes the soaps and detergents.

(a) Soaps. Soaps, if you recall, are the metallic salts of long-chain fatty acids. In the process of saponification, a metallic hydroxide is reacted with the fat, yielding the metallic salt of the fatty acid (soap) and glycerol. Depending upon the metallic hydroxide used in their manufacture, soaps may be either water soluble or oil soluble. We learned previously that group 1 metals and ammonium form water-soluble soaps, and that the group 2 metals (Ca, Mg) form oil-soluble (water-insoluble) soaps. Further, soaps may be considered either hard or soft, hard soaps being those with sodium as the base and soft soaps those with potassium as the base.

1. *Action.* Soaps are effective because of their emulsifying ability. The water-soluble soaps produce oil in water (o/w) emulsions; that is, emulsions in which oil is the internal (dispersed) phase and water is the external phase. In oil-in-water emulsions, the oil globules are broken down into very small particles and are dispersed throughout the water. In water-in-oil (w/o) emulsions, the reverse is true; the water is the internal phase and is surrounded by the oil. Oil-soluble soaps tend to produce water in oil emulsions. Emulsions will be considered in detail in "Manufacturing and Dispensing."

2. *Important soaps.*

- *Hard soap.* Hard soap has the following common names: sapo duris; soap; castile soap. It is a sodium soap. Hard soap is used to render resins soluble and modify harsh actions of certain drugs. As such, it is a common ingredient in pill masses, liniments, and dentifrices. The NF categorizes this preparation as a pharmaceutical necessity for the manufacture of other official preparations.
- *Medicinal soft soap (green soap; sapo mollis medicinalis; soft soap).* Medicinal soft soap is a potassium soap, made by saponification of a suitable vegetable oil (excluding coconut and palm kernel) without removal of the glycerin formed. Although the common name would lead you to believe this soap has a green color, this is no longer true. Long ago, the product was actually green in color due to the chlorophyll contained in the raw vegetable oil. Today, using pure ingredients, the soap has an amber color, but retains the historic common name. Medicinal soft soap is used in the preparation of medicinal soft soap liniment commonly known as tincture of green soap. This tincture is an alcoholic solution which is very

effective as a detergent for cleansing both animate and inanimate objects. It is sometimes employed as a shampoo for scalp conditions.

• *Sodium stearate.* The sodium salt of stearic acid, consisting mainly of sodium stearate and sodium palmitate, is a chemically pure soap. Sodium stearate is a pharmaceutical necessity in the preparation of glycerin suppositories. Inserted rectally, these suppositories cause irritation to the colon and produce evacuation. Some people still refer to these suppositories as "soap sticks."

(b) Synthetic anionic surfactants. Aside from the soaps, there is an ever-increasing variety of related anionic compounds which exhibit similar properties. In the past few years, great strides have been made in this field. The official preparations in this type are:

1. Dioctyl sodium sulfosuccinate, $C_{20}H_{37}NaO_7S$. This product is referred to by the abbreviation DOSS, and is marketed under various trade names. It is neither antibacterial nor detergent in action. It is a wetting agent (reduces surface tension and allows the substance to become wetted by the liquid it contacts). This property has been well utilized by using DOSS as a nonlaxative fecal softener to prevent constipation. By wetting the fecal matter, the bowel is more easily evacuated at regular intervals and without straining. This is very important to the hemorrhoid patient as well as the pregnant patient.

2. Sodium lauryl sulfate. Sodium lauryl sulfate is a true surface active agent and thus a very efficient detergent. Besides being frequently used in household scrubbing and dishwasher products, it is used in such pharmaceutical preparations as toothpastes and shampoos.

(3) The non-ionic surfactants. These surfactants consist of hydrophilic (water-loving) and lipophilic (oil-loving) portions which do not ionize in water. They may consist of high molecular weight alcohols, such as cetyl alcohol, and other substituted long-chain compounds. Although these non-ionic surfactants have not yet widely invaded the detergent field, there is little doubt that, in the near future, developments in this area will lead to better products. Falling into this group are the "spans" and "tweens," two series of solubilizing agents which allow oil and water to mix. These products have their best use in preparations where a flavoring oil tends to precipitate out of a hydroalcoholic solution, such as is the case in phenobarbital elixir and elixir of terpin hydrate with codeine. These spans and tweens will be further explained in "Manufacturing."

17. Dicarboxylic acids and similar compounds. Previously, we discussed the monocarboxylic acids and their derivatives. Polycarboxylic acids, especially the dicarboxylic acids with a normal chain of carbon atoms, are also important. Some of these compounds, naturally occurring and discovered centuries ago, are of pharmaceutical importance. Rather than going into the properties and reactions of the broad group of compounds, many of which are of no particular importance to us, we'll enumerate the official substances and say a few important things about each. The compounds in this area with which you should be familiar are:

a. Oxalic acid, $C_2H_2O_4$. Oxalic acid is the simplest of the dicarboxylic acids, having the formula HOOCCOOH. It is standard in analytical work, a stain remover for rust and iron tannate inks, and an anticoagulant for blood specimens. Being poisonous and caustic in concentrated solution, this preparation is NEVER used as an anticoagulant in vivo, that is, in the living body. Its uses are strictly for use in vitro (in glass).

b. Phosgene, $COCl_2$. Phosgene or carbonyl chloride is a carbonic acid derivative, but is discussed here because its derivatives are more like those of the dicarboxylic acids. Phosgene is a clear, colorless gas, formed by the union of chlorine and carbon monoxide (and compounds yielding these substances). It has a suffocating odor and is highly poisonous. It is classified as a lung irritant among the chemical warfare agents. Phosgene is of importance to the pharmacist only because it is a starting point in the synthesis of urea and the barbiturates.

c. Tartaric acid.

$$\begin{array}{c} \text{HOCHOOH} \\ | \\ \text{HOCHCOOH} \end{array}$$

The chief use of tartaric acid in pharmacy is in the manufacture of effervescent salts. It also imparts a tangy flavor to fruits and drinks.

d. Potassium bitartrate (cream of tartar), KOOCCH(OH)CH(OH)COOH. Besides being used in the preparation of other tartrates and tartaric acid, cream of tartar is a laxative, an ingredient in baking soda (mixed with bicarbonate—on addition of water, CO_2 is liberated).

e. Potassium sodium tartrate (Rochelle salt), KOOCH(OH)-CH(OH)-COONa $4H_2O$. Rochelle salt is a saline cathartic, a pharmaceutical necessity, and an ingredient in compound effervescent powders.

f. Antimony potassium tartrate (tartar emetic), KOOC-CHOH-CHOH-COO (SbO) · $1/2H_2O$. This substance has been used medicinally for its expectorant and emetic action; however, because of the toxicity of antimony, it is now generally reserved for treatment of parasite infections and tropical diseases, such as schistosomiasis, leishmaniasis, and filariasis.

g. Citric acid, $CH_2(COOH)C(OH)$-$(COOH)CH_2COOH$. Sometimes called salt of lemon because it is a natural ingredient in citrus fruits, citric acid is a saturated tricarboxylic acid. It is this substance which imparts the tart flavor to citrus fruits and the beverages using their flavors. Citric acid has the ability to mask undesirable tastes of certain drugs. It is also used in the preparation of citrate of magnesia, a saline cathartic preparation, as well as in effervescent salts.

18. Concepts and terminology of cyclic structures. In the preceding pages, we have been concerned almost exclusively with aliphatic compounds. For clarity and ease of presentation, it was necessary to treat a couple of ring compounds along with the aliphatics. From this point on, the great majority of the compounds presented will be cyclic. Regardless of the words—cyclic compound, ring, closed chain—the structure referred to is distinguished by a nucleus containing no terminal atoms; that is, each element in the structure is joined (bonded) to another member of the ring in an unbroken "fence-like" shape. All ring structures have three or more atoms in the ring.

a. Classification by atoms in the chain. If the atoms in the cycle are all alike, we have an *isocyclic* or *homocyclic* compound. And if these atoms are all carbon atoms, as they often are, the structure is *carbocyclic*. Any ring which includes more than one kind of atom is *heterocyclic*. Some examples should make this clearer.

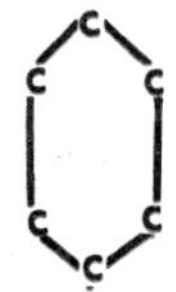

Homocyclic
(Carbocyclic)

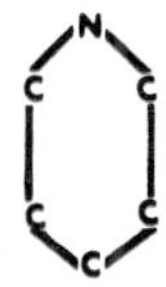

Heterocyclic

b. Classification by number of atoms in the ring. Aside from classifying cyclic compounds into isocyclic or heterocyclic, we also describe them by the number of atoms in the ring. This classification gives us useful information. When talking about a cyclic structure with three atoms in a closed ring, we speak of a three-member ring; four atoms in the cycle is a four-member ring; and so forth. The description, "a three-member, carbocyclic ring," then is very illustrative, telling us that there are three carbon atoms in a closed chain structure. Study the following abbreviated graphic formulas as illustrative of these fundamental principles.

(1) Three-member rings.

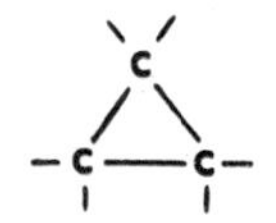

Carbocyclic

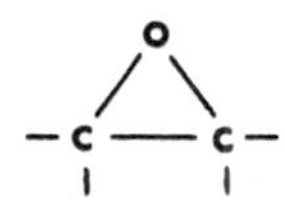

Heterocyclic

(2) Four-member rings.

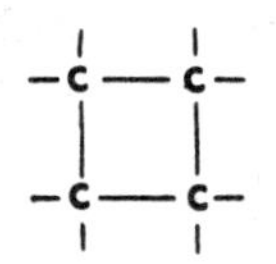

Carbocyclic

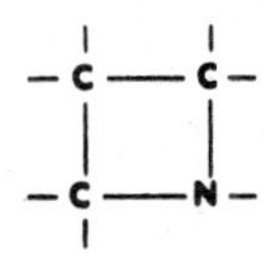

Heterocyclic

(3) Five-member rings.

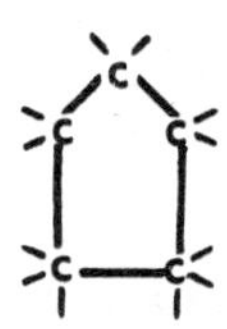

Carbocyclic

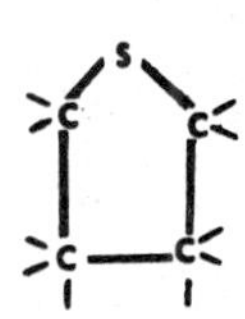

Heterocyclic

(4) Six-member rings.

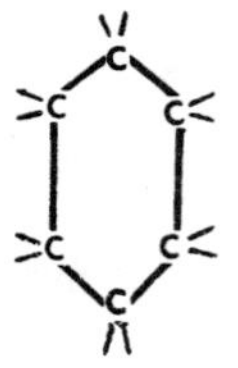

Carbocyclic

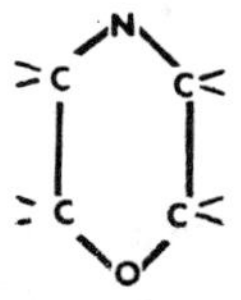

Heterocyclic

c. Alicyclic and aromatic subclasses of carbocyclic structures.

(1) Alicyclic. Alicyclic structures are by far the most common of the carbocyclic structures. They may be saturated, having single bonds as in those formulas shown before, or they may be unsaturated to varying degrees, as represented by the following formulas.

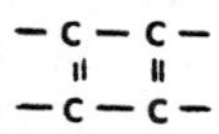

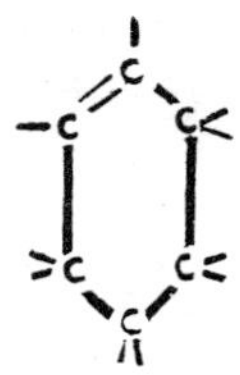

(2) Aromatic. The aromatic compounds are those carbocyclics having six carbon atoms with three double and three single bonds alternated around the cycle. In order to be truly aromatic, all these specifications must be met. In the following graphic formula, benzene, an aromatic compound, is represented.

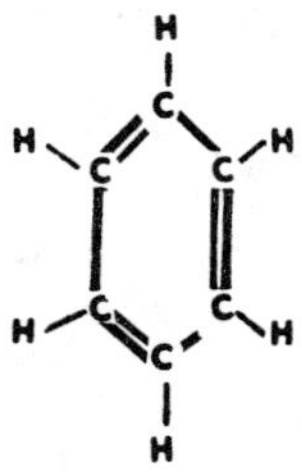

Benzene

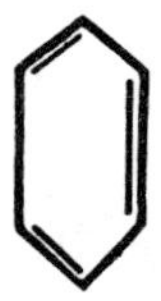

Benzene (simplified formula)

The word "aromatic" in our terminology of cyclic structures can cause considerable trouble if you do not understand its meaning. When aromatic is used in conjunction with organic chemistry, it refers to the specific structure of a group of compounds, NOT to odor!

d. Substitution and isomerism. Benzene, the simplest of the aromatic compounds, can undergo substitution. Because it is the simplest, we will use it as our illustrative device to explain substitution and isomerism.

(1) Monosubstitution. When a single hydrogen is replaced by an element or radical, it is termed monosubstitution. Regardless of which hydrogen is replaced, there is only one possible product–xbenzene (where x equals the substituted radical). Replacement of a hydrogen by a chlorine atom produces chlorobenzene.

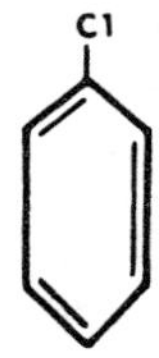

Chlorobenzene

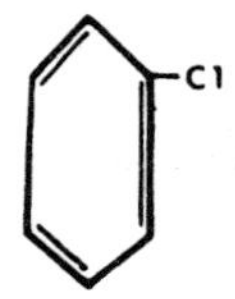

Chlorobenzene

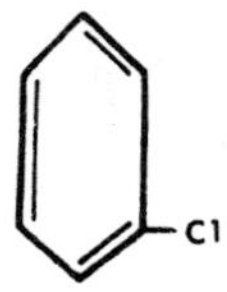

Chlorobenzene

(2) Disubstitution. When two hydrogens are replaced by chlorine, there are three possible isomers, depending upon the positions on the molecule the chlorine assumes. Thus we have–

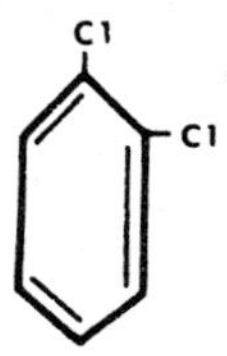

Ortho-Dichlorobenzene

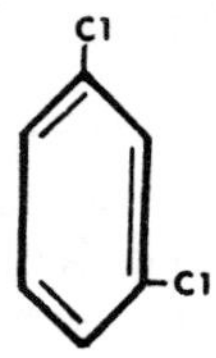

Meta-Dichlorobenzene

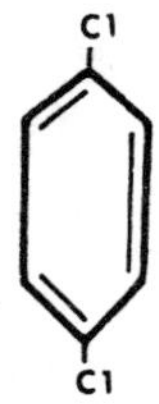

Para-Dichlorobenzene

"Ortho" means "straight line," and as you can see in the structure of ortho-dichlorobenzene, the substitution is in a straight line. "Meta" means "beyond," and in meta-dichlorobenzene, the substitution is beyond or separated by a single carbon. "Para" means "opposite" and in paradichlorobenzene, the chlorine is substituted on carbons at opposite ends of the benzene ring.

(a) Numbering the benzene ring. The benzene ring is numbered in clockwise direction, giving the attached radicals the lowest possible numbers.

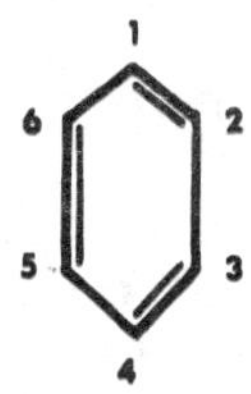

(b) Ortho-dichlorobenzene. Substitution at the 1 and 2 positions yields orthodichlorbenzene (1, 2-dichlorobenzene) which is more commonly written o-dichlorobenzene. It is a liquid used as a solvent and degreasing agent.

(c) Meta-dichlorobenzene. Substitution at the 1 and 3 positions yields meta-dichlorobenzene (1, 3-dichlorobenzene) which is more commonly written m-dichlorobenzene. It is also a liquid which is used as a deodorant in latrines.

(d) Para-dichlorobenzene. Substitution at the 1 and 4 positions yields para-dichlorobenzene (1, 4-dichlorobenzene) which is more commonly written p-dichlorobenzene. It is a crystalline solid used almost exclusively for its ability to kill moths.

(3) Trisubstitution. As with the disubstituted rings, it is possible to have three different configurations with trisubstitution. The following illustrations should serve as adequate explanation of these configurations. You should keep in mind that other representative illustrations, although placed in different positions than shown, will fall into one of the three groups simply by rotation of the molecule.

(4) Tetrasubstitution. Tetrasubstitution is handled in exactly the same manner as trisubstitution. The only difference is that the prefix "tetra" replaces "tri." Thus, four chlorine atoms positioned at the 1, 2, 3, and 5 carbons will be 1, 2, 3, 5-tetrachlorobenzene.

(5) Other types of isomerism. As we progress further into the subject and come to specific instances, other types of isomerism will be illustrated. For the time being, it will serve to mention that isomers are not limited to structural isomers, but also include others such as tautomers, stereoisomers, geometric isomers, optical isomers, and diastereoisomers.

e. *Basic structures.* Certain basic structures will repeatedly show themselves throughout the field of organic chemistry. Since you should be able to recognize the basic portions of various molecules, you should know the structures of the following:

(1) Benzene (benzol), C_6H_6. Benzene is a clear liquid with extremely flammable vapors. It is miscible with alcohol, ether, acetone, chloroform, and oils, but immiscible with water. Therefore, it is a good solvent for fats, resins, and alkaloids. Benzene is very toxic. One teaspoon is lethal orally. In contact with the skin, toxic quantities may be absorbed. Toxicity becomes apparent in patients after prolonged breathing of only one part per million. It has been used medicinally but because of its toxicity and doubtful value, its use, other than as a solvent and starting point in syntheses, is questioned by

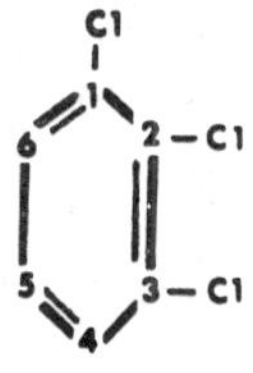

1, 2, 3-trichlorobenzene
(adjacent trichlorobenzene)

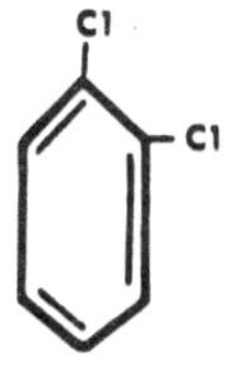

1, 2, 4-trichlorobenzene
(unsymmetrical trichlorobenzene)

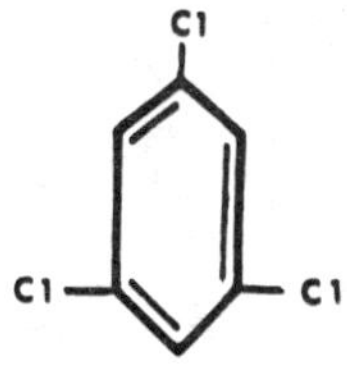

1, 3, 5-trichlorobenzene
(symmetrical trichlorobenzene)

authorities. It has, however, been used as an antispasmodic, antiseptic, parasiticide, and as an agent against trichinosis and leukemia.

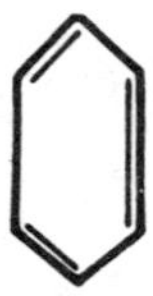

Benzene

(2) Toluene, C_7H_8. Toluene is similar in solvent properties to benzene which it also resembles in color and odor. It is an important solvent and is of great use in the synthesis of many medicinals, industrial chemicals, and dyes. Toluene is a coal tar derivative.

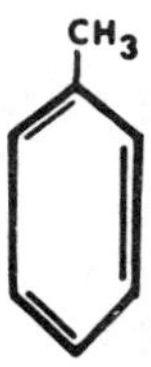

Toluene
(Methylbenzene)

(3) Xylene, C_8H_{10}. Xylene, another derivative of coal tar, is a mixture of the ortho, meta, and para isomers with the meta isomer predominating. It resembles benzene and toluene in its properties. It is used as a solvent, in the synthesis of dyes and other organic substances, and as a cleaning agent for microscope slides. When used as a solvent for Canadian balsam, an oil immersion substance is formed.

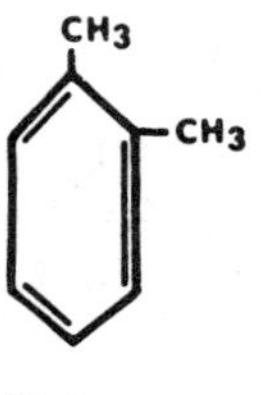

Xylene

(4) Naphthalene, $C_{10}H_8$. Also called tar camphor, napththalene is also obtained from coal tar. It is sold in flakes or balls for use as a moth repellent. It has some value as an antiseptic and anthelmintic. More important, however, is the role of naphthalene as an intermediate in the manufacture of organic preparations.

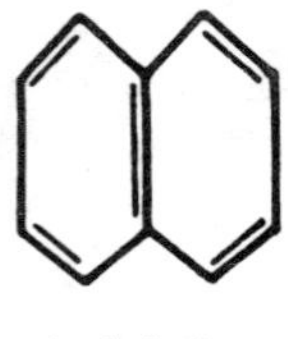

Naphthalene

(5) Anthracene, $C_{14}H_{10}$. Anthracene is a solid obtained from coal tar. It is soluble in the usual organic solvents; less soluble in ether and alcohol than benzene, toluene, xylene, and naphthalene; and insoluble in water. Anthracene is of great importance because of its use in the manufacture of more complex organic compounds, particularly anthraquinone.

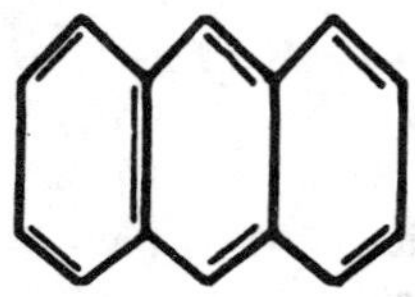

Anthracene

(6) Phenanthrene, $C_{14}H_{10}$. Phenanthrene, a structural isomer of anthracene, has properties similar to anthracene. It is pharmaceutically important because, when reduced, it resembles very closely some of the analgesic alkaloids, the sterols, bile acids, and sex hormones.

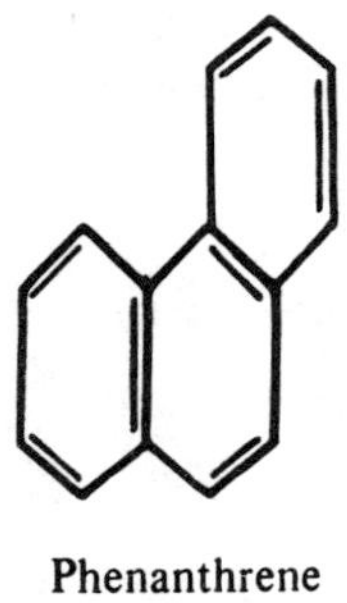

Phenanthrene
(isomer of anthracene)

19. Phenols and related compounds. Up to this point, the presence of a hydroxy group (OH) on a compound has signified that the compound was an alcohol. A hydroxy group attached to an aromatic ring, however, is not an alcohol, but a *phenol.* Phenols, then, are hydroxy derivatives of aromatic rings. Because of the structural similarity of the phenols to the alcohols, many of their properties are similar.

a. Properties. Phenols which contain only the hydroxy group or groups are colorless or white crystals. Those formed from benzene or toluene are soluble in alcohol and to some degree are soluble in water. If the substance is even slightly ionizable, it will exhibit acidity and react with bases. For this reason, phenols are generally incompatible with alkalis. Most phenols are antiseptic and slightly caustic. The medicinal properties of coal tars and wood tar products are attributed to the phenols present in those substances. Phenols, like alcohols, can be esterified, and a large number of useful medicinal agents are esterified phenols.

b. Occurrence and preparation. Some phenols are obtained from the dry distillation of hard wood and coal. Others, particularly some of the very complex molecules, are extracted from plants and animals. Still others are synthesized.

c. Germicidal action and phenol coefficient. Since most of the phenols have germicidal action, a system for rating the efficiency of phenols in germicidal ability has been devised, using as a basis the germicidal action of phenol. The germicidal efficiency of each of the phenols is given a number rating relative to phenol. This number is the phenol coefficient.

d. Pharmaceutically important phenols and their derivatives.

(1) Phenol (carbolic acid), C_6H_5OH.

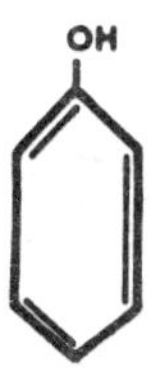

Phenol is a colorless-to-pink, needle-like crystal with a characteristic, antiseptic odor. When heated, the vapors are flammable.

(a) Solubility. Phenol is very soluble in alcohol, ether, chloroform, glycerin, and fixed and volatile oils. It is soluble 1:15 in water. When 90 Gm. of phenol are liquefied by the addition of 10 ml. of water, a permanent liquid results. The addition of more water causes the phenol to recrystallize.

(b) Relationship to acids. Although phenol is called carbolic acid, its only similarity to acids is its ability to neutralize bases. It is much more closely related to alcohol. Both the crystal and the liquefied forms are caustic to organic matter; they are protoplasmic poisons. Unlike acids and bases, phenol's caustic action is not restricted to surface tissue. Left in contact, it is not neutralized but continues to damage deeper tissue. Because of this unusual behavior and the fact that nerve endings are inactivated, deep and severe burns can occur before the victim is aware of it.

(c) Incompatibilities. Phenol is incompatible with camphor, menthol, thymol, phenacetin, and many other compounds, and forms eutectic mixtures with them. When two solids at room temperature are mixed and a liquid results spontaneously, the mixture is said to be eutectic. To illustrate this phenomenon to yourself, pour out equal quantities of phenol crystals and camphor on an ointment slab. With a rubber spatula, rub the two substances together. At first, it will become sticky; after a relatively short period, it will liquefy completely.

(d) Uses. Although officially classified in the USP as an antipruritic, it is further employed as a caustic, disinfectant, antiseptic, preservative, and local anesthetic.

(2) Liquefied phenol (liquefied carbolic acid). This substance contains not less than 88 percent C_6H_6O. An official note in the USP states: "When phenol is to be mixed with a fixed oil, mineral oil or white petrolatum, use crystalline Phenol, not Liquefied Phenol." Liquefied phenol is categorized officially as a caustic to be applied locally in suitable dilution, and then removed with alcohol, but it is used more frequently in a number of preparations for various dermatologic conditions.

(3) Phenolated calamine lotion (compound calamine lotion). In a 1-percent concentration in calamine lotion, the phenol adds a slight anesthetic effect and helps relieve itching.

(4) Dihydroxybenzene, $C_6H_4(OH)_2$. Dihydroxybenzene which occurs in three isomeric forms–ortho, meta, and para–is pharmaceutically important only in its meta isomer. Meta-dihydroxybenzene is official in the USP under the name Resorcinol, common name,

resorcin. It is a white, crystalline powder which acquires a pinkish tint on exposure to light and air. It has a characteristic odor. Resorcinol is soluble in alcohol, water, glycerin, and ether. To illustrate the added solubility of the extra hydroxy group over phenol (with one), phenol is 1:15 water soluble, whereas Resorcinol is soluble 1:1. Resorcinol is antiseptic and antifungal and is very effective against parasitic skin diseases such as eczema and ringworm, and other dermatitides such as psoriasis and seborrhea. It is applied in the form of lotions, pastes, and creams in strengths ranging from 1 to 20 percent; 5 percent is the most widely used concentration.

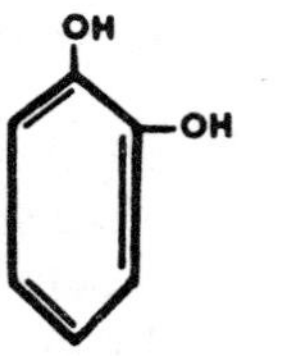

o-dihydroxybenzene
(catechol)

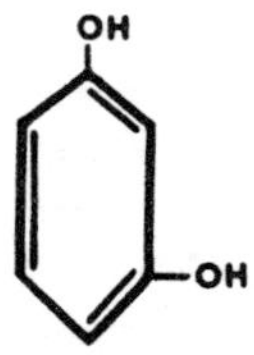

m-dihydroxybenzene
(resorcinol)

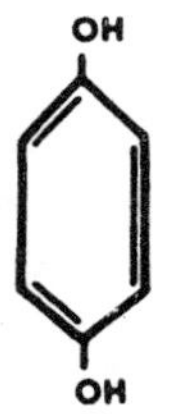

p-dihydroxybenzene
(hydroquinone)

(5) Resorcinol monoacetate (resorcin acetate). By esterifying resorcin with acetic acid, the following reaction occurs to form resorcinol monoacetate.

A common, although not official, name for this medication is Euresol. It is an amber-colored, thick liquid, soluble in alcohol and sparingly soluble in water. Euresol is an antibacterial and antifungal, as well as a local irritant. Although it is used also for psoriasis and eczema, its most common use is in scalp preparations for alopecia (hair loss or baldness). Since alopecia has several causes, you should deduce that resorcinol monoacetate will only be effective in those types caused by a bacterial or fungal infection.

(6) Anthralin (1, 8, 9-anthratriol; 1, 8-dihydroxyanthranol).

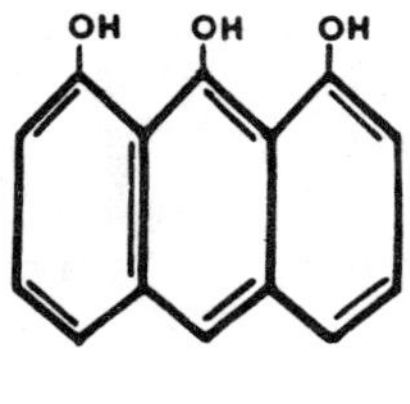

Anthralin is a yellowish-brown, water-insoluble powder, used in the manufacture of skin preparations, particularly anthralin ointment. Anthralin is a local irritant and antieczematic agent. At one time, chrysarobin was a widely used substance, but anthralin has replaced chrysarobin because it is somewhat less irritating and causes less skin discoloration.

(7) Danthron (Dorbane).

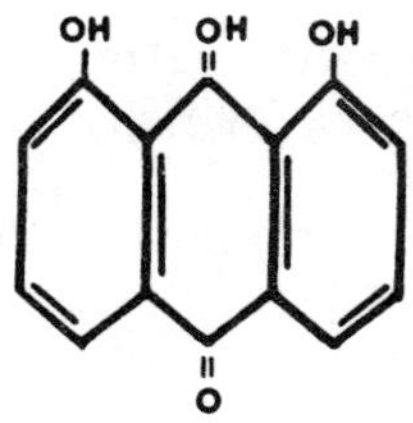

Danthron is a cathartic which appears as a pink dye in alkaline urine. It is most important as an

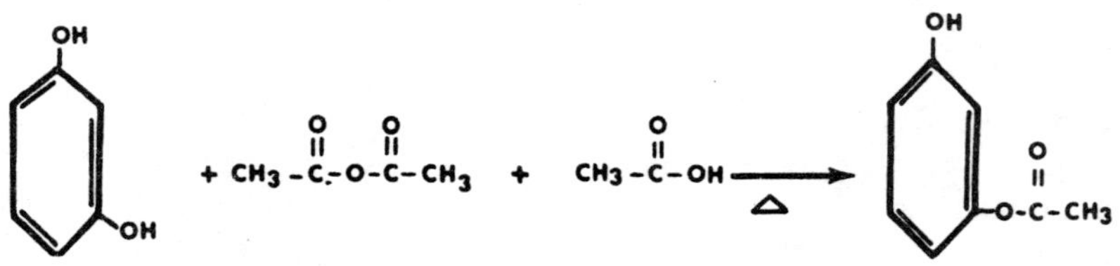

Resorcin   Acetic Anhydride   Acetic Acid   Resorcinol Monoacetate

intermediate in the manufacture of dyes and in veterinary medicine. Its use in human medicine is infrequent, probably because of the demoralizing effect on the patient upon seeing red-colored urine.

(8) Eugenol.

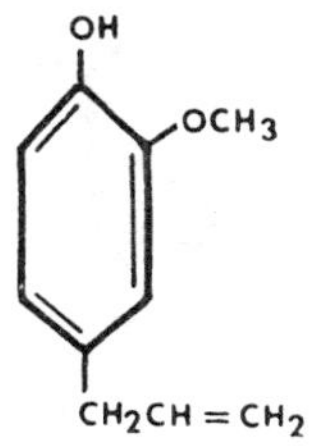

Eugenol is the main constituent in clove oil and, in fact, it is eugenol that is old as artificial oil of cloves. Eugenol occurs naturally in cinnamon oil, sassafras, bay leaves, and pimenta oil. The USP classifies eugenol as a dental obtundant (dulls sensibility to pain) for toothaches; it is applied either on a pledget of cotton or mixed with zinc oxide to form a temporary filling. The basic material used for the synthesis of vanillin is eugenol.

(9) Glyceryl guaiacolate. This stimulating expectorant is incorporated into cough preparations such as Robitussin. It is much easier to tolerate than the plain guaiacol which was previously used.

(10) Hexachlorophene.

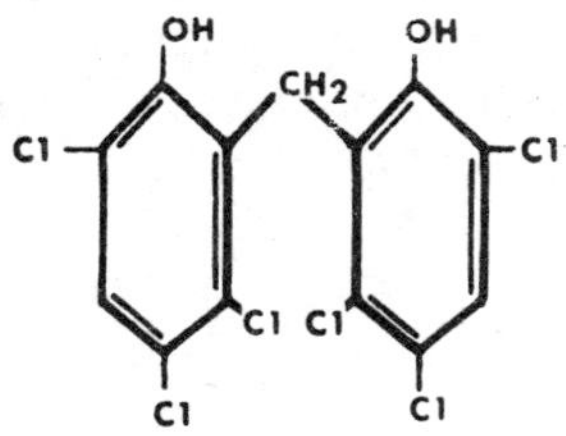

Hexachlorophene is an anti-infective agent. It is incorporated into soaps and surgical scrubs to reduce the bacterial flora. For proper activity it must be left on the skin as a residue to prevent bacterial growth. The protective film is removed when other cleansing agents are used and the bacteriostatic effect is lost. Damage to the nervous system is possible if soaps containing large amounts of hexachlorophene are used improperly over long periods of time. It is now under restricted use.

(11) Hexylresorcinol.

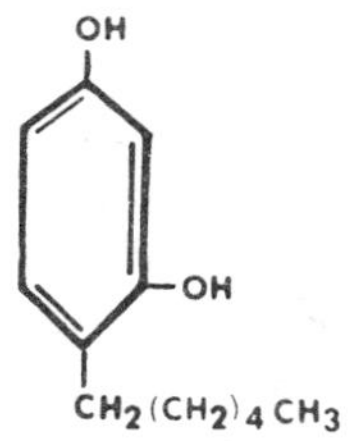

Hexylresorcinol is used in a 1:1000 dilution as an effective antiseptic. It has the advantage of being odorless and nonstaining. It is effective in the treatment internally of many worm infestations. Although relatively nontoxic, it is extremely irritating to the mucous membranes and may cause ulcerations if the capsule containing it is broken in the mouth. Hexylresorcinol is manufactured in the form of a coated pill which resists rupturing, even when chewed.

(12) Thymol.

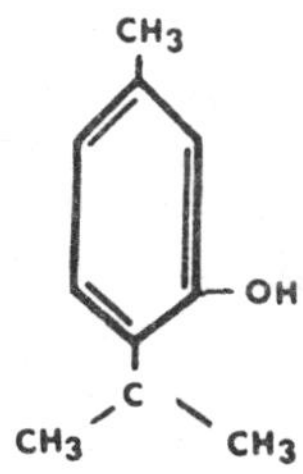

Thymol is an antiseptic, but its action is of short duration. Thymol is mixed with other substances such as camphor and menthol in mouthwashes. These preparations taste nice, but have little effect in sterilizing the field of application.

(13) Cresol.

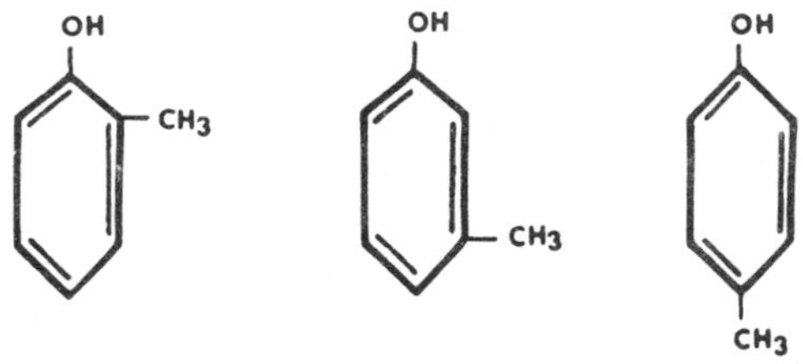

Ortho Meta Para

Cresol is a mixture of o-, m-, and p-cresols obtained from coal tar, containing not more than 5-percent phenol. Cresol is similar to phenol in antiseptic properties and is used as a preservative for injectable solutions.

e. Aromatic alcohols and their derivatives. The aromatic alcohols differ structurally from the phenols in that the hydroxyl group is attached to a side chain of the aromatic ring, rather than to the ring itself. The alcohols resemble the aliphatic alcohols in many respects. Like the aliphatics, they may exist as primary, secondary, and tertiary alcohols. The pharmaceutically important aromatic alcohols include:

(1) Benzyl alcohol (phenylcarbinol).

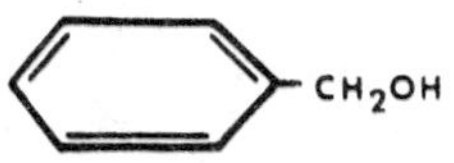

The main action of benzyl alcohol is as a local anesthetic by injection or by application to mucous membranes. It also functions as a bacteriostatic agent in certain injectables.

(2) Benzyl benzoate, C_6H_5-CO-O-CH_2-C_6H_5. Benzyl benzoate is used as a scabacide in the form of a lotion.

20. Aromatic acids and their derivatives. Aromatic acids contain an aromatic ring and a carboxyl group. This acid group may be attached either directly to the ring or to a side chain. The aromatic acids are important mainly because of the physiologically active agents produced by their esterification. Among these are analgesics, antispasmodics, antiseptics, and local anesthetics. The pharmaceutically important aromatic acids and their derivatives include–

a. Benzoic acid, C_6H_5COOH.

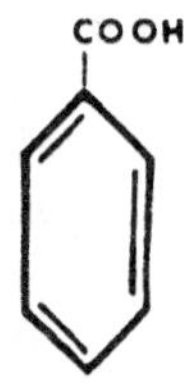

Benzoic acid occurs free in nature and esterified in balsams. It is quite soluble in alcohol but only about 3:1000 in water. It is used in external antiseptic preparations and as a preservative in mucilages and suspensions. Sodium benzoate is used as a food preservative. Derivatives and salts of benzoic acid are important pharmaceutically and these will be considered in later portions of this chapter under "anesthetic amines, amides, and vitamins."

b. Salicylic acid (O-hydroxybenzoic acid).

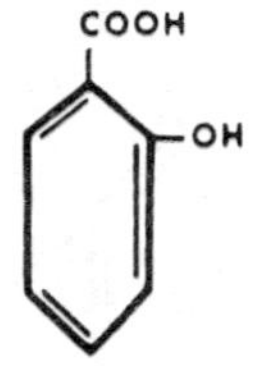

Salicylic acid is a phenol, as well as an aromatic acid, but is much less caustic than phenol. It has antiseptic and germicidal properties, and in stronger concentrations it acts as a keratolytic.

(1) Uses. Not used internally because of its irritating nature, salicylic acid is mainly employed in external preparations for the treatment of warts, corns, fungus infections, and some eczemas. Tissue cells swell, soften, and peel off after repeated or prolonged contact with salicylic acid.

(2) Whitfield's ointment. Whitfield's ointment, used topically as a fungicide, is a combination of benzoic and salicylic acids in polyethylene glycol ointment.

c. Methylparaben; propylparaben. Two different but very closely related derivatives of benzoic acid are the parabens. These substances are used singly or in combination as preservatives in many pharmaceutical preparations and cosmetics. Combining the two produces a synergistic effect; that is, the antiseptic effect of the combination is greater than the total effect of the individual components.

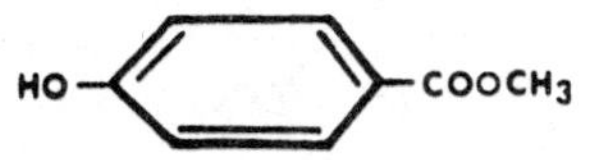

Methylparaben
(Methyl p-Hydroxybenzoate)

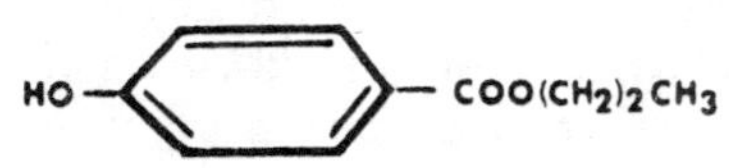

Propylparaben
(Propyl p-Hydroxybenzoate)

d. Sodium salicylate.

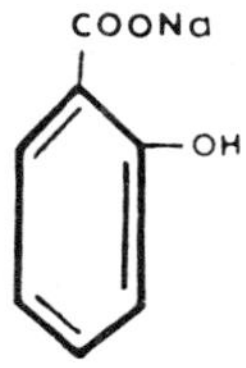

Sodium salicylate is widely employed as an analgesic and antipyretic.

e. Methyl salicylate (oil of wintergreen).

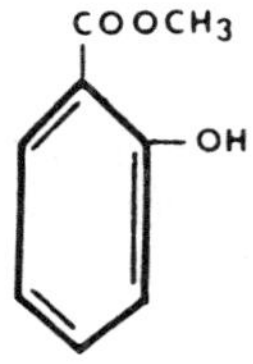

Methyl salicylate is used as a flavoring agent and as a counterirritant.

f. Phenyl salicylate (Salol).

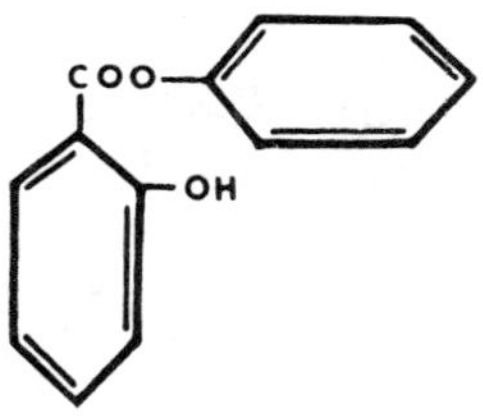

Phenyl salicylate is used as an extemporaneous enteric coating for tablets and capsules. This substance is not soluble in the acid media of the stomach but rapidly dissolves in the alkaline intestine. No more than necessary should be used for coating the tablets, as salol breaks down into phenol and salicylic acid in the body.

g. Aspirin (acetylsalicylic acid, ASA).

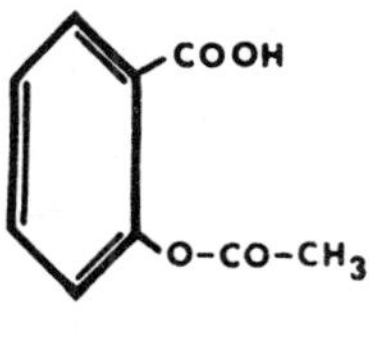

Like the other salicylates we have discussed, aspirin is analygesic and antipyretic and has some value in relieving pain of almost any origin. Aspirin is not soluble in water; it must be administered as a tablet, capsule, or suppository. It may be solubilized to some extent, but the solutions are not stable and hydrolyze within a few days to salicylic and acetic acids. Hydrolyzed aspirin has a strong odor of acetic acid and tablets may display crystals of salicylic acid on their surface; they should not be used.

21. **Aromatic halogenated compounds and similar structures.** At the beginning of our discussion of cyclic structures, we illustrated some substitution possibilities of benzene, showing specifically chlorine mono, di, tri, and tetra substitution. In all these cases, the halogenation was directly on the benzene ring. It is also possible to halogenate a side chain; this was described in the aliphatic portion of this chapter. Since we have already discussed the reactions, let us look at some specific compounds resulting from halogenation of cyclic structures.

a. Gamma benzene hexachloride (benzene hexachloride; 1, 2, 3, 4, 5, 6-hexachlorocyclohexane; Lindane) $C_6Cl_6H_6$.

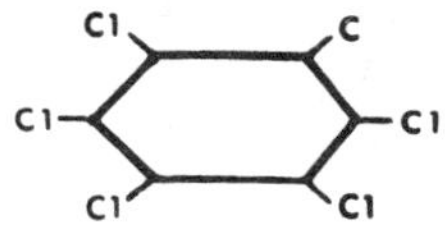

Gamma benzene hexachloride is the gamma isomer of hexachlorocyclohexane. It exists as a white crystalline powder with a musty odor. It is used as an insecticide and in the treatment of scabies and lice of the head, pubic area, and feet.

b. Chlordane. Chlordane is a nearly odorless liquid used as an insecticide. It is equal to DDT in its effectiveness as an insecticide and is superior to many other insecticides. It is used particularly against cockroaches, ants, grasshoppers, and some animal parasites. It is of no medical value to humans.

c. Halazone tablets (p-dichlorosulfamoylbenzoic acid).

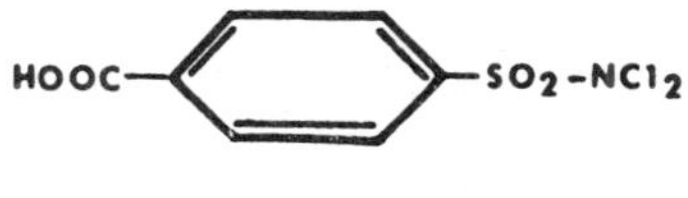

Halazone tablets, containing 4 mg. of active ingredient, produce a concentration of 2-5 parts per million when dissolved in a quart of water.

Water which has been treated with halazone tablets and allowed to stand for 30 minutes is safe for drinking although it may not taste pleasant. This is an adequate and convenient method for the extemporaneous purification of water for drinking purposes when your water supply is contaminated or its potability is doubtful.

d. Merbromin (Mercurochrome).

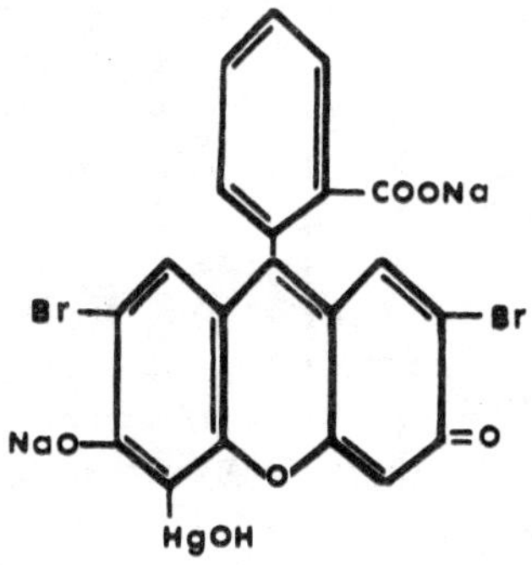

Merbromin is a weak antiseptic and acts as a bacteriostatic agent. It owes most of its activity to the mercury and, in tinctures, to the alcohol present.

e. Povidone-iodine (Betadine). By tying iodine into a very complex molecule (povidone), its sting is almost eliminated and the duration of its action is increased. Although basically not as effective as iodine, its sustained action and absence of sting are desirable qualities, and in minor cuts and abrasions it is a suitable antiseptic. It is also an effective throat gargle and douche.

f. Diiodohydroxyquin (Floraquin).

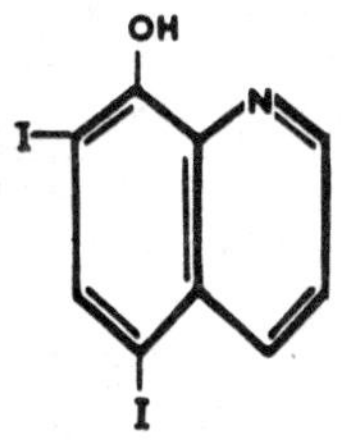

Diiodohydroxyquin is used in the treatment of intestinal amebiasis and certain fungal infections. It is administered as an enteric coated tablet and also applied topically.

g. Iodochlorhydroxyquin (Vioform). This compound is similar in structure and activity to diiodohydroxyquin.

22. **Amines and amides (the nitrogen-containing compounds).** In this broad class of substances are the alkaloids, antihistamines, sulfa drugs, barbiturates, analgesics, and local anesthetics. The majority of the medications prescribed in today's medicine are of the amine-amide group. No differentiation will be made here between amine derivatives or amide derivatives. It is important that you remember they are related, but different: and they all contain nitrogen. For further simplification, these products will be covered in groups with related action, rather than with related structure. The pharmacology of these compounds is treated in detail in chapter 9.

a. General structure. Below are shown the general structures of primary, secondary, and tertiary amines, and primary amides. We are limiting our coverage to primary amides because only they are of medical significance.

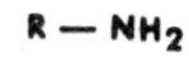

Primary Amine

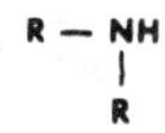

Secondary Amine

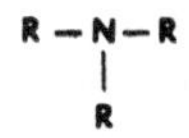

Tertiary Amine

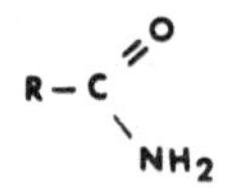

Primary Amide

b. The analgesic amines and amides. Agents which alleviate pain are termed analgesics. They are covered in chapter 9. Below are two members of this group; notice the similarities and differences in these compounds. Use this section in conjunction with your study of their pharmacology.

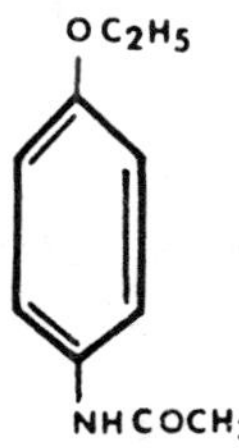

Phenacetin (Acetophenetidin)

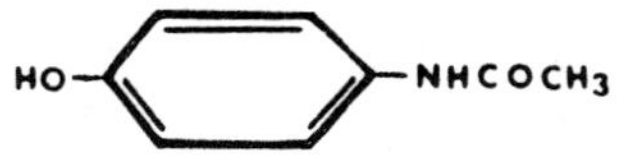

Acetaminophen (Tylenol)

c. Local anesthetic amines and amides. Loss of feeling and sensation to a localized portion of the body is known as local anesthesia. Such action may be caused by freezing, protoplasmic poisoning, or specific action on a nerve ending to prevent impulses from passing. Below are the names and structures of drugs that block nerve impulses.

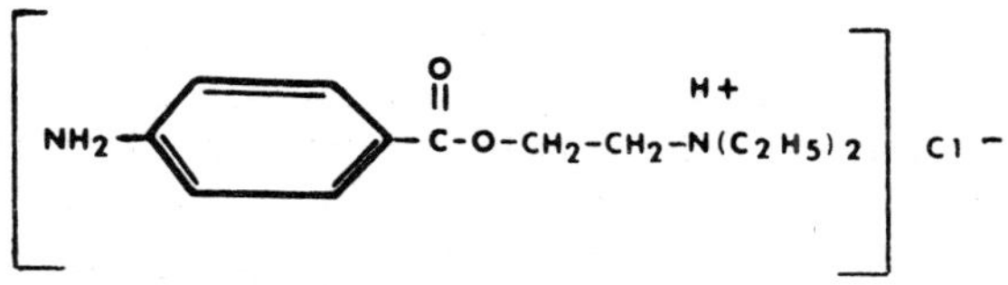

Procaine Hydrochloride (Procaine: Novocaine)

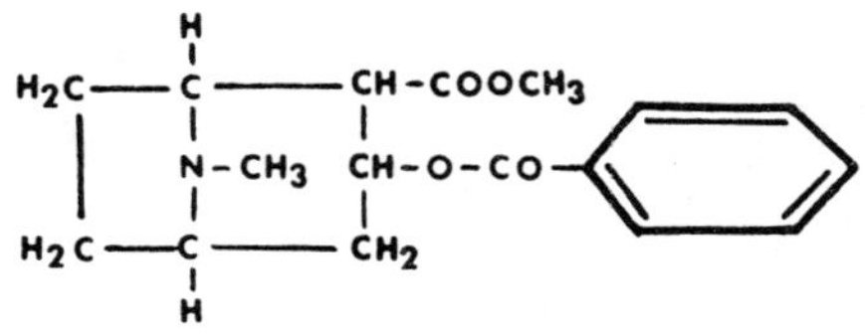

Cocaine

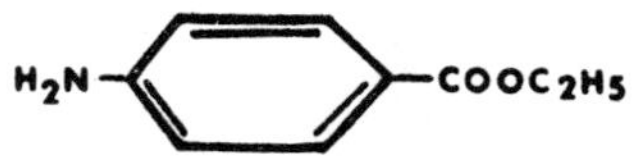

Ethylaminobenzoate (Benzocaine)

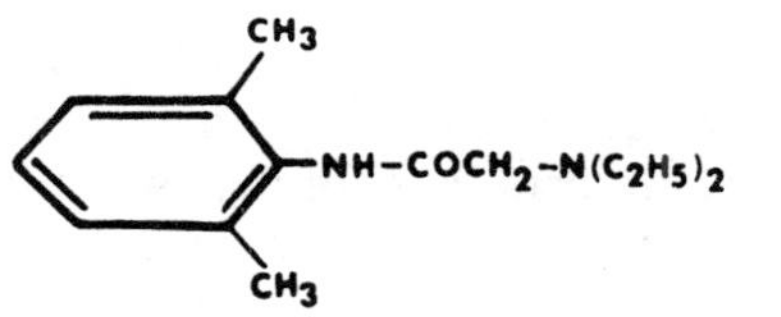

Lidocaine (Xylocaine)

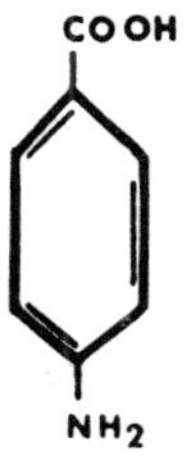

p-Aminobenzoic Acid

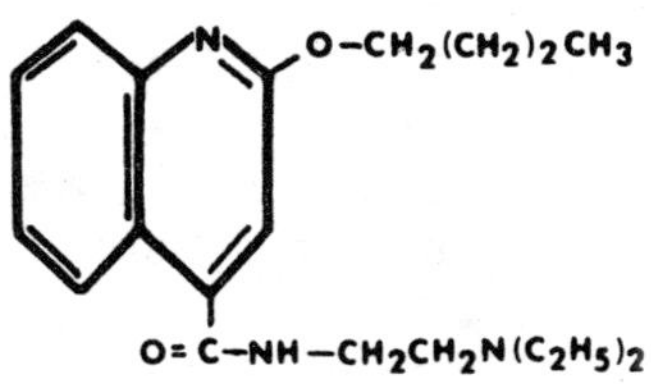

Dibucaine (Nupercaine)

NOTE

By itself, p-aminobenzoic acid has no anesthetic properties. Its derivatives, however, do. Many of the important local anesthetics are closely related chemically to p-aminobenzoic acid.

d. Sedative and hypnotic amines and amides. Hypnotic, soporific, and somnifacient are synonymous terms, all referring to agents which produce sleep. Sleep may be produced by this class of drugs when there is no specific stimulus such as pain, coughing, or severe itch preventing it. Sedative drugs have a quieting effect. They produce relaxation, lessen excitement, and generally slow motor activity without producing sleep. Hypnotic and sedative properties are generally inherent in the same drug. Small doses produce sedation; larger doses produce hypnosis.

(1) Barbiturates. The barbiturates are a class of compounds called ureides, very closely related to amines and amides, and the most widely used sedatives and hypnotics. This class encompasses hundreds of compounds. The parent structure, barbituric acid or malonylurea, is formed by the combination of malonic acid and urea. As shown in the formulas below, barbituric acid exists as a mixture of two forms, the "keto" form and the "enol" form.

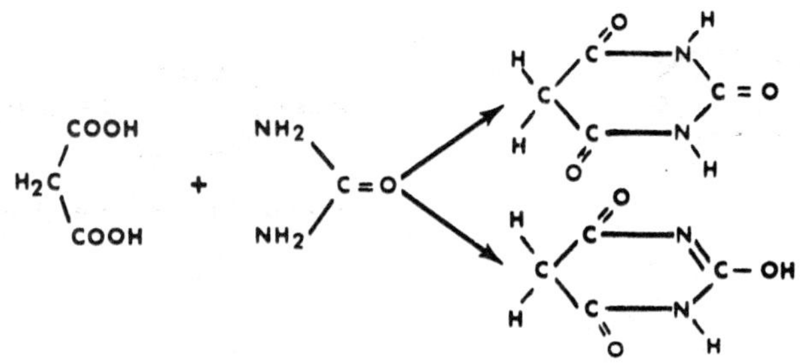

Keto Form

Enol Form

Malonic Acid Urea Malonylurea (Barbituric Acid)

(a) Barbituric acid. Barbituric acid itself is not active as a hypnotic or sedative. These properties are acquired through substitution of the hydrogens attached to the carbon atom. When organic groups are substituted for these hydrogens, the compounds become sedative and hypnotic. By replacing the hydrogen of the hydroxyl group in the enol form with sodium or potassium, soluble salts are produced. These soluble salts are important in the making of internal liquid preparations and injectables.

(b) Classes. Classes have been selected on the relative duration of action. The classes are: long-acting, intermediate-acting, short-acting, and ultra-short acting. Chapter 9 gives descriptions of these classes and detailed information about the individual agents.

(c) Long-acting barbiturates. The long-acting barbiturates are mainly used as sedatives. The more important members of this group are—

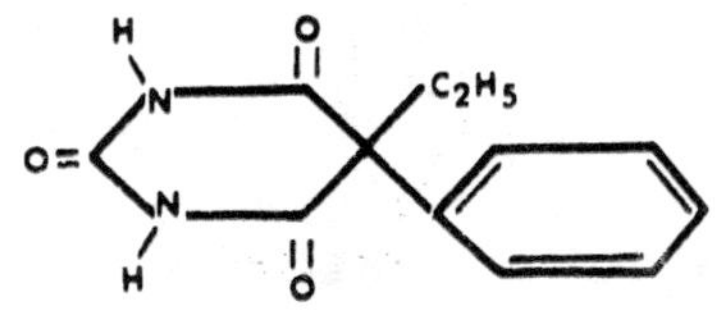

Phenobarbital (Luminal)

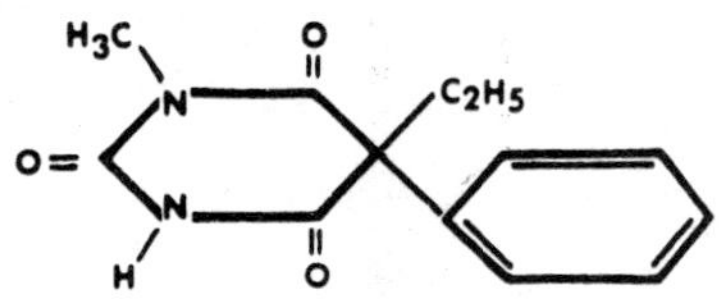

Mephobarbital (Mebaral)

(d) *Intermediate-acting barbiturates.*

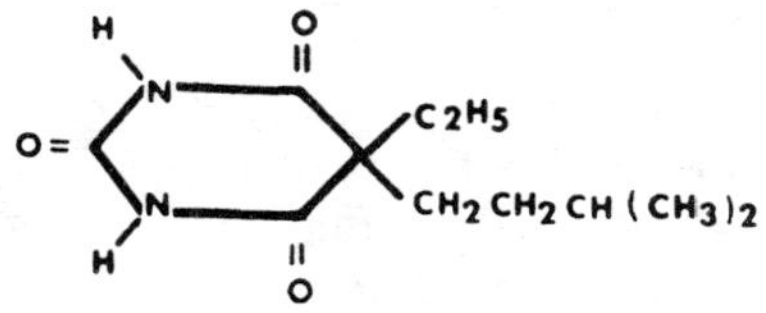

Amobarbital (Amytal)

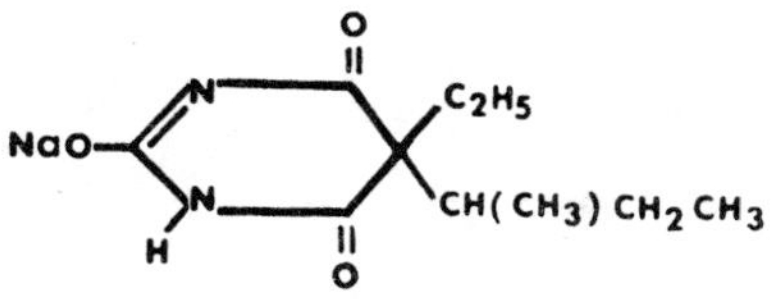

Butabarbital Sodium (Butisol)

(e) *Short-acting barbiturates.* The short-acting barbiturates are almost exclusively applied for their hypnotic rather than their sedative effects. Combinations of the short-acting and intermediate-acting are popular.

1. *Pentobarbital sodium (Nembutal).*

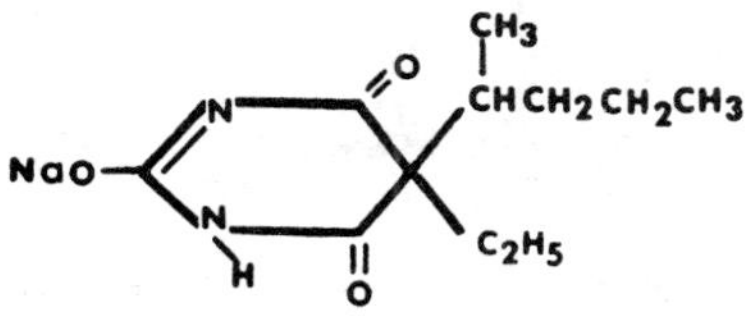

2. *Secobarbital (Seconal).*

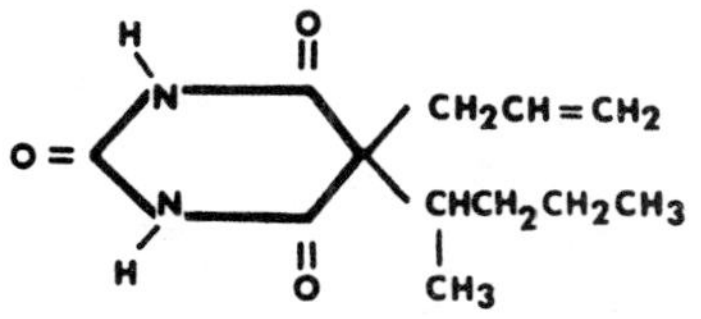

(f) *Ultra short-acting barbiturates.*

1. *Thiopental sodium (Pentothal sodium).*

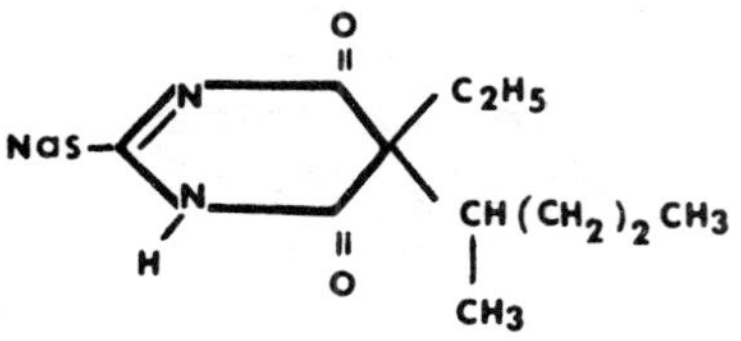

Here, for the first time in the barbiturate class of drugs, we find a sulfur atom in the molecule, and hence this barbiturate is called a thiobarbiturate (thio = sulfur).

2. *Thiamylal sodium (Surital sodium).*

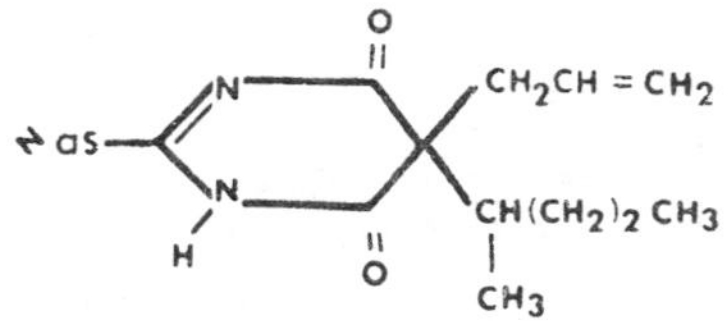

3. *Hexobarbital sodium (Evipal sodium).*

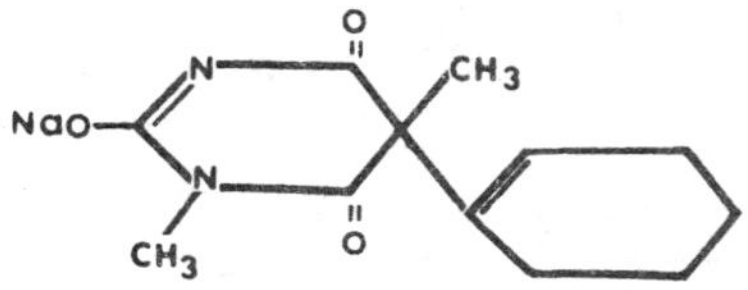

Notice in the molecular structure that an atom of oxygen replaces the sulfur. Certain authorities say that the substitution of oxygen for sulfur produces a safer drug.

(2) *Other ureides.* The hydantoins are ureides and are also central nervous system depressants but with selective activity. They depress the area of the brain where epileptic seizures originate but do not depress other areas. Epilepsy is a disease caused by unusual electric brain impulses. Generally, epilepsy is of four types, the two most important of which are grand mal and petit mal. Diphenylhydantoin (Dilantin), is the most widely used of this group.

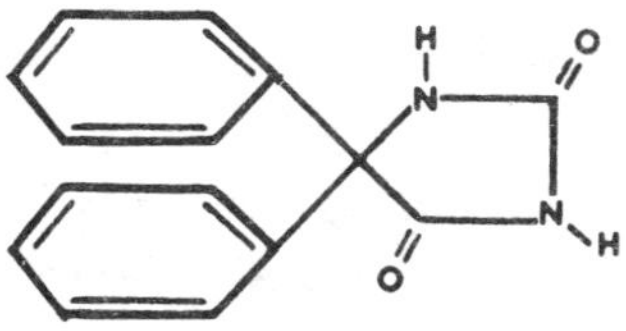

Diphenylhydantoin

e. *Antimicrobial amines and amides.* In 1908 a compound, p-aminobenzenesulfonamide, was synthesized. But it was not discovered until almost 30 years later that it had medicinal value. In 1935, a red dye discovered three years earlier was found to have wonderful curative powers. This compound was named Prontosil. Shortly thereafter it was determined that Prontosil was effective because of the p-aminobenzenesulfonamide portion of its molecule. Since then over 3300 sulfonamides have been used clinically. Other agents, unrelated to the sulfa drugs, have been discovered which display antimicrobial properties of the sulfa drugs.

(1) Sulfonamides.

(a) General formula. The general formula for the sulfonamides is–

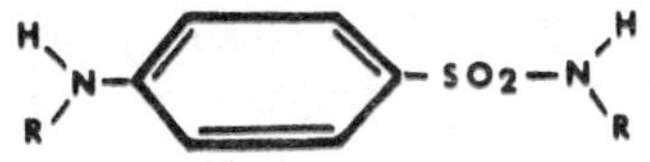

As we proceed from one specific sulfa to another, observe the very slight changes in this formula. In some, a hydrogen may replace the radical (R). In others, ring structures or aliphatic side chains may be the radical. Each of the sulfas, however, is very closely related to the rest.

(b) Important sulfonamides.

1. Sulfanilamide.

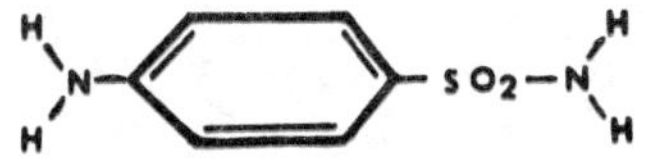

Learn the formula for sulfanilamide, for all the other sulfas are related to it. Although sulfanilamide itself has fallen into disuse in human medicine because of its toxicity, it is important as the parent compound of the other sulfonamides.

2. Sulfadiazine.

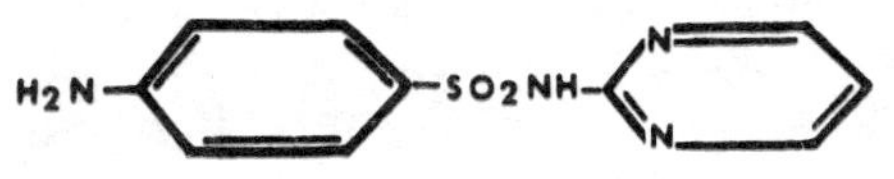

3. Sulfisoxazole.

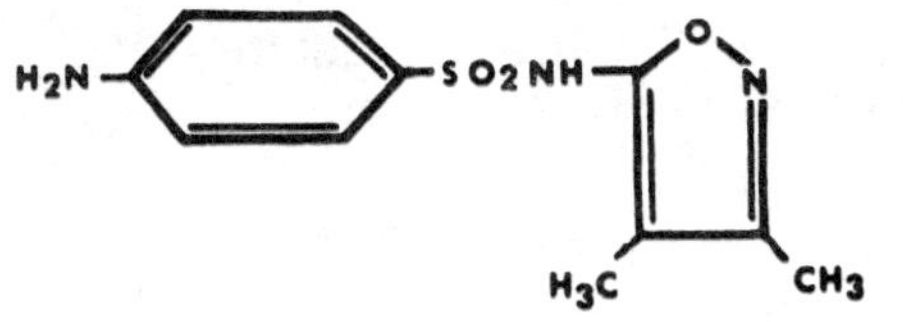

A big breakthrough in sulfonamide therapy came with the discovery of sulfisoxazole. It is safer than the others and is effective in urinary tract infections.

(c) Incompatibilities. Most of the incompatibilities encountered with the sulfa drugs are of an acid-base nature. Aqueous solutions of the sodium salts of sulfonamides have a pH between 9 and 10. They precipitate on exposure to air because they absorb CO_2. Sulfonamides are precipitated from solution by mineral acid salts of the local anesthetics (Procaine HCl, Tetracaine HCl), the sympathomimetic amines (ephedrine HCl), and by many other substances yielding an acid pH.

(2) Antimicrobial agents not related to the sulfonamides. Other than the nitrofurans, each member of this group is so widely different from the next that we will treat each member individually without any generalizations. Chapter 9 will give descriptions and actions of these agents.

(a) Isoniazid [isonicotinic acid hydrazide (INH)].

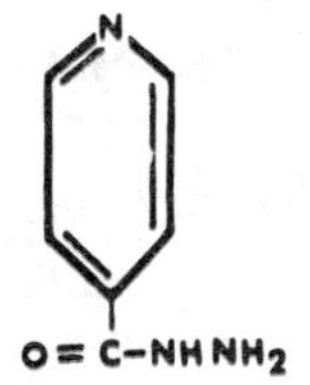

This potent and selective drug is a specific in the treatment of tuberculosis.

(b) Aminosalicylic acid [p-aminosalicylic acid (PAS)].

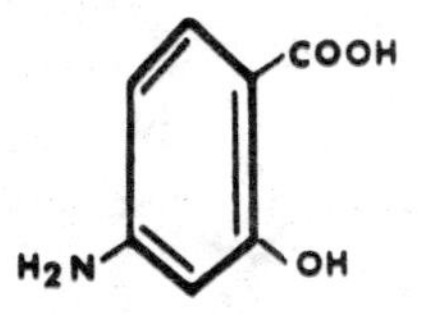

PAS is another antibacterial with selective action against the tubercle bacillus. When used alone, it is not as effective as either isoniazid or streptomycin.

(c) Methenamine mandelate (Mandelamine).

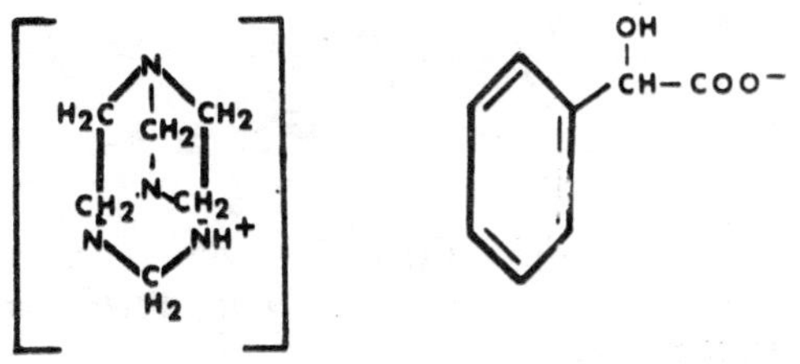

Methenamine is a urinary antiseptic. Because methenamine is effective in an acid pH (6 or below), it is generally administered in combination with mandelic acid or sodium acid phosphate. Thus methenamine mandelate is an efficient combination.

(d) Nitrofurans.

1. Nitrofurazone (Furacin).

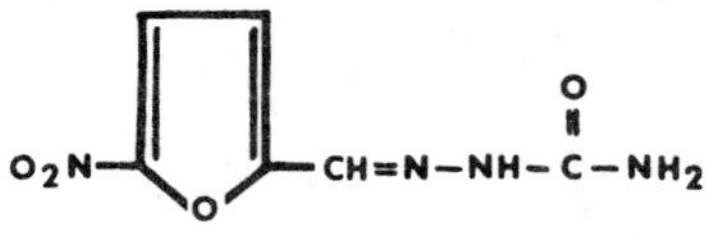

Nitrofurazone is a *local* antibacterial agent applied in the form of solutions or ointments.

2. Furazolidone (Furoxone).

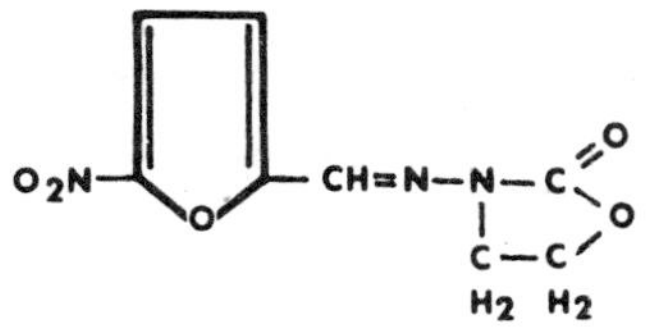

Furazolidone is an anti-infective agent employed for local activity in the intestinal tract and vagina.

3. Nitrofurantoin (Furadantin, Macrodantin).

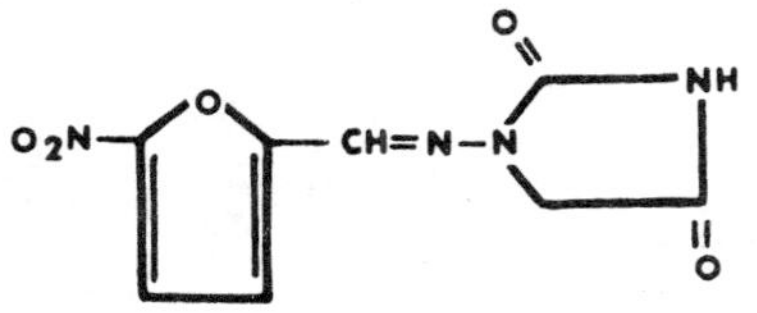

Nitrofurantoin is an anti-infective which is generally limited in therapeutic usage to infections of the urinary tract.

f. Antihistamines. Generally speaking, all the antihistamines are alike in action, differing only in potency and dosage. A few, however, have antinauseant properties, and may be agents of choice for motion sickness. A more detailed discussion of the antihistamines is covered in chapter 9. The most widely used antihistamine preparations are–

(1) Diphenhydramine hydrochloride (Benadryl HCl).

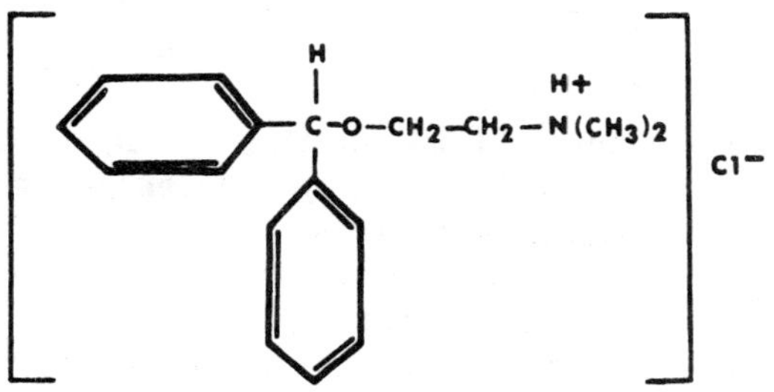

Diphenhydramine hydrochloride is a general antihistamine.

(2) Tripelennamine hydrochloride [Pyribenzamine HCl (PBZ)].

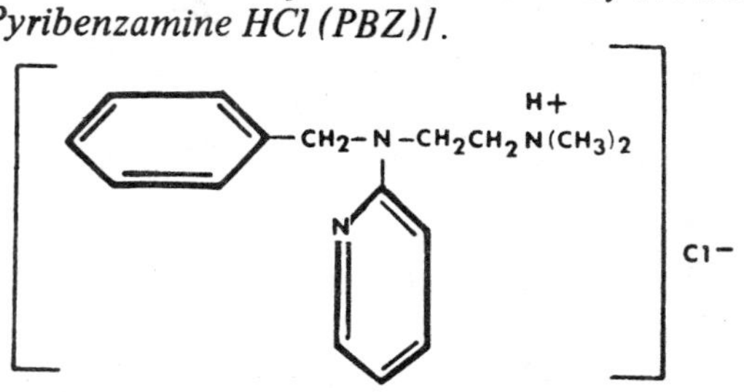

Tripelennamine is a general antihistamine.

(3) Chlorpheniramine maleate (Chlor-Trimeton maleate; Teldrin).

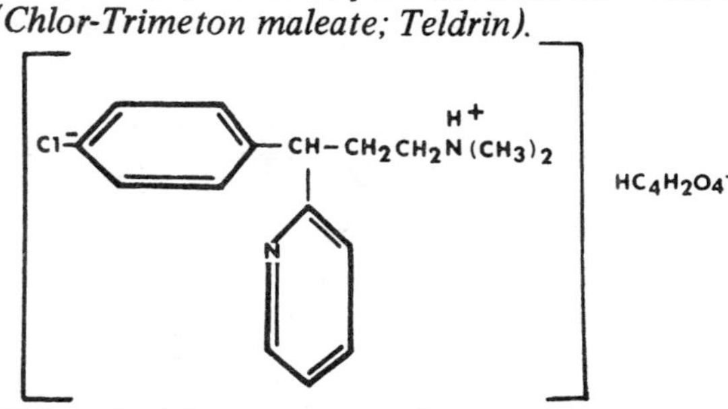

Chlorpheniramine maleate is a general antihistamine.

(4) Promethazine hydrochloride (Phenergan).

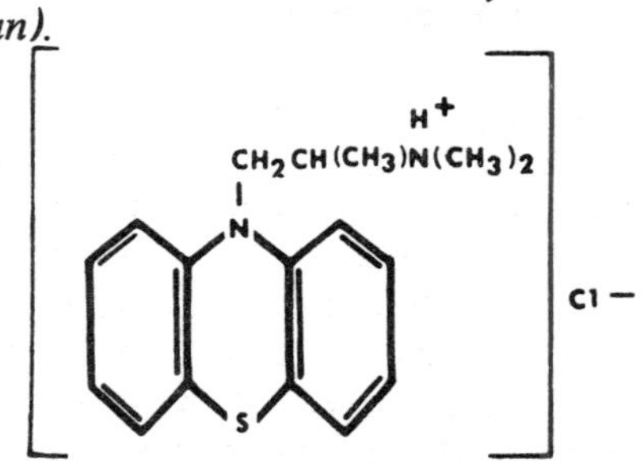

Promethazine is used as a general antihistamine and sedative in cough preparations.

(5) Dimenhydrinate (Dramamine).

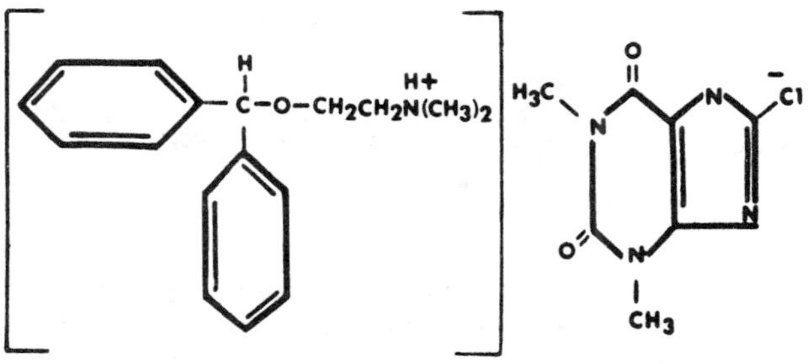

Dimenhydrinate is a combination of diphenhydramine (Benadryl) and 8-chlorotheophylline. Dimenhydrinate does not have very good antihistamine properties, but is antinauseant in action. It is mainly used for its antimotion sickness effects.

(6) Cyclizine hydrochloride (Marezine HCl).

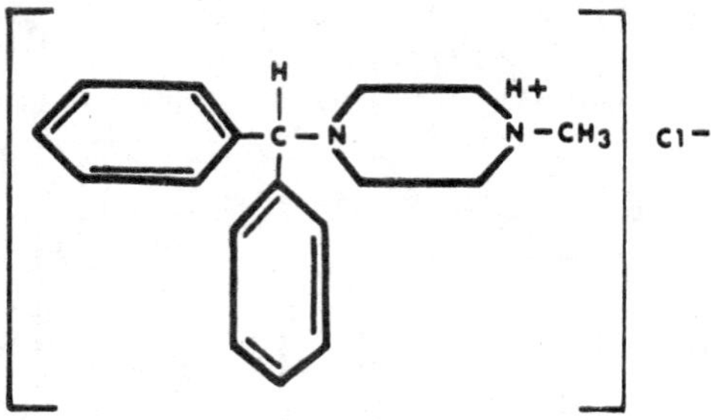

Cyclizine is effective in the prevention and relief of the dizziness, nausea, and vomiting associated with motion sickness.

(7) Meclizine hydrochloride (Bonine).

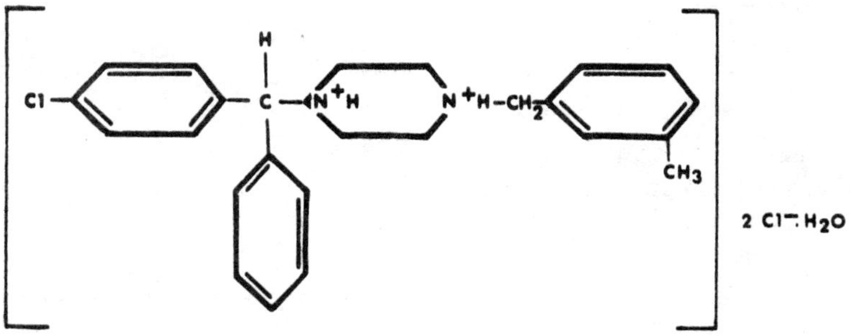

Meclizine is effective in motion sickness.

g. Autonomic nervous system amines and amides. Drugs which affect the action of the autonomic nervous system (covered in detail in chapter 9) are classified as sympathomimetic, parasympathomimetic, sympatholytic, or parasympatholytic, depending upon their action.

(1) Sympathomimetic amines. The sympathomimetic amines have actions in the body comparable to epinephrine, and it is this compound which is considered as the prototype of the group.

(a) Epinephrine (Adrenalin).

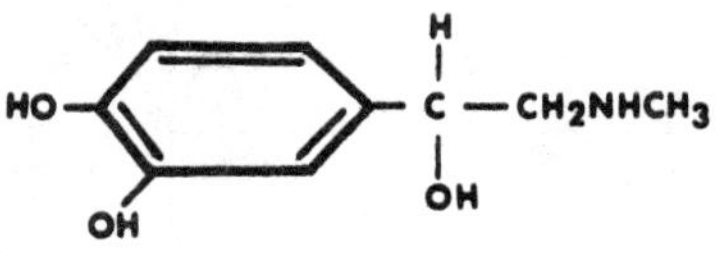

In the presence of oxidizing agents and sunlight, epinephrine decomposes, first turning pink and then showing a brown sediment. Preparations which are brown in color or contain a precipitate should not be used.

(b) Ephedrine.

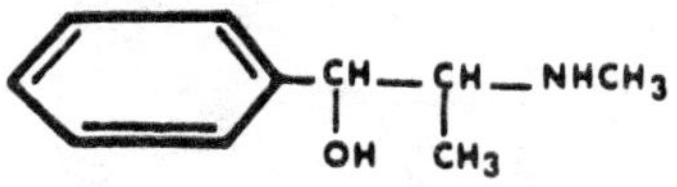

(c) Amphetamine sulfate (Benzedrine sulfate).

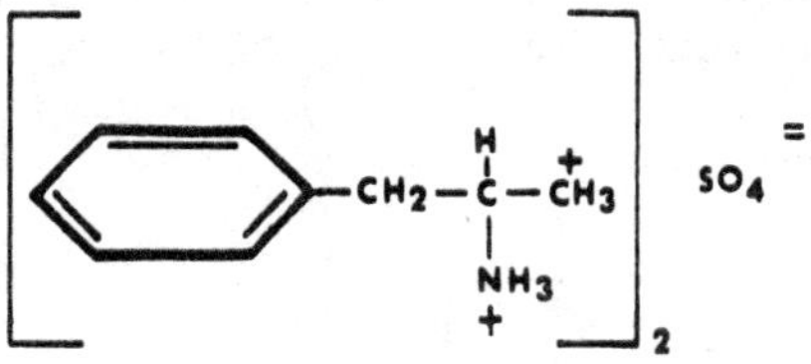

(d) Phenylephrine hydrochloride (Neo-Synephrine hydrochloride).

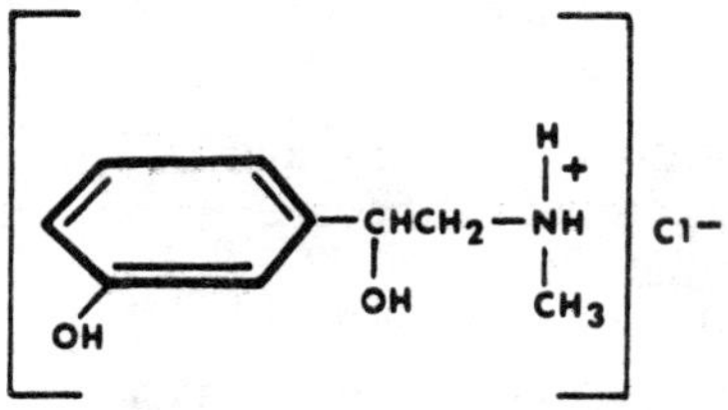

Phenylephrine is used as a decongestant in nose drops.

(e) Naphazoline hydrochloride (Privine HCl).

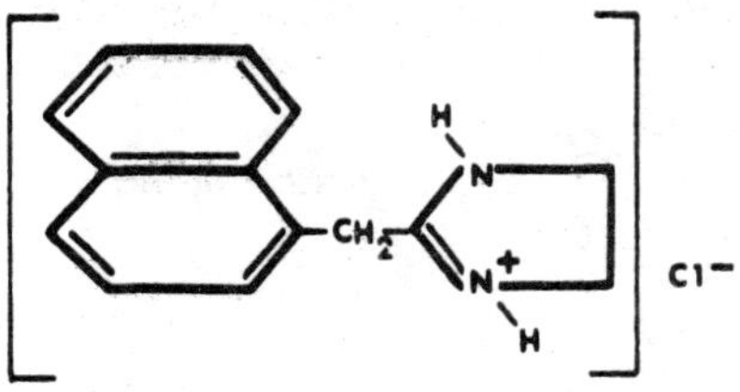

Although they differ greatly in structure, naphazoline, epinephrine, and phenylephrine have similar vasoconstrictor properties.

(2) Parasympathomimetic amines. Acetylcholine is the natural parasympathetic amine occurring in the body. Since it is almost

immediately inactivated in the body by cholinesterase, it is of no therapeutic significance. Pilocarpine shares many of the actions of acetylcholine, as does bethanechol.

(a) Acetylcholine.

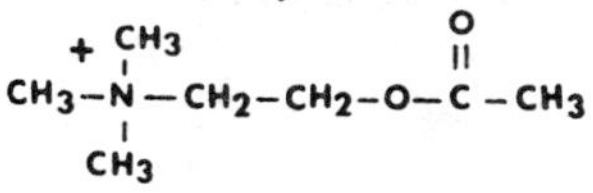

(b) Pilocarpine hydrochloride.

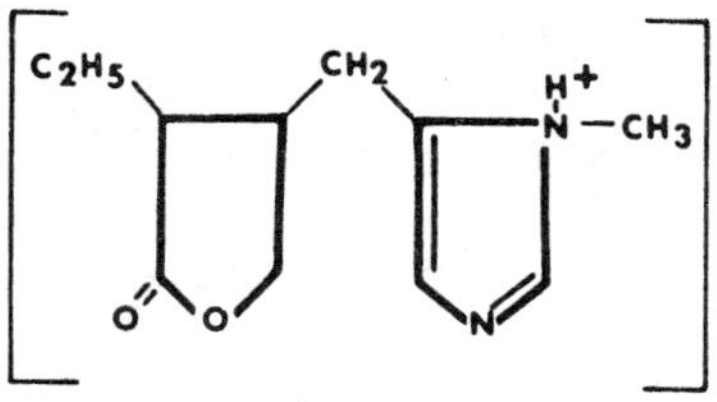

(c) Bethanechol chloride (Urecholine).

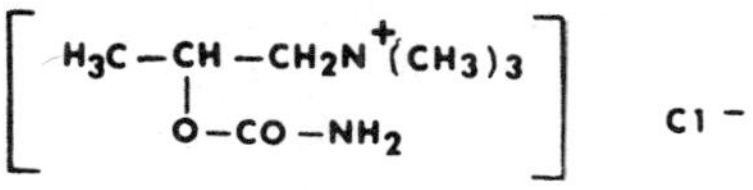

(3) Sympatholytic agents. The sympatholytic agents block the action of the sympathetic stimuli by their presence at the nerve receptor.

(a) Phenoxybenzamine hydrochloride (Dibenzyline HCl).

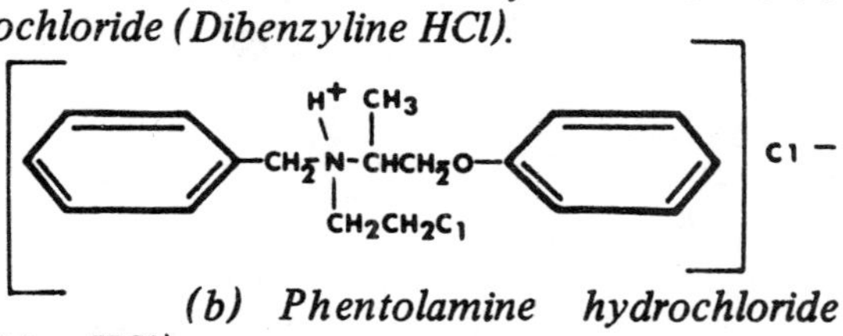

(b) Phentolamine hydrochloride (Regitine HCl).

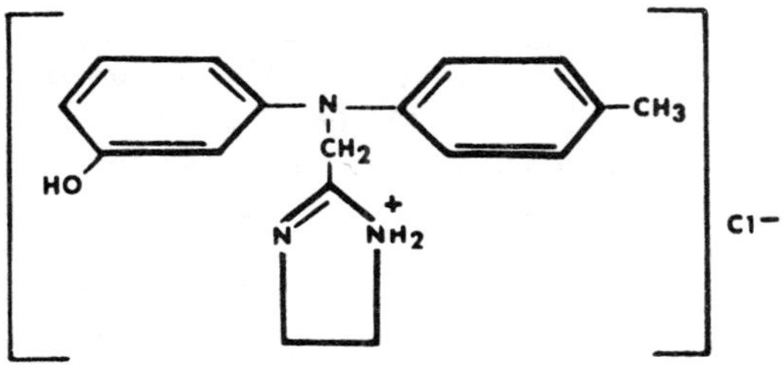

(4) Parasympatholytic agents. These agents cause actions opposite to the parasympathomimetic drugs previously discussed. The two prototypes are atropine and propantheline.

(a) Atropine.

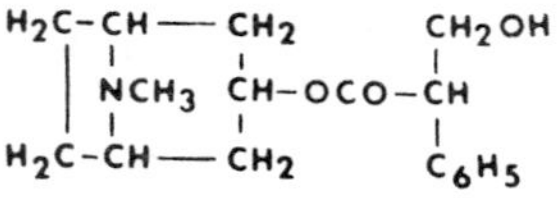

(b) Propantheline bromide (Pro-Banthine).

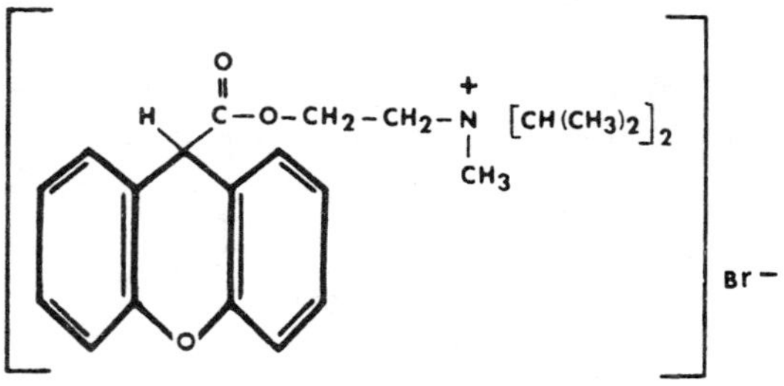

23. Amino acids, peptides, and proteins.

a. Amino acids. Amino acids are difunctional organic compounds containing an amino group and a carboxylic acid.

(1) General formula. The general formula for the amino acids is—

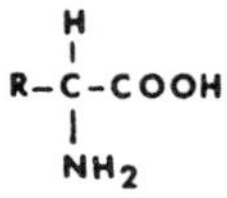

(2) Glycine. Glycine, the simplest of the amino acids, conforms to the general formula—

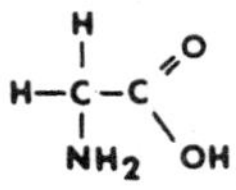

(3) Essential amino acids. Twenty-one different amino acids are found in the body and all are necessary for proper body function. Most amino acids can be manufactured in the body; however, ten are not. These amino acids must be included in the diet and are known as "essential amino acids."

Threonine	Phenylalanine
Methionine	Tryptophan
Lysine	Histidine
Arginine	Leucine
Valine	Isoleucine

b. Peptides. Two or more amino acids may combine to form a peptide and water. During digestion, amino acids are liberated from complex protein structures and condense together to form polypeptides. The formula below shows a typical dipeptide with the molecule of water before it is eliminated.

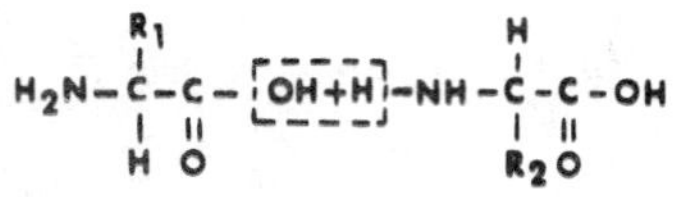

c. Proteins. Proteins are polymers of amino acids. They are important food substances. Proteins are extremely high molecular weight (10,000 to 1 million) polypeptides. In the following formula for a very small part of a protein molecule, you should be able to distinguish the individual amino acids making up the complex structure.

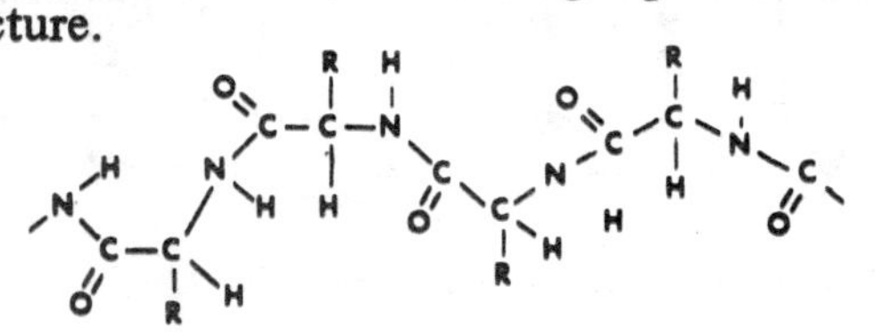

(1) Properties. Unlike many organic materials, particularly those of high molecular weight, a considerable number of the proteins are soluble in water and insoluble in the general organic solvents. All proteins contain carbon, hydrogen, oxygen, and nitrogen; many contain sulfur and phosphorus.

(2) Precipitation and salting-out. Precipitation and salting-out are similar in that both result in a substance coming out of the solution. Salting-out, however, is a particular kind of precipitation in which the substance is thrown out of solution because another has been dissolved. Protein precipitants and substances causing salting-out include alcohol, acetone, neutral salts, heavy metal salts, and some acids. In some instances, addition of excess solvent will cause a redissolution of the protein; in other instances, the precipitation is not reversible.

(3) Coagulation. Irreversible precipitation of proteins is known as coagulation. This reaction is preceded by denaturation in which some of the bonds of the protein are ruptured, forming an insoluable substance. We have previously described the coagulation of proteins in inorganic chemistry with the experiment of a heavy metal salt introduced into egg white. Frying or boiling an egg demonstrates the effect of heat on proteins.

(4) Classification. The classification of proteins is based upon their solubility and upon the results of their hydrolysis. Proteins cannot be isolated as pure individual compounds with distinct properties, so a really satisfactory chemical classification is impossible.

(a) Simple proteins. These are the proteins which yield only alpha amino acids or derivatives of alpha amino acids when broken down into simpler compounds. In this class fall:

- Albumins (egg albumin, blood serum albumin).
- Globulins (serum globulin of blood).
- Glutelins (glutenin in wheat).
- Prolamines (gliadin from wheat).
- Albuminoids (elastin in tendons; keratin in hair; collagen in connective tissue).
- Histones (histone from the thymus gland).
- Protamines (salmin in salmon sperm).

(b) Conjugated proteins. These are combinations of simple proteins and other nonprotein groups.

- Chromoproteins (hemoglobin in red corpuscles).
- Glycoproteins (mucin from saliva).
- Phosphoproteins (casin in milk).
- Nucleoproteins (nuclein from cell nuclei).
- Lipoproteins (lecithin + protein).

(c) Derived proteins. These are proteins produced by chemical action on naturally occurring proteins.

1. Primary protein derivatives:

- Proteans.
- Metaproteins.
- Coagulated proteins.

2. Secondary protein derivatives:

- Proteoses.
- Peptones.
- Peptides.

(5) The importance of proteins. Proteins supply the specific amino acids important to life and health which cannot be manufactured in the body. They are essential to growth and repair of tissues. Industrially, proteins are used in the manufacture and processing of leather, gelatin, glue, ice cream, cheese, textiles, and plastics.

(6) Pharmaceutically important amino acids and proteins.

(a) Fibrinogen (Human Fibrinogen) is a blood plasma clotting factor.

(b) Gelatin, obtained from the skin, connective tissue, and bones of animals, is a pharmaceutical necessity for capsules, emulsions, and suppositories, as well as a nutritive substance.

(c) Gelfoam, a sterile, pliable, nonantigenic surgical sponge prepared from gelatin,

is used by itself or saturated with thrombin, as a hemostat.

(d) Glutamic acid hydrochloride is a gastric acidifier which is used in conditions where insufficient or no acid is naturally secreted, as in the achlorhydria of pernicious anemia.

(e) Infant formulas. The prepared liquid and powdered formulas used for feeding infants during their first few months of life are mainly protein portions of milk.

(f) Methionine (Meonine) is a sulfur-containing amino acid used in the prevention and treatment of liver damage.

(g) Protamine sulfate is an antidote for an overdose of heparin (an anticoagulant).

(h) Protein hydrolysates are solutions of amino acids and short chain peptides. They are used as nutritive agents where oral intake of proteins is limited. They are generally administered IV and only in severely ill patients.

(i) *Others.* Many other official products contain proteins but are placed in their more specific categories. Such compounds are enzymes, some hormones, biologicals, surgical sutures, and mild silver protein.

24. Volatile oils. The volatile or essential oils are found in various plant organs and tissues. Generally, they are the odorous and taste-bearing principles of the plants in which they occur. Volatile oils may contain hydrocarbons, alcohols, acids, esters, aldehydes, ketones, phenols, lactones, nitrogen compounds, and sulfur compounds.

a. *Properties.* Volatile oils differ widely in taste, smell, composition, density, and boiling range.

- Pure oils are colorless, becoming varicolored on exposure to air.
- The most distinctive property of the individual oil is its odor.
- The taste of volatile oils varies from sweet to mild, pungent, hot, acrid, caustic, or burning.
- The majority of the volatile oils are lighter than water; their specific gravity varies from about 0.8 to 1.17.
- Most of the oils are optically active (dextro or levorotatory).
- Most oils are not water soluble, but on contact with water they dramatically flavor and scent it. They are soluble in alcohol, ether, chloroform, oils, fats, and resins.
- Because of their volatility, these oils should be stored in well-filled, tightly stoppered amber bottles, away from light and heat.

b. *Preparation.* Volatile oils are generally obtained from plants through distillation, steam distillation, expression, or extraction. These four processes are explained in chapter 6.

c. *Important pharmaceutical volatile oils and preparations.*

(1) Oils used almost exclusively for their flavoring ability are—

• Lavender oil	• Rose oil
• Peppermint oil	• Lemon oil
• Spearmint oil	• Orange oil
• Cinnamon oil	• Anise oil
• Sassafras oil	• Caraway oil
• Cherry juice	• Fennel oil
• Raspberry juice	• Cardamon oil

(2) *Other oils.* Other oils are used as carminatives, germicides, diuretics, perfumes, condiments, stimulants (local), astringents, preservatives, antiseptics, toothache drops, expectorants, and inhalants for bronchial infections.

25. Carbohydrates. We have discussed in the preceding parts of this chapter two types of food substances, the fats and oils, and the proteins. The third food substance, the carbohydrates, is at least as important as the others.

a. *Composition.* Chemically, the carbohydrates are polyhydroxy aldehydes or ketones, or organic compounds which on hydrolysis yield polyhydroxyaldehydes or ketones. They are definite chemical compounds, not merely hydrated forms of carbon. Widely distributed in nature, they are obtained from the plant kingdom and used by the animal kingdom.

b. *Classification.* The diagrammatic breakdown of the carbohydrate class of compounds shown in figure 1 will be helpful to you in understanding the relative position of the various subclasses involved. The diagrammatic breakdown of the carbohydrate family illustrates that it is subdivided first into two broad categories, the sugars and the nonsugars. The sugars are sweet and water soluble.

(1) *Monosaccharides.* Within the subclass of sugars is a group which contains three

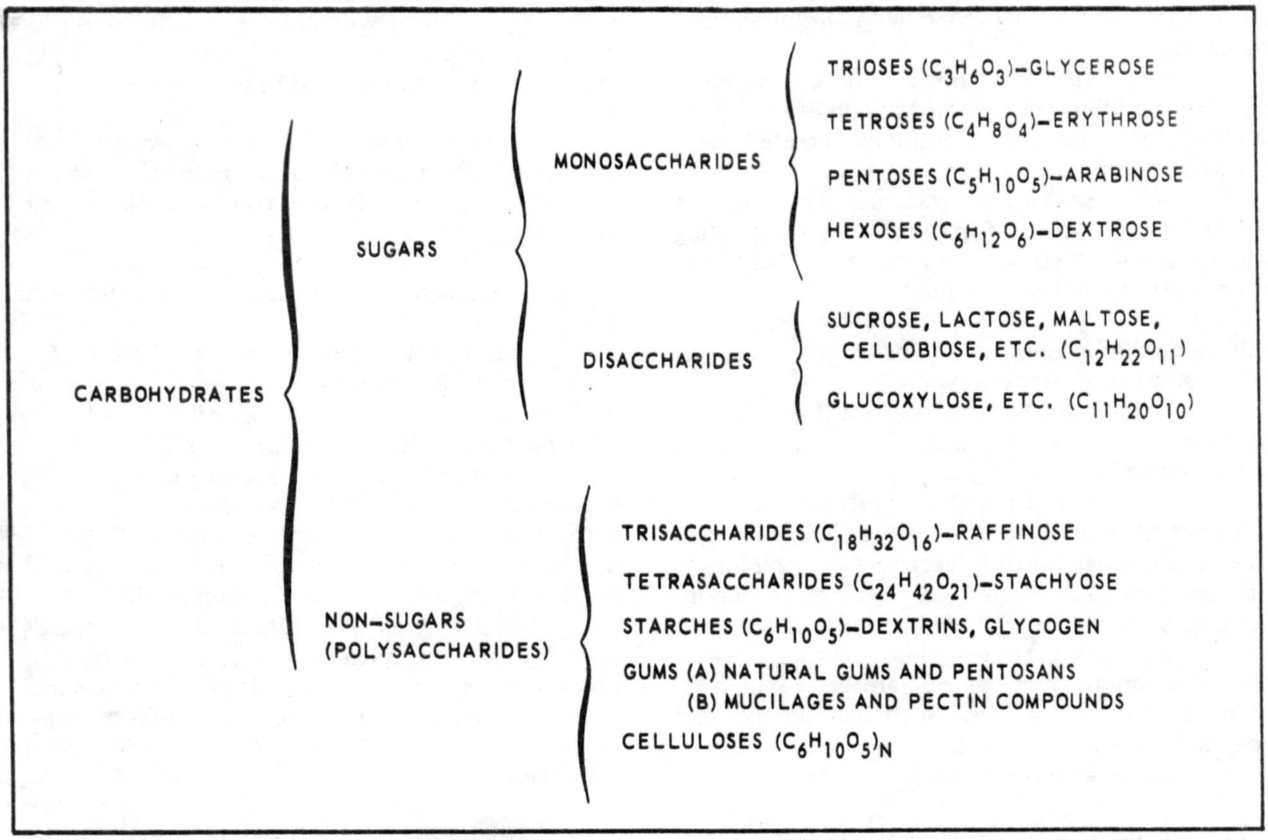

Figure 1. Diagrammatic breakdown of the carbohydrates.

or more carbons and cannot be hydrolyzed. These are the monosaccharides. These sugars are naturally occurring.

(2) Disaccharides. Sugars which are made up of two molecules of monosaccharides are called disaccharides. Upon hydrolysis, these disaccharides are broken down into the two separate monosaccharides of which they are composed.

(3) Polysaccharides. The more complex carbohydrates, which on hydrolysis are broken down into three, four, or more monosaccharide units, are the polysaccharides.

c. *Stereoisomerism.* Stereoisomerism is a long and complex idea involving many different types of isomers. It will serve our purposes adequately to explain that stereoisomerism is due to spatial rather than structural arrangement and that the two most common forms of stereoisomerism are geometric and optical.

(1) Geometric isomerism. Isomers are formed because some factor, such as double bond, prevents free rotation of the atoms within the molecule. The isomers formed by geometric isomerism are termed cis- and trans- and the difference is shown below in the diagrams of the two geometric forms of butenedioic acid.

cis-form trans-form

The double bond illustrated holds the atoms from rotating, and thus there are two distinctly different geometric possibilities.

(2) Optical isomerism. In optical isomerism, the isomers differ in their ability to rotate polarized light, due to asymmetrical structure or crystalline structure.

(a) Asymmetric atom. An asymmetric atom (in our study it will always be a carbon atom) is one which has four different atoms or radicals attached to it. Glyceraldehyde has one asymmetric carbon atom. This carbon has attached to it a hydrogen, a hydroxyl group, an aldehyde group, and an alcohol group.

(b) Mirror images. Hold your hands up in front of you with the palms turned in. What you see are two identical five-fingered extremities. They are identical in every respect except that they are mirror images of each other. The isomers formed in optical isomerism are similarly mirror images of each other.

(c) Polarized light. A film or crystal that allows only light vibrating in one direction to pass is a polarizer. The lenses of polaroid sunglasses are an example. Light vibrating in every direction approaches the lens, but only light vibrating in one plane passes; the remainder is stopped by the lens. A second polarizer placed crosswise to the first will exclude the light passed by the first. The illustration in figure 2 shows light being polarized.

(d) Optical rotation. When polarized light is passed through a solution of an optically active substance, it will be diverted either to the left or to the right. A substance which rotates the light to the right is called the dextro (d-) or (+) isomer. That which rotates the light to the left is the levo- (l-) or (-) isomer. A mixture of 50 percent each of the d- and l-isomers will produce no rotation. Such a mixture is called a racemic mixture.

(e) Enantiomorphs. Looking again at glyceraldehyde, you see that there are two optical isomers, each the mirror image of the other. Such isomers are called enantiomorphs (from the Greek meaning "opposite form").

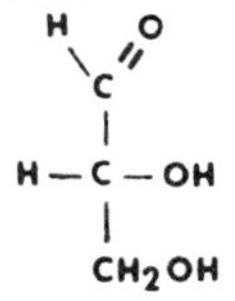

d-glyceraldehyde

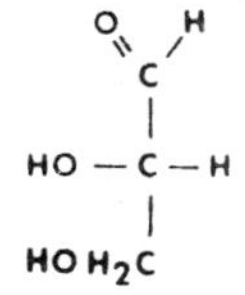

l-glyceraldehyde

(f) Nomenclature. In naming optical isomers, we wish to know two things: the spatial arrangement of the atoms (configuration) and the direction of optical rotation. If the OH group nearest the end opposite the carbonyl group is on the right, it has the D configuration. If on the left, it has the L configuration.

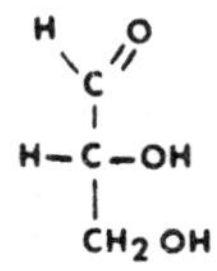

Glyceraldehyde

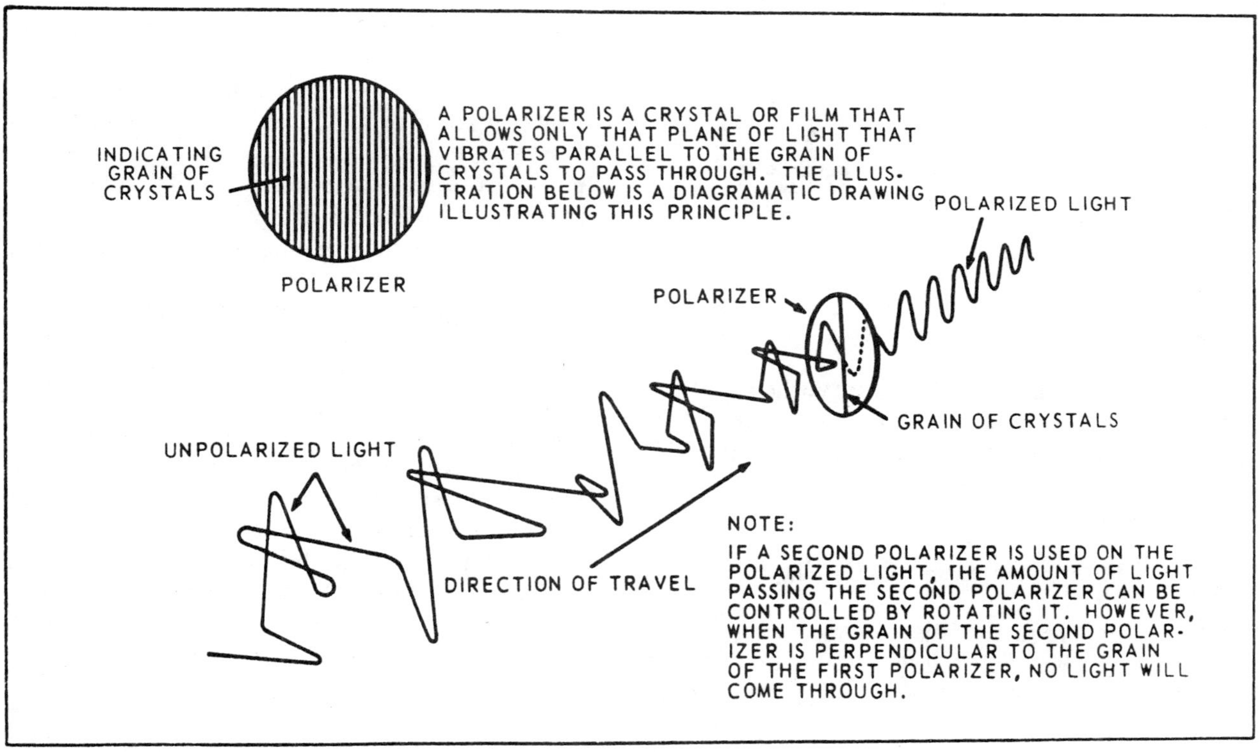

Figure 2. Principle of polarization.

Under this system, the compound above becomes D-(+) glyceraldehyde. The OH on the carbon farthest from the carbonyl group is on the right side, thus the D-. By experiment, this compound is found to rotate the light to the right, thus the (+). If the compound were to rotate the light to the left, it would have been called D-(-) glyceraldehyde.

(g) Number of enantiomorphs. Each asymmetric carbon atom can yield two enantiomorphs, and as the number of asymmetric carbons increases, the number of isomers increases. The possible number of enantiomorphs for a compound is 2^x, in which the x stands for the number of asymmetrical carbons.

d. Monosaccharides. The simplest carbohydrates are the monosaccharides. They cannot be broken down by hydrolysis. Monosaccharides are classified according to the number of carbon atoms they contain. If a monosaccharide contains five carbon atoms it is known as a pentose; one containing six carbons is a hexose. These are the most common types of monosaccharides. Carbohydrates are further classified as aldoses or ketoses to indicate whether they are aldehydes or ketones. The most common monosaccharide, glucose, is an aldohexose, a six-carbon sugar containing an aldehyde group.

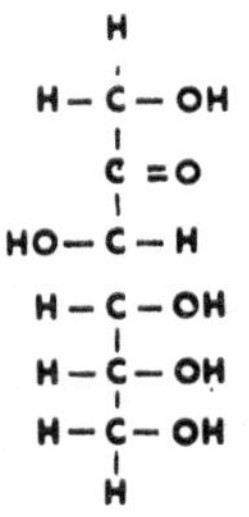

D-Fructose, a ketohexose

(1) Glucose. In photosynthesis, plants take carbon dioxide and water, in the presence of sunlight, and manufacture glucose. As a byproduct of this reaction, oxygen is liberated into the atmosphere.

$$\text{Energy} + 6CO_2 + 6H_2O \longrightarrow C_6H_{12}O_6 + 6O_2\uparrow$$

In man and animals, the reverse takes place; glucose is broken down into carbon dioxide and water, and in the process usable energy is liberated.

(a) Formula.

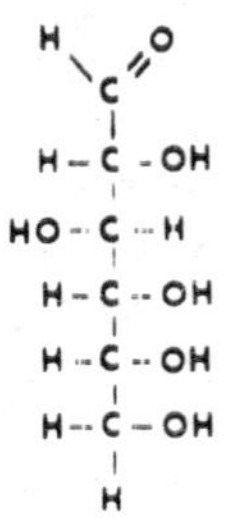

D (+) Glucose

(b) Occurrence and preparation. Glucose, which is also known as dextrose, is widely distributed in nature, and made commercially by the breakdown of starch. It is the carbohydrate used by the body tissues and is the sugar most commonly found in blood and other body fluid. In sugar diabetes (diabetes mellitus), it is dextrose that appears in large quantities in the blood and urine.

(c) Uses. Glucose is used as a food substance and a sweetening agent. Patients who, for one reason or another, cannot be fed by the normal oral route are given intravenous feedings of sterile glucose solution.

(d) Preparations.

- Dextrose (D-glucose; grape sugar) a sweetish granular crystalline substance, is the principal source of energy in the human body. It is stored in the liver in the form of glycogen. Dextrose may be either hydrous or anhydrous; the container's label must specify the type.
- Dextrose injection is a sterile solution of dextrose intended for intravenous administration. It may be used, depending upon the purpose, in concentrations ranging from 5 to 50 percent. The 5-percent solution is isotonic with the blood and is intended as a blood volume replenisher. Higher concentrations are intended as nutrients and diuretics. Bacteriostatic agents are not allowed in this preparation because it is given in large quantities which could provide the patient with excessive doses of the bacteriostatic agent at the same time. Because of the absence of any bacteriostatic agent, this preparation must be meticulously sterilized and that portion which is not immediately used when the container is opened should be discarded. Units showing any sign of turbidity should not be used.

• Dextrose and sodium chloride injection is a nutrient and fluid and electrolyte replenisher.

(2) Fructose (levulose).

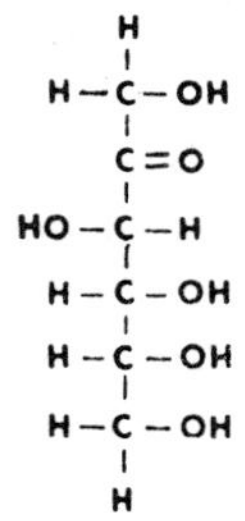

Fructose is a monosaccharide and the only official ketone sugar. It is levorotatory.

(a) Occurrence. Fructose occurs naturally, chemically united with glucose in our common table sugar and in honey. It is the sweetest sugar known.

(b) Uses. Fructose is commonly employed as a nutrient and sweetening agent.

(c) Preparations.

• Fructose injection is used as a parenteral nutrient, as it is more rapidly metabolized than dextrose. Fructose can be injected in concentrations twice as strong as dextrose without ill effects. It is especially useful in nutrition or hydration of diabetics as they can tolerate fructose almost normally.

• Fructose and sodium chloride injection is used either as a nutrient or as an electrolyte replenisher for patients in bad states of nutrition.

e. Disaccharides. Chemically, disaccharides are "double sugars," that is, two molecules of monosaccharides linked chemically.

(1) Sucrose (saccharum; sugar; cane sugar; beet sugar). Sucrose is a combination of the monosaccharide units, glucose and fructose. It is commercially obtained from sugar cane, sugar beet, and sorghum. Upon hydrolysis, sucrose yields a mixture of glucose and fructose; the combination is frequently referred to as invert sugar. Invert sugar is sweeter, more easily digested, and more rapidly assimilated than sucrose. Sucrose is a nutrient and is subject to contamination by molds and bacteria. In very high concentrations, as in syrup, the osmotic pressure is so high that it acts as bactericide by dehydrating the organisms which it contacts. Pharmaceutically, sucrose is of major importance in the preparation of syrup which is an 85-percent solution of sugar in water. Syrup is used as a sweet vehicle.

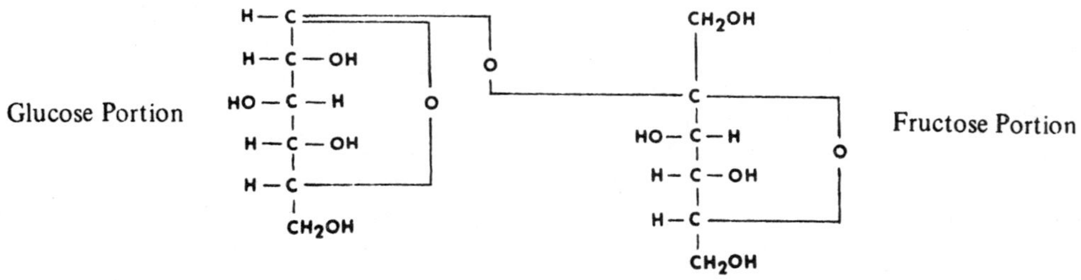

(2) Lactose (saccharum lactis; milk sugar). Lactose is the disaccharide most commonly found in both human and cow's milk and is commonly called milk sugar. Upon hydrolysis it breaks down into the two monosaccharides, glucose and galactose. Though not as sweet tasting as some of the other sugars, lactose is easily digested and is a common ingredient in baby formulas. Milk sugar is used in pharmacy as a diluting agent in most capsules, tablets, and hypodermic tablets. Specially refined, beta-lactose is more soluble than ordinary lactose and is preferred, especially for the hypodermic tablets. Lactose is often an ingredient in the nutrient medium used in the culture of the *Penicillium notatum* organism.

Glucose Portion

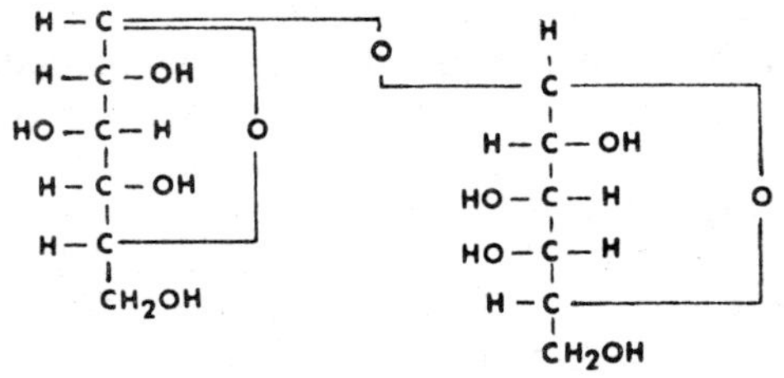

Galactose Portion

(3) Relative sweetness. In discussing the sugars, we have indicated that they vary in sweetness. It may be interesting for you to note the relative sweetness of some of the sugars. The formulation below shows the relative sweetness of several of the sugars compared to sucrose, which has been given the arbitrary value of 100.

Fructose	173
Invert sugar	123
Sucrose	100
Glucose	74
Maltose	32
Galactose	32
Lactose	16

f. Polysaccharides. At the beginning of our discussion of the carbohydrate family, we subdivided carbohydrates into sugars and nonsugars; the sugars were further subdivided into monosaccharides and disaccharides, which we have already discussed. The nonsugars, or polysaccharides, are actually broken down into starches, gums, and celluloses. Rather than going into discussion of the nonsugars by class, we will merely mention and state some facts about the more important substances and agents which will fall into this category of nonsugars.

(1) Starch (amylum; corn starch):

(a) Occurrence. Starch is naturally occurring in plants such as corn, potatoes, rice, tapioca, and wheat. Plants store starch for the same reason animals store glycogen, that is, as a reserve source of energy. Glycogen is often called animal starch. Starch occurs as small granules which, under microscope, reveal a very distinct shape which varies with the source from which it is obtained.

(b) Properties. Starch is not soluble in cold water, but in boiling water it forms a milky solution or paste. When heated alone, starch breaks down into gummy dextrins. In the ironing of clothes treated with starch, the dextrins formed give the material a stiff, shiny finish. Dextrins in water solution are used as adhesives. Iodine is a test for starch, yielding a bright blue color.

(c) Uses. Starch is categorized as a pharmaceutical necessity and is an ingredient in many official preparations. It is a good absorbent, filling agent, dusting powder, and tablet disintegrator. On contact with the liquids in the stomach, the starch grains absorb the moisture, swell, and physically disintegrate the tablet.

(2) Cotton. Cotton is a complex polysaccharide of natural origin. It is not soluble or digestible, and is of no food value. It is the most widely used surgical absorbent. It is official in the USP and must meet very specific requirements. Official cotton must be free of impurities, have no fatty matter, must be bleached white, and be sterilized in its final container. It must meet strenuous standards for fiber length, and water absorbability. There are specific instructions for its storage and labeling.

(3) Acacia (gum arabic). Acacia may be in the form of flakes or powder and is used in the

pharmacy as a suspending or emulsifying agent and as a demulcent. Acacia is soluble in water, producing a colloidal solution known as a mucilage. Such solutions are incompatible with high alcoholic solutions and other organic solvents.

(4) Pectin. Pectin is a purified carbohydrate from citrus fruit and apple pulp. It is a coarse or fine powder and slightly yellowish in color. It dissolves in about 20 times its weight in water and forms a thick colloidal solution. Pectin is not digested in the human alimentary canal and forms a thick protective coating on the intestinal wall. In combination with kaolin, it is usually efficacious in symptomatic treatment of diarrhea. Pectin is used commercially as a jelling agent in making jellies and has further pharmaceutical application as an emulsion stabilizer.

(5) Agar (agar-agar). Agar, when dissolved in water, forms a gel which can absorb five or more times its weight of water. The gel is used as a culture medium for bacteria and as a stabilizer in emulsions.

(6) Tragacanth. Tragacanth absorbs water and swells to form a soft adhesive mucilage which is used in the base for sterile lubricants and nasal jellies. It is also used as an adhesive in pills and troches; as a suspending agent; as an adjuvant to emulsifiers to retard creaming and to increase consistency; and as a soothing application or demulcent.

(7) Plantago seed (psyllium seed). Plantago seed is indigestible and mucilaginous and acts as a mild cathartic. Metamucil makes use of the actions of the plantago seed.

(8) Methylcellulose (Methocel). Methylcellulose, a neutral, odorless, tasteless, and inert substance, is a synthetic substitute for gums and mucilages. It is used as a dispersing, thickening, emulsifying, and coating agent, and as a bulk laxative. It is used in eye drops, nose drops, creams, lotions, burn preparations, and in cosmetics and dentifrices. Tablets of methylcellulose taken internally with water produce a normal, non-straining bowel evacuation for chronic constipation. Its bulking ability is also of value in satisfying the empty feeling of diet patients.

26. Glycosides. Glycosides are organic compounds consisting of a combination of sugars with nonsugar molecules. The pharmaceutically important glycosides are naturally occurring in plants and are only rarely found in animals.

a. Structure. Upon hydrolysis, the glycosides break down into one or more sugar molecules and one or more nonsugar molecules. The nonsugar portion is termed the aglycone. The most commonly occurring sugar found in glycoside molecules is glucose, and those compounds containing glucose are called glucosides. Glycosides, including glucosides, may be alpha or beta, and as shown in the graphic formulas below, the alpha form is that in which the OR group (OCH_3 in this case) is on the same side as the OH of the second carbon atom.

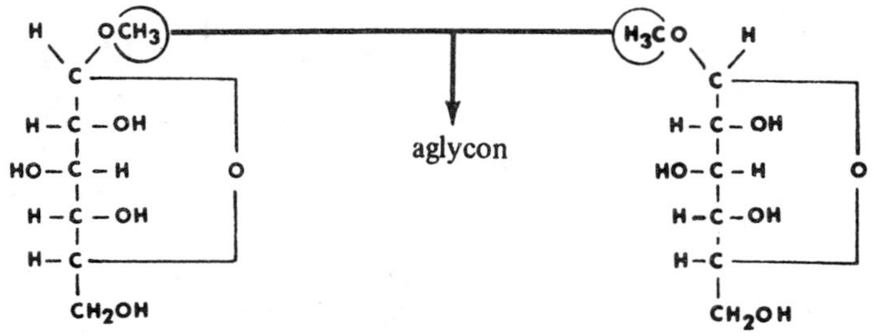

a–Methylglucoside *β–Methylglucoside*

b. Properties. Generally, the glycosides are colorless or white, optically active, alcohol or dilute-alcohol soluble extracts. They may be classified by a number of methods, based upon chemical grouping, occurrence, or therapeutic application.

c. Classes of glycosides. The two most important classes of glycosides, pharmaceutically, are the cardiac and the cathartic glycosides.

(1) Cardiac glycosides. Often referred to as the digitaloid drugs, the cardiac glycosides are not all glycosides, nor are they all derived from digitalis. However, the aglycone portions of the molecules are all very similar chemically and the actions are almost identical except for the onset and duration of action. These medications strengthen the contraction of heart muscle and are sometimes called cardiotonic drugs. Their main application is in the treatment of congestive heart failure. Digitalis is the prototype of this class.

(a) Digitalis (foxglove; digitalis leaf). Digitalis is the dried leaf of *Digitalis purpurea.* It is biologically standardized, one USP unit being the smallest quantity necessary to kill a pigeon. One hundred mg. of the powder equals one unit. After exhaustive investigation, scientists agree that the most important constituents of digitalis are digitoxin, gitoxin, digoxin, and lanatoside C.

(b) Digitoxin (Crystodigin; Purodigin).

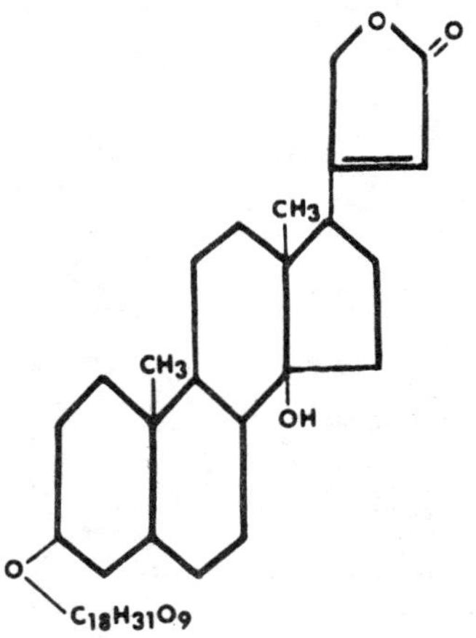

Digitoxin is the primary active glycoside in official digitalis and its action is similar tc that of digitalis.

(c) Digoxin (Lanoxin).

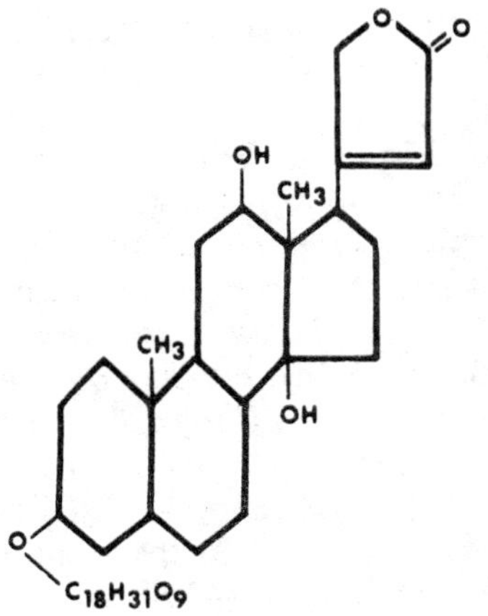

Digoxin is the cardiac glycoside from the leaves of *Digitalis lanata.* Its action, although of less duration, is similar to digitalis.

(d) Lanatoside C (Cedilanid).

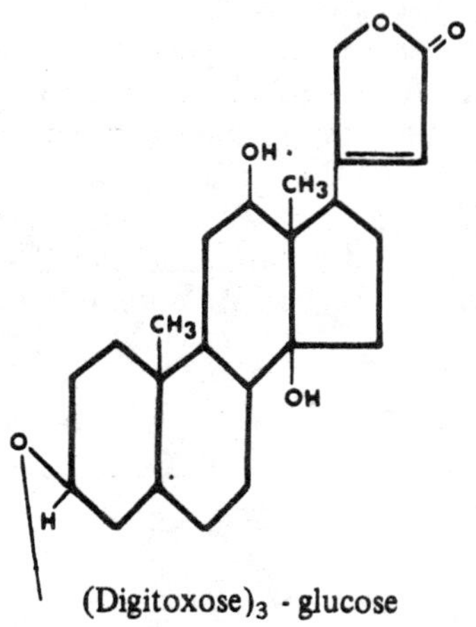

Lanatocide C is a cardiotonic glycoside from *Digitalis lanata.* As you can see, the aglycone is identical with that of digoxin.

(2) Cathartic glycosides. The cathartic glycosides or the anthroquinone purgatives, as they are sometimes called, are contained in such official drugs as cascara and senna. Upon ingestion, these drugs are assimilated in the GI tract, circulated through the blood stream, and are carried to the large intestine where, through their irritant action, they produce catharsis.

(a) Cascara sagrada.

(b) Senna (senna leaf).

(c) Danthron (Dorbane).

Danthron is a synthetic cathartic derived from anthraquinone.

27. Steroids. The steroids are a class of compounds found in both plants and animals with cyclopenta-phenanthrene as their basic structure. These include sterols, bile acids, sex hormones, adrenocortical hormones, and some miscellaneous substances.

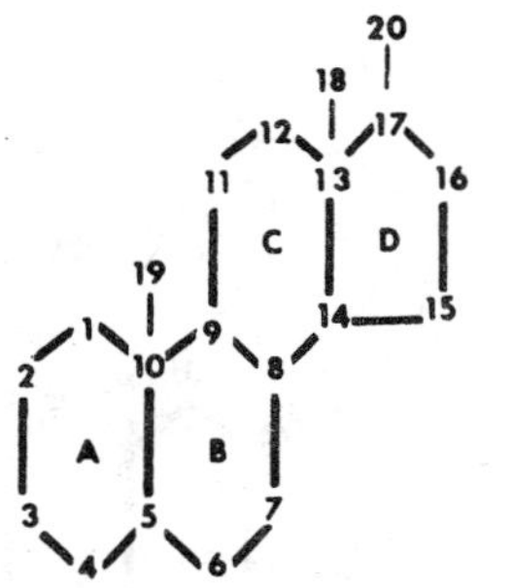

Perhydro-cyclopenta-phenanthrene

a. Sterols. The sterols have been previously mentioned in the discussion of fats, fixed oils, and waxes. Chemically, they have the cyclopenta-phenanthrene nucleus, with an aliphatic side chain at the 20 position, a CH_3 at the 18th and 19th carbon, and an alcohol (OH) group at the 3d carbon. They are secondary alcohols. The most important sterol is cholesterol (or cholesterin), a zoosterol. It is a component of gallstones and brain and spinal cords. The brain and spinal cords of animals are first saponified; the remaining unsaponifiable matter yields cholesterol. In recent years there has been much concern over the significance of cholesterol in the body and human diet. Normal human blood contains cholesterol in colloidal solution. If the concentration becomes too high, the cholesterol precipitates out of its colloidal solution and deposits on the walls of the arteries and heart to cause a type of sclerosis.

b. Bile salts. The bile salts are a group of very similar acids, the bile acids, chemically joined to glycine and taurine (amino acids). The parent compound of this group is cholic acid, shown below.

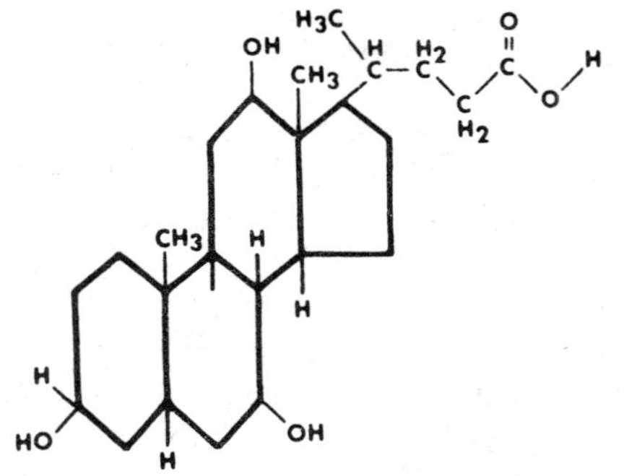

Bile salts emulsify the fats consumed in our diet and make them more readily reactive with the natural enzymes. The bile salts are necessary for the proper absorption of the fat-soluble vitamins. Dehydrocholic acid (Decholin) is the oxidation product of cholic acid. It causes an increase in biliary secretion when given in the form of a tablet, or the soluble salt (sodium dehydrocholate) by injection.

c. Sex hormones. Hormones are secreted by glands into the blood stream. They regulate other organs. The anterior lobe of the pituitary gland secretes a gonadotropic substance which causes the gonads to develop, both in the male and in the female. These glands, in response, manufacture and secrete their own hormones.

(1) Female hormones.

(a) Estradiol.

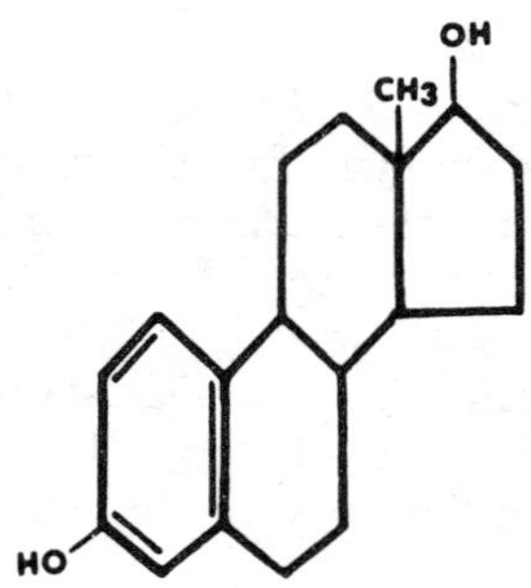

Estradiol is the basic female hormone. Notice that the A ring in this tetracyclic compound is aromatic and thus the OH group is a phenolic, rather than an alcohol group, giving the compound the stability and chemical reactivity of a phenol.

(b) Estrone. Estrone is closely related chemically to estradiol.

(c) Diethylstilbestrol (Stilbestrol).

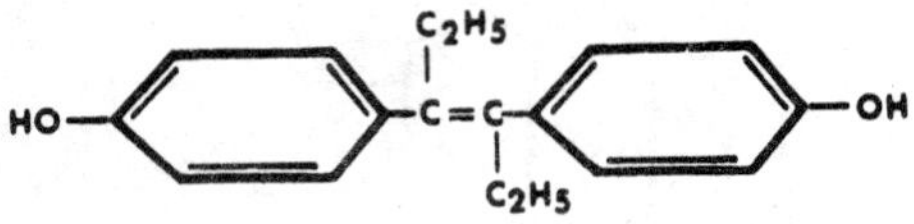

Diethylstilbestrol is one of the most popular and most widely used of preparations of this type. It is frequently used after childbirth to treat engorgement of the breasts and suppress lactation. Diethylstilbestrol is synthetic.

(2) Male hormones. The male hormones, called androgens, are also steroids. Testosterone is the basic hormone of this group of agents and is graphically represented below.

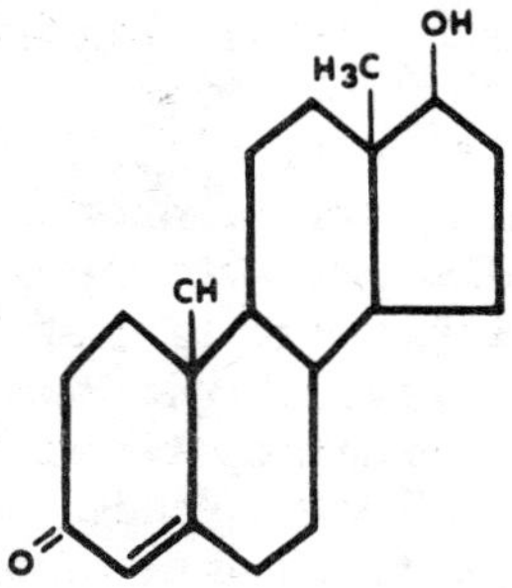

Other agents are methyltestosterone and norethandrolone.

d. Adrenal cortex hormones. Although it is possible for the human to survive without the adrenal cortex and the hormones produced by it, serious repercussions are displayed. Over 44 steroids have been isolated from the adrenal cortex, 7 of which elicit a biological effect. Notice the structural similarity between the corticosteroids in the opposite column and on the following page.

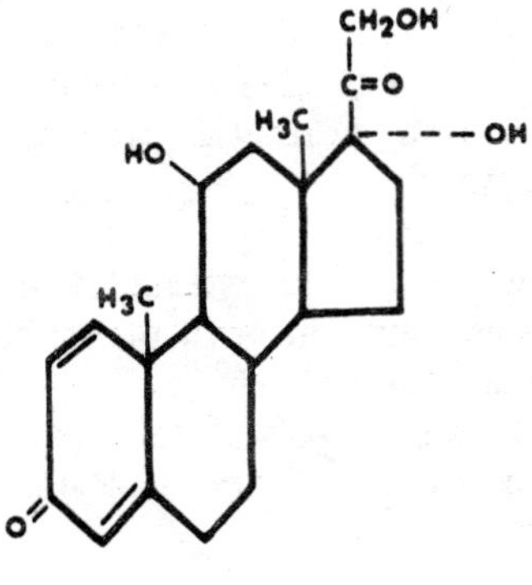

Prednisone

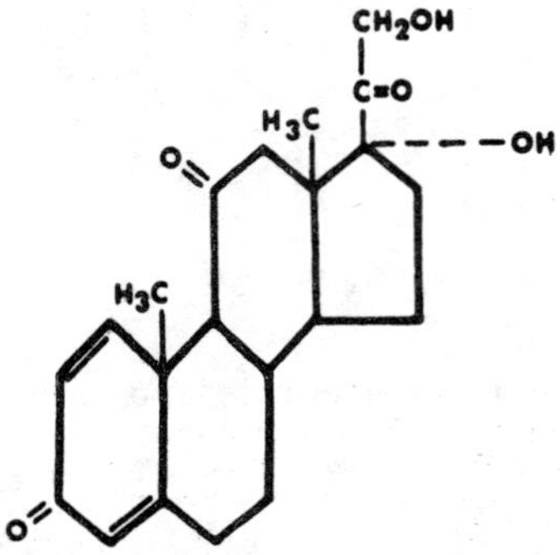

Prednisolone

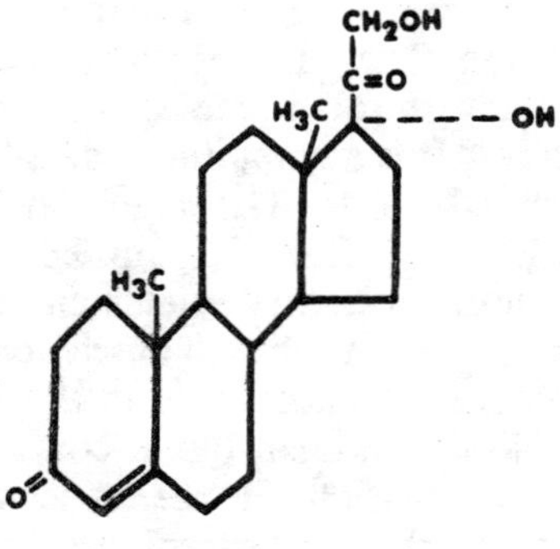

Cortisone

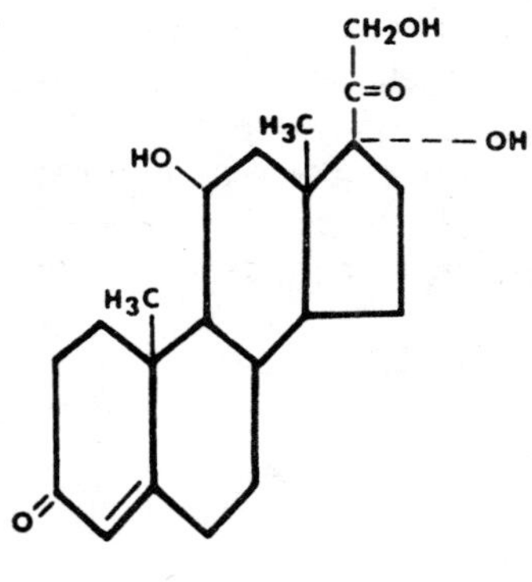

Hydrocortisone

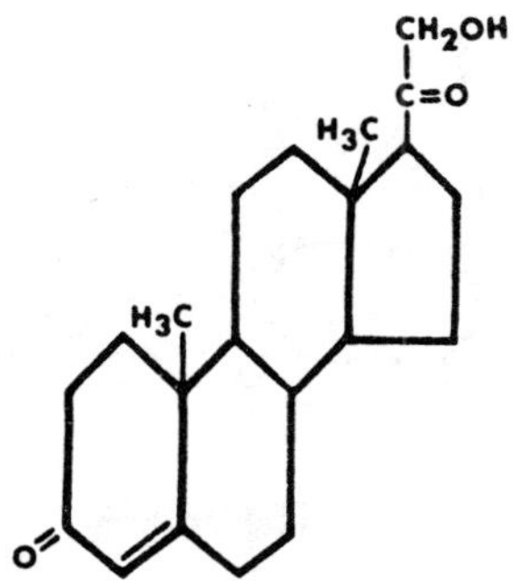

Desoxycortisone

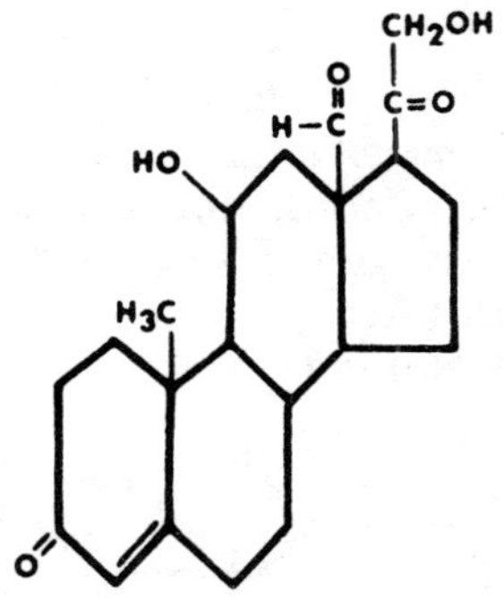

Aldosterone

28. **Plant drugs.** The plant drugs were first called vegetable alkalies, but later renamed alkaloids, meaning alkali-like. These are the active principles in plants. Centuries ago, crude plants were used as poisons; these included plants such as poison hemlock and deadly nightshade. Others were made into teas and extracts for curative uses. In the early 1800's, it was found that the alkaloidal content was the effective ingredient of these plants. Since then hundreds of alkaloids have been isolated, including some of the most important pharmaceutically. Despite the large number of alkaloids already in use, only about 5 percent of the plant kingdom has been explored for medicinal value. At present a systematic screening process has been initiated to identify new and therapeutically useful agents in the plant world. Although most of the alkaloids are physiologically active, their responses are greatly varied. Some depress, while others stimulate. Some are miotic, others mydriatic. Some raise blood pressure, others lower it.

a. General properties of the alkaloids.

(1) Alkaloids are complex organic compounds containing nitrogen and it is the nitrogen which confers the alkali-like property to them.

(2) The vast majority of the alkaloids are of plant origin, but a few are derived from the animal kingdom.

(3) The majority are naturally occurring. A few, however, are either completely or partially synthetic.

(4) Most are physiologically active; their responses vary.

(5) Almost all of the alkaloids are white or colorless crystalline powders. Nicotine is a liquid; sanguanarine and berberine are red and yellow, respectively.

(6) Most of the alkaloids are chemical compounds which are comprised of carbon, hydrogen, nitrogen, and oxygen. The liquid alkaloids contain no oxygen.

(7) Alkaloidal solutions are alkaline in reaction and therefore react with acids to form salts.

(8) Alkaloids are generally insoluble in water, but their salts are water soluble. Sulfates and hydrochlorides are the most widely used salts.

(9) Most of the alkaloids are optically active.

(10) Most have a bitter taste, and many are violently poisonous.

(11) The alkaloids have many incompatibilities. Preparations containing them should be carefully scrutinized for the possibility of incompatibility. Some alkaloidal precipitants are the heavy metals, tannic acid, and the tannins.

b. Nuclei (or fragments of nuclei) common to the alkaloids.

in the Orient where, in many areas, it grows wild. The capsules of the Papaver somniferum (opium poppy) are slit and the exudate collected, air-dried, and powdered to yield opium. From the opium plant can be extracted more than 20 different alkaloids, of which only a few are important to the physician and pharmacist. Powdered opium contains 9.5 percent of anhydrous morphine. It is

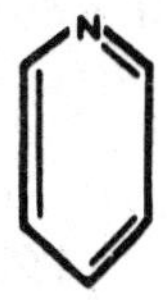

Pyridine

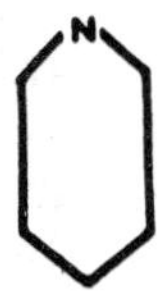

Piperidine

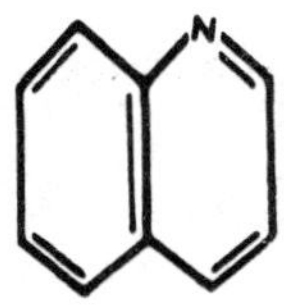

Quinoline

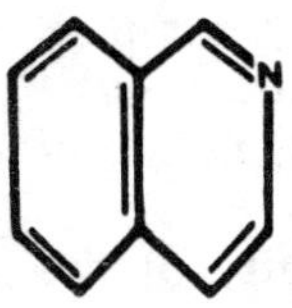

Isoquinoline

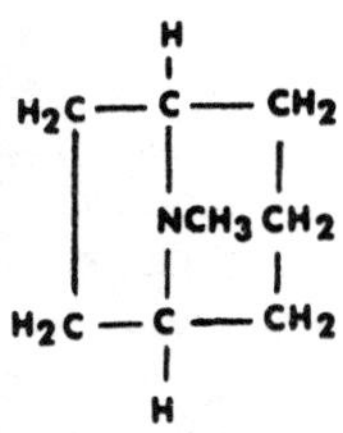

Tropane

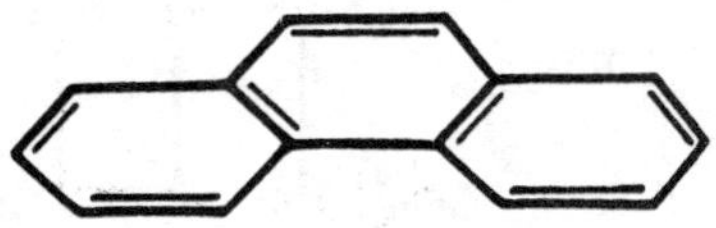

Phenanthrene

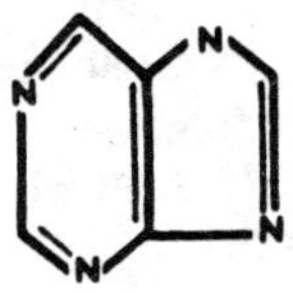

Purine

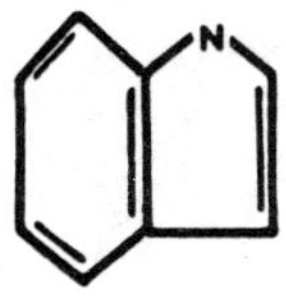

Indole

c. Pharmaceutically important alkaloids. The pharmaceutically important alkaloids can be conveniently divided into seven subcategories: opium alkaloids, cinchona alkaloids, tropane alkaloids, xanthine alkaloids, ergot alkaloids, rauwolfia alkaloids, and miscellaneous alkaloids.

(1) Opium alkaloids. Opium is one of the oldest medications known to man. The plant from which it is obtained has long been cultivated

used mainly in the manufacture of the two more commonly prescribed forms, opium tincture and paregoric. Opium is firmly regulated by the Controlled Substances Act.

(a) Morphine.

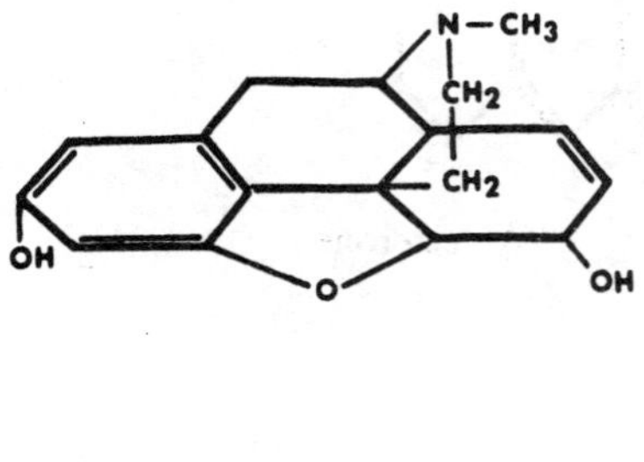

Morphine, the first opium alkaloid to be discovered, is a member of the phenanthrene group. It is of tremendous importance to the physician and the patient and, used properly, is an effective analgesic, sedative, hypnotic, and respiratory depressant. However, addiction is one of its drawbacks. Morphine is generally used in the form of soluble salts, particularly the sulfate. It cannot be stressed too often that morphine is a potent, addicting drug which must be rigidly controlled. The penalties for mishandling this and related drugs are very severe.

(b) Codeine.

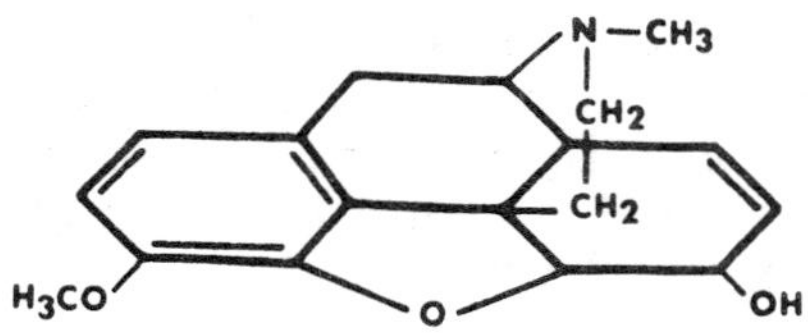

Codeine may be obtained either from the opium plant or made by methylating morphine. It is also official in the form of its phosphate and sulfate salts. The phosphate is more soluble. It is used as an analgesic and cough suppressor.

(c) Dihydrocodeinone bitartrate (Hydrocodone; Hycodan). Dihydrocodeinone is a semisynthetic agent prepared from codeine. It has the same antitussive qualities as codeine and is equally addicting.

(d) Dextromethorphan hydrobromide (Romilar).

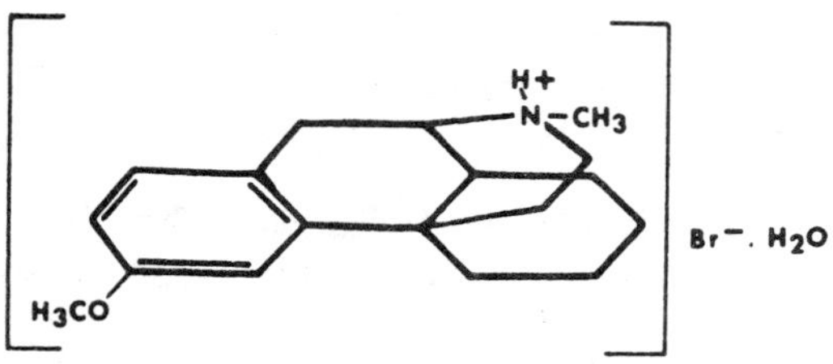

Dextromethorphan is a synthetic morphine derivative with no addicting qualities. It is effective against the cough reflex for which it is used exclusively. Dextromethorphan has no analgesic action.

(e) Propoxyphene hydrochloride (Darvon).

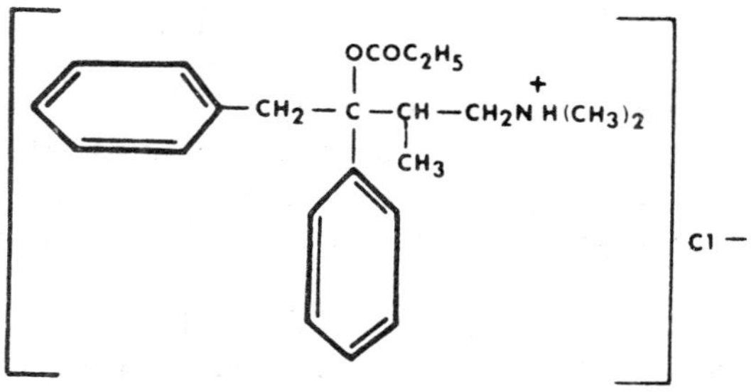

Dextropropoxyphene is a synthetic analgesic which is not addicting and has no antitussive properties.

(f) Levopropoxyphene (Novrad). Levopropoxyphene, an isomer of d-propoxyphene, has been recently found to have excellent antitussive properties and no analgesic or antipyretic properties.

(g) Meperidine hydrochloride (Demerol HCl).

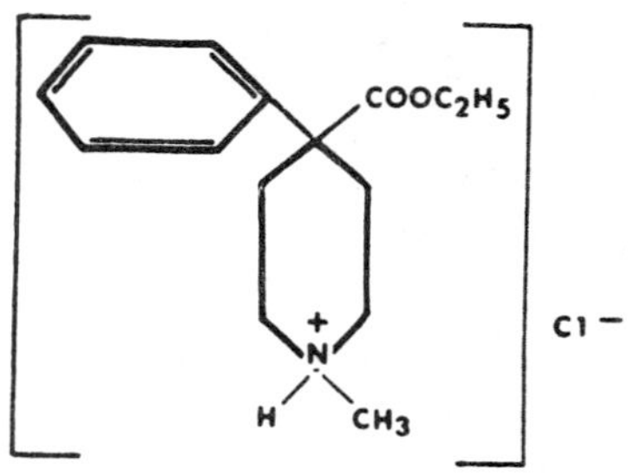

Meperidine produces sedation and analgesia.

(h) Papaverine hydrochloride.

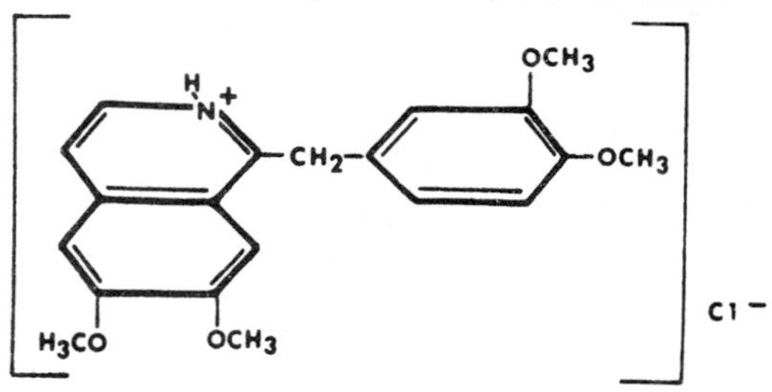

Papaverine is obtained from opium or prepared synthetically. It is an isoquinoline derivative. Papaverine is a smooth muscle relaxant. It is nonaddicting and not controlled as a narcotic drug.

(i) Other natural and synthetic derivatives.

- Hydromorphone (Dilaudid).
- Diacetylmorphine (heroin).
- Apomorphine hydrochloride.
- Methadone hydrochloride (Dolophine HCl).

(2) Cinchona alkaloids. The cinchona tree is indigenous to the Far East and Latin America. Its bark contains useful alkaloids related to quinoline. The crude drug, cinchona, also known as cinchona bark, Peruvian bark, and Jesuits' bark, is rarely used today except as a cheap substitute for the alkaloids it contains. It is antimalarial, antipyretic, and analgesic in action. It contains the following pharmaceutically important alkaloids:

(a) Quinine. Over 100 salts of quinine have been listed. The actions and uses of this drug are more thoroughly considered in chapter 9.

(b) Quinidine sulfate. Quinidine is the stereoisomer of quinine but is a heart drug rather than an antimalarial.

(c) Quinacrine hydrochloride (Atabrine).

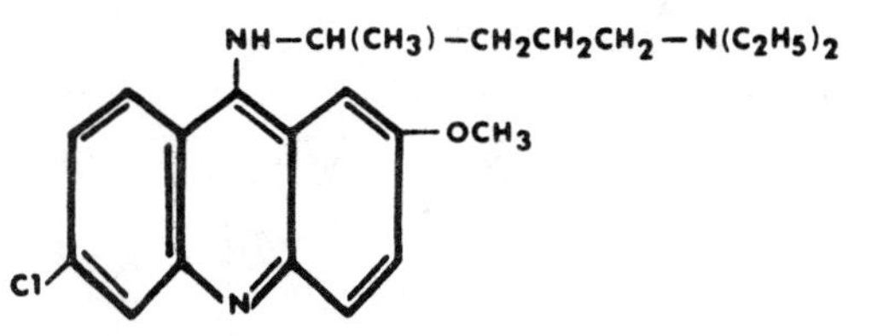

Quinacrine

(d) Chloroquine phosphate (Aralen phosphate).

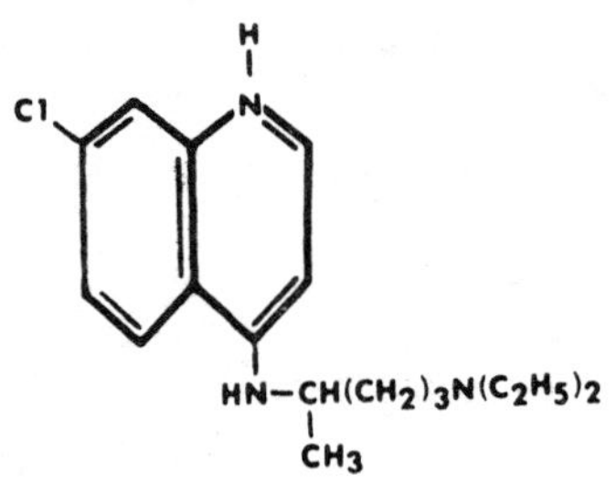

Chloroquine

(e) Primaquine phosphate.

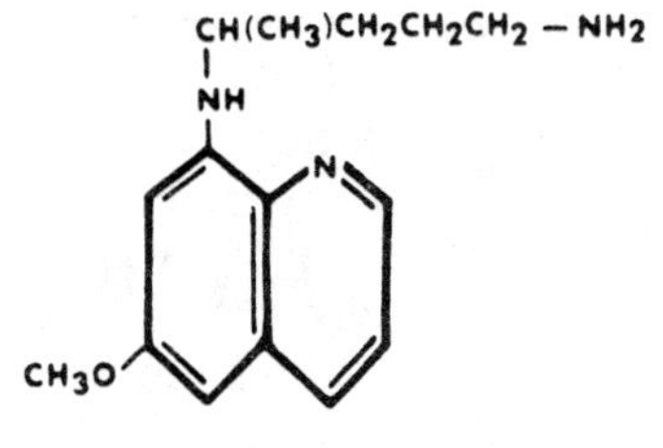

Primaquine

(f) Comparison of cinchona alkaloid structures. In the comparison of the cinchona alkaloid structures below, notice the relationship between the agents; quinine and quinidine are structurally identical but stereoisomers of each other.

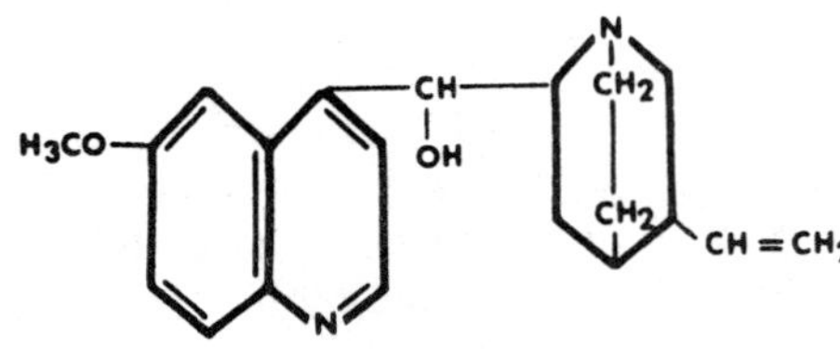

Quinine

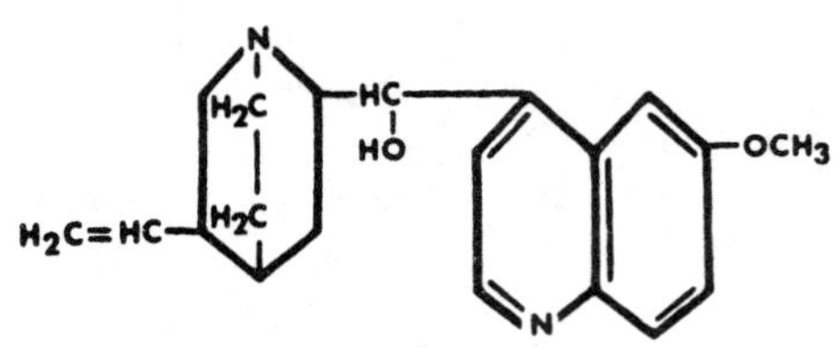

Quinidine

(3) The tropane alkaloids. The tropane alkaloids actually consist of two groups: the solanaceous (nightshade) members which are atropine and related substances, and cocaine which is derived from the coca leaf. Although these two terms are used together, you should understand the difference between them.

(a) Cocaine.

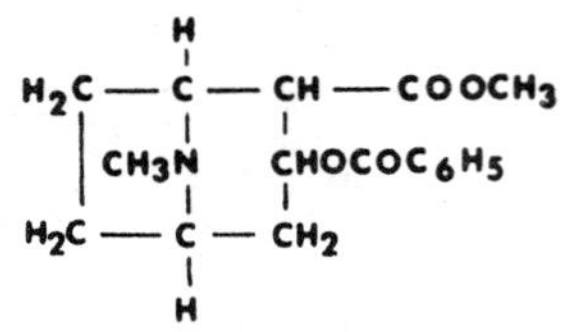

Cocaine is an alkaloid from the coca leaf. Compare its structure with that of the members of the nightshade family which follow.

(b) Tropane alkaloids from the nightshade family. The tropane alkaloids from the nightshade family are referred to as the solanaceous alkaloids. Of this group, atropine is the most important and is the prototype. Below are the formulas for these alkaloids. The nightshade or solanaceous family consists of belladonna plant (deadly nightshade), hyoscyamus, strammonium, and other plants. Belladonna derives its name from Italian "bella + donna" meaning "beautiful lady," because squeezings from this plant were used by the elegant women of the time as an eye wash to dilate the pupils.

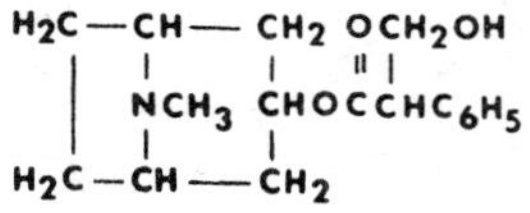

Atropine
(l-hyoscyamus)

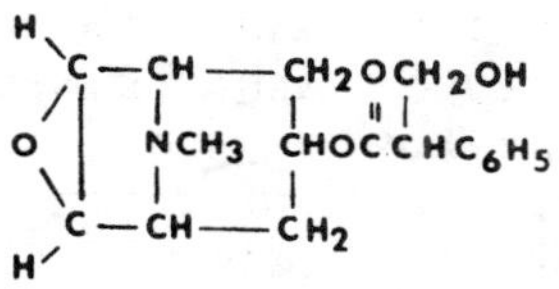

Scopolamine
(Hyoscine)

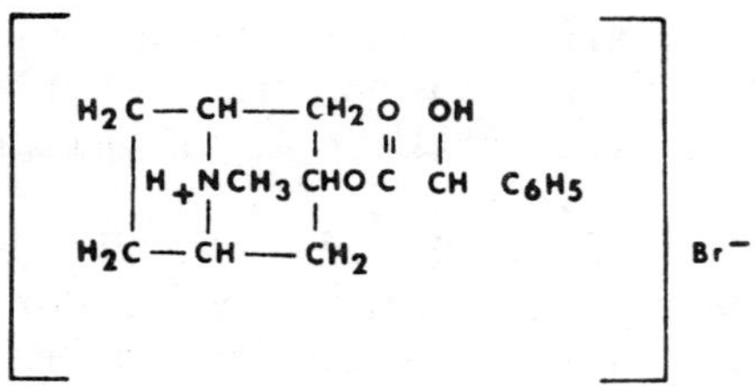

Homatropine Hydrobromide

(4) Xanthine alkaloids. The xanthine alkaloids and their derivatives all contain the parent molecule, purine, which is graphically depicted below.

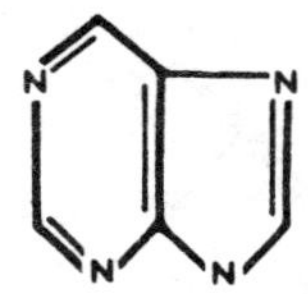

Caffeine, theophylline, and theobromine all contain the same (purine) base, but occur naturally in different plants. Generally, all the xanthine derivatives can be said to be central nervous system stimulants, diuretics, and smooth muscle relaxants.

(a) Theophylline.

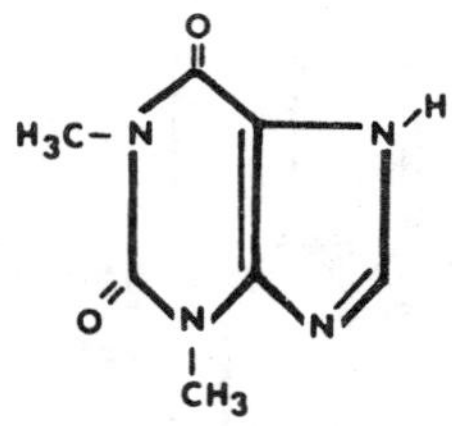

Theophylline

(1, 3-Dimethylxanthine)

(b) Caffeine.

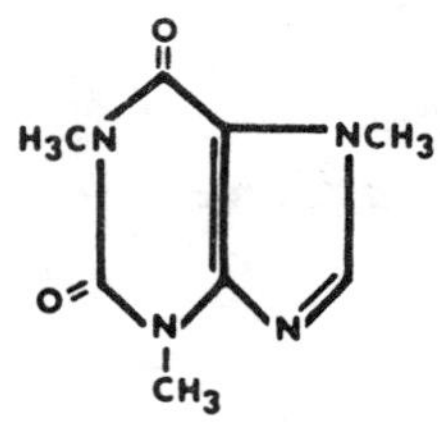

Caffeine

(1, 3, 7-Trimethylxanthine)

(c) Theobromine.

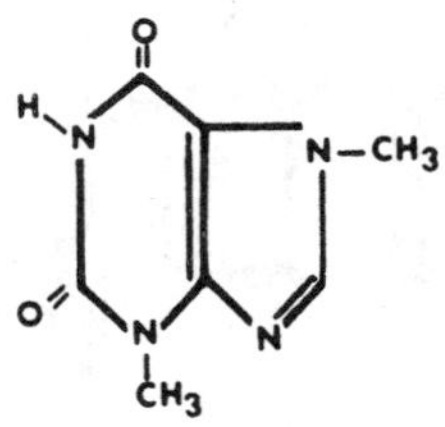

Theobromine

(3, 7-Dimethylxanthine)

(5) Ergot alkaloids. Ergot is a growth produced by a fungus growing on grains such as rye, wheat, oats, barley, and rice. The official ergot is that growth from the rye plant.

(a) Constituents. Ergot is made up of a number of different chemical substances which include alkaloids, carbohydrates, sterols, glycerides, amino acids, and coloring principles. Of

these constituents, we will be concerned only with the alkaloidal principles, all of which are substituted amides of lysergic acid.

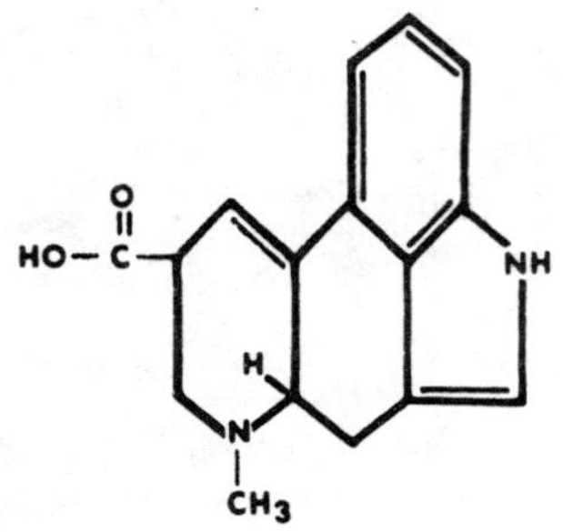

Lysergic Acid

(b) Ergonovine maleate (Ergotrate maleate).

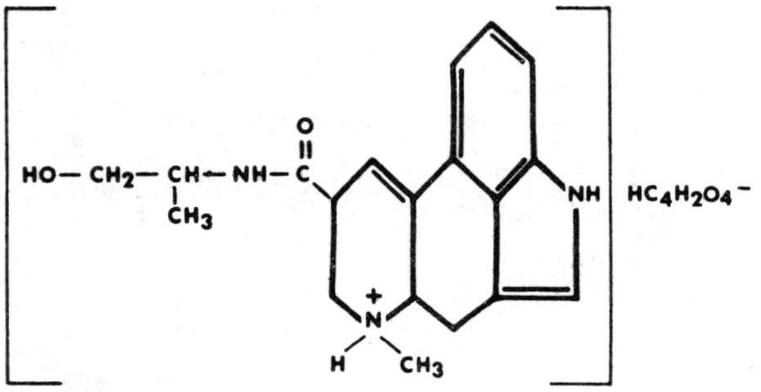

(c) Ergotamine tartrate (Gynergen).

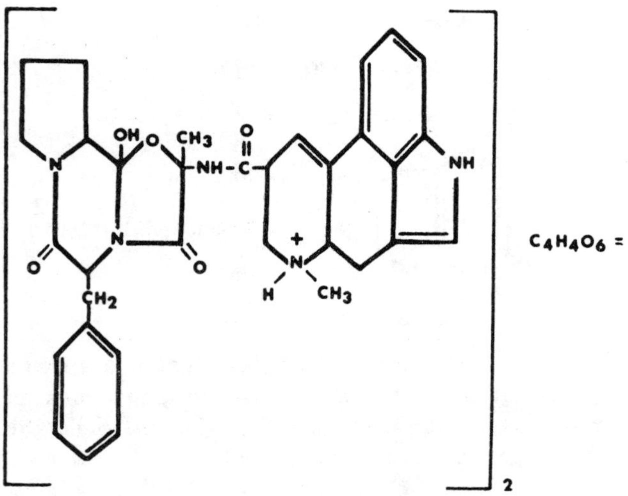

(6) Rauwolfia alkaloids. It was not until 1931 that the first crystalline alkaloid was isolated from the rauwolfia plant, a plant used since ancient times as a remedy. With the recognition of this alkaloid, reserpine, an entirely new field of endeavor sprang into operation. It is through research on rauwolfia, reserpine, and other similar agents that the entire field of tranquilizers and psychotherapeutics has emerged. The rauwolfia alkaloids are intended primarily for reducing high blood pressure.

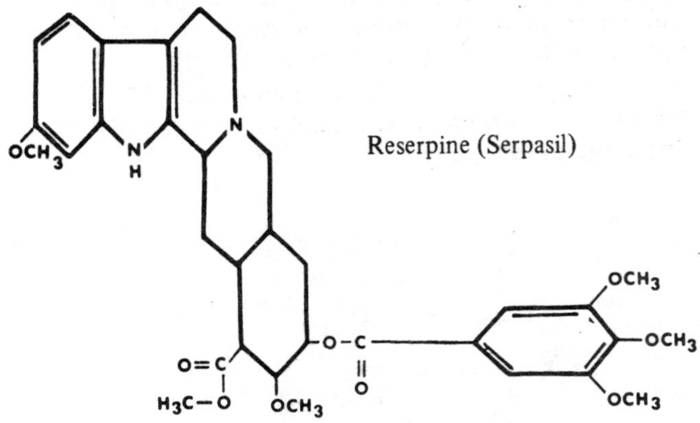

Reserpine (Serpasil)

29. Antibiotics. In a broad sense, and from the derivation of their name, antibiotics are agents against life. From a more restricted medical and pharmaceutical sense, however, they are chemical substances produced by microorganisms and are capable of inhibiting the growth of or destroying other bacteria and microorganisms. Before the birth of Christ, the Chinese used moldy soybean curd as a curative application for boils and furuncles, and yet it was not until 1929 that Sir Alexander Fleming discovered penicillin. Even then antibiotic investigation was slow because of the considerable attention being paid to the sulfonamides. It was not until the 1940's that they really began to find their place in medicine.

a. Methods of antibiotic production. Antibiotics which cannot as yet be synthesized, or are too costly to obtain by synthesis, may be produced by two methods: the surface process and the submerged process.

(1) Surface process. In this method, the organisms producing the antibiotic grow in pad-like formation on the surface of a liquid or divided solid medium. This process is adequate only for producing the small amounts required for laboratory use.

(2) Submerged process. The submerged process is the only natural method for producing

antibiotics in the vast quantities necessary for clinical use. It is a much faster and more efficient process than the surface method. Steel tanks, with capacities up to 30,000 gallons, are filled with a sterilized nutrient medium and inoculated with a master culture. After 50 to 90 hours of culturing under rigid temperature and sterile controls, the batch is extracted and concentrated.

b. Penicillins. By substituting various groups for the R in the following general formula, we arrive at a number of different penicillins.

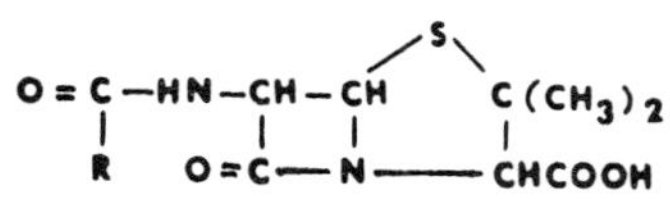

(1) Penicillin G (Benzyl penicillin). The R =

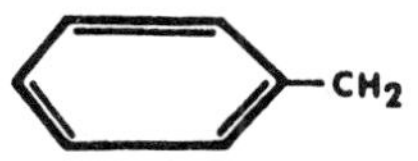

(2) Penicillin V (phenoxymethyl penicillin). The R =

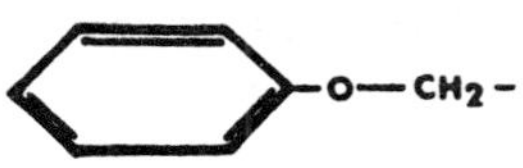

(3) Methicillin (Staphcillin). The R =

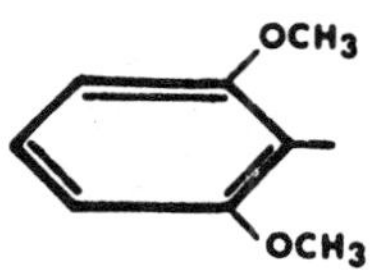

(4) Oxacillin (Prostaphlin). The R =

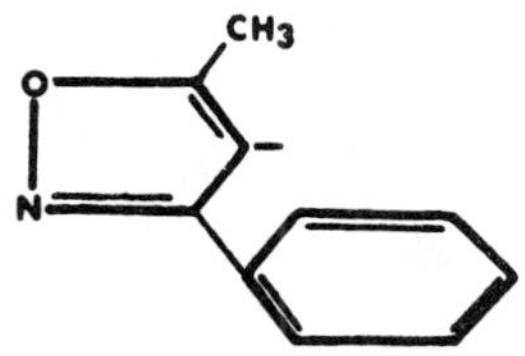

(5) Ampicillin (Polycillin). The R =

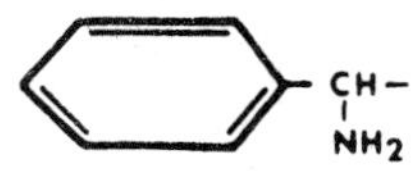

(6) Carbenicillin (Geopen).

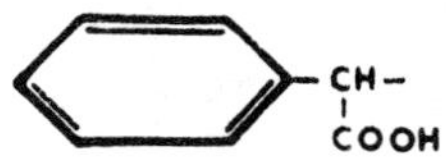

c. Chloramphenicol (Chloromycetin).

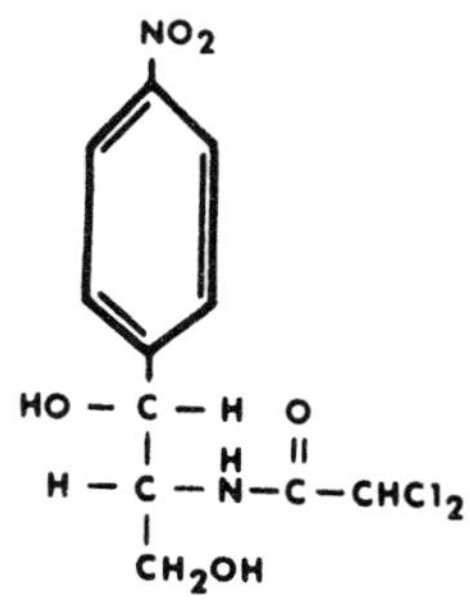

d. Tetracyclines.
(1) Tetracycline (Achromycin).

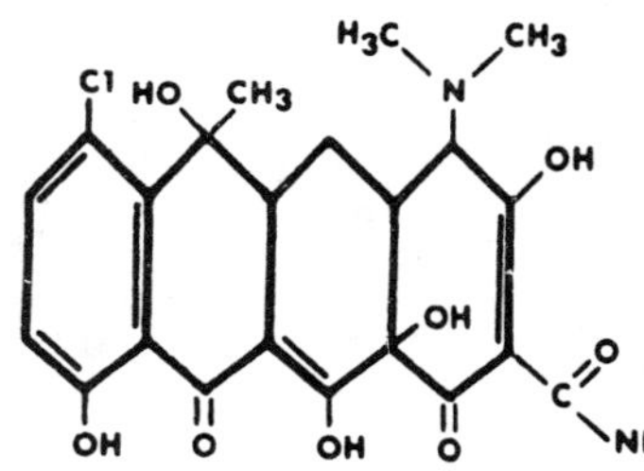

(2) Chlortetracycline (Aureomycin).
(3) Oxytetracycline (Terramycin).

e. Cephalothin (Keflin).

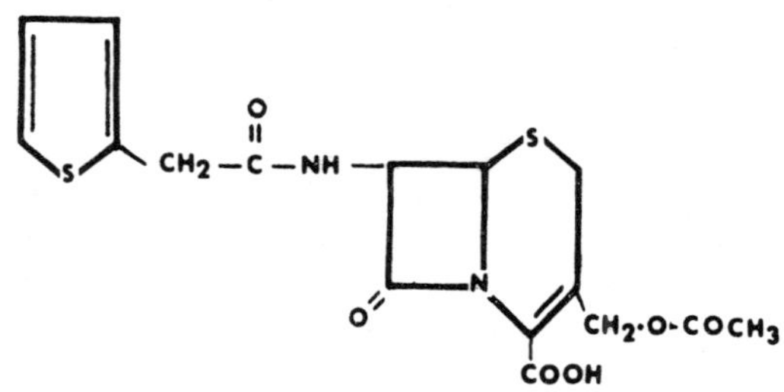

f. *The "Mycins."*

(1) Gentamicin (Garamycin).

(2) Kanamycin (Kantrex).

(3) Neomycin.

(4) Streptomycin.

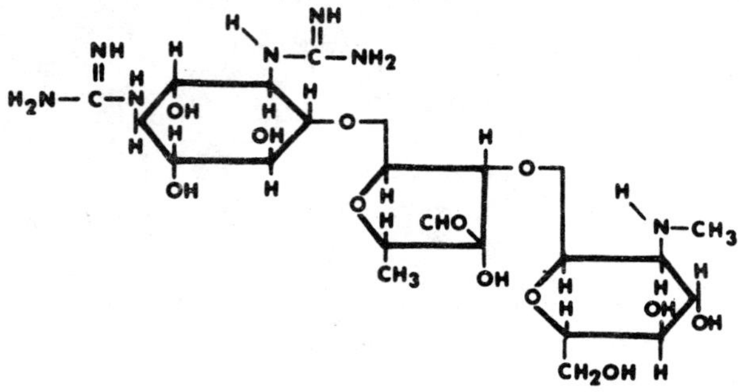

ANSWER SHEET

T NO. ________________ PART ________ TITLE OF POSITION ____
(AS GIVEN IN EXAMINATION ANNOUNCEMENT - INCLUDE OPTION, IF ANY)

CE OF EXAMINATION ____ DATE ____________
(CITY OR TOWN) (STATE)

RATING

USE THE SPECIAL PENCIL. MAKE GLOSSY BLACK MARKS.

1 A B C D E	26 A B C D E	51 A B C D E	76 A B C D E	101 A B C D E
2 A B C D E	27 A B C D E	52 A B C D E	77 A B C D E	102 A B C D E
3 A B C D E	28 A B C D E	53 A B C D E	78 A B C D E	103 A B C D E
4 A B C D E	29 A B C D E	54 A B C D E	79 A B C D E	104 A B C D E
5 A B C D E	30 A B C D E	55 A B C D E	80 A B C D E	105 A B C D E
6 A B C D E	31 A B C D E	56 A B C D E	81 A B C D E	106 A B C D E
7 A B C D E	32 A B C D E	57 A B C D E	82 A B C D E	107 A B C D E
8 A B C D E	33 A B C D E	58 A B C D E	83 A B C D E	108 A B C D E
9 A B C D E	34 A B C D E	59 A B C D E	84 A B C D E	109 A B C D E
10 A B C D E	35 A B C D E	60 A B C D E	85 A B C D E	110 A B C D E

Make only ONE mark for each answer. Additional and stray marks may be counted as mistakes. In making corrections, erase errors COMPLETELY.

11 A B C D E	36 A B C D E	61 A B C D E	86 A B C D E	111 A B C D E
12 A B C D E	37 A B C D E	62 A B C D E	87 A B C D E	112 A B C D E
13 A B C D E	38 A B C D E	63 A B C D E	88 A B C D E	113 A B C D E
14 A B C D E	39 A B C D E	64 A B C D E	89 A B C D E	114 A B C D E
15 A B C D E	40 A B C D E	65 A B C D E	90 A B C D E	115 A B C D E
16 A B C D E	41 A B C D E	66 A B C D E	91 A B C D E	116 A B C D E
17 A B C D E	42 A B C D E	67 A B C D E	92 A B C D E	117 A B C D E
18 A B C D E	43 A B C D E	68 A B C D E	93 A B C D E	118 A B C D E
19 A B C D E	44 A B C D E	69 A B C D E	94 A B C D E	119 A B C D E
20 A B C D E	45 A B C D E	70 A B C D E	95 A B C D E	120 A B C D E
21 A B C D E	46 A B C D E	71 A B C D E	96 A B C D E	121 A B C D E
22 A B C D E	47 A B C D E	72 A B C D E	97 A B C D E	122 A B C D E
23 A B C D E	48 A B C D E	73 A B C D E	98 A B C D E	123 A B C D E
24 A B C D E	49 A B C D E	74 A B C D E	99 A B C D E	124 A B C D E
25 A B C D E	50 A B C D E	75 A B C D E	100 A B C D E	125 A B C D E

ANSWER SHEET

TEST NO. ____________ PART ______ TITLE OF POSITION ____________________________
(AS GIVEN IN EXAMINATION ANNOUNCEMENT - INCLUDE OPTION, IF ANY)

PLACE OF EXAMINATION ______________________________ DATE ____________
(CITY OR TOWN) (STATE)

RATING

USE THE SPECIAL PENCIL. MAKE GLOSSY BLACK MARKS.

1 A B C D E	26 A B C D E	51 A B C D E	76 A B C D E	101 A B C D E
2 A B C D E	27 A B C D E	52 A B C D E	77 A B C D E	102 A B C D E
3 A B C D E	28 A B C D E	53 A B C D E	78 A B C D E	103 A B C D E
4 A B C D E	29 A B C D E	54 A B C D E	79 A B C D E	104 A B C D E
5 A B C D E	30 A B C D E	55 A B C D E	80 A B C D E	105 A B C D E
6 A B C D E	31 A B C D E	56 A B C D E	81 A B C D E	106 A B C D E
7 A B C D E	32 A B C D E	57 A B C D E	82 A B C D E	107 A B C D E
8 A B C D E	33 A B C D E	58 A B C D E	83 A B C D E	108 A B C D E
9 A B C D E	34 A B C D E	59 A B C D E	84 A B C D E	109 A B C D E
10 A B C D E	35 A B C D E	60 A B C D E	85 A B C D E	110 A B C D E

Make only ONE mark for each answer. Additional and stray marks may be counted as mistakes. In making corrections, erase errors COMPLETELY.

11 A B C D E	36 A B C D E	61 A B C D E	86 A B C D E	111 A B C D E
12 A B C D E	37 A B C D E	62 A B C D E	87 A B C D E	112 A B C D E
13 A B C D E	38 A B C D E	63 A B C D E	88 A B C D E	113 A B C D E
14 A B C D E	39 A B C D E	64 A B C D E	89 A B C D E	114 A B C D E
15 A B C D E	40 A B C D E	65 A B C D E	90 A B C D E	115 A B C D E
16 A B C D E	41 A B C D E	66 A B C D E	91 A B C D E	116 A B C D E
17 A B C D E	42 A B C D E	67 A B C D E	92 A B C D E	117 A B C D E
18 A B C D E	43 A B C D E	68 A B C D E	93 A B C D E	118 A B C D E
19 A B C D E	44 A B C D E	69 A B C D E	94 A B C D E	119 A B C D E
20 A B C D E	45 A B C D E	70 A B C D E	95 A B C D E	120 A B C D E
21 A B C D E	46 A B C D E	71 A B C D E	96 A B C D E	121 A B C D E
22 A B C D E	47 A B C D E	72 A B C D E	97 A B C D E	122 A B C D E
23 A B C D E	48 A B C D E	73 A B C D E	98 A B C D E	123 A B C D E
24 A B C D E	49 A B C D E	74 A B C D E	99 A B C D E	124 A B C D E
25 A B C D E	50 A B C D E	75 A B C D E	100 A B C D E	125 A B C D E